THE
MELATONIN HYPOTHESIS

Breast Cancer and Use of Electric Power

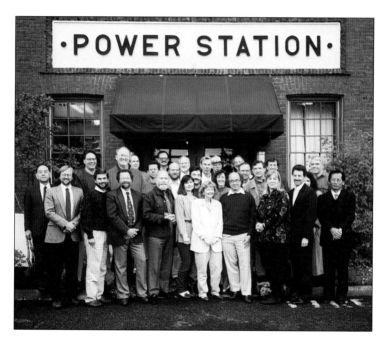

Pictured are attendees of "The Melatonin Summit" which took place at the Edgefield Manor in Troutdale, Oregon, in May of 1995. This summit was convened with the express intention of generating new collaborations among the diverse group of participants, and to produce a book on a subject of common interest: to wit, an objective assessment of the effects of light and EMF on neuroendocrine function, and how these effects might relate to risk of breast cancer. The U.S. Department of Energy sponsored this meeting, which included scientists from Japan, Sweden, Germany, and the United States. The location of the summit, the Edgefield Manor, was built in 1917 as the country home for indigent citizens. Electricity for the manor was produced by a coal-fired generator in the "Power Station."

THE MELATONIN HYPOTHESIS

Breast Cancer and Use of Electric Power

THE
MELATONIN HYPOTHESIS

Breast Cancer and Use of Electric Power

EDITED BY
Richard G. Stevens
Bary W. Wilson
Larry E. Anderson

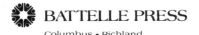

BATTELLE PRESS
Columbus • Richland

DISCLAIMER

Funding for the publication of this volume and funding for a portion of the research discussed in this volume was provided by the United States Department of Energy (DOE). The views and opinions of the authors expressed herein do not necessarily state or reflect those of the DOE. Neither the DOE, nor Battelle Memorial Institute, nor any of their employees, makes any warranty, express or implied, or assumes any legal liability or responsibility for the accuracy, completeness, or usefulness of any information, apparatus, product, or process disclosed, or represents that its use would not infringe privately owned rights. Reference herein to any specific commercial product, process, or service by trade name, trademark, manufacturer, or otherwise does not necessarily constitute or imply its endorsement, recommendation, or favoring by the DOE or Battelle Memorial Institute. Trademarks belong to their various owners, and are not specifically identified herein. The DOE encourages wide dissemination of the technical information contained herein, with due respect for the Publisher's rights regarding the complete volume.

PACIFIC NORTHWEST NATIONAL LABORATORY
operated by
BATTELLE MEMORIAL INSTITUTE for the
UNITED STATES DEPARTMENT OF ENERGY
under Contract DE-AC06-76RL0 1830

Library of Congress Cataloging-in-Publication Data

The melatonin hypothesis : breast cancer and use of electric power /
    edited by Richard G. Stevens, Bary W. Wilson, Larry E. Anderson.
        p.   cm.
    Includes bibliographical references and index.
    ISBN 1-57477-020-9 (hardcover)
        1. Breast—Cancer—Etiology.   2. Carcinogenesis.   3. Melatonin—Pathophysiology.
    4. Electromagnetic fields—Physiological effect.   5. Light—Physiological effect.
    6. Pineal gland—Pathophysiology.
    I. Stevens, Richard G., 1951– .   II. Wilson, Bary W., 1945– .
    III. Anderson, Larry E., 1943–   .
    RC280.B8M443   1997   96-27522
    616.99´449071—dc20   CIP

Printed in the United States of America

Battelle Press
505 King Avenue
Columbus, Ohio 43201-2693
614-424-6393; 1-800-451-3543
FAX: 614-424-3819
Home page: http://www.Battelle.org

Contents

Preface ix

Contributors xi

1. **Overview**—*Richard G. Stevens, Bary W. Wilson,
   and Larry E. Anderson* 1

PART I. Introduction

2. Breast Cancer—*Richard G. Stevens and
   Stephanie J. London* 9

3. Melatonin Biosynthesis, Regulation, and Effects
   —*Russel J. Reiter* 25

4. Overview of Electromagnetic Field Exposure and
   Dosimetry—*Douglas L. Miller* 49

5. Understanding Dose: Implications for
   Bioelectromagnetics Research—*Norman H. Hansen* 81

PART II. Issues in Field Perception

6. Magnetoreception in Terrestrial Vertebrates:
   Implications for Possible Mechanisms of EMF
   Interaction with Biological Systems—*John B. Phillips
   and Mark E. Deutschlander* 111

7. Action of Melatonin in Magnetic Field Inhibition of Nerve-
   Growth-Factor-Induced Neurite Outgrowth
   in PC-12 Cells—*Carl F. Blackman, Shawnee G. Benane,
   and Dennis E. House* 173

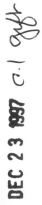

PART III. Circumstantial Case

Section 1. Melatonin Effects on Breast Cancer

8. Systemic, Cellular, and Molecular Aspects of
   Melatonin Action on Experimental Breast Carcinogenesis
   —*David E. Blask* 189

Section 2. Light Effects on Melatonin

9. Light and Melatonin in Humans—*Lennart Wetterberg* . . 233

10. Signal Transduction of Light for Melatonin
    Regulation in Humans—*George C. Brainard* 267

11. Response of Mammalian Pineal Gene Expression to
    Light and Magnetic Field Exposure—*Wendy Haggren* . . 297

12. Daytime Melatonin in Postmenopausal Japanese-
    American Women—*Michinori Kabuto* 319

Section 3. EMF Effects on Melatonin

13. Effects of 50-Hz Magnetic Fields on Pineal Function
    in the Rat—*Masamichi Kato and Tsukasa Shigemitsu* 337

14. In Search of a Direct Effect of Weak (50-Hz) Magnetic
    Fields on the Pineal Gland of Djungarian Hamsters—
    Alexander Lerchl, Michael Niehaus, Petra Niklowitz 377

15. Studies of Melatonin, Cortisol, Progesterone, and
    Interleukin-1 in Sheep Exposed to EMF from a 500-kV
    Transmission Line—*Jack M. Lee Jr., Fred Stormshak, James
    Thompson, David L. Hess, and Steve Hefeneider* 391

16. Effects of Exposure to 60-Hz EMF on Melatonin in
    Nonhuman Primates Might Depend on Specific
    Aspects of Field Exposure—*Walter R. Rogers,
    Russel J. Reiter, and John L. Orr* 429

17. Human Exposure to Magnetic Fields: Effects on
    Melatonin, Hormones, and Immunity—*Charles Graham
    and Michael Gibertini* 479

18. 60-Hz Magnetic Field Exposure Effects on the Melatonin Rhythm in the Djungarian Hamster—*Steven M. Yellon* . 503

19. Effect of EMF Exposure on the Neuroendocrine System—*Bary W. Wilson and Kathleen S. Matt* 527

PART IV: Direct Evidence

20. Magnetic Fields and Breast Cancer: Experimental Studies on the Melatonin Hypothesis—*Wolfgang Löscher and Meike Mevissen* 555

21. Laboratory Studies on Extremely Low Frequency (50/60-Hz) Magnetic Fields and Carcinogenesis— *Robert P. Liburdy and Wolfgang Löscher* 585

22. Magnetic Fields, Melatonin, Tamoxifen, and Human Breast Cancer Cell Growth—*Robert P. Liburdy and Joan D. Harland* 669

23. Epidemiologic Studies of EMF and Breast Cancer Risk: A Biologically Based Overview—*Thomas C. Erren* 701

PART V. Synthesis and Conclusions

24. Synthesis and Conclusions—*Richard G. Stevens, Bary W. Wilson, and Larry E. Anderson* 739

Glossary 749

Index 755

Preface

Beginning in the late 1970s, our laboratory conducted experiments which showed a suppression of the normal nocturnal rise in melatonin production in rats exposed to an AC electric field. These experiments required an unusual degree of commitment, even by the demanding standards of success in science. This was due to the fact that melatonin, the "Dracula" of hormones, only comes out at night; excision of pineal glands from the experimental rats had to occur at midnight and continue until 2 or 3 in the morning. Sleep-deprivation euphoria and bloodshot eyes were a common sight in our laboratory.

At the time, the observations of lowered melatonin from field exposure seemed scientifically interesting, but it was unclear what, if any, implications it might have for human health. Over the years, our research group continued to actively participate in the larger scientific communication of information and ideas on bioeffects of exposure to electric and magnetic fields. This has included collegial interactions at many national and international meetings, and hosting of innumerable visiting scientists. Our group itself has, by design, included researchers from a wide range of disciplines. From this rich diversity of experience came the "Melatonin Hypothesis." With its basis in the modest and, at the time, arcane nocturnal experiments of almost 20 years ago, this hypothesis has become one of the salient hypotheses on breast cancer etiology in the main cancer research community.

The work on development of the Melatonin Hypothesis was substantively advanced in 1995 in a conference at the Edgefield Manor in Troutdale, Oregon, attended by most of our authors (as pictured and described on the overleaf). This book is, therefore, the product of much effort on the part of a large number of people, and long-term core funding from the U.S. Department of Energy. In particular, taking good ideas from many people and transforming them into a good-looking and coherent document requires at least one person who passionately follows all aspects of writing and production. We the editors are very fortunate to have had Ms. Kathy Lumetta tackle this book as technical editor. It is rare to find someone with superior technical skill who is also so effective in personal communication with the editors and scientific contributors.

—The Editors

Contributors

Larry E. Anderson, Ph.D., Pacific Northwest National Laboratory, Richland, Washington, USA

Shawnee G. Benane, B.S., National Health and Environmental Effects Research Laboratory, US Environmental Protection Agency, Research Triangle Park, North Carolina, USA

Carl F. Blackman, Ph.D., National Health and Environmental Effects Research Laboratory, US Environmental Protection Agency, Research Triangle Park, North Carolina, USA

David E. Blask, Ph.D., M.D., Laboratory of Experimental Neuro-endocrinology/Oncology, Mary Imogene-Bassett Research Institute, Cooperstown, New York, USA

George C. Brainard, Ph.D., Department of Neurology, Jefferson Medical College, Thomas Jefferson University, Philadelphia, Pennsylvania, USA

Mark E. Deutschlander, B.S., Department of Biology, Indiana University, Bloomington, Indiana, USA

Thomas C. Erren, MD, MPH, Institut und Poliklinik für Arbeits- und Sozialmedizin der Universität zu Köln, Germany

Michael Gibertini, Ph.D., Midwest Research Institute, Kansas City, Missouri, USA

Charles Graham, Ph.D., Midwest Research Institute, Kansas City, Missouri, USA

Wendy Haggren, Ph.D., Pettis Veterans Affairs Medical Center, Loma Linda, California, USA

Norman H. Hansen, M.S.E.E., Pacific Northwest National Laboratory, Richland, Washington, USA

Joan D. Harland, Ph.D., Life Sciences Division, Lawrence Berkeley National Laboratory, University of California, Berkeley, California, USA

Steve Hefeneider, Ph.D., Portland Veterans Affairs Medical Center and Oregon Health Sciences University, Portland, Oregon, USA

David L. Hess, Ph.D., Oregon Regional Primate Research Center, Beaverton, Oregon, USA

Dennis E. House, M.S., National Health and Environmental Effects Research Laboratory, US Environmental Protection Agency, Research Triangle Park, North Carolina, USA

Michinori Kabuto, D.H.Sc., Environmental Risk Research Division, National Institute for Environmental Studies, Tsukuba City, Japan

Masamichi Kato, M.D., Department of Physiology, Hokkaido University School of Medicine, Sapporo, Japan

Jack M. Lee, Jr., Ph.D., Bonneville Power Administration, Portland, Oregon, USA

Alexander Lerchl, Priv.-Doz., Dr. rer. nat., Institute of Reproductive Medicine of the University, Münster, Germany

Robert P. Liburdy, M.Sc., Ph.D., Life Sciences Division, Lawrence Berkeley National Laboratory, University of California, Berkeley, USA

Stephanie J. London, M.D., Dr.P.H., National Institute of Environmental Health Sciences, Research Triangle Park, North Carolina, USA

Wolfgang Löscher, Dr.Med.Vet., Department of Pharmacology, Toxicology, and Pharmacy, School of Veterinary Medicine, Hannover, Germany

Kathleen S. Matt, Ph.D., Arizona State University, Tempe, Arizona, USA

Meike Mevissen, Dr.Med.Vet., Department of Pharmacology, Toxicology, and Pharmacy, School of Veterinary Medicine, Hannover, Germany

Douglas L. Miller, Ph.D., Pacific Northwest National Laboratory, Richland, Washington, USA

Michael Niehaus, Dipl. Biol., Institute of Reproductive Medicine of the University, Münster, Germany

Petra Niklowitz, Dr. rer. nat., Institute of Reproductive Medicine of the University, Münster, Germany

John L. Orr, Ph.D., D.A.B.T., Department of Biosciences and Bioengineering, Southwest Research Institute, San Antonio, Texas, USA

John B. Phillips, Ph.D., Department of Biology, Indiana University, Bloomington, Indiana, USA

Russel J. Reiter, Ph.D., D.Med., Department of Cellular and Structural Biology, The University of Texas Health Science Center, San Antonio, Texas, USA

Walter R. Rogers, Ph.D., D.A.B.T., Department of Biosciences and Bioengineering, Southwest Research Institute, San Antonio, Texas, USA

Tsukasa Shigemitsu, D.Eng., Abiko Research Laboratory, Central Research Institute of Electric Power Industry, Abiko, Chiba, Japan

Richard G. Stevens, Ph.D., Pacific Northwest National Laboratory, Richland, Washington, USA

Fred Stormshak, Ph.D., Department of Animal Sciences, Oregon State University, Corvallis, Oregon, USA

James Thompson, Ph.D., Department of Animal Sciences, Oregon State University, Corvallis, Oregon, USA

Lennart Wetterberg, M.D., Ph.D., Department of Psychiatry at St. Göran's Hospital, Karolinska Institute, Stockholm, Sweden

Bary W. Wilson, Ph.D., Pacific Northwest National Laboratory, Richland, Washington, USA

Steven M. Yellon, Ph.D., Loma Linda University School of Medicine and Center for Perinatal Biology, Loma Linda, California, USA

THE
MELATONIN HYPOTHESIS

Breast Cancer
and Use of
Electric Power

1 Overview

RICHARD G. STEVENS
BARY W. WILSON
LARRY E. ANDERSON
Pacific Northwest National Laboratory,
Richland, Washington

FORMAT OF THE BOOK

The organization of this book is the editors', but the style and content of the chapters belong to the authors. There was no attempt to press each chapter into a uniform writing style. Indeed, it was the editors' express intent that each of the authors present material in his/her own style. As a result, styles and content vary. Some chapters present extremely focused accounts of experiments conducted in a single laboratory. Other chapters present broad reviews of a topic pertinent to the theme of the book. Clarity in writing and organization was the literary goal. Information and objectivity was the scientific goal.

THE MYSTERY OF BREAST CANCER

Breast cancer is a disease of modern life. As societies industrialize, risk increases; for example, the historically low risk in Japan has been rising fast in recent decades. Yet it is unclear which of the myriad changes coming with industrialization account for this increase. There is little consensus among researchers on the primary causes of breast cancer; although reproductive factors are acknowledged to be important, the debate on dietary fat continues to rage (*Epidemiol. Rev.* 15:110–132, 1993).

One hallmark of modern life in industrialized societies is the pervasive use of electric power. Electric power produces light at night (LAN) as well as anthropogenic electric and magnetic fields (EMF), both relatively new exposures in the human environment. The "Melatonin Hypothesis" states that exposure to LAN and/or EMF may disrupt the function of the pineal gland and its primary hormone melatonin, and that this disruption lowers melatonin production, a consequence that may lead to an increase in the long-term risk of breast cancer.

The circumstantial case for the hypothesis has three aspects to it: (1) light effects on melatonin, (2) EMF effects on melatonin, and (3) melatonin effects on breast cancer. The best-understood of these aspects is light effects on melatonin. It is clear that the normal nocturnal melatonin rise in humans can be suppressed by light of sufficient intensity. (It is unknown whether ambient nighttime illumination in homes can affect melatonin in women. It is also unknown whether the artificial electric lighting in buildings typical of the daytime environment for workers in modern societies can alter circadian rhythms of melatonin.) The evidence for an effect of melatonin on breast cancer in experimental animals is strong, but the evidence in humans is scant and difficult to gather. The least-understood aspect of the circumstantial case is EMF effects on melatonin. Whereas a half-dozen independent laboratories have published findings of melatonin suppression in animals, there are inconsistencies. More importantly, there are no published data which clearly demonstrate an EMF-induced suppression in humans.

The direct evidence bearing on the hypothesis is sparse but provocative. Two laboratories have published data reporting substantial increases in chemically induced breast cancer in rats by a weak AC magnetic field (*Cancer Lett.* 61:75–79, 1991; *Cancer Lett.* 71:75–81, 1993; *Carcinogenesis* 16:119–125, 1995), and one has reported an EMF-induced reversal of melatonin's oncostatic action (*J. Pineal Res.* 14:89–97, 1993). The epidemiologic evidence is also very limited, showing some support of the hypothesis (*J. Natl. Cancer Inst.* 86:921–925, 1994; *Am. J. Epidemiol.* 142:446–448, 1995) as well as negative findings (*J. Natl. Cancer Inst.* 86:885–886, 1994). Results from the first two large epidemiologic studies to be focused specifically on the hypothesis will be reported in early 1997 from the Fred Hutchinson Cancer Research

Center in Seattle and the Karolinska Institute in Stockholm. Several more large studies are just getting under way.

Putting two lines of evidence together yielded the electric power–breast cancer hypothesis. First, Bary Wilson and colleagues published work reporting a suppression of the normal nocturnal rise in melatonin in rats by exposure to a 60-Hz electric field (*Bioelectromagnetics* 1:236, 1980; *Bioelectromagnetics* 2:371–380, 1981), analogous to work by Peter Semm et al. showing an effect of an artificial static magnetic field on pineal activity in guinea pigs (*Nature* 288:607–608, 1980). Second, melatonin, in turn, may be important in breast cancer etiology (*Cancer Res.* 41:4432–4436, 1981; *Cancer Res.* 48:6121–6126, 1988; *J. Cancer Res. Clin. Oncol.* 117:526–532, 1991). In addition, other factors that might disrupt pineal function—such as alcohol, shift work, and the lighted environment in buildings—might also be surmised to affect long-term risk of breast cancer.

To date, the body of evidence is sufficient to bind electric power over for trial, but not nearly adequate to render a verdict. Though the hypothesis is in its early stages of evaluation, it may be resolved within 5 years because, sadly, breast cancer is so common in industrialized societies that many large studies can be conducted simultaneously.

THE BOOK

This book is intended to examine in detail the electric power–breast cancer hypothesis with contributions from many of the original researchers in the areas bearing on the hypothesis. The book is divided into five parts, as seen in the table of contents.

Part I contains four chapters intended to give a contextual basis for what follows. Stevens and London provide a short description of breast cancer and what is known about its pathogenesis and causes. Reiter describes melatonin: what it is and what it does. Miller then provides a background on EMF in terms not requiring an advanced degree in physics. And finally, Hansen describes the EMF found in typical human environments, and features various aspects of EMF exposure and models of interaction that are currently receiving attention in the bioelectromagnetics community.

Part II includes a detailed discussion by Phillips and Deutschlander of mechanisms of magnetic field perception. They draw the distinction between the radical pair-based mechanism and the magnetite-based mechanism of magnetoreception. Drawing from studies in migratory birds and shore-seeking newts, they present evidence for a magnetic sensing mediated by the visual system, and describe the role of light. They tackle straight-on, from a biophysical, physiological, and behavioral perspective, the plausibility of detecting EMF at the levels typically encountered in the environment. Blackman et al. present a discussion of the effects of a 230-mG, 50-Hz magnetic field on neurite outgrowth from PC-12 cells. This system has been used by these authors to test a variety of biophysical hypotheses of interaction between weak AC magnetic fields and biological systems.

Part III presents the circumstantial case for investigating electric power's involvement in breast cancer risk. In Section 1, Blask reviews the evidence, much of which he and his colleagues have generated, that melatonin inhibits breast cancer cell proliferation. Melatonin administration reduces mammary tumor yield in rodents given chemical carcinogens, whereas pinealectomy enhances yield. Melatonin also can slow the growth of certain human breast cancer cell lines in culture. In humans, however, there is very little direct evidence on whether and to what extent melatonin levels affect breast cancer risk. The question is difficult to address in humans due to the fact that melatonin is produced primarily at night.

Section 2 includes four chapters about light and melatonin. Wetterberg presents a historical and scientific review of the role of light on pineal function, and then delves, in some detail, into melatonin and depression. Brainard gives specific details on effects of light intensity and wavelength on melatonin in humans. He highlights the emerging area of low-light effects. Haggren discusses gene expression in response to light as it relates to those genes involved in pineal function and the circadian clock. Kabuto presents data on the relationship of daytime urinary melatonin levels and 24-hour production, and the effect of light on this relationship. He also compares Japanese and American women in levels of melatonin and estradiol.

Section 3 presents chapters from many of the original researchers working on EMF effects on melatonin. Kato and Shigemitsu have conducted an extensive series of experiments examining the effect of exposure to a 50-Hz magnetic field on melatonin production in rats; they summarize these results in their chapter. Lerchl et al. have performed experiments, reviewed here, using rapid changes of a static field. Lee et al. performed an experiment with sheep housed under a large transmission line in the countryside, and another group of sheep away from the line in an open field. They then compared nighttime melatonin levels of these two experimental groups. Rogers et al., as elucidated in their chapter, are the first to report on the possible effects of a magnetic field on melatonin production in a nonhuman primate—the baboon. Graham and Gibertini describe their experiments with human volunteers. They are in the process of determining whether or not exposure to a 60-Hz magnetic field can lower melatonin in humans. The chapters by Yellon and by Wilson and Matt both discuss the use of hamsters to examine EMF effects on pineal and neuroendocrine function in general.

Part IV contains four chapters that present direct evidence bearing on the electric power–breast cancer hypothesis. Löscher and Mevissen provide details on their experiments with magnetic fields and chemically induced mammary cancer in rats. They discuss both the gross tumor yield data, and focused experiments designed to determine the underlying mechanisms for the mammary tumor results they have observed. Liburdy and Löscher then present a broad overview of potential EMF biological effects that may be related to carcinogenesis in general. Liburdy and Harland focus on their results with a magnetic field-induced reversal of melatonin's oncostatic action in the MCF-7 human breast cancer cell line. Finally, Erren reviews the limited epidemiologic evidence on EMF and breast cancer, and provides a meta analysis of the existing studies in women and in men.

Part V is the synthesis and conclusions, in which the editors pull together main themes, and suggest future lines of inquiry.

PART I
Introduction

2   Breast Cancer

RICHARD G. STEVENS
   Pacific Northwest National Laboratory,
   Richland, Washington
STEPHANIE J. LONDON
   National Institute of Environmental Health Sciences,
   Research Triangle Park, North Carolina

CONTENTS

THE BREAST CANCER BURDEN
HISTOLOGY AND ESTROGEN RECEPTOR STATUS
SCREENING
ESTROGEN
RISK FACTORS
   Age
   Genetic Predisposition
   Personal Characteristics and the Environment
NEW AVENUES
REFERENCES

Breast cancer has a range of nearly 10-fold among countries: from a low of ~1 case per 10,000 women per year (e.g., Algeria) to a high of ~1 case per 1,000 women per year (e.g., the United States). The reason for these vast differences in risk is a mystery.

THE BREAST CANCER BURDEN

Every review of breast cancer begins with a recitation of the distressing facts: Breast cancer is the leading cause of cancer morbidity and mortality in women in industrialized societies, and the number of new cases diagnosed in the United States in 1995 was approximately 182,000, with 46,000 deaths (Wingo et al. 1995). The cumulative lifetime risk of a woman developing breast cancer in the United States by age 85 is one in nine (Feuer et al. 1993). Risk is higher in urban than in rural communities (Blot et al. 1977), and highest in the northeast portion of the country (Sturgeon et al. 1995) due, in part, to a high concentration of urban centers.

There are large international differences in rates of breast cancer incidence and mortality (MacMahon et al. 1973; Parkin et al. 1992). Rates are low in Africa and Asia, intermediate in southern Europe and South America, and high in northern Europe and North America (Parkin et al. 1992). Race does not appear to account for the geographic variation in rates. Rates are low in Japan, intermediate in Japanese living in Hawaii, and high in Japanese living in California (Buell 1973; Haenszel and Kurihara 1968). Incidence has increased dramatically, particularly since 1980, when screening became widely available (Kelsey and Horn-Ross 1993). Since 1911, rates in Iceland have risen from a low level such as found in Asia, to a level approaching that of the United States (Bjarnason et al. 1974); incidence in Sweden is rising rapidly as well (Ranstam et al. 1990). Risk of breast cancer in Japan has historically been much lower than in the United States and northern Europe; however, in recent decades, that risk has been rising (Wakai et al. 1995; Ursin et al. 1994; Wynder et al. 1991). In Japan, age-adjusted mortality has increased from 4.1 per 100,000 women in 1950 to 6.6 in 1991; incidence has increased from 13.5 per 100,000 in 1975 to 24.3 in 1985 (Wakai et al. 1995).

Breast cancer mortality has been increasing in much of the world (Ursin et al. 1994; Hoel et al. 1992; Davis et al. 1990), although not in the United States. Percent increases between 1970 and 1985 ranged from 7% in England to 63% in Singapore. Increases in incidence and mortality have followed cohort patterns that are similar among countries despite differences in absolute risk (Stevens et al. 1982). As first observed by MacMahon (1958), birth cohorts of women born near the turn of the century have had the lowest lifetime risk, and risk has increased with each successive birth cohort. This trend continued in the United States at least up until about the cohorts of 1926–1930 (Tarone and Chu 1992).

HISTOLOGY AND ESTROGEN RECEPTOR STATUS

The majority of breast cancers at diagnosis are infiltrating ductal carcinomas, usually adenocarcinomas (Harris et al. 1992). Other histologic types include lobular, tubular, medullary, and mucinous. Regardless of histology, most tumors arise in the terminal section of the ducts (Russo et al. 1990). Tumors also can be divided into estrogen receptor positive (ER$^+$) and estrogen receptor negative (ER$^-$). The ER$^+$ tumors are believed to require estrogen for growth. They often respond to treatment with agents, such as tamoxifen, that compete for estrogen receptors, thereby depriving the tumor cells of the estrogen they require for growth. ER$^+$ tumors appear also to be better-differentiated and not as virulent as ER$^-$ tumors.

If risk increases as societies industrialize, it is unclear which aspects of life in industrialized societies account for the increase. Options include personal characteristics, diet, and the environment, each of which will be discussed in this chapter. The first question, however, is whether the reported increases in incidence are real, or are an artifact of screening programs.

SCREENING

The extent to which widespread mammographic screening accounts for the increasing incidence of breast cancer is not clear. Ursin et al. (1994) have taken the view that the constancy of mortality rates in women of ages 35–64 in the United States and western Europe adds to the argument that increases in incidence are due to screening, but they also concluded that the increased mortality in older women (65–74) cannot be explained by increased screening. White et al. (1990) evaluated the potential effects of screening on the increase in breast cancer incidence from 1974–1987 using SEER registry data and concluded that screening can account for the increases among perimenopausal women (ages 45–64) but not for younger (ages 25–44) or older (ages over 65) women.

In contrast, Harris et al. (1992) pointed out that mammographic screening has been shown to decrease long-term mortality from breast cancer. Their position is that breast cancer screening causes at most a transient rise in incidence, and since its use was not widespread at least through the early 1980s, it can explain little of the long-term increase in the incidence of breast cancer. However, if aggressive screening programs detect lesions that are classified as malignant but are actually indolent and would not have been detected otherwise, then the apparent rise in incidence is not meaningful (Fox 1979).

Glass and Hoover (1990) analyzed trends in breast cancer incidence from 1960–1985 in a large population-based tumor registry (Kaiser Permanente) in Portland, Oregon. They reported a 131% increase in ER^+ breast cancer between the mid-1970s and the mid-1980s. In contrast, there was only a 22–27% increase in ER^- tumor incidence. According to the authors, these increases in reported breast cancer incidence were unlikely to arise solely from improved screening and diagnosis. The authors speculated that the greater increase in ER^+ tumors might be due to "hormonal influences." However, although ER status has clear treatment implications, it is not clear that ER^+ and ER^- tumors are different etiologically. They have similar known risk factors, and ER^- tumors may simply reflect a more advanced malignant state of the same underlying disease. In addition, tumors detected on screening may be less aggressive, and more likely ER^+.

There is a controversy whether known risk factors can account for the distribution of breast cancer cases or whether important, unidentified influences are affecting risk. Madigan et al. (1995) estimated that 41% of cases in the United States are accounted for by known risk factors, leaving 59% unaccounted for. It could be, however, that many of these unaccounted-for cases also are due to known risk factors but have eluded estimation by the limited ability of relatively crude data sources available.

It is open to debate whether there has in fact been a long-term increase in breast cancer risk above the already-high rates in the United States and other industrialized societies. If the increases are real, what might be the causes?

ESTROGEN

Estrogen and estrogen metabolism are thought to be crucial to understanding breast cancer etiology (Henderson et al. 1988). Estrogen stimulates turnover of the breast epithelial cells at risk of malignant transformation, which is expected to influence risk (Moolgavkar et al. 1980). Under this view, any personal characteristic (e.g., age at menarche, age at birth of first child) or factor in the environment that affects estrogen metabolism or production can be expected to influence breast cancer risk. Though study results have been mixed (Thomas 1984), recent epidemiologic evidence supports the hypothesis that estrogen availability in blood is greater in postmenopausal women who later develop breast cancer than in those who do not (Toniolo et al. 1995).

A hypothesis to account for lower risk in Japan was that Japanese in Japan have lower blood levels of estrogen and thereby lower risk. Studies to test this hypothesis found no difference in estrogen levels between Japanese and American women (Bulbrook et al. 1976). However, these early studies examined Japanese women in and around Tokyo who would be expected to be more westernized in lifestyle than women in rural parts of Japan. Indeed, Shimizu et al. (1990) deliberately chose Japanese women from a rural agricultural area and found them to have estradiol levels 35% lower than the American women of similar age in their study.

RISK FACTORS

Age

The strongest risk factor for breast cancer is age. The relative risk of mortality for ages 50–54 compared to age 25–29 is ~50 (Wakai et al. 1995); for ages 80–84 it is ~100. The relationship of age to risk of breast cancer is unique. For most solid tumors, the log of incidence increases linearly with the log of age [i.e., linear on a log-log plot (Cook 1969)]; slopes range from 4 for melanoma to 10 for prostate cancer. In contrast, breast cancer incidence rises rapidly prior to menopause, then levels off before again increasing into old age, but at a slower pace than the rate before menopause (Moolgavkar et al. 1979). The idea that breast cancer might in fact be two different diseases—one premenopausal form and another postmenopausal—was in part based on the observation that low-risk societies lacked the rise in risk after menopause (de Waard 1979). However, after adjustment for cohort effects, the rise into old age is common to all populations studied regardless of the absolute level of risk; e.g., the pattern is very similar in Japan and the

United States though the absolute risks are three- to fourfold lower in Japan (Wakai et al. 1995). This unique relationship of risk to age is consistent with models for carcinogenesis that take account of the growth characteristics of the breast tissue (Moolgavkar et al. 1980; Pike et al. 1983); whereas most epithelial tissue continues to shed and replenish cells throughout life, breast tissue involutes during menopause.

Genetic Predisposition

There is growing evidence that cancer arises from the malignant conversion of a single cell (Wainscoat and Fey 1990). Currently, there is great excitement about the biology of oncogene and tumor suppressor gene action, and how these classes of genes might transform a single normal cell into a malignant cell that will grow to become a clinically detectable neoplasm (Weinberg 1989, 1991). For breast cancer, several genes have been identified that segregate with disease in high-risk families (Ford and Easton 1995). BRCA1 and BRCA2 appear to confer a lifetime risk approaching 100%, and germinal mutation of them may account for as much as 5% of cases in the population. Ford and Easton (1995) state, "The fact that many mutations are clearly inactivating suggests that BRCA1 acts as a tumor-suppressor gene. Under this model, cancers in BRCA1-linked families result from the inheritance of an inactivating mutation in one copy of the gene followed by a somatic loss of the non-mutant (wildtype) gene on the other chromosome." Women with a family history of breast cancer are at increased risk themselves, and this association may be explained by one or more of the breast cancer susceptibility genes (Peto et al. 1996). In addition, cases of breast cancer found in families with other affected women (i.e., hereditary breast cancer) typically appear at a considerably younger age than cases without a family history (Marcus et al. 1996).

Germinal mutation of one or more of these "cancer" genes may explain inherited high susceptibility; somatic mutation may explain all other cases. If this is true, then a genotoxic agent such as ionizing radiation will cause breast cancer by directly mutating the relevant genes. Agents that are not directly genotoxic, but that increase proliferation or turnover of the cells at risk, also will increase risk by increasing the chances that one mutated homologue, by whatever means, will become homozygous. Pitot and Dragan (1991) argue that proliferation-stimulating agents (promoters are one class) account for a greater proportion of cancer cases than strictly genotoxic agents in the environment. With regard to breast cancer, perhaps all cases are caused at the cellular level by homozygosity for an abnormal "cancer" gene, but the differences in risk among societies may be accounted for more by factors that affect cell turnover kinetics and tissue proliferation (e.g., hormonal influences) than by factors that directly mutate DNA.

Personal Characteristics and the Environment

The most clearly understood risk factors for breast cancer are reproductive. The pioneering work of MacMahon and colleagues first shed light on the role of reproductive history in breast cancer epidemiology (MacMahon et al. 1973; Trichopoulos et al. 1972). The evidence is that early age at menarche and late age at menopause increase risk, and that early age at first full-term pregnancy and a large number of children decrease risk (Kelsey et al. 1993). These effects are consistent with models of breast carcinogenesis that take account of tissue turnover kinetics (Moolgavkar et al. 1980; Pike et al. 1983). Early menarche and late menopause prolong the period in which estrogen is produced and the breast tissue is actively proliferating. Early age at first full-term pregnancy is thought to lead to terminal differentiation of breast cells for the production of milk, and thereby removes them from the susceptible pool; each subsequent pregnancy may further this process.

The most frustrating risk factors to disentangle are dietary. In rats, many experiments in which the subjects are fed a high-fat diet have shown increased yield of chemically induced mammary tumors (Welsch 1985). Whether dietary fat explains the high rates of breast cancer in industrialized societies, however, is hotly disputed. Prentice and Sheppard (1990) argue that the high correlation of per-capita fat consumption and breast cancer risk among countries, and the strong animal model, taken together, support an important role for fat, and that the epidemiologic studies done within countries lack power to detect an effect because of the narrow within-country range of fat intake. Willett and Stampfer (1990) argue that the international correlation is hopelessly confounded with other risk factors and therefore is the weakest of evidence, and that the large cohort studies which have shown no effect (e.g., Willett et al. 1992) do have power to detect effects of the magnitude claimed by Prentice and Sheppard (1990), at least if fat consumption in adulthood is important (Hunter et al. 1996). Energy (caloric) intake in childhood, which is intimately related to fat intake, may well be an important determinant of lifetime risk, as reflected in the association of height with risk (Micozzi 1987; Tretli 1989). However, it is very difficult to obtain persuasive evidence one way or the other on childhood energy intake, because it occurs so long before disease and can only be inferred through the association of risk with adult height.

Studies of diet and breast cancer are hampered by the possibility that it is the diet early in life that influences risk. However, childhood diet is difficult to assess in studies of adults. To some extent, height provides a surrogate for childhood energy intake in that caloric restriction during childhood limits attained height. Japanese people have experienced a dramatic increase in attained height in this century as childhood energy intake has increased; breast cancer rates have risen in tandem (Hirohata et al. 1985). In general, the literature suggests that adult height is a modest risk factor for breast cancer (Hunter and Willett 1993). This association is observed even in populations for whom caloric restriction in childhood is unlikely to have been widespread, including the United States. The association between height and breast cancer risk in generally well-nourished populations has lead to speculation regarding other mechanisms (Hunter and Willett 1993). For example, adult height may be related to mammary gland mass. In turn, dense breast tissue on mammography, a correlate for mammary gland mass, is strongly related to breast cancer risk (Oza and Boyd 1993). Nonetheless, the relation between lifestyle factors in childhood and attained height has not been fully explored. Intakes of fat, protein, and/or micronutrients may play a role. Physical activity and adiposity also may play a role in attained height, as well as the timing of menarche, which is an independent risk factor for breast cancer. There is some evidence that strenuous physical activity in adulthood may lower risk by as much as half (D'Avanzo et al. 1996), but the evidence on this point is sparse.

There are other areas of research on diet that have been investigated. The possibility that the lower rates of breast cancer among Asian women might be related to their much higher intake of soya is

currently under investigation. Soya contains large amounts of the isoflavones daidzein and genistein which may act as anti-estrogens by competing with endogenous estrogens in binding to receptors (Lu et al. 1996). While epidemiologic data on soy protein intake are few, an inverse association with breast cancer risk was observed among pre-menopausal women in Singapore (Lee et al. 1992). Daily intake of soya for one month decreased estradiol levels and increased cycle length in premenopausal women, providing suggestive evidence for a role of soya intake in breast cancer prevention (Lu et al. 1996). There is sug-gestive evidence that higher intake of vitamin A (including caro-tenoids), but not vitamins E or C, may afford a very small level of pro-tection against breast cancer (Hunter and Willett 1993). Initial interest in the possibility that selenium might decrease breast cancer risk has not been confirmed in a number of studies (Hunter and Willett 1993).

Ionizing radiation is directly genotoxic and has been shown to increase risk of breast cancer in women exposed to high doses, partic-ularly in early life (Land et al. 1980). For specific groups, such as chil-dren treated by radiation for Hodgkin's disease, there can be large increases in breast cancer risk in survivors (Bhatia et al. 1996). However, the impact of background radiation and medical applica-tions on the population at large is undoubtedly very small (Doll and Peto 1981; UNSCEAR 1994) and does not account for high rates in industrialized societies.

Oral contraceptives appear to increase risk of breast cancer in young women who have a long history of use (Thomas 1993). However, oral contraceptive use cannot explain the international dif-ferences in breast cancer rates that existed prior to their introduction.

A history of benign breast disease on biopsy increases a women's risk of breast cancer by about 50%. When specific types of benign breast disease are considered, the increase in risk is three- to fivefold for atypical hyperplasia and slightly less than twofold for any evi-dence of proliferation on the biopsy (Bodian 1993). However, even lesions without proliferation appear to increase the risk of breast can-cer. Thus it appears that benign breast disease defines a group of women, including those with and without a family history, who have increased susceptibility. The underlying mechanism explaining why these diverse pathologic entities increase risk is not well understood.

Alcohol consumption increases risk (Hiatt and Bawol 1984; Longnecker et al. 1988; Blot 1992). There is some evidence that alcohol intake may result in an increase in estrogen production (Reichman et al. 1993), possibly through an effect on pineal melatonin production (Stevens and Hiatt 1987). Chronic increase in estrogen burden then might increase long-term risk of breast cancer.

Some environmental chemicals, notably organochlorine pesticide residues, can have estrogenic activity and may therefore influence breast cancer risk. However, the extent to which environmental exposure to these chemicals actually affects risk in women is unclear based on the existing evidence (Wolff et al. 1993; Krieger et al. 1994; Safe 1995). More studies of this possibility are under way.

NEW AVENUES

Many candidate exposures, in addition to the known risk factors, have been suggested that might help explain why risk of breast cancer is so high in industrialized societies. The subject of this book is electric power and its possible effects on melatonin synthesis (Stevens et al. 1992). Other candidate explanations include early energy intake (Micozzi 1987; Tretli 1989; Willett et al. 1992), and in utero exposure to estrogen (Trichopoulos 1990; Trichopoulos and Lipman 1992; Yuen et al. 1994). These candidate exposures are not mutually exclusive. Taken together, along with known risk factors and other potential etiologic agents, they may eventually help explain the high rates of breast cancer in industrialized countries. At this point, however, there is no agreement on which, if any, of these exposures are important—and so the mystery remains.

REFERENCES

Bhatia, S., L.L. Robison, O. Oberlin, M. Greenberg, G. Bunin, F. Fossati-Bellani, A.T. Meadows. 1996. Breast cancer and other second neoplasms after childhood Hodgkin's disease. *New Engl. J. Med.* 334:745–751.

Bjarnason, O., N. Day, G. Snaedal, H. Tulinius. 1974. The effect of year of birth on the breast cancer age-incidence curve in Iceland. *Int. J. Cancer* 13:689–696.

Blot, W.J. 1992. Alcohol and cancer. *Cancer Res. Suppl.* 52:2119s–2123s.

Blot, W.J., J.F. Fraumeni, B.J. Stone. 1977. Geographic patterns of breast cancer in the United States. *J. Natl. Cancer Inst.* 59:1407–1411.

Bodian, C.A. 1993. Benign breast diseases, carcinoma in situ, and breast cancer risk. *Epidemiol. Rev.* 15:177–187.

Buell, P. 1973. Changing incidence of breast cancer in Japanese-American women. *J. Natl. Cancer Inst.* 51:1479–1483.

Bulbrook, R.D., M.C. Swain, D.Y. Wang, J.L. Hayward, S. Kumaoka, O. Takatani, O. Abe, J. Utsunomiya. 1976. Breast cancer in Britain and Japan: Plasma oestradiol, oestrone and progesteron, and their urinary metabolites in normal British and Japanese women. *Eur. J. Cancer* 12:725–735.

Cook, P.J., R. Doll, S.A. Fellingham. 1969. A mathematical model for the age distribution of cancer in man. *Int. J. Cancer* 4:93–112.

D'Avanzo, B., C. Nanni, C. La Vecchia, S. Franceschi, E. Negri, A. Giacosa, E. Conti, M. Montella, R. Talamini, A. Decarli. 1996. Physical activity and breast cancer risk. *Cancer Epidemiol. Biomark. Prev.* 5:155–160.

Davis, D.L., D. Hoel, J. Fox, A. Lopez. 1990. International trends in cancer mortality in France, West Germany, Italy, Japan, England and Wales, and the USA. *Lancet* 336:474–481.

de Waard, F. 1979. Premenopausal and postmenopausal breast cancer: One disease or two? *J. Natl. Cancer Inst.* 63:549–552.

Doll, R., R. Peto. 1981. The causes of cancer: Quantitative estimates of avoidable risks of cancer in the United States today. *J. Natl. Cancer Inst.* 66:1191–1308.

Feuer, E.J., L.-M. Wun, C.C. Boring, W.D. Flanders, M.J. Timmel, T. Tong. 1993. The lifetime risk of developing breast cancer. *J. Natl. Cancer Inst.* 85:892–897.

Ford, D., D.F. Easton. 1995. The genetics of breast and ovarian cancer. *Br. J. Cancer* 72:805–812.

Fox, M.S. 1979. On the diagnosis and treatment of breast cancer. *J. Am. Med. Assoc.* 241:489–494.

Glass, A.G., R.N. Hoover. 1990. Rising incidence of breast cancer: Relationahip to stage and receptor status. *J. Natl. Cancer Inst.* 82:693–696.

Haenszel, W., M. Kurihara. 1968. Studies of Japanese migrants. *J. Natl. Cancer Inst.* 40:43–68.

Harris, J.R., M.E. Lippman, U. Veronesi, W. Willett. 1992. Breast cancer (in three parts). *New Engl. J. Med.* 327:319–28, 327:390–398, 327:473–480.

Henderson, B.E., R. Ross, L. Bernstein. 1988. Estrogens as a cause of human cancer: The Richard and Hinda Rosenthal Foundation award lecture. *Cancer Res.* 48:246–253.

Hiatt, R.A., R.D. Bawol. 1984. Alcoholic beverage consumption and breast cancer. *Am. J. Epidemiol.* 120:676–683.

Hirohata, T., T. Shigemitsu, A.M. Nomura, Y. Nomura, A. Horie, I Hirohata. 1985. Occurrence of breast cancer in relation to diet and reproductive history: A case–control study in Furuoka, Japan. *Natl. Cancer Inst. Monogr.* 69:187–190.

Hoel, D.G., D.L. Davis, A.B. Miller, E.J. Sondik, A.J. Swerdlow. 1992. Trends in cancer mortality in 15 industrialized countries, 1969–86. *J. Natl. Cancer Inst.* 84:313–320.

Hunter, D.J., W.C. Willett. 1993. Diet, body size, and breast cancer risk. *Epidemiol. Rev.* 15:110–132.

Hunter, D.J., D. Spiegelman, H.-O. Adami, L. Beeson, P.A. van den Brandt, A.R. Folsom, G.E. Fraser, R.A. Goldbohm, S. Graham, G.R. Howe, L.H. Kushi, J.R. Marshall, A. McDermott, A.B. Miller, F.E. Speizer, A. Wolk, S.-S. Yaun, W. Willett. 1996. Cohort studies of fat intake and the risk of breast cancer—a pooled analysis. *New Engl. J. Med.* 334:356–361.

Kelsey, J.L., P.L. Horn-Ross. 1993. Breast cancer: Magnitude of the problem and descriptive epidemiology. *Epidemiolog. Rev.* 15:7–16.

Kelsey, J.L., M.D. Gammon, E.M. John. 1993. Reproductive factors and breast cancer. *Epidemiol. Rev.* 15:36–47.

Krieger, N., M.S. Wolff, R.A. Hiatt, M. Rivera, J.Vogelman, N. Orentreich. 1994. Breast cancer and serum organochlorines: A prospective study among white, black, and Asian women. *J. Natl. Cancer Inst.* 86:589–599.

Land, C.E., J.D. Boice, R.E. Shore, J.E. Norman, M. Tokunaga. 1980. Breast cancer risk from low-dose exposures to ionizing radiation: Results of parallel analysis of three exposed populations of women. *J. Natl. Cancer Inst.* 65:353–376.

Lee, H.P., L. Gourley, S.W. Duffy, J. Esteve, J. Lee, N.E. Day. 1992. Risk factors for breast cancer by age and menopausal status: A case-control study in Singapore. *Cancer Causes & Control* 3:313–322.

Longnecker, M.P., J.A. Berlin, M.J. Orza, T.C. Chalmers. 1988. A meta-analysis of alcohol consumption in relation to risk of breast cancer. *J. Am. Med. Assoc.* 260:652–656.

Lu, L.W., K.E. Anderson, J.J. Grady, M. Nagamain. 1996. Effects of soya consumption for one month on steriod hormones in premenopausal women: Implications for breast cancer risk reduction. *Cancer Epidemiol Biomark. Prev.* 5:63–70.

MacMahon, B. 1958. Cohort fertility and increasing breast cancer incidence. *Cancer* 11:250–254.

MacMahon, B., P. Cole, J. Brown. 1973. Etiology of human breast cancer. *J. Natl. Cancer Inst.* 50:21–42.

Madigan, M.P., R.G. Ziegler, J. Benichou, C. Byrne, R.N. Hoover. 1995. Proportion of breast cancer cases in the United States explained by well-established risk factors. *J. Natl. Cancer Inst.* 87:1681–1685.

Marcus, J.N., P. Watson, D.L. Page, S.A. Narod, G.M. Lenoir, P. Tonin, L. Linder-Stephenson, G. Salerno, T.A. Conway, H.T. Lynch. 1996. Hereditary breast cancer. *Cancer* 77:697–709.

Micozzi, M.S. 1987. Cross-cultural correlation of childhood growth and adult breast cancer. *Am. J. Phys. Anthropol.* 73:525–537.

Moolgavkar, S.H., R.G. Stevens, J.A.H. Lee. 1979. Effect of age on incidence of breast cancer in females. *J. Natl. Cancer Inst.* 62:493–501.

Moolgavkar, S.H., N.E. Day, R.G. Stevens. 1980. Two-stage model for carcinogenesis: Epidemiology of breast cancer in females. *J. Natl. Cancer Inst.* 65:559–569.

Oza, A.M., N.F. Boyd. 1993. Mammographic parenchymal patterns: A marker of breast cancer risk. *Epidemiol. Rev.* 15:196–208.

Parkin, D.M., C.S. Muir, S.L. Whelan, Y.T. Gao, J. Ferlay, J, Powell, eds. 1992. *Cancer Incidence in Five Continents*, Vol. 6, Publication No. 120. International Agency for Research on Cancer: Lyon, France.

Peto, J., D.F. Easton, F.E. Matthews, D. Ford, A.J. Swerdlow. 1996. Cancer mortality in relatives of women with breast cancer: The OPCS study. *Int. J. Cancer* 65:275–283.

Pike, M.C., M.D. Krailo, B.E. Henderson, J.T. Casagrande, D.G. Hoel. 1983. "Hormonal" risk factors, "breast tissue age" and the age-incidence of breast cancer. *Nature* 303:767–770.

Pitot, H.C., Y.P. Dragan. 1991. Facts and theories concerning the mechanisms of carcinogenesis. *FASEB J.* 5:2280–2286.

Prentice, R.L., L. Sheppard. 1990. Dietary fat and cancer: Consistency of the epidemiologic data, and disease prevention that may follow from a practical reduction in fat consumption. *Cancer Causes & Control* 1:81–97.

Ranstam, J., L. Janzon, H. Olsson. 1990. Rising incidence of breast cancer among young women in Sweden. *Br. J. Cancer* 61:120–122.

Reichman, M.E., J.T. Judd, C. Longcope, A. Schatzkin, B.A. Clevidence, P.P. Nair, W.S. Campbell, P.R. Taylor. 1993. Effects of alcohol consumption on plasma and urinary hormone concentrations in premenopausal women. *J. Natl. Cancer Inst.* 85:722–727.

Russo, J., B.A. Gusterson, A.E. Rogers, I.H. Russo, S.R. Wellings, M.J. van Zwieten. 1990. Biology of disease: Comparative study of human and rat mammary tumorigenesis. *Lab Invest.* 62:244–278.

Safe, S.H. 1995. Environmental and dietary estrogens and human health: Is there a problem? *Environ. Health Perspect.* 103:346–351.

Shimizu, H., R.K. Ross, L. Bernstein, M.C. Pike, B.E. Henderson. 1990. Serum oestrogen levels in postmenopausal women: Comparison of American whites and Japanese in Japan. *Br. J. Cancer* 62:451–453.

Stevens, R.G., R.A. Hiatt. 1987. Alcohol, melatonin, and breast cancer. *New Engl. J. Med.* 317:1287.

Stevens, R.G., S.H. Moolgavkar, J.A.H. Lee. 1982. Temporal trends in breast cancer. *Am. J. Epidemiol.* 115:759–777.

Stevens, R.G., S. Davis, D.B. Thomas, L.E. Anderson, B.W. Wilson. 1992. Electric power, pineal function, and the risk of breast cancer. *FASEB J.* 6:853–660.

Sturgeon, S.R., C. Schairer, M. Gail, M. McAdams, L.A. Brinton, R.N. Hoover. 1995. Geographic variation in mortality from breast cancer among white women in the United States. *J. Natl. Cancer Inst.* 87:1846–1853.

Tarone, R.E., K.C. Chu. 1992. Implications of birth cohort patterns in interpreting trends in breast cancer rates. *J. Natl. Cancer Inst.* 84:1402–1410.

Thomas, D.B. 1984. Do hormones cause breast cancer? *Cancer Suppl.* 53:595–604.

Thomas, D.B. 1993. Oral contraceptives and breast cancer. *J. Natl. Cancer Inst.* 85:359–364.

Toniolo, P.G., L. Mortimer, A. Zeleniuch-Jacquotte, S. Banerjee, K.L. Koenig, R.E. Shore, P. Strax, B.S. Pasternack. 1995. A prospective study of endogenous estrogens and breast cancer in post-menopausal women. *J. Natl. Cancer Inst.* 87:190–197.

Tretli, S. 1989. Height and weight in relation to breast cancer morbidity and mortality: A prospective study of 570,000 women in Norway. *Int. J. Cancer,* 44:23–30.

Trichopoulos, D. 1990. Hypothesis: Does breast cancer originate in utero? *Lancet* 335:939–940.

Trichopoulos, D., R.D. Lipman. 1992. Mammary gland mass and breast cancer risk. *Epidemiology* 3:523–526.

Trichopoulos, D., B. MacMahon, P. Cole. 1972. Menopause and breast cancer risk. *J. Natl. Cancer Inst.* 48:605–613.

UNSCEAR. 1994. *Sources and Effects of Ionizing Radiation.* UNSCEAR Report to the General Assembly. United Nations Publication E.94.IX.11.

Ursin, G., L. Bernstein, M.C. Pike. 1994. Breast cancer. In: *Cancer Surveys, Imperial Cancer Research Fund,* Vol. 19/20:241–264. Cold Spring Harbor Laboratory Press: Plainview New York.

Wainscoat, J.S., M.F. Fey. 1990. Assessment of clonality in human tumors: A review. *Cancer Res.* 50:1355–1360.

Wakai, K., S. Suzuki, Y. Ohno, T. Kawamura, A. Tamakoshi, R. Aoki. 1995. Epidemiology of breast cancer in Japan. *Int. J. Epidemiol.* 24:285–291.

Weinberg, R.A. 1989. Oncogenes, antioncogenes, and the molecular basis of multistep carcinogenesis. *Cancer Res.* 49:3713–3721.

Weinberg, R.A. 1991. Tumor suppressor genes. *Science* 254:1138–1146.

Welsch, C.W. 1985. Host factors affecting the growth of carcinogen-induced rat mammary carcinomas: A review and tribute to Charles Brenton Huggins. *Cancer Res.* 45:3415–3443.

White, E., C.Y. Lee, A.R. Kristal. 1990. Evaluation of the increase in breast cancer incidence in relation to mammography use. *J. Natl. Cancer Inst.* 82:1546–1552.

Willett,W.C., M.J. Stampfer. 1990. Dietary fat and cancer: Another view. *Cancer Causes & Control* 1:103–109.

Willett, W.C., D.J. Hunter, M.J. Stampfer, G. Colditz, J.E. Manson, D. Spiegelman, B. Rosner, C. Hennekens, F.E. Speizer. 1992. Dietary fat and fiber in relation to risk of breast cancer. *J. Am. Med. Assoc.* 268:2037–2044.

Wingo, P.A., T. Tong, S. Bolden. 1995. Cancer statistics. *CA Cancer J. Clin.* 45:8–30.

Wolff, M.S., P.G. Toniolo, E.W. Leel, M. Rivera, N. Dubin. 1993. Blood levels of organochlorine residues and risk of breast cancer. *J. Natl. Cancer Inst.* 85:648–652.

Wynder, E.L., Y. Fujita, R.E. Harris, T. Hirayama, T. Hiyama. 1991. Comparative epidemiology of cancer between the United States and Japan. *Cancer* 67:746–763.

Yuen, J., A. Ekbom, D. Trichopoulos, C.-C. Hsieh, H.-O. Adami. 1994. Season of birth and breast cancer risk in Sweden. *Br. J. Cancer* 70:564–568.

3 Melatonin Biosynthesis, Regulation, and Effects

Russel J. Reiter
Department of Cellular and Structural Biology,
The University of Texas Health Science Center,
San Antonio, Texas

Contents

Introduction
Mechanisms of Pineal Melatonin Synthesis
Changes in Melatonin Levels Throughout Life
Alterations in the Normal Melatonin Rhythm
Theoretical Relationships of Free Radicals,
    Melatonin, and Disease Processes
Melatonin in Relation to Reproduction
Concluding Remarks
References

Introduction

Originally thought to be exclusively produced in the pineal gland, melatonin was subsequently found to be synthesized in several other tissues as well, most notably in the retina (Pang and Allen 1986) and possibly in the Harderian glands as well (Gern and Karn 1983). Although there are several organs that may produce melatonin, it is the pineal gland which provides the bulk of the melatonin that escapes into the blood. Thus, surgical removal of the pineal reduces circulating melatonin concentrations to low or undetectable levels in the blood (Reiter 1991b), even though other organs continue to produce it.

The production of melatonin within the pineal gland is unique in that its synthesis is under control of the sympathetic fibers which innervate it from the superior cervical ganglia (King and Steinlechner 1985; Ebadi and Govitrapong 1986). Hormones secreted by endocrine organs, a category into which the pineal gland falls, are typically regulated by hormones from other glands. In the case of the pineal, however, hormones from a variety of endocrine glands play only a minor role in determining the rate and/or quantity of melatonin produced.

The postganglionic sympathetic fibers that terminate among the pinealocytes, the hormone-producing cells of the pineal, make synaptic-like contacts with these cells. The firing rate of the incoming neurons varies according to the phase of the light:dark cycle. During the night, the sympathetic neurons entering the pineal gland exhibit an increased rate of firing; this induces the release of the neurotransmitter norepinephine from the intrapineal nerve terminals, eventually leading to a rise in melatonin production (Reiter 1991a; Stehle 1995). In contrast to what occurs during the night, in the day the firing rate of the sympathetic neurons destined for the pineal gland is quelled and, as a result, melatonin synthesis and secretion remain low. The differential firing of the neurons between the day and night accounts for the circadian rhythm in melatonin production, whereby the level of melatonin synthesis is higher at night than during the day. This day:night variation in pineal melatonin synthesis is characteristic of all mammalian species, including man.

The sympathetic neurons that innervate the pineal gland are driven by the intrinsic activity of the biological clock—a group of neurons, known as the suprachiasmatic nuclei, located in the hypothalamus of the brain behind the eyes (Grosse et al. 1994). The clock governing the intrinsic activity of the suprachiasmatic nuclei is not precise and runs with a period of slightly more than 24 hours. This being the case, a synchronizer of the biological clock is necessary so that the rhythmic activity of the suprachiasmatic nuclei is precisely 24 hours in duration. This is the function of the regularly recurring light:dark cycle as it is perceived by the eyes. Messages about light are transferred to the suprachiasmatic nuclei, via the retinohypothalamic tract, where they suppress the electrical activity of the clock, thereby ensuring low activity in the neurons innervating the pineal gland. Conversely, in the absence of light (i.e., during darkness), the suprachiasmatic nuclei are relieved of the inhibitory influence of light, the neurons entering the pineal gland are activated, and melatonin synthesis and secretion follow.

Once released into the blood, melatonin has a variety of actions. It clearly interacts with membrane receptors located on specific cells in the central nervous system (Reppert et al. 1994) and elsewhere (Morgan et al. 1992). The signal-transduction mechanisms in these cells involve the intracellular second messenger cyclic AMP (cAMP). Besides this, there are nuclear binding sites for melatonin (Acuña-Castroviejo et al. 1994) that are linked to gene expression (Carlberg and Weisenberg 1995). In addition to the receptor-mediated actions of melatonin, the indole has direct intracellular effects after its binding to calmodulin (Huerto-Delgadillo et al. 1994; Bettahi et al. 1996), and it has the ability to directly scavenge free radicals (Hardeland et al. 1995; Reiter et al. 1995).

MECHANISMS OF PINEAL MELATONIN SYNTHESIS

As already noted, organs other than the pineal gland synthesize the indole hormone. The melatonin found in the blood, however, is primarily derived from the pineal. Melatonin is a product of tryptophan metabolism; tryptophan is an amino acid taken up from circulation by the pinealocytes. It is quickly converted to 5-hydroxytryptophan in a reaction catalyzed by tryptophan hydroxylase (Reiter 1991a). The enzyme aromatic L-amino acid decarboxylase promotes the conversion of 5-hydroxytryptophan to serotonin; the latter compound is in very high concentrations within the pineal gland (Giarman et al. 1960). The metabolic pathway by which serotonin is converted to melatonin initially involves the N-acetylation of serotonin to N-acetylserotonin and O-methylation of the latter compound by the enzyme hydroxyindole-O-methyl transferase (HIOMT) (Fig. 1). The

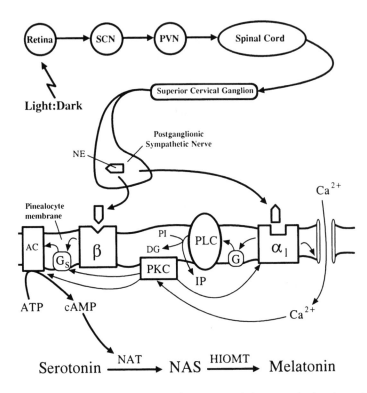

Fig. 1. Neural connections between the eyes and the pineal gland, and intra-cellular mechanisms that lead to the generation of melatonin. SCN= suprachiasmatic nuclei (biological clock); PVN = paraventricular nuclei; NE = norepinephrine; β = β-adrenergic receptor; Ca^{2+} = calcium; NAT = N-acetyl transferase; HIOMT = hydroxyindole-O-methyl transferase.

acetylation of serotonin, which is catalyzed by the enzyme N-acety-transferase (NAT), is generally considered rate-limiting in melatonin production. The gene regulating NAT has recently been cloned (Borjigin et al. 1995; Coon et al. 1995). Once produced, melatonin quickly escapes into the systemic circulation; the mechanism of release of melatonin from pinealocytes is presumably by simple diffusion. Because of the close association of pineal and blood melatonin levels, the levels of melatonin in the blood are accepted as an index of the synthetic activity of the pineal gland at virtually the same time (Reiter 1991b).

Melatonin production within the pineal gland occurs in a distinctly circadian manner, with the bulk of the synthesis occurring during the night, as described previously. Because melatonin synthesis is essentially restricted to the daily dark period in every species in which it has been studied, it has been referred to as the chemical expression of darkness (Reiter 1991a). To reiterate, the nocturnal production of melatonin is a consequence of a neural message that arrives in the pineal gland from the suprachiasmatic nuclei of the hypothalamus. The activity of the suprachiasmatic nuclei, an endogenous circadian rhythm generator, is capable of activating the pineal at night; light, detected by the eyes, is inhibitory to the suprachiasmatic nuclei (Fig. 1). Therefore, the acute exposure of animals or man to light at night causes a rapid decline in pineal melatonin production and a drop in circulating levels of the hormone (Lewy et al. 1980). Likewise, the extension of light into the normal period of darkness, provided the light is sufficiently bright, prevents the nighttime increase in pineal melatonin synthesis; therefore, blood melatonin concentrations remain low. The degree of suppression of nocturnal melatonin synthesis by acute light exposure at night is light-intensity dependent, with bright light being most inhibitory (McIntyre et al. 1989). Also, experimentally limiting the daily dark period with the use of artificial light determines the duration of elevated melatonin, because the length of time melatonin levels remain elevated at night is proportional to the length of the dark period (DeVries et al. 1993). Thus, light can be used as a "drug" to manipulate or totally suppress the circadian melatonin rhythm and, therefore, the quantity of melatonin produced.

The neural connections between the eyes and the pineal gland have been defined in a variety of mammals (Grosse et al. 1994), and it is assumed that the same pathway exists in humans (Kneisley et al. 1978; Bruce et al. 1981). This pathway involves photoreceptor cells in the retina, projections via the retinohypothalamic tract to the suprachiasmatic nuclei, connections to the intermediolateral cell column of the upper thoracic cord, preganglionic sympathetic fibers to the superior cervical ganglia, and postganglionic projections to the pineal gland (Fig. 1). Although the receptors in the retinas presumably mediate the inhibitory effects of light on melatonin synthesis, even in some totally blind subjects who have no light perception, acute light exposure still reduces circulating melatonin levels. Some of the neurotransmitters in the pathway include the excitatory amino acid glutamate at the retinohypothalamic tract–suprachiasmatic nuclei interface, and norepinephrine at the level of the postganglionic sympathetic neuron–pinealocyte interface (Fig. 1). Norepinephrine released from the postganglionic neurons within the pineal act via well-described metabolic pathways to promote the nocturnal rise in NAT activity and melatonin synthesis (King and Steinlechner 1985; Reiter 1991b). Messenger RNA levels for NAT increase proportional to the rise in melatonin production (Roseboom et al. 1996). The reduction of NAT and melatonin, which occurs normally during the late dark period, is the consequence of a protein that specifically attenuates NAT transcription (Stehle 1995).

Shortly after its production, melatonin quickly escapes from the pinealocytes, presumably by simple diffusion, to enter the blood. This release generates a nighttime rise in blood melatonin levels similar to that seen in the pineal gland itself (Fig. 2). Presumably because of its high lipid solubility, melatonin also gains access to every other bodily fluid, in which it exhibits a circadian rhythm, albeit at a reduced amplitude, like that in the blood. Likewise, it is believed that melatonin is taken up by every cell, where it may be partially compartmentalized (Menendez-Pelaez and Reiter 1993; Menendez-Pelaez et al. 1993). In particular, preliminary findings suggest that, intracellularly, highest concentrations of melatonin exist in the nucleus. None of the morphophysiological barriers that exist in the body (e.g., the blood–brain barrier) is an impediment to the passage of melatonin. Its ability to enter every cell is important for melatonin's function as an antioxidant (Reiter et al. 1995; Reiter 1996). Presumably, intracellular levels of melatonin vary in a circadian manner as they do in the pineal gland and in bodily fluids.

Besides light at night, pharmacological agents can be used to manipulate melatonin production. At least in nonhuman mam-

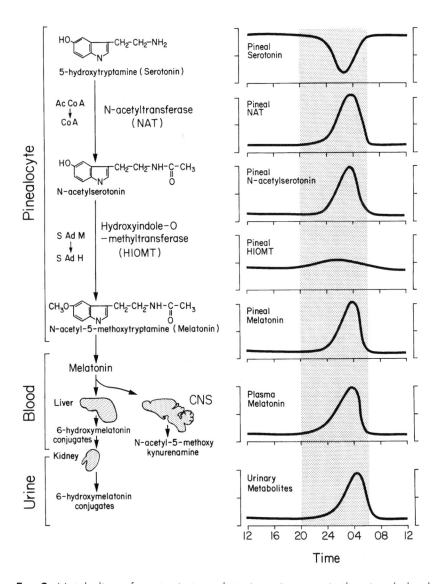

FIG. 2. Metabolism of serotonin to melatonin as it occurs in the pineal gland. After its release from the pineal, melatonin is metabolized in the liver and the brain, with the metabolites being excreted in the urine. On the right are the 24-hour rhythms of each of the constituents; the shaded area represents nighttime. CNS = central nervous system.

mals, the administration of MK-801, an N-methyl-D-aspartate (NMDA) receptor blocker at the level of the suprachiasmatic nuclei, prevents light from inhibiting pineal melatonin production (Colwell et al. 1991; Poeggeler et al. 1995). Agents that block the interaction of norepinephrine with its receptors on the pinealocyte membrane (e.g., propranolol) depress melatonin synthesis (Arendt et al. 1985; Brismar et al. 1988). Conversely, β-adrenergic receptor agonists (e.g., isoproterenol) and drugs that delay norepinephrine re-uptake into postganglionic sympathetic neurons in the pineal (e.g., disimpramine) promote melatonin production (Demisch 1993) in the rat pineal, although this finding has been difficult to document in the human. Other drugs which alter circulating melatonin levels in humans include benzodiazepines (Monteleone et al. 1989) and methoxypsoralen (Mauviard et al. 1991); the former depresses melatonin levels while the latter increases them. It is likely that a variety of neurally active drugs also may impact the ability of the pineal gland to synthesize and secrete melatonin in a circadian manner, although these have rarely been endpoints in studies where such drugs were used (Demisch 1993).

CHANGES IN MELATONIN LEVELS THROUGHOUT LIFE

In utero, the fetus is believed to receive a circadian melatonin message from the maternal pineal via its placental transfer (Kennaway et al. 1991); following parturition, the newborn is deprived of the significant rhythm for several months, during which the infant pineal produces little melatonin. The circadian melatonin cycle in the newborn human gradually develops beginning at 3–4 months of age such that in 1-year-old infants, the melatonin cycle is characteristically circadian (Gupta 1988). Children who die of sudden infant death syndrome (SIDS) reportedly have a poorly developed pineal gland (Sparks and Hunsaker 1988) and low levels of melatonin (Sturner et al. 1994). Typically, children who die of SIDS do so at the age their melatonin rhythms should be developing; however, whether the reported observations in pineal development and the melatonin cycle relate to SIDS is unknown, although this speculation has been rendered (Maurizi 1988).

During childhood (i.e., 1–10 years of age), the melatonin rhythm is generally believed to be robust; the largest day:night differences in melatonin that individuals will ever experience are present at this time. In general, children have been rather sparingly studied in terms of their circadian melatonin cycle. There may be one group of children in which a melatonin rhythm may be absent— children with infantile lipofuscinosis, or Batten's disease (Gupta 1993). Lipofuscin, which is a product of lipid peroxidation, abundantly accumulates in children with this condition, suggesting that the low levels of melatonin may relate to the disease. Melatonin is known to be a potent scavenger of the hydroxyl radical (•OH) (Tan et al. 1993a) and may neutralize the peroxyl radical (Pieri et al. 1994) as well. These radicals initiate and propagate, respectively, lipid peroxidation (Kehrer 1993); thus, low melatonin levels would be expected to be related to lipofuscin accumulation. However, whether the low levels are in fact related to the extensive lipid damage these children sustain remains unknown. Low levels of melatonin during childhood, because of the indole's ability to protect DNA from oxidative damage (Tan et al. 1993b), may also increase the likelihood of cancer in these children.

Over the 3- to 5-year period when individuals are undergoing sexual maturation, there is substantial reduction in nocturnal melatonin levels (Waldhauser et al. 1993). The reduction in circulating melatonin levels during puberty may be due to reduced melatonin synthesis in the pineal gland and secondary to the large increase in body mass at this time. This reduction in melatonin may be permissive to normal sexual maturation. Certainly, the maintenance of a very exaggerated circadian melatonin rhythm beyond the normal age of puberty has been associated with delayed sexual maturation, a condition that was overcome when melatonin levels were reduced to the normal adult values (Puig-Domingo et al. 1992). A definitive relation between melatonin and pubertal onset in humans has not yet been established.

After adulthood is achieved, most individuals maintain a circadian melatonin cycle. The amplitude of the nocturnal melatonin peak varies widely (Fig. 3), although there is no gender difference in mean blood melatonin levels. The melatonin rhythm is

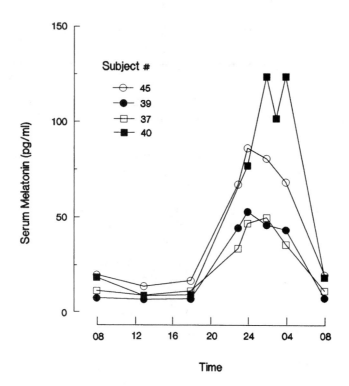

FIG. 3. The 24-hour melatonin rhythm in four adult human subjects. While males and females exhibit similar average rhythms, individually there are great variations in the nighttime melatonin rise.

genetically determined (Wetterberg et al. 1983), with the amplitude of the nighttime peak being highly reproducible from night to night. Thus, if a person is seen to have an attenuated melatonin cycle at an early age, it is believed that this low amplitude rhythm will be maintained throughout life. This means that the pineal gland of some individuals produces much less melatonin during a lifetime than does the gland of another person.

There seems to be no life event that is associated with the loss of the circadian melatonin cycle during aging; rather, it is accepted that after puberty the melatonin rhythm gradually wanes, with the eventual consequence that in advanced age a day:night difference in melatonin levels may be barely discernible (Reiter 1992, 1995b). The drop in melatonin during aging is likely due to a reduction in its production in the pineal gland, since the enzymes that catalyze melatonin's formation, as well as the levels of this constituent in the gland, are reduced in old animals (Reiter et al. 1980, 1981).

The human pineal gland exhibits a fate similar to that of animals in advanced age (Fig. 4). Because the biosynthetic activity of the human pineal deteriorates during adulthood, blood levels of melatonin also falter (Iguchi et al. 1982). The age-related drop in melatonin in the blood is reflected in a similar depression in the levels of its chief urinary metabolite, 6-hydroxy melatonin sulfate (Sack et al. 1986). Besides a reduction in nighttime maximal levels of melatonin, the duration of time melatonin remains elevated at night is also lessened (Nair et al. 1986). These reductions may be important because both the duration of elevated melatonin as well as the maximal level achieved determine the total quantity of melatonin produced.

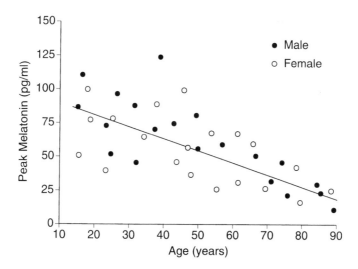

FIG. 4. Gradual reduction in nighttime melatonin levels in the blood of humans throughout life. Males and females exhibit a similar decline.

Few experimental attempts have been made to maintain a youthful melatonin rhythm into advanced age. In Fisher 334 rats, which are often used for experimental studies on aging, calorie restriction (by 25–40%) that prolongs life also substantially maintains the melatonin rhythm well past the age it is normally lost (Stokkan et al. 1991). Although melatonin functions as an antioxidant, whether the preserved rhythm has any functional significance for the old animals in protecting against oxidative damage remains unknown.

ALTERATIONS OF THE NORMAL MELATONIN RHYTHM

The condition of jet lag typically develops when individuals quickly cross several time zones, creating a situation in which the body's circadian rhythms are temporarily not properly synchronized to the prevailing light:dark cycle (Bellamy 1986). During the period when the rhythms are being re-adjusted to the new time zone, humans experience several signs, among them difficulty sleeping. Considering melatonin's sleep-enhancing property (Dawson and Encel 1993), it is believed that a disturbance of the melatonin rhythm is partially responsible for the phenomenon of jet lag (Arendt et al. 1987); as a result, taking melatonin to combat the condition has been examined and found to be effective (Pietie et al. 1989). Like jet lag, shift work, which compromises endogenous circadian rhythms, also disturbs the melatonin cycle (Madakoro et al. 1993). Thus, supplemental melatonin also may be useful in treating these individuals, because it has acute sleep-promoting effects as well as rhythm-entraining effects, with the latter consequence following a phase-response curve which is opposite to that induced by light (Lewy et al. 1992).

Besides the conditions described above, melatonin may be useful in a large number of other sleep disorders, including delayed sleep-phase syndrome, altered sleep:wake cycles in blind individuals, sleep disorders associated with dysynchronized circadian rhythms, and age-related sleep inefficiency. Melatonin is easily administered by a variety of means and it has a seemingly wide margin of safety as a drug (Norlund and Lerner 1977). Indeed, virtually no toxicity has been described.

THEORETICAL RELATIONSHIPS OF
FREE RADICALS, MELATONIN, AND DISEASE PROCESSES

Whereas another chapter in this book (Chapter 8, by Blask) reviews the actions of melatonin as an oncostatic agent, briefly summarized below is the association of free radicals with DNA damage, with the transformation of benign to malignant cells, and with the promotion of tumor growth. Since melatonin has been demonstrated to possess free radical scavenging and antioxidant activity (Reiter et al. 1995), changes in its production may relate to each of these aspects of cancer.

   The most toxic of the free radicals, particularly the •OH, are readily capable of inflicting damage to nuclear DNA (Fig. 5); thereby they have been associated with cancer initiation (Ames and Shigenaga 1993). Melatonin, on the other hand, has been shown to reduce the ability of free radicals to damage DNA, thus potentially decreasing the likelihood that they will initiate cancer. Once initiated, DNA-altered cells undergo a number of transformations before a tumor is established. Recently, it was speculated and evidence was provided for the fact that the transformation of

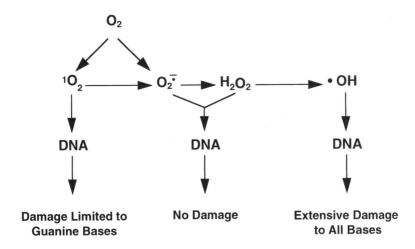

FIG. 5. Whereas singlet oxygen ($^1O_2$) has a limited capacity to damage DNA, extensive damage to DNA bases occurs when hydroxyl radicals (•OH) are produced in the vicinity of the nucleotide.

benign cancer cells into malignant cells is a consequence of progressive damage to cellular DNA (Malins et al. 1996). If this is defin-
itively established, antioxidants such as melatonin would be
important in curtailing this biotransformation of cancer cells.
Finally, cell proliferation and tumor cell growth are known to be
accelerated by free radicals (Poot and Joenje 1993). This being the
case, again, antioxidants such as melatonin would be expected to
slow tumor growth.

These three aspects of free radical biology are summarized here
because there is evidence that magnetic field exposures may in fact
reduce melatonin (Reiter and Richardson 1992; Reiter 1993). This
reduction could theoretically at least hasten all aspects of tumor
growth, because free radicals would be in higher concentrations as
a result of the reduction in melatonin.

If a reduction of melatonin were to be accompanied by an
increased free radical production, the problem could be even more
serious; for example, in a situation in which magnetic fields increase
free radical concentrations by reducing termination reactions
(Scaiano 1995; Walleczek 1995), the likelihood of oxidative damage
is also elevated. As a result of the combination of reduced antioxidant protection due to a reduction in melatonin (Reiter 1993) and
an increased number of free radicals being available to damage
DNA, the possibility of an increased cancer risk may be realized.

While this theory may have relevance to the reported rise in can-
cer incidence in individuals living in the vicinity of high power lines
(Wertheimer and Leeper 1979; London et al. 1991; Feychting and
Ahlbom 1993), at this point there is no evidence that it has validity.
On the other hand, it is a plausible explanation for the reported
observations, and could be experimentally tested in the laboratory.

Since free radicals are involved in a variety of neurological diseases of aging (Reiter 1995a), and inasmuch as melatonin has been
shown to reduce free radical-induced damage to the brain (Reiter
et al. 1995), magnetic field exposure may also, theoretically at least,
be associated with an earlier onset or a higher frequency of some
of these age-related conditions, as noted herein. In this context, it
is of interest that Sobel and colleagues (1995) reported a higher frequency of Alzheimer's disease in women exposed to higher-than-

normal magnetic fields. More studies of this type may turn up additional correlations between electric and magnetic field (EMF) exposure and disease processes. Under any circumstances, if magnetic field exposure produces biological or clinical changes that involve melatonin, these changes may be related to melatonin's efficacy as a free radical scavenger and antioxidant.

MELATONIN IN RELATION TO REPRODUCTION

Even better known than the effects of melatonin on free radical metabolism is its influence on reproductive physiology. In photoperiodic mammals, the changing light:dark cycle, because of its influence on the circadian production of melatonin, regulates seasonal changes in reproductive capability (Reiter 1980). This action of melatonin applies to a large number of species that breed only periodically throughout the year, with the duration of elevated nocturnal melatonin usually being considered the important message that the pineal imparts to the neuroendocrine–reproductive axis (Bartness et al. 1993). While the duration hypothesis of melatonin action is widely accepted and has the most experimental support, there are other features of the circadian melatonin rhythm that could also cue the reproductive system as to the status of the prevailing light:dark environment (Reiter 1987).

The specific effects of melatonin in terms of its regulation of the hypothalamo–hypophysial–reproductive axis are likely a consequence of an interaction of the indole with membrane receptors (Reppert et al. 1994) located in the hypophysiotrophic region of the hypothalamus. The primary site of these receptors is the suprachiasmatic nucleus (Reppert et al. 1994), but, additionally, the pars tuberalis of the anterior pituitary gland is rich in membrane receptors for melatonin (Morgan et al. 1992). Both these groups of receptors may be involved in mediating reproductive changes that are a consequence of melatonin administration. The action of melatonin on these cells results in a reduction in the intracellular levels of cAMP, but how this change relates to a suppression of the appropriate hypothalamic releasing hormones remains to be established.

In many but not all species, an increase in melatonin production leads to a reduction in the secretion from the anterior pituitary gland of trophic hormones (e.g., luteinizing hormone, follicle stimulating hormone, and prolactin) that normally support high reproductive activity (Reiter 1980). As a result of these reductions, spermatogenesis and ovulation are compromised in males and females, respectively, and steroid hormone production and secretion from the gonads similarly fall. The reduced testosterone secretion in males and lowered estrogen secretion in females leads to a collapse of the accessory sex organs as well. Thus, the sum of a stimulation of melatonin production in photosensitive mammals frequently is a total involution of the neuroendocrine–reproductive axis such that the animals are no longer reproductively competent. In humans, it is generally believed that melatonin also has a negative impact on reproductive physiology (Puig-Domingo et al. 1992), although the sexual changes that occur as a result of perturbations of the melatonin cycle are usually considered to be slight compared to those observed in experimental mammals (Garcia-Patterson et al. 1996).

The reported associations between reproductively active hormones and melatonin has a number of implications in terms of the EMF–cancer issue. If increased melatonin levels reduce reproductive hormones, then a reduction of melatonin would reasonably be expected to lead to a rise in the levels of these same constituents. This information was used by Stevens (1987) to develop a theory, which was subsequently refined by Stevens and Davis (1996), in which a possible reduction in melatonin as a consequence of EMF exposure may increase the incidence of breast cancer in particular. In the theory, the lower melatonin levels lead to an augmentation of prolactin and estrogen levels, which then act at the level of hormone-sensitive cells in the breast, thereby increasing their growth and proliferation. If the cells in question have been transformed into cancer cells, the result would be an increased tumor growth. This theory has garnered a great deal of interest, and these associations are currently being tested. These important relationships are summarized in greater detail elsewhere in this book (see Chapter 2).

CONCLUDING REMARKS

A great deal is known about how the environmental light:dark cycle affects and regulates melatonin production by the pineal gland. The pineal is the only endocrine organ in the body whose primary regulatory control is an environmental variable. Likewise, it is the only endocrine organ whose function depends essentially exclusively on a neural input.

The electromagnetic spectrum, particulary in the visible range, suppresses melatonin synthesis in the pineal gland of all vertebrates, including man. Thus, electromagnetic energy has an important function in controlling the internal milieu of vertebrates. This being the case, perturbations of the photoperiod would be expected to alter organismal physiology in predictable ways. Research is now defining the changes that occur, and there is little doubt that the changes are complex and multifaceted.

Melatonin clearly has a wide range of effects in animals. Although initially discovered as a hormone that regulates reproductive physiology, the indole now has been linked to a large number of functions. A major challenge of future research is to define the health effects of changes in melatonin production, and to determine whether wavelengths outside the visible range reproducibly alter the circadian synthesis of this important chemical mediator.

REFERENCES

Acuña-Castroviejo, D., R.J. Reiter, A. Menendez-Pelaez, M.I. Pablos, A. Burgos. 1994. Characterization of high-affinity melatonin binding sites in purified cell nuclei of rat liver. *J. Pineal Res.* 16:100–112.

Ames, B.N., M.K. Shigenaga. 1993. Oxidants are a major contributor to cancer and aging. In: *DNA and Free Radicals*, B. Halliwell, O. Aruoma, eds., pp. 1–18. London: Ellis Horwood.

Arendt, J., C. Bojkowski, C. Franey. 1985. Immunoassay of 6-hydroxymelatonin sulfate in human plasma and urine: Abolition of the urinary 24 hour rhythm with atenolol. *J. Clin. Endocrinol. & Metab.* 60:1166–1173.

Arendt, J., M. Aldhous, J. English. 1987. Some effects of jet lag and their alleviation by melatonin. *Ergonomics* 30:1379–1383.

Bartness, T.J., J.B. Powers, M.H. Hastings, E.L. Bittman, B.D. Goldman. 1993. Timed infusion paradigm for melatonin delivery: What has it taught us about the melatonin signal, its reception and the photoperiodic control of seasonal responses? *J. Pineal Res.* 15:161–190.

Bellamy, N. 1986. The jet lag phenomenon: Etiology, pathogenesis, clinical features and management. *Modern Med. Can.* 41:717–732.

Bettahi, I., D. Pozo, C. Osuna, R.J. Reiter, D. Acuña-Castroviejo, J.M. Guerrero. 1996. Melatonin reduces nitric oxide synthase activity in rat hypothalamus. *J. Pineal Res.* 20:205–210.

Borjigin, J., M.M. Wang, S.H. Snyder. 1995. Diurnal variation in mRNA encoding serotonin N-acetyltransferase in pineal gland. *Nature* 378:783–785.

Brismar, K., B. Hylander, K. Eliasson. 1988. Melatonin secretion related to side-effects of beta-blockers from the central nervous system. *Acta Med. Scand.* 223:525–530.

Bruce, J., L. Tamarkin, C. Riedel. 1981. Sequential cerebrospinal fluid and plasma sampling in humans: 24-hour melatonin measurements in normal subjects and after peripheral sympathectomy. *J. Clin. Endocrinol. & Metab.* 72:819–823.

Carlberg, C., I. Weisenberg. 1995. The orphan receptor family RZR/ROR, melatonin and 5-lipoxygenase: An unexpected relationship. *J. Pineal Res.* 18:171–178.

Colwell, C.S., R.G. Foster, M. Menaker. 1991. NMDA receptor antagonists block the effects of light on circadian behavior in the mouse. *Brain Res.* 554:105–110.

Coon, S.L., P.H. Roseboom, R. Baler, J.L. Weller, M.A.A. Namboodiri, E.V. Koonin, D.C. Klein. 1995. Pineal serotonin N-acetyltransferase: Expression cloning and molecular analysis. *Science* 270:1681–1683.

Dawson, D., N. Encel. 1993. Melatonin and sleep in humans. *J. Pineal Res.* 15:1–12.

Demisch, C. 1993. Chemical pharmacology of melatonin regulation. In: *Melatonin. Biosynthesis, Physiological Effects, and Clinical Applications*, H.-S. Yu and R.J. Reiter, eds., pp. 513–540. Boca Raton, Florida: CRC Press.

DeVries, M.J., B.N. Cardozo, J. Van der Want. 1993. Glutamate immunoreactivity in terminals of the retinohypothalamic tract of the Norwegian rat. *Brain Res.* 506:231–234.

Ebadi, M., P. Govitrapong. 1986. Orphan transmitters and their receptor sites in the pineal gland. *Pineal Res. Rev.* 4:1–54.

Feychting, M., A. Ahlbom. 1993. Magnetic fields and cancer in children residing near Swedish high-voltage power lines. *Am. J. Epidemiol.* 138:467.

Garcia-Patterson, A., M. Puig-Domingo, S.M. Webb. 1996. Thirty years of human pineal research: Do we know its clinical relevance? *J. Pineal Res.* 20:1–6.

Gern, W.A., C.M. Karn. 1983. Evolution of melatonin's functions and effects. *Pineal Res. Rev.* 1:49–91.

Giarman, N.J., D.X. Freedman, L. Picard-Ami. 1960. Serotonin concentration of the pineal of man and monkey. *Nature* 186:480–482.

Grosse, J., A. Loudon, M.H. Hastings. 1994. The effect of light pulses on the activity rhythms and expression of c-*fos* in the SCN of tau mutant hamsters. *Adv. Pineal Res.* 8:89–94.

Gupta, D. 1988. Pathophysiology of pineal function in health and disease. *Pineal Res. Rev.* 6:261–300.

Gupta, D. 1993. The role of melatonin in human pathophysiology. In: *Melatonin. Biosynthesis, Physiological Effects, and Clinical Applications*, H.-S. Yu and R.J. Reiter, eds., pp. 417–446. Boca Raton, Florida: CRC Press.

Hardeland, R., I. Balzer, B. Poeggeler, B. Fuhrberg, H. Uria, G. Behrmann, R. Wolf, T.J. Meyer, R.J. Reiter. 1995. On the primary functions of melatonin in evolution: Mediation of photoperiodic signals in a unicell, photooxidation, and scavenging of free radicals. *J. Pineal Res.* 18:104–111.

Huerto-Delgadillo, L., F. Anton-Tay, G. Benitez-King. 1994. Effects of melatonin on microtuble assembly depend on hormone concentration: Role of melatonin as a calmodulin antagonist. *J. Pineal Res.* 17:55–62.

Iguchi, H., K.I. Kato, H. Ibayashi. 1982. Age-dependent reduction in serum melatonin concentrations in healthy human subjects. *J. Clin. Endocrinol. & Metab.* 55:27–29.

Kehrer, J.P. 1993. Free radicals, mediators of tissue injury and disease. *Crit. Rev. Toxicol.* 23:21–48.

Kennaway, D.J., C.D. Mathews, R.P. Seamark. 1991. On the presence of melatonin in pineal gland and plasma of foetal sheep. *J. Steroid Biochem.* 8:559–564.

King, T.S., S. Steinlechner. 1985. Pineal indolealkylamine synthesis and metabolism: Kinetic considerations. *Pineal Res. Rev.* 3:69–114.

Kneisley, L.W, M.A. Moskowitz, H.J. Lynch. 1978. Cervical spinal cord lesions disrupt the rhythm in human melatonin secretion. *J. Neural Transm. Suppl.* 13:325–338.

Lewy, A.J., T.A. Wehr, F.K. Goodwin, D.A. Newsome, S.P. Markey. 1980. Light suppresses melatonin secretion in humans. *Science* 210:1267–1269.

Lewy, A.J., S. Ahmed, J.M. Jackson. 1992. Melatonin shifts human circadian rhythms according to a phase response curve. *Chronobiol. Int.* 9:380–392.

London, S.J., D.C. Thomas, J.D. Bowman, E. Sobel, T.-C. Cheng, J.M. Peters. 1991. Exposure to residential electric and magnetic fields and risk of childhood leukemia. *Am. J. Epidemiol.* 134:923–937.

Madakoro, S., H. Nakagawa, K. Misaka. 1993. Melatonin rhythms in irregular shift workers. *Jap. J. Psychiatry & Neurol.* 47:466–467.

Malins, D.C., N.L. Polissar, S.J. Gunzelman. 1996. Progression of human breast cancers to the metastatic state is linked to hydroxyl radical-induced DNA damage. *Proc. Nat. Acad. Sci. USA* 93:2557–2563.

Maurizi, C.P. 1988. Could supplementary dietary tryptophan prevent sudden infant death syndrome? *Med. Hypotheses* 17:149–154.

Mauviard, F., P. Pevét, P. Forlat. 1991. 5-Methoxyproralen enhances plasma melatonin concentrations in the mole rat: Non-noradrenergic stimulation and lack of effect in pinealectomized animals. *J. Pineal Res.* 11:35–41.

McIntyre, I.M., T.R. Norman, G.D. Burrows. 1989. Human melatonin suppression by light is intensity dependent. *J. Pineal Res.* 6:149–159.

Menendez-Pelaez, A., R.J. Reiter. 1993. Distribution of melatonin in mammalian tissues: The relative importance of nuclear verses cytosolic receptors. *J. Pineal Res.* 15:59–69.

Menendez-Pelaez, A., B. Poeggeler, R.J. Reiter, L.R. Barlow-Walden, M.I. Pablos, D.-X. Tan. 1993. Nuclear localization of melatonin in different mammalian tissues: Immunocytochemical and radioimmunoassay evidence. *J. Cell. Biochem.* 53:392–382.

Monteleone, P., D. Forzeati, C. Orazzo, M. Maj. 1989. Preliminary observations on the suppression of nocturnal melatonin levels by short-term administration of diazepam. *J. Pineal Res.* 6:253–258.

Morgan, P.J., P. Barrett, G. Davidson, W. Lawson. 1992. Melatonin regulates the synthesis and secretion of several proteins by pars tuberalis cells of the ovine pituitary. *J. Neuroendocrinol.* 4:557–563.

Nair, N.V.P., N. Hariharasubramanian, C. Pilapil, I. Isaac, J.X. Thavundayil. 1986. Plasma melatonin—An index of brain aging in humans. *Biol. Psychiatry* 21:141–150.

Norlund, J.J., A.B. Lerner. 1977. The effects of oral melatonin on skin color and the release of pituitary hormones. *J. Clin. Endocrinol. & Metab.* 45:768–774.

Pang, S.F., A.E. Allen. 1986. Extra-pineal melatonin in the retina: Its regulation and physiological function. *Pineal Res. Rev.* 4:55–96.

Pieri, C., M. Marra, F. Moroni, F. Recchioni, F. Marcheselli. 1994. Melatonin: A peroxyl radical scavenger more effective than vitamin E. *Life Sci.* 55:271–276.

Pietie, K., J.V. Conaglem, L. Thompson. 1989. Effect of melatonin on jet lag after long haul flights. *Br. Med. J.* 298:705–707.

Poeggeler, B., L.R. Barlow-Walden, R.J. Reiter, S. Saarela, A. Menendez-Pelaez, K. Yaga, L.C. Manchester, L.D. Chen, D.-X. Tan. 1995. Red light-induced suppression of melatonin synthesis is mediated by NMDA receptor activation in retinally normal and retinally degenerate rats. *J. Neurobiol.* 28:1–8.

Poot, M., H. Joenje. 1993. Oxidative stress and cell proliferation in vitro. In: *DNA and Free Radicals*, B. Halliwell, O.I. Aruoma, eds., pp. 211–228. London: Ellis Horwood.

Puig-Domingo, M., S.M. Webb, J. Serrano, M.A. Peinado, R. Corcoy, J. Ruscolleda, R.J. Reiter, A. deLeiva. 1992. Melatonin-related hypogonadotrophic hypogonadism. *New Eng. J. Med.* 327:1356–1359.

Reiter, R.J. 1980. The pineal and its hormones in the control of reproduction in mammals. *Endocrine Rev.* 1:109–131.

Reiter, R.J. 1987. The melatonin message: Duration versus coincidence hypotheses. *Life Sci.* 46:2119–2131.

Reiter, R.J. 1991a. Melatonin: The chemical expression of darkness. *Mol. Cell. Endocrinol.* 79:C153–C158.

Reiter, R.J. 1991b. Pineal melatonin: Cell biology of its synthesis and of its physiological interactions. *Endocrine Rev.* 12:151–180.

Reiter, R.J. 1992. The aging pineal gland and its physiological consequences. *BioEssays* 14:169–175.

Reiter, R.J. 1993. Static and extremely low frequency electromagnetic field exposure: Reported effects on the circadian production of melatonin. *J. Cell. Biochem.* 51:394–403.

Reiter, R.J. 1995a. Oxidative processes and antioxidative defense mechanisms in the aging brain. *FASEB J.* 9:526–533.

Reiter, R.J. 1995b. The pineal gland and melatonin in relation to aging: A summary of the theories and of the data. *Exp. Gerontol.* 30:199–212.

Reiter, R.J. 1996. Melatonin: Its intracellular and genomic actions. *Trends Endocrinol. Metab.* 7:22–27.

Reiter, R.J., B.A. Richardson. 1992. Magnetic field effects on pineal indoleamine metabolism and possible biological consequences. *FASEB J.* 6:2283–2287.

Reiter, R.J., B.A. Richardson, L.Y. Johnson, B.N. Ferguson, D.T. Dinh. 1980. Pineal melatonin rhythm: Reduction in aging Syrian hamster. *Science* 210:1372–1373.

Reiter, R.J., C.M. Craft, J.E. Johnson Jr., T.S. King, B.A. Richardson, G.M. Vaughan, M.K. Vaughan. 1981. Age-associated reduction in nocturnal melatonin levels in rats. *Endocrinology* 109:1295–1297.

Reiter, R.J., D. Melchiorri, E. Sewerynek, B. Poeggeler, L. Barlow-Walden, J. Chuang, G.G. Ortiz, D. Acuña-Castroviejo. 1995. A review of the evidence supporting melatonin's role as an antioxidant. *J. Pineal Res.* 18:1–11.

Reppert, S.M., D.R. Weaver, T. Ebisawa. 1994. Cloning and characterization of a mammalian receptor that mediates reproductive and circadian responses. *Neuron* 13:1177–1185.

Roseboom, P.H., S.L. Coon, R. Baler, S.K. McCune, J.C. Weller, D.C. Klein. 1996. Melatonin synthesis: Analysis of more than 150-fold nocturnal increase in serotonin. N-acetyltransferase messenger ribonuclei acid in the rat pineal gland. *Endocrinology* 137:1906–1909.

Sack, R.L., A.J. Lewy, D.L. Erb, W.M. Vollmer, C.M. Singer. 1986. Human melatonin production decreases with age. *J. Pineal Res.* 3:379–388.

Scaiano, J.C. 1995. Exploratory laser flash photolysis study of free radical reactions and magnetic field effects in melatonin chemistry. *J. Pineal Res.* 19:189–195.

Sobel, E., Z. Davanipour, R. Sulkava, T. Erkinjuntti, J. Wikstrom, V.W. Henderson, G. Buckwalter, J.D. Bowman, P.J. Lee. 1995. Occupations with exposure to electromagnetic fields: A possible risk factor for Alzheimer's disease. *Am. J. Epidemiol.* 142(5):515–524 .

Sparks, D.L., J.C. Hunsaker III. 1988. The pineal gland in sudden infant death syndrome: Preliminary observations. *J. Pineal Res.* 5:111–118.

Stehle, J.H. 1995. Pineal gene expression: Dawn in a dark matter. *J. Pineal Res.* 18:179–190.

Stevens, R.G. 1987. Electric power use and breast cancer: A hypothesis. *Am. J. Epidemiol.* 125:556–561.

Stevens, R.G., S. Davis. 1996. The melatonin hypothesis: Electric power and breast cancer. *Environ. Health Persp.* 104:135–140.

Stokkan, K.-A., R.J. Reiter, K.O. Nonaka, A. Lerchl, B.P. Yu, M.K. Vaughan. 1991. Food restriction retards aging of the pineal gland. *Brain Res.* 545:66–72.

Sturner, W.Q., H.J. Lynch, M.H. Deng, R.J. Wurtman. 1994. Circadian rhythm in SIDS: Melatonin levels in body fluids. *Abstr. Int. Assoc. Forensic Sci.* 8:120.

Tan, D.-X., L.-D. Chen, B. Poeggeler, L.C. Manchester, R.J. Reiter. 1993a. Melatonin: A potent, endogenous hydroxyl radical scavenger. *Endocr. J.* 1:57–60.

Tan, D.-X., B. Poeggeler, R.J. Reiter, L.-D. Chen, S. Chen, L.C. Manchester, L.R. Barlow-Walden. 1993b. The pineal hormone melatonin inhibits DNA-adduct formation induced by the chemical carcinogen safrole in vivo. *Cancer Lett.* 70:65–71.

Waldhauser, F., B. Ehrhart, E. Forster. 1993. Clinical aspects of melatonin action: Impact on development, aging and puberty, involvement of melatonin in psychiatric disease and importance of neuroimmunoendocrine interactions. *Experientia* 49:671–681.

Wallaczek, J. 1995. Magnetokinetic effects on radical pairs: A paradigm for magnetic field interactions with biological systems at lower than thermal energy. In: *Electromagnetic Fields: Biological Interactions and Mechanisms*, M. Blank, ed., pp. 395–420. Washington, D.C.: American Chemical Society.

Wertheimer, N.W., E. Leeper. 1979. Electrical wiring configurations and childhood cancer. *Am. J. Epidemiol.* 109:273.

Wetterberg, L., L. Iselius, J. Lindsten. 1983. Genetic regulation of melatonin excretion in urine. *Clin. Genet.* 24:403–406.

4   Overview of Electromagnetic Field Exposure and Dosimetry

Douglas L. Miller
Pacific Northwest National Laboratory,
Richland, Washington

Contents

Introduction
Relationships of Static and ELF Fields to the
    Electromagnetic Spectrum
Exposure to Static and ELF Electromagnetic Fields
Internal Dosimetry of Static and ELF
    Electromagnetic Fields
Relationship of Dosimetry to Mechanisms and Bioeffects
Summary and Context
References

Introduction

Electricity and magnetism have fascinated us throughout human history. From early observations of lightning originating in the heavens, and the use of the mysterious magnetic field of the Earth for navigation, man's knowledge and skill in using electric charge and current have grown to today's detailed understanding and technological mastery. Electricity and magnetism originate at the atomic level with charged electrons orbiting around an oppositely charged nucleus. On a macroscopic scale, electric charges (i.e., electrons) can accumulate as

49

static charge, and may flow through conductors to produce electric current. Electromagnetic fields define their existence by their physical effects on electrical charges and currents. The electric field strength at a point in space can be specified by the force experienced by an electric charge at that point (see, for example, Halliday and Resnick 1966). Likewise, the magnetic field can be specified by the force on a moving electric charge (e.g., a current in a wire), which is perpendicular to its direction of motion. In everyday experience, these two fields and their associated phenomena seem quite different, and they were not shown to be related until the work of Oersted in the early 1800s. Many scientists contributed to deciphering the complex nature of static and oscillating electromagnetic fields, which was put into the form of mathematical laws—the famous Maxwell's Equations—toward the end of the last century. These laws show that oscillating electric and magnetic fields are strongly interdependent and can be radiated from a source as electromagnetic radiation. The spectrum of electromagnetic radiation of increasing oscillation frequency is now understood to include AM broadcast radio waves at roughly a megahertz, microwaves at a few gigahertz, visible light at frequencies around a petahertz [10^{15} Hertz (Hz)], and even X-rays or gamma rays at exahertz (10^{18} Hz) or higher frequencies. The range of frequencies and associated spectral ranges and wavelengths are illustrated in Figure 1.

Over this tremendous range of frequencies, the physical properties and interactions of electricity and electromagnetic fields with matter provide richly varied subjects for scientific inquiry. Interaction mechanisms that might operate on biological subjects are particularly intriguing with regard to potentially harmful, or beneficial, biological effects. Since the beginning of the physical understanding of electricity and magnetism, attempts have been made to explore any associated bioeffects on humans, especially in regard to exploiting any effects for medicinal purposes (Rowbottom and Susskind 1984). For example, Galvanni discovered in the late 1700s that electricity stimulated muscles to contract, and this work led to many attempts to invent therapeutic applications of electricity and electromagnetic fields. In general, consideration of the biological effects of electromagnetic fields are quite different for different regions of the electromagnetic spectrum. Each region

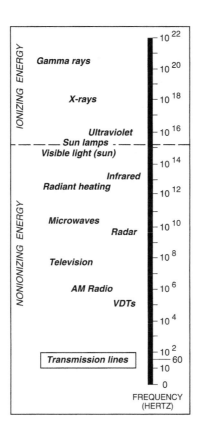

FIG. 1. Illustration of the electromagnetic frequency spectrum, with 60 Hz at the bottom. Static (DC) fields do not appear on this graph, because it is plotted on a logarithmic scale (i.e., the next lower frequency would be 3 Hz). (Reprinted from EPRI 1994 with permission from the Electric Power Research Institute, Palo Alto, California.)

has characteristic features relating to the physical exposure of a biological subject; to the dosimetry of fields within the subject; to the mechanisms by which the interaction leads to biological effects; and to the nature, consequences, and interpretation of the effects. Microwave radiation, for example, is radiated from manmade sources to which humans can be exposed. In the familiar microwave oven, the exposure is manipulated through shielding to give high exposure inside the oven with very low exposure outside the oven. The microwaves penetrate an exposed subject to a short distance as the electromagnetic energy is absorbed, giving a "dose." The absorbed energy appears as heat, which is a universal mechanism for biological effects. At high absorption rates, this can produce dramatic thermal effects, such as the familiar cooked dinner in the microwave oven. At low absorption rates, there are no apparent effects at all when temperature elevations are insignificant, such as in the cook.

This overview primarily considers static and extremely low frequency (ELF) electric and magnetic fields (EMF), with emphasis on the 60-Hz magnetic fields that are of interest in other chapters of this volume. As with other regions of the electromagnetic spectrum, this low-frequency region has a number of unique features, considerations, and interpretations. In this chapter, ELF fields will be described and placed into the context of the rest of the electromagnetic spectrum. The sources and typical exposures of humans and other subjects are then discussed, with attention to the remarkable complexity of low-level exposure. The dosimetric interaction of ELF EMF exposure with the body or other subjects is then presented, primarily in terms of the electrical fields and currents induced in biological subjects. Possible mechanisms for effects and their relation to the dosimetry problem are then considered, including some issues related to low signal-to-noise ratios. The overview concludes with a discussion of the relationship of these physics and engineering considerations to the general question of the biological effects of ELF EMF.

RELATIONSHIPS OF STATIC AND ELF FIELDS TO THE ELECTROMAGNETIC SPECTRUM

A static electric field surrounds any charged object with an electric potential proportional to the charge. Within the field E, the electric potential varies from point to point, and it is convenient to define

$$E = V/d \qquad\qquad \text{(Eq. 1)}$$

in which V is the difference in electrical potential, or voltage, between the two points separated by a distance d. This provides the normal mathematical units for the electric field of volts (V) per meter. For example, a flashlight battery with a 1.5-V potential difference between its terminals fills the surrounding space with static electric field with strengths up to about 30 V/m near the battery (i.e., d = 5 cm), and declining to zero at infinity. In general, the field is three-dimensional and has direction as well as a magnitude. Equation 1 defines the field in one dimension along the line passing through the two points. The resultant direction of the field at a point is the direction of the force exerted on a charged particle. The static electric field may exist in the absence of any magnetic field, and does not represent electromagnetic radiation.

If the terminals of a flashlight battery are connected by a conductor, electrons flow continuously from one terminal to the other under the action of the electromagnetic force (equal to the product of E and the charge) as a direct current (DC). This electric current density J in amperes (A) per square meter is given by

$$J = \sigma E \qquad \text{(Eq. 2)}$$

in which σ in siemens (S) per meter specifies the conductivity of the conductor. The proportionality constant may alternatively be specified as a resistivity (the inverse of conductivity) in ohm–meters. If the conductor is a wire, then the integrated total quantities are normally given, so that the total current in amperes equals the total voltage across the distance of wire divided by its total resistance. A new field, the magnetic field, arises from the motion of the electrons in the wire, which is proportional to the current in the wire, and inversely proportional to the distance from the wire. The magnetic field is in the form of loops around the wire, that is, in a direction perpendicular to the wire. The magnetic field strength H has units of amperes per meter. For nonmagnetic materials, the magnetic induction B is given by

$$B = \mu_0 H \qquad \text{(Eq. 3)}$$

in which $\mu_0 = 1.26 \times 10^{-6}$ H/m and is the permeability constant of free space. In practice, B is normally specified in Tesla (T) or Gauss

(G) units, and the conversion between these quantities is that 80 A/m equals 0.1 mT or 1 G. The magnetic field exerts a force on other moving electrons (i.e., electric currents) which is perpendicular to their direction of motion and proportional to their speed. There is no magnetic monopole (analogous to the electric charge), and the simplest magnetic object is a dipole. Magnetic dipoles are formed by current loops, such as occur in a completed electrical circuit, and can be characterized by a magnetic dipole moment. At the atomic level, electrons orbiting an atomic nucleus form current loops with dipole moments. In ferromagnetic material, the magnetic dipole moments of the atoms can be permanently aligned, as in the familiar bar magnet. For magnetic material, Equation 3 has an additional term on the right side involving the magnetization of the material. This phenomenon can be reproduced macroscopically; for example, a coil of wire carrying an electric current forms an electromagnet. The static magnetic field may exist independent of the electric field, and, again, does not represent electromagnetic radiation.

When the electric and magnetic fields vary with time, new phenomena appear that result from the fundamental relationship between the two fields. Of course, fields can vary with time in many ways, such as a transient step when a circuit is switched on, or an oscillation when the field varies sinusoidally with time at a specific frequency. Sinusoidal variation is particularly important because this alternating current (AC), at 50 or 60 Hz, is the form of electric power most commonly used in modern society. For example, a sinusoidally varying magnetic field expressed as a function of time t can be expressed as

$$B(t) = B_0 sin(\omega t) \qquad \text{(Eq. 4)}$$

in which ω is the angular frequency (equal to 2π times frequency) and B_0 is the amplitude of the oscillation. A changing magnetic field induces an electric field and current in a conductor. The total voltage induced around, say, a circular loop of radius r, is given by the rate of change of the field expressed as a time derivative dB/dt (pronounced de-bee-de-tee) times the area of the loop:

$$V(t) = \frac{\pi r^2 \, dB(t)}{dt} = \pi r^2 \omega B_0 cos(wt) \qquad \text{(Eq. 5)}$$

This equation represents the basis for measurement of AC magnetic fields by the voltage induced in a loop or coil of wire. For example, a 60-Hz field of 0.1-mT (1-G) amplitude induces an AC voltage of amplitude 0.12 V in a 1-m loop of wire. In addition, the magnetic induction of electric fields, such as expressed by Equation 5, represents the basis of induced-field dosimetry for biological subjects (see section on Internal Dosimetry, p. 62).

A changing electric field produces a magnetic field, a phenomenon which is the counterpart to magnetic induction of electric fields. This effect is generally quite small for ELF frequencies, because the proportionality constant is one over the square of the speed of light. At higher frequencies, the symmetrical nature of the mutual induction of electric and magnetic fields becomes important, because an electromagnetic disturbance self-propagates as electromagnetic radiation at the speed of light c = 300,000 km/second in free space. This important physical constant specifies proportionality between the electric and magnetic fields in the wave, E=cB, and also defines the wavelength λ = c/f for a given frequency f. In regard to interaction with objects exposed to an electromagnetic wave, the wavelength sets the size scale of receiving or radiating objects: An antenna is capable of efficiently radiating or receiving only when its size approaches a wavelength. At, say, 3 GHz microwave frequency, the wavelength is only 10 cm, and microwaves are radiated efficiently from small antennae, or even manipulated into narrow beams (e.g., radar). At 60 Hz, the wavelength is 5,000 km, so that 60-Hz fields generally are not radiated. In this case, the electric and magnetic fields are considered separately as quasi-static fields for virtually any situation encountered in the normal human environment (also known as the "near-field" of the emitting object). That is, ELF fields are considered to be time-varying static fields, rather than electromagnetic radiation, and the ratio E/B = c does not apply.

For static fields, there is no propagation of energy through space, although the fields have a static energy density proportional to the square of E or B. For radiated fields, in the "far-field" of an emitting object, energy is transmitted from point to point. The Poynting vector specifies the direction and rate of transfer of energy in an electromagnetic wave in terms of the vector product of the E and B fields, divided by μ_0, in units of watts (W) per square meter. This relation, together with the fixed ratio E/B = c, allows the calculation of the electric and magnetic fields in an electromagnetic wave. For example, if the intensity of an electromagnetic wave is 1 W/m², then E would be 19.4 V/m and B would be 64.8 nT.

For some situations, the quantum nature of electromagnetic waves must be considered, as first deduced by Einstein in explaining the photoelectric effect. The energy in an electromagnetic wave is concentrated in bundles called photons, each of which has energy equal to Plank's constant (6.625×10^{-34} joule-second) times the frequency. Each photon has a very small energy, which is conveniently specified in units of electron volts (eV) equal to 1.6×10^{-19} joule. This concept becomes important for very short wavelength radiation, which efficiently interacts with individual molecules. A relevant application of these concepts is to the phenomenon of vision. Visible-light wavelengths extend from about 400 nm (violet) to about 750 nm (red). The corresponding frequencies and energies range from 7.5×10^{14} Hz and 3.1 eV for violet light to 4×10^{14} Hz and 1.65 eV for red light. Vision is accomplished via the interaction of photons of light with the rhodopsin molecule contained in sensitive retinal cells in the eye; low-light vision would not be possible except for this quantized interaction on the molecular scale. As few as seven photons of yellow (507 nm) light absorbed during a flash can be registered by the brain as being seen (see, for example, Hobbie 1988). Below about 1 eV, the photon concept becomes less useful, because the energies become too low (or, wavelengths too long) for direct molecular interaction. At 60 Hz, for example, the photon energy would be only 2.45×10^{-13} eV.

The quantized nature of photons becomes the dominant characteristic for ionizing electromagnetic radiation. An X-ray of 10^{18} Hz consists of 4,140 eV photons, and these concentrated energy packets can knock loose an electron and ionize a molecule. Each photon contains only a small amount of energy; for example, 1.51×10^{15} of the 4.14 keV photons would be needed to deliver 1 joule of energy to a square meter of surface each second, which is 1 W/m². Yet, only one ionizing photon would be required to alter an otherwise stable molecule such as DNA, and ultimately lead to a detectable bioeffect. The interaction of ionizing radiation with matter is therefore discussed in terms of ionizations, and the roentgen unit (R) is defined by the electric charge produced by ionization in air (2.58×10^{-4} C/kg). There is a threshold of roughly 10 eV below which photons can no longer cause ionization.

EXPOSURE TO STATIC AND ELF EMF

EMF exist in the human environment, and interaction of humans with these fields can be considered to be field exposures. Exposure of humans and all other living things to static EMF is ubiquitous due to static electric charges and to the geomagnetic field of the Earth. Static electric charges built up on insulating materials such as carpet and clothing can produce potentials of thousands of volts, and can be painfully discharged into conductive objects. Manmade high-voltage systems present a hazard potential, primarily from the electrical discharge and electric shocks (rather than from electric fields). The Earth's magnetic field varies somewhat with position on the planet, and forms the basis of compass-guided navigation. At high latitudes, the field impinges nearly vertically with about 50 μT (0.5 G) flux density. This field may be perturbed by permanent magnets, metal objects, or mineral deposits in some locations. Because these fields expose essentially all people on the Earth, and have done so throughout human existence, there are no unexposed populations. Certain instances of manmade exposure, such as for magnetic resonance imaging (MRI) with static fields of several Tesla, can represent a source of concern for potential health risks. These high-field exposures have received significant attention and evaluation, with setting of exposure limits of 20 mT for long-term exposure, or 2 T for medical exposure (WHO 1987).

Exposure to time-varying EMF is also ubiquitous in the industrialized world due to the development of electric power and its widespread utilization for human activity. The use of time-varying fields for this purpose evolved as a result of their efficiency in power delivery. All distribution wires have some resistance, and the power lost during transmission is given by the resistance times the square of the current. Simply increasing current to increase power delivery rapidly runs afoul of resistive loss and wire heating. Thus, in order to maximize the transmitted power, given by the product of the voltage and the current, it is advantageous to minimize the current by raising the voltage. When DC and AC systems were considered during the development of electrical energy for commercial use, the AC systems quickly won out, because AC voltages can be easily manipulated with transformers. Transformers are used to increase voltages for transmission, and then to decrease them again for use. Coils of wire within transformers generate large AC magnetic fields in iron cores, and then induce AC current in a second coil with a different number of turns. The ratio of turns of the coils provides the different ratios of current to voltage for a given power level. With regard to human exposure, these differing ratios of current to voltage result in different ratios of electric and magnetic fields. In power transmission, electric fields are related to the potential difference between the wire and electrical ground, and magnetic fields are related to the current in the wire. In the modern environment, a person encounters a range of exposure situations related to electric power generation and use (EPRI 1994). These include transmission lines using voltages of 100–500 kV, distribution lines and transformers at about 20–70 kV, and end-use sources (e.g., motors and appliances) at 115–240 V. All these sources of EMF oscillate at the power-generation frequency of 50 (e.g., in Europe) or 60 Hz (e.g., in North America). Magnetic fields near high-voltage power lines are illustrated in Figure 2. Some sources and typical 60-Hz exposure levels are listed in Table 1. In contrast to the natural background DC field of the Earth, the natural background level of 60-Hz EMF is very low. However, the typical background level created by manmade sources in the modern human environment, such as in the home, is roughly 100 nT (1 mG) (Kaune et al. 1987; Silva et al. 1989).

In general, then, sources and levels of human exposure to ELF EMF are fairly well-known. In practice, however, the measurement and characterization of the exposure of specific humans to power-frequency magnetic fields poses some significant problems. A nonexposed control group is essentially impossible to assemble. In addition, the definition of exposure in the exposed group is

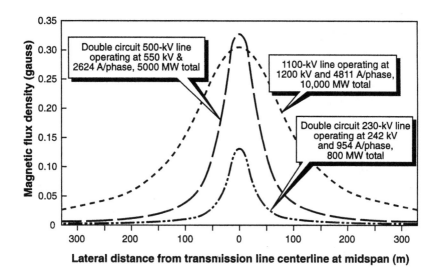

FIG. 2. Magnetic fields near electric transmission lines of various sizes. (Reprinted from EPRI 1994 with permission from the Electric Power Research Institute, Palo Alto, California.)

TABLE 1
Typical Exposure Levels Associated with Sources Found in the Modern Environment[a]

Source	60 Hz Fields	
	Electric (V/m)	Magnetic (μT)
Under 500-kV power line	7800	30
Near conventional electric blanket	250	2.2
30 cm from television	30	0.04–2.0
Near electric shaver	–	0.8–9.0
Near electric iron	60	0.12–0.3
Typical residential	0.8–13	0.09-0.2

[a] Adapted from EPRI (1994) and DOE (1995).

problematic. A simple specification might be the product of the field magnitude and the exposure duration. However, this type of specification does not have the same meaning in terms of interaction energy as, for example, intensity times duration for radiated waves. A better specification might be the square of the exposure times duration, because this measure would be related to the energy levels of the interaction. Another factor is the extreme variability of the exposure to 60-Hz fields, illustrated in Figure 3. Because everyone is exposed for long periods to the background of roughly 100 nT, the detailing of brief, relatively high field exposures under power lines or near appliances might be a more meaningful characterization of exposure. Typical appliances can yield a wide range of exposures (Gauger 1985), including some of fairly long duration, such as from electric blankets (Florig and Hoburg 1990).

These problems are especially acute for retrospective characterization of exposure for the purpose of epidemiology, and a significant research effort has been devoted to assessing human exposure

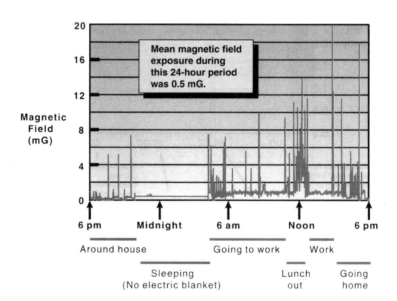

FIG. 3. An example of the variable magnetic field levels encountered in a day in modern life as recorded by a recording field meter. (From DOE 1995.)

to power-frequency fields (Kaune 1993). Because everyone is exposed to some extent, the normal scientific comparison of exposed versus unexposed control groups is precluded, and subjects must be placed into categories of relatively high or low exposure. Exposure must be classified on the basis of a few measurements, since truly complete measurements of large groups is impossible. Alternatively, surrogate exposure measures have been developed to provide an estimate of long-term differences in exposure in the absence of actual measurement of each subject's total exposure history. Surrogate measures can be developed most readily for relatively constant sources, such as power lines. For example, wire-code classification of nearby power lines has been utilized to characterize exposure at residences (Wertheimer and Leeper 1979). The characterization of occupations as "electrical" or "nonelectrical" has been used for classifying exposure groups, such as utility workers (see, for example, Savitz and Loomis 1995). These measures are useful, but are even farther removed from true exposure characterization, and the differentiation of exposures remains a key uncertainty in epidemiological research.

Typically, the distinction between different groups is blurred and their exposure ranges overlap. When an association is found between exposure and some effect, this problem becomes more acute, because it is unknown whether better exposure characterization would lead to a more definite association, or eliminate the association. For this reason, considerable research effort has gone into evaluating the validity of surrogate measures of exposure by correlating the measure both with actual field measurements, and with potential confounding factors. For example, wire coding has been compared to spot measurements of actual fields in residences, and observed endpoints have been more closely associated with wire coding than with the spot measurements of actual fields (Savitz et al. 1988; London et al. 1991). Unfortunately, it is impossible to know if the wire codes might better represent the historical exposure record (supporting the exposure–effect association), or if the codes might be correlated with some confounding factor such as age of residential housing, or density (weakening the exposure–effect association) (Pearson and Wachtel 1995). If successful, the search for confounding factors could be very important, because these new risk factors could provide alternative explanations of the reported association of field with disease.

Humans are also subjected to field exposure over other regions of the electromagnetic spectrum, particularly to radiated electromagnetic waves (Fig. 1). As noted previously, significant energy can be transmitted at frequencies well above the ELF range, and this energy can be absorbed by exposed subjects. Radio and microwaves fall into this category, and have received significant research and regulatory attention in regard to the heating mechanism. Since these fields are radiated, exposure can be discussed in terms of incident intensity (i.e., W/m^2), which is an important distinction from the case of quasi-static fields. Visible light also falls under this category, although many different units are used for specification of exposure to light. Electromagnetic waves whose photon energies exceed about 10 eV are considered ionizing radiation. Exposure to ionizing electromagnetic radiation is specified in terms of the formation of ions, owing to the dominant interaction mechanism.

INTERNAL DOSIMETRY OF STATIC AND ELF EMF

Electric and magnetic fields interact with physical objects according to their size, shape, and electrical properties. Biological tissue is not a magnetic material and has a permeability equal to that of empty space (except in regard to the presence of magnetic particles in tissue, as noted on p. 74). Many materials conduct electric charge when an electric field is applied, and are characterized by the property conductivity measured in siemens per meter. In animals, most tissues are moderately good conductors of electricity; some values of tissue conductivities are listed in Table 2. For comparison, copper has a conductivity of 59×10^6 S/m. Insulating materials (also called dielectrics) have very low conductivities, and when subjected to an electric field experience a displacement of electric charge (displacement current) that is characterized by the relative dielectric constant (relative to the permittivity of free space $\varepsilon_o = 8.85 \times 10^{-12}$ F/m). This displacement results in the induction of surface charges and

TABLE 2
Electrical Properties of Some Biological
Tissues in the ELF Range[a]

Tissue	Conductivity σ (S/m)	Permittivity ε (relative)[b]
Isotonic saline	1.34	—
Blood	0.6	—
Muscle (parallel to fibers)	0.52	1.1×10^6
Muscle (perpendicular to fibers)	0.076	3.2×10^5
Liver	0.13	8.5×10^5
Lung	0.092	4.5×10^5
Fat	0.02–0.07	1.5×10^5
Bone	0.013	3800

[a] Adapted from Foster and Schwan (1987).
[b] ε is relative to $\varepsilon_o = 8.9 \times 10^{-12}$ F/m.

displacement currents proportional to the time rate of change of the electric field. For sinusoidal fields, this phenomenon is proportional to the frequency times the amplitude of the electric field, and therefore becomes increasingly important for increasing frequencies. The relative dielectric constants of some biological tissues are also listed in Table 2.

The internal dosimetry of static EMF is relatively simple. A static electric field interacts with biological objects by inducing surface charge. This can be relevant to bioeffects considerations in regard to forces between charged structures. For example, buildup of surface charges can cause hair to stand up. In addition, static charge buildup can lead to a potential for discharges to conductors. Because tissue is conductive, the static electric field is essentially excluded from inside the body. Static magnetic fields can cause magnetic objects to orient with the field; for example, as a compass needle aligns with the Earth's geomagnetic field. A static magnetic field penetrates the body unperturbed, and does not induce electric fields within the body, as may be determined from Equation 5 for a frequency of zero. Thus, as a practical matter, the internal dosimetry of static EMF is immaterial. A noteworthy exception to this conclusion arises when a conductive subject moves within a nonuniform static field, as discussed below.

Time variation as for ELF fields results in the induction of electric fields and currents within any conductive object, such as the body. The characterization of these fields and currents represents the internal dosimetry of an external exposure (Tenforde and Kaune 1987). Although this internal characterization of EMF interaction is termed dosimetry, it should be noted that there is no established dose-quantity for ELF fields (i.e., a better term might be internal "exposimetry"). Oscillating electric fields result in the reversal of the surface charges with each cycle, which yield a small oscillating current within the body. The internal electric fields and currents are related according to Equation 2, and the induced currents are proportional to the frequency of the exposure field. Determination of the induced-current dosimetry for electric fields can be a complex process that involves two steps: determination of the surface charge and, subsequently, determination of the resulting internal currents. An idea of the dosimetry for ELF electric field exposure can be gained by considering the model situation of a grounded homogeneous human standing beneath a 60-Hz power line in a vertical, 1-kV/m field (Fig. 4A). The induced surface charges distort the external field, creating a local surface field up to 18 kV/m at the head. The flow of charge through the body yields current densities, independent of the conductivity, of about 200 μA/m^2 in the torso, increasing up to 2 mA/m^2 in the ankles. Assuming an average conductivity of 0.2 S/m, the current density in the torso is accompanied by an induced electric field of 1 mV/m. Thus, the unperturbed external field of 1 kV/m is reduced by a factor of about 1 million inside the body.

Determination of the induced field dosimetry for ELF magnetic field exposure is somewhat simpler than for electric fields in that only one step is required, but can be difficult for complex shapes and structures. One useful, if oversimplified, model is the homogeneous cylinder. For a time-varying magnetic field directed along the axis of the cylinder, the induced current flows in circular loops around the axis. For magnetic field induction, the induced electric field is independent of conductivity (in this homogeneous model), and the magnitude of the induced field E in a cylinder is given by:

$$E_\theta = \pi frB \qquad \text{(Eq. 6)}$$

in which r is the radial distance from the axis of the cylinder, and the subscript θ denotes the circumferential direction. The induced field is zero for zero frequency (DC field), and increases in proportion to frequency. The relative induced field level for different frequencies can readily be estimated by using Equation 6 as a basis; for example, 60-Hz exposure fields produce slightly higher induced fields than 50-Hz exposure fields, other factors being equal. The field induced in the cylinder is zero at the axis and increases to a maximum at the surface of the cylinder. Applying this model to a human of 1 m circumference (about 15 cm radius) in a vertical, 0.1-mT (1-G), 60-Hz field (Fig. 4B) yields a maximum

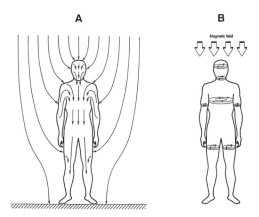

FIG. 4. Illustrations of the internal induced field dosimetry of electric **(A)** and magnetic **(B)** fields. For the electric field, the contact of the body with the electrical ground is important for the internal flow of current. For the magnetic field, the induced current flows in loops lying in planes perpendicular to the field direction, and contact with electrical ground is not important. (Adapted from Reilly1992 and reprinted with permission from Cambridge University Press.)

induced field of 3 mV/m. This maximum value on the surface of the torso is somewhat higher than for the case of the electric field considered previously, but decreases to comparable values inside the "chest." The cylinder model is useful for this simple estimate, but for more accurate calculations, other orientations and more complex models, such as ellipsoidal or anatomically based shapes, are required.

Induced-field dosimetry allows a coherent analysis of the general problem of ELF exposure and dosimetry. One valuable application is to the calculation of scaling factors for comparing exposure levels in different subjects. For example, a researcher might wish to expose laboratory rats to the magnetic field level, which would yield equivalent induced electric fields in the animals. As is evident from Equation 6, the induced field is expected to be roughly proportional to the size (radius) of an animal. Thus a 0.1-mT field produces an induced field of approximately 3 mV/m in the torso of a man as noted previously, but only about 0.6 mV/m in a rat (assuming a 3-cm radius). A researcher would need to expose the rat to about 0.5 mT to obtain roughly equivalent internally induced fields. Several examples of the external exposure fields needed for inducing internal fields roughly equivalent to those within a human standing in a vertical, 0.1-mT magnetic field are listed in Table 3. Because laboratory studies allow exquisite control of exposure and of exposure groups, definitive animal models of a reported human effect could clear up many uncertainties regarding the cause-and-effect relationship. However, laboratory animal studies have not yet firmly established a clearly reproducible effect even for field levels many times higher than those encountered in the human environment.

This concept of equivalent exposure can be extended to in vitro experiments, which provide a rational basis for comparison to in vivo exposure. Assuming that the induced electric field is the critical dosimetric factor, a wide variety of in vivo EMF exposures can be simulated in vitro simply by applying an electric field to the cell medium. Alternatively, in vitro electric fields can be induced by magnetic field exposure. (A few examples of equivalent exposures for cell suspensions in test tubes or culture dishes are also listed in

TABLE 3
Approximate Scaling Factors for Several In Vivo and In Vitro
Subjects Specified as the 60-Hz Magnetic Field
Needed to Induce Equal Maximum Internal Electric Fields[a]

Subject	Diameter	Magnetic field (mT)
Human	30	0.1
Rat	6	0.5
Mouse	2.5	1.2
Petri dish	8	0.38
Test tube	1.5	2.0

[a] To a human in a vertical, 0.1-mT magnetic field.

Table 3.) However, the induced field in such arrangements is highly nonuniform, since the induced electric field is zero at the center (see Eq. 6). In some in vitro experiments, this factor is taken into account by using dishes with a ring-shaped volume to provide more uniform induced field exposure (Misakian et al. 1993). Although such considerations can help to place in vitro exposure in perspective, many other differences exist between in vitro and in vivo conditions that complicate the interpretation of in vitro results.

Homogeneous fields simplify the consideration of internal dosimetry, but more accurate and realistic assessment may require consideration of inhomogeneity. Situations involving inhomogeneous fields may be considered in terms of homogeneous models of the subject. As noted previously, one important situation arises for the motion of a subject in an inhomogeneous static magnetic field. Since the frequency dependence of induced fields is a consequence of the dependence on dB/dt, this aspect of the relation can be used to evaluate induced field dosimetry of situations in which an object moves within a spatially varying field DC field. This situation pertains, for example, to motion within the Earth's magnetic field. Thus, the body is constantly subjected to induced electric fields due to the dB/dt associated with moving or turning in the Earth's field or other DC fields encountered in the human environment. AC fields can have complex patterns in space, a situation which presents problems for dosimetric characterization. Fields may have rapid spatial variation over parts of the body, such as near electric tools, appliances, or wires. Induced fields for these situations may be considered using simple homogeneous models. A rough approximation of maximum induced fields in such conditions may be obtained by considering the average of the exposure field over the body and the resulting simplified induced fields (Robertson-deMers and Miller 1992). Complex computer calculations may be needed for more accurate dosimetry in such situations; for example, these are used for consideration of medical treatment with AC magnetic fields (D'Inzeo et al. 1995).

Inhomogeneities also occur in the exposed subject and have recently begun to be addressed in dosimetric models and experiments. All animals are complex assemblies of organized tissues which have different conductivities (see Table 2), and these variations must influence the flow of electrical current. For example, the pattern of electrical burn injuries indicates that current follows low resistance paths such as blood vessels and muscle (Reilly 1992). As a first approximation, inhomogeneities in tissues appear to reduce the induced fields from those expected from consideration of homogeneous models (Hart 1993). The conductivity variations can be modeled from detailed anatomical descriptions for numerical calculations of induced fields from environmental exposures (Gandhi and Chen 1992) or medical treatment planning (D'Inzeo et al. 1995). Another important source of inhomogeneity are biological membranes, which can act as insulating barriers to current flow and alter the pattern of induced fields. In a simple example of this phenomenon, 60-Hz induced fields inside an egg yolk are greatly reduced relative to the white by the vitelline membrane (Miller 1991); this tendency also may apply even for larger membranes such as the peritoneum (Miller 1996).

The dosimetric consideration of EMF interactions can be carried to the microscopic scale of individual cells. A specific cell is subjected to the local electric field induced in the overall subject (e.g., an animal or cell suspension). The cellular membrane is a good insulator (dielectric) so that the overall conductivity S should be expressed as a complex quantity

$$S = \sigma + i\omega\varepsilon\varepsilon_0 \qquad \text{(Eq. 7)}$$

in which i = |-1 and represents the mathematical imaginary unit, indicating that the conduction and displacement currents are 90° out of phase for sinusoidal fields. In the simplest model, a rectangular cell presents resistance and capacitance to the flow of electrical current (Barnes 1992). A cellular membrane has a high resistance (i.e., the conductivity is quite low, of the order of 10^{-8} S/m) and a capacitance of about 5 mF/m^2, which reflects a permittivity constant of about 5. At 60 Hz, the permittivity part of the complex conductivity in Equation 7 roughly equals the conductivity part. Since the liquid medium around the cells in suspension or in tissue has a conductivity of about 1 S/m, essentially all the induced current at low frequencies flows around the cell rather than through it. Although cells can be very nonspherical in shape (e.g., elongated neuronal cells) and can communicate through extended assemblies via gap junctions, which represent significant deviations from the simple cell models used in most calculations, this insulating property of the membrane is so large relative to the external medium that it remains an important consideration at low frequencies. At the radio-frequency range, far above the ELF range, the permittivity part of the overall conductivity increases such that some current flows through the cells. This feature of the microscopic dosimetry of induced fields has important consequences for dosimetry. The bulk properties of tissue are partly determined by the properties of the extracellular space at low frequencies, but these bulk properties change above roughly 1 MHz such that the overall permittivity is reduced. At microwave or higher frequencies, the capacitance of the cell membrane becomes unimportant in this context.

Because no induced current penetrates to the interior of cells in the ELF frequency range, direct effects of induced current on intracellular processes seem unlikely. This point has been the subject of intense scrutiny, because it appears to have a bearing on the validity of any cellular bioeffects reported at low levels. The cellular membrane is not a passive element in an electrical circuit. Living cells have a transmembrane resting potential of the about 50 mV, which is much larger than any expected ELF field-induced perturbation in membrane potential (McLeod 1992). Fields applied directly to the medium must be very high to cause effects by transmembrane voltage perturbations; for example, 300–500 V/m in studies with plant roots (Robertson et al. 1981). Such high fields would be essentially impossible to generate in the body by electric field induction with external EMF.

Another aspect of dosimetry at the cellular level relates to fundamental thermal noise. A background "noise" potential exists across any resistor, including cells, due to random thermal agitation, which limits the applied electric field to which molecules could possibly respond to about 20 mV/m (Adair 1991). This noise level implies that any biologically effective influence from a very low voltage-induced field must relate to its relatively coherent nature as a "signal" at 60 Hz relative to the random background noise. That is, a much smaller coherent signal at a specific frequency may be detectable by the system (Weaver and Astumian 1990). These considerations illustrate the difficulty in absolutely ruling out low-level effects (i.e., proving the negative), and have led to the exploration of various "resonance" models of ELF field interaction mechanisms for which biological systems might be "tuned" to the ELF signal, as discussed briefly on page 74.

In living animals, normal electrophysiology has a bearing on the interpretation of induced-field dosimetry. Brain, heart, and various muscles all have electrical activity that produces internal electric fields throughout the body. These stray fields are exploited in medical practice for diagnostic purposes in the electroencephalogram, electrocardiogram, and electromyogram, all of which have components in the ELF range. When an external exposure to EMF occurs, the resulting induced fields add to the existing electrophysiological fields. The largest natural fields are due to the heart action, for which the electrocardiogram signal represents potential differences between parts of the body. The local electric fields created in rat chest-wall tissues by the cardiac fields and induced by a 1-mT

(10-G) magnetic field exposure from the front at 60 Hz can be measured simultaneously (Miller et al. 1994), as illustrated in Figure 5. In a frequency spectrum of the signal during exposure, the peak at 60 Hz due to the external exposure is evident above the background of the spectrum of the cardiac signal. The induced and endogenous field levels were comparable in this experiment: The

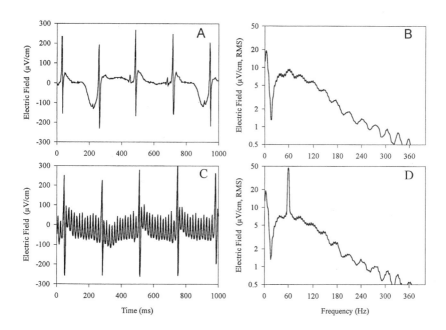

FIG. 5. Trace of the electric field **(A)** versus time and **(B)** the frequency spectrum of this signal detected in the direction of the longitudinal axis of the animal, at the chest of a large anesthetized rat lying on its side. The trace **(A)** resembles an electrocardiogram waveform, except for the baseline fluctuations (evident at about 200 and 900 milliseconds in this trace) which are associated with the animal's breathing motion. The spectrum **(B)** has relatively high readings at about 4 Hz, which represent the fundamental heartbeat frequency, and a broad peak extending from about 30–95 Hz. When 60-Hz magnetic field exposure is applied at 1 mT from the front, the time trace **(C)** has an added sinusoidal wave on the baseline due to the induced electric field, and the spectrum **(D)** includes a spike at 60 Hz.

cardiac field had a peak-to-peak (QRS complex) field of about 30 mV/m, and a 60-Hz root-mean-square (RMS) component of about 0.6 mV/m; the induced field had a peak-to-peak value of about 14 mV/m and a 60-Hz RMS component of about 5 mV/m. Near the heart, the cardiac fields were relatively large, up to 2.5 V/m peak-to-peak with a 60-Hz component of 25 mV/m RMS, and the induced fields were not detectable. The physiological electric fields have an important bearing on the interpretation of induced-field dosimetry. Since the body normally has apparently harmless electric fields in the ELF range, induced ELF electric fields seem unlikely to be harmful unless they exceed the natural fields in some respect. That is, weak ELF exposure fields would produce induced electric-field signals which would be lost in the normal electrophysiological "noise" fields in the body.

At frequencies well above the ELF range, electromagnetic waves are radiated from various devices and pose different dosimetric problems. These electromagnetic waves strongly interact with biological materials and the energy they carry is rapidly absorbed (i.e., converted into heat). For example, microwave exposures are considered in terms of the intensity and the specific absorption rate in watts per kilogram. The absorption depends on the strength of the interaction of the electromagnetic wave with the body, and is enhanced for wavelengths comparable to the size of the body, which essentially acts as a receiving antenna (Gandhi 1990). Electromagnetic waves decline exponentially inside the body due to the absorption, with an exponential constant known as the "skin depth" and given by

$$\delta = \frac{1}{\sqrt{\pi f \mu \sigma}}$$

(Eq. 8)

for good conductors (Reilly 1992). For average tissue ($\sigma = 0.2$ S/m) and normal permeability ($\mu = \mu_0 = 1.26 \times 10^{-6}$ H/m), the skin depth is 0.035 m at 1 GHz. An instructive comparison calculation can be made for ELF magnetic fields (even though these are quasi-static): The skin depth would be 145 m at 60 Hz. Thus, in the ELF range, a magnetic field penetrates the body of even very large animals virtually unperturbed. One consequence of these considerations is that heating due to absorbed energy is an important dosimetric consideration at microwave frequencies, but irrelevant at 60 Hz for any conceivable exposure levels.

RELATIONSHIP OF DOSIMETRY TO MECHANISMS AND BIOEFFECTS

The next step in the etiology of EMF effects, beyond consideration of exposure and the internal dosimetry, would be consideration of how the induced fields could cause a biological change; that is, what are the mechanisms of bioeffects? Aside from burns due to very high fields in electrical shock, there are very few viable and substantiated mechanisms for bioeffects of EMF, particularly in the ELF range. Nerve stimulation may be important at relatively high levels and can be used therapeutically (Reilly 1992). However, even for established effects, the exact details of the connection between induced fields and the resulting effect can be elusive. For example, the sensation of light can be generated by exposure to ELF electric or magnetic fields; this reversible effect is called "phosphenes" (Tenforde 1987). The thresholds for seeing magnetophosphenes are as low as 10 mT at 20 Hz, with a slowly increasing threshold at higher frequencies. Internal field induction is thought to be responsible for magnetophosphenes, but the induced fields appear to be too small to stimulate nerves directly: The detailed mechanism remains unknown (Reilly 1992). All of these biophysical dosimetric considerations seem to indicate that bioeffects should not occur at relatively low levels of exposure such as are encountered in the everyday human environment.

In stark contrast to this conclusion, epidemiological studies have associated serious disease, such as cancer, with residential-level magnetic field exposure. The epidemiological results do not provide a demonstration of causality and may not be completely convincing (Carstensen 1995). Nevertheless, the association of harmful effects with the low magnetic fields encountered in everyday life, and the lack of physical explanation through conventional induced-field dosimetry, has stimulated a search for alternative dosimetric hypotheses.

The coherence of the exposure field may be an important consideration for avoiding the thermal noise problem; Litovitz et al. (1991) report that coherence times of at least 10 seconds are needed for an in vitro effect (even though this time was too short to solve the thermal noise problem). An important mechanism for enhancing the effectiveness of weak exposure is that of resonance; that is, the tuning of a biological process to the 60-Hz power-line frequency. For example, "ion cyclotron resonance" has been proposed as a mechanism of interaction of ELF magnetic fields with specific molecules (Liboff 1985). The cyclotron frequency is given by the ratio of the charge of an ion to its mass, times the local DC magnetic field. A correspondence of this frequency with the power-line frequency for important ions like Ca^{2+} was suggested in this hypothesis to have biological significance. Changes in diatom mobility and other effects have been reported which appear to follow this idea (Smith et al. 1987). Subsequently, significant theoretical problems with this concept have been noted (see for example, Halle 1988) and some observed effects have proven difficult to reproduce, such as those observed with diatoms (Parkinson and Sulick 1992). However, the idea that some sort of resonance mechanism could help to explain various reported effects persists, and new models and tests remain under consideration. Lednev (1991) has provided new interpretation of the model, but problems remain (Adair 1992). Further modifications have been proposed by Blanchard and Blackman (1994), and some experimental tests of their ion parametric resonance theory appear to support the model (Blackman et al. 1994). Such models pose many difficulties in interpretation, particularly in relation to typical human exposure and the epidemiological question. Attempts to apply resonance models to epidemiological studies has recently begun, and provide a different approach for analyzing the results (Bowman et al. 1995).

Another important alternative dosimetric hypothesis questions the assumption that no direct magnetic field interaction occurs with tissue. For example, magnetite particles have been found in human tissues, and the possibility of a direct interaction mechanism based on this ferromagnetic mineral has been suggested (Kirschvink et al. 1992). Strings of single-domain magnetite crystals of about 50 nm orient in the Earth's magnetic field and are present, for example, in magnetotaxic bacteria. However, ELF magnetic fields have to compete in consideration of this mechanism with the background geomagnetic fields of about 50 μT, which apparently limits the exposure levels capable of influencing the particles (Adair 1993; Polk 1994). Several other interactions and mechanisms have been discussed in this regard, such as magnetic field interactions with free radicals (Polk 1992), but thus far none have proved to be the key to connecting low-level ELF EMF exposure with effective biological perturbation.

SUMMARY AND CONTEXT

In this chapter, basic physical considerations related to the question of bioeffects associated with ELF EMF have been briefly outlined. At each step in the logical progression from external exposure to internal dosimetry and physical mechanisms for influencing biological subjects, uncertainty and problems with signal-to-noise ratios consistently appear for the small field levels normally encountered in the environment. Quite real and measurable fields exist throughout our modern environment, and our day-to-day activity results in exposure to all of us. Yet, consideration of how to describe this exposure for the purpose of evaluating possible associations with bioeffects and disease have currently defied resolution. The dosimetry of ELF EMF in terms of internally induced electric fields and currents represents theoretically and experimentally definitive physics and biophysics. However, this information seems only to limit any possible roll for the minute fields induced by residential-level exposure. The well-known mechanisms of heating and nerve stimulation appear to be irrelevant to the central problem of low-field effects, but attempts at developing alternative hypotheses often run afoul of classical physics principles. A major problem is that the "signals" represented by ELF EMF exposure, dosimetry, and mechanisms of action at low levels are lost in the "noise" of source complexity, normal electrophysiology, and ordinary phenomena. Even in instances in which the signal approaches or exceeds the noise, one can only conclude that some influence is not impossible. In summary, there currently exists no established physical pathway connecting the exposure experienced in everyday life to diseases which have been associated with ELF EMF.

This perplexing situation has led to some level of polarization in the bioelectromagnetics research community. On the one hand, forceful arguments appear to limit any possibility of effects of low-level EMF exposure (see, for example, Adair 1991). On the other hand, it is difficult in a logical sense to rule out the unknown. At the same time, equally elegant biological and epidemiological studies continue to indicate potential health effects, but with a tantalizing irregularity which does not seem to lend itself to physical analysis and resolution of the problem of the missing physical connection. The problem is vexing. Clearly, the biophysics should be continuously re-evaluated while alternative explanations are sought for association of low-level exposures with significant bioeffects. The ubiquitous nature of ELF magnetic field exposure and the magnitude of potential health effects urges open-minded and full reconciliation by the scientific process.

REFERENCES

Adair, R.K. 1991. Constraints on biological effects of weak extremely-low-frequency electromagnetic fields. *Physiol. Rev.* A43:1039–1048.

Adair, R.K. 1992. Criticism of Lednev's mechanism for the influence of weak magnetic fields on biological systems. *Bioelectromagnetics* 13:231–235.

Adair, R.K. 1993. Effects of ELF magnetic fields on biological magnetite. *Bioelectromagnetics* 14:1–4.

Barnes, F.S. 1992. Some engineering models for interactions of electric and magnetic fields with biological systems. *Bioelectromagnetics* Suppl.1:67–88.

Blackman, C.F., J.P. Blanchard, S.G. Benane, D.E. House. 1994. Empirical test of an ion parametric resonance model for magnetic field interactions with PC-12 cells. *Bioelectromagnetics* 15:239–260.

Blanchard, J.P., C.F. Blackman. 1994. Clarification and application of an ion parametric resonance model for magnetic field interactions with biological systems. *Bioelectromagnetics* 15:217–238.

Bowman, J.D., D.C. Thomas, S.J. London, J.M. Peters. 1995. Hypothesis: The risk of childhood leukemia is related to combinations of power-frequency and static magnetic fields. *Bioelectromagnetics* 16:48–59.

Carstensen, E.L. 1995. Magnetic fields and cancer. *IEEE Eng. Med. Biol.* 1995:362–369.

D'Inzeo, G., K.P. Esselle, S. Pisa, M.A. Stuchly. 1995. Comparison of homogeneous and heterogeneous tissue models for coil optimization in neural stimulation. *Radio Sci.* 30:245–253.

Department of Energy (DOE). 1995. *Questions and Answers about EMF Electric and Magnetic Fields Associated with the Use of Electric Power.* DOE/EE-0040, Washington, D.C.: U.S. Government Printing Office.

Electric Power Research Institute (EPRI). 1994. *Electric and Magnetic Field Fundamentals.* BR-103745, Palo Alto, California: Electric Power Research Institute.

Florig, H.K., J.G. Hoburg. 1990. Power-frequency magnetic fields from electric blankets. *Health Phys.* 58:493–502.

Foster, K.R., H.P. Schwan. 1987. Dielectric properties of tissues. In: *Handbook of Biological Effects of Electromagnetic Fields*, C. Polk, E. Postow, eds., pp. 27–96. Boca Raton, Florida: CRC Press.

Gandhi, O.P. 1990. Electromagnetic energy absorption in humans and animals. In: *Biological Effects and Medical Applications of Electromagnetic Energy*, O.P. Gandhi, ed., Chapter 8. Englewood Cliffs, New Jersey: Prentice Hall Inc.

Gandhi, O.P., J.Y. Chen. 1992. Numerical dosimetry at power-line frequencies using anatomically based models. *Bioelectromagnetics* Suppl. 1:43–60.

Gauger, J.R. 1985. Household appliance magnetic field survey. *IEEE Trans. PAS* 104:2436–2444.

Halle, B. 1988. On the cyclotron resonance mechanism for magnetic field effect on transmembrane ion conductivity. *Bioelectromagnetics* 9:381–385.

Halliday, D., R. Resnick. 1966. *Physics.* New York: John Wiley & Sons, Inc.

Hart, F.X. 1993. Current–density distribution induced in a two-dimensional inhomogeneous human model by a time-varying magnetic field. In: *Electricity and Magnetism in Biology and Medicine,* M. Blank, ed., pp. 572–574. San Francisco: San Francisco Press.

Hobbie, R.K. 1988. *Intermediate Physics for Medicine and Biology,* 2nd ed. New York: John Wiley & Sons Inc.

Kaune, W.T. 1993. Assessing human exposure to power-frequency electric and magnetic fields. *Environ. Health Perspect.* 101(Suppl. 4):121–133.

Kaune, W.T., R.G. Stevens, N.J. Calahan, R.K. Severson, D.B. Thomas. 1987. Residential magnetic and electric fields. *Bioelectromagnetics* 8:315–335.

Kirschvink, J.L., A. Kobayashi-Kirschvink, J.C. Diaz-Ricci, S. Kirschvink. 1992. Magnetite in human tissues: A mechanism for the biological effects of weak ELF magnetic fields. *Bioelectromagnetics* Suppl. 1:101–114.

Lednev, V.V. 1991. Possible mechanism for the influence of weak magnetic fields on biological systems. *Bioelectromagnetics* 12:71–75.

Liboff, A.R. 1985. Cyclotron resonance in membrane transport. In: *Interactions Between Electromagnetic Fields and Cells,* A. Chiabrera, C. Nicolini, H P. Schwann, eds., pp. 181–196. New York: Plenum Press.

Litovitz, T.A., D. Krause, J.M. Mullins. 1991. Effect of coherence time of the applied magnetic field on ornithine decarboxylase activity. *Biochem. Biophys. Res. Commun.* 178:862–865.

London, S., D.C. Thomas, J.D. Bowman, E. Sobel, T.C. Cheng, J.M. Peters. 1991. Exposure to residential electric and magnetic fields and risk of childhood leukemia. *Am. J. Epidemiology* 134:932–937.

McLeod, K.J. 1992. Microelectrode measurements of low frequency electric field effects in cells and tissues. *Bioelectromagnetics* Suppl.

1:161–178.

Miller, D.L. 1991. Electric fields induced in chicken eggs by 60-Hz magnetic fields and the dosimetric importance of biological membranes. *Bioelectromagnetics* 12:349–360.

Miller, D.L. 1996. Miniature-probe measurements of electric fields induced by 60 Hz magnetic fields in rats. *Bioelectromagnetics* 17:167–173.

Miller, D.L., J.A. Creim, L.E. Anderson. 1994. Comparison of cardiac and 60 Hz magnetically induced electric fields in rats. In: Abstracts of the 16th Annual Bioelectromagnetics Society Meeting, Copenhagen, Denmark, June 12–17, p. 129. Frederick, Maryland: The Bioelectromagnetics Society.

Misakian, M., A.R. Sheppard, D. Krause, M.E. Frazier, D.L. Miller. 1993. Biological, physical, and electrical parameters for in vitro studies with ELF magnetic and electric fields: A primer. *Bioelectromagnetics* Suppl. 2:1–73.

Parkinson, W.C., G.L. Sulik. 1992. Diatom response to extremely low-frequency magnetic fields. *Radiat. Res.* 130:319–330.

Pearson, R.L., H. Wachtel. 1995. Childhood cancer risk in relation to residential environment and lifestyle factors that are associated with wire codes. In: Abstracts of the 17th Annual Bioelectro-magnetics Society Meeting, Boston, Massachusetts, pp. 87–88. Frederick, Maryland: The Bioelectromagnetics Society.

Polk, C. 1992. Dosimetry of extremely-low-frequency magnetic fields. *Bioelectromagnetics Suppl.* 1:209–235.

Polk, C. 1994. Effects of extremely low frequency magnetic fields on biological magnetite. *Bioelectromagnetics* 15:261–270.

Reilly, J.P. 1992. *Electrical Stimulation and Electropathology.* Cambridge, Massachusetts: Cambridge University Press.

Robertson, D., M.W. Miller, E.L. Carstensen. 1981. Relationship of 60-Hz electric-field parameters to the inhibition of growth of *Pisum sativum* roots. *Radiat. Environ. Biophys.* 19:227–233.

Robertson-De Mers, K.A., D.L. Miller. 1992. Measurement of mag-netically induced electric fields in conductive media near a 60-Hz current-carrying wire. *Bioelectromagnetics* 13:209–221.

Rowbottom, M., C. Susskind. 1984. *Electricity and Medicine: History of Their Interaction.* San Francisco: San Francisco Press.

Savitz, D.A., D.P. Loomis. 1995. Magnetic field exposure in relation to leukemia and brain cancer mortality among electric utility workers. *Am. J. Epidemiol.* 141:123–134.

Savitz, D.A., F.A. Wachtel, F.A. Barnes, E.M. John, J.G. Tvrdik. 1988. Case–control study of childhood cancer and exposure to 60-Hz magnetic fields. *Am. J. Epidemiol.* 128:21–38.

Silva, M., N. Hummon, D. Rutter, C. Hooper. 1989. Power frequency magnetic fields in the home. *IEEE Trans Power Deliv.* 4:465–478.

Smith, S.D., B.R. McLeod, A.R. Liboff, K.E. Cooksey. 1987. Calcium cyclotron resonance and diatom motility. *Bioelectromagnetics* 8:215–227.

Tenforde, T.S. 1987. Interaction of ELF magnetic fields with living matter. In: *Handbook of Biological Effects of Electromagnetic Fields*, C. Polk, E. Postow, eds., pp. 197–225. Boca Raton, Florida: CRC Press.

Tenforde, T.S., W.T. Kaune. 1987. Interaction of extremely low frequency electric and magnetic fields with humans. *Health Phys.* 53:585–606.

Weaver, J.C., R.D. Astumian. 1990. The response of living cells to very weak electric fields: The thermal noise limit. *Science* 247:459–462.

Wertheimer, N., E. Leeper. 1979. Electrical wiring configuration and childhood cancer. *Am. J. Epidemiol.* 109:273–284.

World Health Organization (WHO). 1987. Magnetic fields. *Environmental Health Criteria 69*, WHO, Geneva.

5 Understanding Dose: Implications for Bioelectromagnetics Research

NORMAN H. HANSEN
Pacific Northwest National Laboratory,
Richland, Washington

CONTENTS

THE CONCEPT OF "DOSE" IN BIOELECTROMAGNETICS
COMMON EMF DOSE METRICS
THEORIES OF BIOEFFECTS CAUSAL MECHANISMS
 AND PROPOSED METRICS
 Coherence
 Transient Signal-to-Noise
 Ion Parametric Resonance
EMF MEASUREMENTS THAT SUPPORT BIOEFFECTS
 METRIC EXTRACTION
EXPOSURE ASSESSMENT IN THE REAL WORLD
 A Real-World Example
 A Second Look at Laboratory Measurements
SUGGESTIONS FOR STUDY DESIGN
SUMMARY
ACKNOWLEDGMENTS
REFERENCES

THE CONCEPT OF "DOSE" IN BIOELECTROMAGNETICS

Long-term studies to investigate the possible association between exposure to electric and magnetic fields (EMF) and risk for certain diseases are now being conducted in several countries. Of greatest interest in the context of dose metrics are studies in the United States and Sweden which will determine the association, if any, between EMF exposure and risk of breast cancer. A key element in such studies is the methodology used for estimating dose. Two questions immediately arise:

1. What constitutes dose in bioelectromagnetics?
2. How can a useful definition of dose be factored into practical exposure assessment studies?

Both questions have far-reaching implications with regard to study design, data acquisition, and data interpretation. Before examining these in detail, let us first arrive at a working definition. The word, "dose," originates from the Greek *dosis*, meaning "something given." This usage of the word applies to a measured quantity of a remedy such as, in the ancient Greek period, an herbal extract, or, in modern times, an over-the-counter or prescription medication. For the treatment of headache, the maximum over-the-counter therapeutic dose of acetylsalicylic acid, the active ingredient in aspirin, is 1000 mG for adults. We also talk of therapeutic doses of ionizing radiation in the treatment of cancers. It is important to note from these examples that dose is a measurable quantity of an identifiable, active agent such as acetylsalicylic acid or gamma radiation. Hence, the following definition:

dose   *A measurable quantity of an identifiable, active agent or of a surrogate for that agent.*

A surrogate can be anything that is strongly correlated to the measurement of the primary active agent. For example, if the buffering ingredient in a buffered aspirin is calcium carbonate, we could establish a fixed ratio between the quantity of calcium carbonate and the quantity of acetylsalicylic acid in a specific brand of aspirin. The amount of calcium carbonate consumed could serve as a surrogate, albeit not a practical one, for measuring the dose of acetylsalicylic acid. A simple, practical surrogate for dose of acetylsalicylic acid would be the number of tablets taken. This would yield excellent estimates for dose if we knew whether the tablets contained 325 mg or 500 mg of acetylsalicylic acid. Lacking that information, our choice of tablet count as a surrogate for dose still offers what may be a reasonable approximation. We will see how surrogate measures are used in bioeffects studies.

In the discipline of bioelectromagnetics, *non*ionizing doses of extremely low frequency (ELF) EMF radiation may be applied to cell cultures or other living organisms to study possible biological effects. It has been shown that small doses (12 mG for 3 days) of 60-Hz magnetic fields can inhibit the growth rate of in vitro human breast cancer cells (MCF-7) (Liburdy et al. 1993). This result, replicated by Blackman et al. (1996), is quite remarkable when one realizes that this exposure induces voltage changes that are small compared to the naturally occurring thermal noise within the cells.

In common usage, the word "dose" also refers to the measured quantity *received*. In the context in which we will consider EMF exposure, this implies a means for measuring how much EMF nonionizing radiation a living organism has taken in. It is important to note that the properties of the EMF actually measured in a determination of dose will depend on our concept of what initiates a biological effect. In the following section, we will discuss common means for estimating dose to humans.

Consider now the first question: *What constitutes dose in bioelectromagnetics?* In the simple example cited above (Liburdy et al. 1993), a dose of 12 mG [AC root mean square (RMS)] for 3 days was sufficient to cause an observable biological effect in a culture of human breast cancer cells. Because dose, in this case, is a measure of average field strength, we imply that the "active ingredient" of the applied magnetic field is *field strength*. However, there are other features of the field, such as transients and intermittence, that vie as potential "active ingredients" for biological effects. Until such time as one or more causal mechanisms for EMF-induced bioeffects have been substantiated, our concept of dose is necessarily imprecise.

How can a useful definition of dose be factored into practical exposure assessment studies? A major driving consideration in large epidemiologic studies is cost. Comprehensive EMF exposure measurements that take into account all theoretical causal mechanisms are time-consuming and expensive. Therefore, it is common practice to use inexpensive dose measures such as AC RMS spot measurements. It is also common to attempt to find inexpensive surrogates for actual measurements. For example, in a Finnish garment industry study, which will be discussed herein, the sewing machine motor model could be used as a surrogate for actual field measurements. This approach is quite reasonable if one assumes that field strength or transients are likely sources of bioeffects, because motor model is strongly correlated with field strength and transient metrics. On the other hand, if coherence or resonance are suspected as causal factors, motor model is a poor surrogate because of its poor correlation with the corresponding metrics. Coherence metrics depend more strongly on operator duty cycles and background noise than on motor brand. Resonance metrics have a strong dependence on contours in the static magnetic field shaped by auxiliary objects such as ferrous table legs. A widely known example is the use of wire codes as a surrogate for magnetic field strength measurements. The apparent increased odds ratios for cancer in VHCC-wired homes may be attributed to various confounding factors such as air pollution and nighttime light levels (Wachtel et al. 1996). The value of wire code as a surrogate for magnetic field strength is being debated.

The trend to use simple dose metrics or simple surrogate metrics presents the risk of hiding a potential correlation between EMF exposure and observable health effects. Wherever possible, data-acquisition protocols should be designed to support the testing of multiple causal-mechanism hypotheses. Defaulting to the least expensive dose metric may leave unanswered the question of what causes EMF bioeffects.

COMMON EMF DOSE METRICS

EMF dose metrics currently in common use can be examined for how well they function as measures of dose. We also can investigate their limitations and identify which characteristics of EMF they adequately portray.

The most commonly used metric in bioelectromagnetics research is AC RMS flux density ($B_{AC,RMS}$). Popular instruments such as the EMDEX II® employ this metric using various stratagems. The simplest is to capture a single spot measurement as an estimate of subject dose. Alternatively, an individual's dose can be estimated by asking him or her to wear a sampling exposure meter throughout the workday. $B_{AC,RMS}$ may be sampled at intervals and recorded for subsequent downloading to a computer where secondary metrics such as rate of change (RoC) may be extracted.

The extraction of $B_{AC,RMS}$ from an EMF waveform is an integration process that yields a single positive value by calculating the RMS of the waveform over a certain period. In integral form, it is given by

$$B_{AC,RMS} = \left(\frac{1}{\tau} \int_0^\tau B^2(t)dt \right)^{1/2} \text{ [eq.1]} \tag{Eq.1}$$

where τ is the period, nominally 40 milliseconds, and B(t) is the flux-density waveform. In discrete form, it is given by

$$B_{AC,RMS} = \left(\frac{1}{n} \sum_{i=0}^{n-1} B_i^2 \right)^{1/2} \text{ [eq. 2]} \tag{Eq.2}$$

where n is the number of samples, nominally covering 40 milliseconds of the flux-density waveform; and B_i represents the equally spaced samples. While the synthesis of complex data into simple metrics is desirable, it is important to recognize which information is being discarded to achieve this simplicity. Even if our sampling meter were capable of recording $B_{AC,RMS}$ every 40 milliseconds, the output signal would have an effective bandwidth of only 12.5 Hz. Single, higher-frequency transient events tend to be missed or averaged out. Thus, one might suspect a poor correlation between $B_{AC,RMS}$ and high-frequency transient metrics.

$B_{AC,RMS}$ measurements form the basis for dose estimation in many epidemiologic studies. The Case–Control Study of Breast Cancer conducted by the Fred Hutchinson Cancer Research Center in Seattle (Stevens, personal communication) makes use of the EMDEX II meter for collecting nighttime exposure estimates. $B_{AC,RMS}$ is sampled every

30 seconds. For every 10-minute interval, metrics are calculated and stored from the sampled $B_{AC,RMS}$ values. The metrics (Table 1) extracted for this study illustrate the useful information that can be obtained from periodically sampled AC RMS values. Number of samples above a threshold ($N_{B>Thresh}$) can be extracted to test the hypothesis that field strength must be above a certain threshold for a certain minimum amount of time before a particular bioeffect occurs.

TABLE 1
Metrics Extracted from Periodically Sampled AC RMS Flux Density

Metric	Description
Mean, median, standard deviation, minimum, maximum, 90TH percentile, 10TH percentile	Standard statistical values
$N_{B>2mG}$	Number of $B_{AC,RMS}$ samples exceeding 2 mg
RoC	Rate of change metric

RoC (Lee et al. 1992), also called "variability," is a secondary metric that can be extracted from a series of sampled $B_{AC,RMS}$. The following definition yields a value in G/second.

$$RoC = \left[\frac{1}{n-1} \sum_{1}^{n-1} \left(\frac{B_{AC,RMS_i} - B_{AC,RMS_{i-1}}}{\Delta t} \right)^2 \right]^{1/2} \quad \text{[eq. 3]} \qquad \text{(Eq. 3)}$$

where Δt is the period between samples and the $B_{AC,RMSi}$ are determined by Equation 2. Equation 3 is a discrete form of the RMS and, thus, this implementation of the RoC is, in effect, an RMS value calculated from RMS values. The RoC metric is a measure of low-frequency variation in the steady-state magnetic waveform. High-frequency components are ignored unless their energy contributes significantly to the original (Eq. 2) RMS calculations.

We will discuss transients in greater detail in the next section, but we introduce here a few common metrics applicable to higher-frequency transients. The flux-density time-rate-of-change (dB/dt) is significant in electromagnetic theory because of its voltage-inducing properties. In agreement with Faraday's law, coils are voltage-sensitive to changes in flux density and, therefore, can be used to directly measure dB/dt. The dB/dt waveform can be summarized using various metrics. One simple metric is dB/dt(max), the maximum value of the dB/dt waveform. Although it is a useful comparative figure, dB/dt(max) only characterizes a single event. Additional information is available from metrics such as $N_{dB/dt>Thresh}$, the number of dB/dt events exceeding a threshold.

It is evident from this discussion that metrics in common use implicitly assume certain aspects of the EMF waveform to be more significant than others. Because some field characteristics are ignored, it may not be possible to test certain bioeffects hypotheses.

THEORIES OF BIOEFFECTS CAUSAL MECHANISMS AND PROPOSED METRICS

A significant controversy has existed over the validity of reported EMF-induced biological effects. The primary basis for this controversy has been the evident lack of a plausible physical mechanism for biological effects resulting from EMF exposure. Several causal-mechanism theories have been proposed and work is ongoing to test various hypotheses. It is beyond the scope of this chapter to exhaustively tabulate and discuss all current theories for EMF bioeffects. Instead, we will look at three popular theories and examine relevant dose metrics that have been proposed for each (Hansen and Wilson 1995).

Coherence

Litovitz et al. (1991) postulate that cells may be able to discriminate voltages induced by external fields from thermal noise based on coherence. Coherence time is loosely defined as the time during which frequency, phase, and amplitude of the field are held constant. Their studies indicate that exposure to a magnetic field exhibiting temporal coherence enhances enzyme ornithine decarboxylase (ODC) activity in murine L929 fibroblasts. By shifting the signal between 55 and 65 Hz, they were able to test coherence times ranging from 0.1–50.0 seconds; ODC activity was found to vary with coherence time. Also, the superposition of temporally incoherent magnetic fields (ranging from 30–90 Hz) mitigates biological response to the coherent signal (Litovitz et al. 1994a). They argue that this temporally incoherent, externally applied noise is differentiated from internal thermal noise based on *spatial* coherence. At receptor cites in the cell membranes, the externally applied noise is perceived as spatially coherent, whereas internal thermal noise is perceived as spatially incoherent (Litovitz et al. 1994b). Thus, external noise can suppress the effect while internal thermal noise cannot.

A dose metric proposed to test the coherence hypothesis is percent time in coherence ($\%t_{coh}$). For purposes of extracting a quantitative metric, we define coherence time as that time during which the signal (B) remains constant for at least 10 seconds without interruptions greater than 100 milliseconds. A 200-second flux-density waveform is examined by comparing 100-millisecond segments. As long as the DC offset and the AC RMS of the field for all three axes remain constant within ± 10% for longer than 10 seconds, this time is accumulated as the total time in coherence. Durations of less than 10 seconds are not added to the total. After all 200 seconds of waveform data are examined, the total time in coherence is divided by the total period (200 seconds) and multiplied by 100 to arrive at $\%t_{coh}$.

Flux-density waveform activity such as that caused by an operator cycling equipment on and off tends to make $\%t_{coh}$ small. A steady-state waveform such as that associated with a harmonically pure (free from asynchronous transients), constantly loaded transformer will result in a high value for $\%t_{coh}$.

Transient Signal-to-Noise

One argument against the plausibility of EMF-initiated biological effects is based on the question of a signal-to-noise ratio (Adair 1991). Typical amplitudes of AC power-frequency magnetic fields do not induce cellular voltages that are greater than thermal (Nyquist-

Johnson) noise. It is argued that if induced cellular signals are "lost in the noise," then cellular processes cannot detect them and, hence, no effects can occur.

This may not be the case for transients. Sastre et al. (in press) have shown that residential transients can induce transmembrane voltages with a signal-to-noise ratio > 1. This is significant because it offers a viable path for the initiation of bioeffects based on well-established physics.

A dose metric proposed for transients is simply the signal-to-noise ratio for the maximum flux-density transient (S/N_{trans}). The Nyquist-Johnson noise (N) is given by

$$N = \sqrt{4R_m kTf_{BW}} \tag{Eq. 4}$$

where k is Boltzman's constant, T is temperature in degrees Kelvin, and f_{BW} is the cellular response bandwidth. R_m is the membrane resistance and can be expressed in terms of the membrane conductance and cell radius:

$$R_m = \frac{1}{G_m 4\pi r_{cell}^2} \tag{Eq. 4b}$$

The cellular transmembrane voltage response is defined by the following equation, an adaptation by Sastre of an expression from Foster and Schwan (1989):

$$\Delta V(\omega) = \frac{j0.75\omega B(\omega) r_{loop} r_{cell}}{1 + G_m r_{cell}\left(0.5\rho_a + \rho_i\right) + j\omega r_{cell} C_m\left(0.5\rho_a + \rho_i\right)} \tag{Eq. 5}$$

where $B(\omega)$ is the Fourier transform of the flux-density waveform, r_{loop} is the current-loop radius taken to be the radius of the adult male human chest, r_{cell} is the cell radius, G_m is the membrane conductance, C_m is the membrane capacitance, ρ_a is the external resistivity, and ρ_i is the internal resistivity. For the purpose of extracting S/N_{trans}, typical mammalian cell values are used (see Table 2).

In the calculation of $\Delta V(\omega)$, $B(\omega)$ is bandwidth limited to the cellular response bandwidth (f_{BW}). The inverse Fourier transform is calculated to obtain $\Delta V(t)$, and signal (S) is taken to be the difference between the maximum and minimum excursions.

TABLE 2
Typical Mammalian Cell Parameters

Parameter	Typical mammalian value
C_m	0.01 Farads/m^2
G_m	1.0×10^4 siemens/m^2
r_{cell}	10 micrometers
r_{loop}	10 cm (male human chest)
ρ_a	2 m/siemen
ρ_i	2 m/siemen
f_{BW}	160 kHz

It is interesting to note that transients from some sources such as electric motor brushes have frequencies extending into the low megahertz. S/N_{trans} for such transients approaches zero because of the bandwidth limit of the cellular response.

Ion Parametric Resonance

Blackman et al. (1984) observed that calcium ion efflux in chick brain (in vitro) is enhanced for specific combinations of ELF AC magnetic fields and DC fields of the same order of magnitude as the geomagnetic field. This is suggestive of a mechanism initiated by nuclear magnetic resonance, but the frequencies are too low. To explain these effects, Liboff (1985) proposes that these changes in ion flux are attributable to a mechanism tied to cyclotron resonances. Changes in the motility of calcium (Ca^{2+}) in diatoms were also believed to be linked to cyclotron resonances (McLeod et al. 1987; Smith et al. 1987). Based on the work of Podgoretskii (1960) and Podgoretskii and Khrustalev (1964) in atomic spectroscopy, Lednev (1991) postulated the following theory for the reaction rate of Ca^{2+} binding with a protein:

An applied static field (B_{DC}) splits an excited energy level of the Ca^{2+}-protein complex into two sublevels. The application of a collinear alternating field (B_{AC}) at the appropriate (ion cyclotron) resonance frequency modulates the sublevels. The on-resonance probability that transitions will occur from the sublevels to a lower level is given by

$$P = A_1^2 + A_2^2 + 2A_1 A_2 J_n\left(\frac{nB_{AC}}{B_{DC}}\right) \text{ [eq. 6a]} \qquad \text{(Eq. 6a)}$$

where A_1 and A_2 are the amplitudes of emission for transitions from the two sublevels, and $J_n(nB_{AC}/B_{DC})$ is the Bessel function of order n with n integer. The B_{AC} of Equation 6a is a peak-to-peak value. The frequency index, n, is given by

$$n = f_c / f_{AC} \qquad \text{(Eq. 6b)}$$

where the cyclotron resonance frequency, f_c, is given by

$$f_c = \frac{qB_{DC}}{2\pi m} \qquad \text{(Eq. 6c)}$$

Each ion will have a unique charge-to-mass ratio. The cyclotron resonance frequency is set by the magnitude of the Zeeman splitting under the applied static field B_{DC}. Equation 6a predicts maximum responses for specific ratios of B_{AC} to B_{DC}. Physicists have criticized the Liboff and Lednev theories for violation of basic physical principles (Halle 1988; Sandweiss 1990; Adair 1992).

The ion parametric resonance (IPR) model proposed by Blanchard and Blackman (1994) is a modification of the Lednev model which, they assert, "corrects mathematical errors in the earlier Lednev model and extends that model to give explicit predictions of biological responses to parallel AC and DC magnetic fields caused by field-induced changes in combinations of ions within the biological system." The probability of observable biological responses takes on the following form:

$$P = K_1 + K_2 (-1)^n J_n\left(\frac{2 \cdot nB_{AC}}{B_{DC}}\right) \text{ [eq. 7]} \qquad \text{(Eq. 7)}$$

where the K_1 and K_2 are selected to fit experimental data. Specifically, K_1 is selected to fit the no-exposure, or "sham," data, and K_2 scales the equation to fit the magnitude of the measured response in the exposure data. The selection of K_1 and K_2 does not affect the ratios of B_{AC} to B_{DC} for which maximum responses occur. It is important to note that the B_{AC} of Equation 7 are measured as peak values, not as RMS. The factor of 2 in this equation would be omitted if peak-to-peak values were used. Equation 7 contains a factor of $(-1)^n$ not found in the Lednev equation (Eq. 6a).

Two dose metrics have been proposed for the IPR model. One is percent volume of body in resonance ($\% V_{res}$); the other is the nominal probability (P_{nom}). Percent volume in resonance can be calculated separately for any ion of interest. We assess this metric for ions having biological significance (listed here in order of decreasing charge-to-mass ratio): H^+, S^{6-}, Li^+, Mn^{7+}, S^{4-}, Cr^{6+}, Mn^{6+}, Mg^{2+}, Mn^{4+}, Cr^{3+}, Mn^{3+}, Fe^{3+}, Ca^{2+}, Na^+, Cr^{2+}, Mn^{2+}, Fe^{2+}, Cu^{2+}, Zn^{2+}, Cl^-, K^+, and Cu^+. To arrive at the metric, lines of constant B corresponding to resonances for the ion of interest are determined from volumetrically sampled flux-density data. A $\pm 10\%$ tolerance is applied, creating a thick, three-dimensional surface that intersects a human model. The percentage of body volume intersected is calculated. The dimensions of the human-body model were determined by outlining digitized cross-sections of a human cadaver.

The P_{nom} is derived from Equation 7 with $K_1 = 0$ and $K_2 = 1.719640$, or

$$P_{nom} = 1.719640 \cdot \left| J_n\left(\frac{2 \cdot n B_{AC}}{B_{DC}} \right) \right| \quad \text{eq. 8} \tag{Eq. 8}$$

Note also that the sign of the expression is eliminated. This metric represents a relative probability of an effect occurring; the direction of the effect (enhancement versus suppression) is not represented. P_{nom} ranges from 0–1.

Other valid metrics can be developed to test these three proposed mechanisms. In addition, there are several more hypothetical bioeffects mechanisms for which metrics could be developed.

EMF MEASUREMENTS THAT SUPPORT BIOEFFECTS METRIC EXTRACTION

We have already discussed the potential problems that can arise when simple, inexpensive metrics are chosen for use in an exposure assessment study. It is important to remember that certain proposed bioeffects mechanisms may be eliminated from consideration when simplistic metrics are chosen to represent exposure. The concept of dose in bioelectromagnetics is imprecise, because a dose–response model is yet to be determined. Such a model is more likely to be determined if metrics are chosen which adequately represent those features of the electromagnetic waveform that are proposed initiators for biological effects.

A practical limitation on metric selection is cost. The major factor affecting cost with regard to metrics is the complexity of data acquisition required to support desired metric extraction. It is desirable to attempt to capture "everything," meaning to perform high-bandwidth, high-dynamic-range, long-duration data acquisitions. These acquisitions would need to be repeated at finely spaced grid points in a three-dimensional volume. It is obviously advantageous to have such an all-inclusive data set, which would enable the extraction of nearly any imaginable metric. Nevertheless, the time required to gather such data and the astronomical storage requirements needed for so much information would be prohibitive from a cost standpoint.

To support metric extraction for the three mechanisms discussed previously using one all-inclusive data acquisition would be a daunting prospect. It is more practical to develop a protocol that employs several less ambitious measurements, each addressing the special requirements of one or more metrics. The set of measurements found in Table 3 are being used in the U.S. Department of Energy's EMF RAPID Appliance Study (Hansen et al. 1996) to support metric extraction for the above mechanisms. They have also been tested in exposure assessment in the Finnish garment industry.

Successful exposure assessment requires more than taking data sufficient for metric extraction. It is essential that a measurement protocol be developed that takes into account all factors which affect the accuracy and integrity of the measurements. For example, if the protocol calls for the mapping of a three-dimensional volume, then the protocol must call out the steps needed to assure that a steady-state condition is maintained over the duration of the measurements. Notably, the spatial map would be discontinuous if a piece of equipment were switched off right in the middle of the acquisition. The protocol must

TABLE 3
Bioeffects Mechanism-Centered Magnetic Field Measurements

Magnetic field acquisition	Metric extraction
ELF (DC-3kHz) spot measurements	B_{DC}, $B_{AC,RMS}$, B_{PK}, dB/dt_{PK}
Operator-envelope, 3-dimensional ELF grid data (nominally acquired at a spacing of 20 cm)	$\%V_{res}$, P_{nom}
ELF operator exposure data (200 seconds of flux-density data acquired from a sensor strapped to an operator performing normal equipment operation)	$\%t_{coh}$, S/N_{trans}, RoC (all spot measurement metrics may also be extracted)
High-frequency (< 1.5 MHz) dB/dt data	dB/dt_{PK}, S/N_{trans}

also assure adequate documentation so that the data can be properly associated with its source and no relevant information is lost. The details of a well-designed data-acquisition protocol are beyond the scope of the current discussion. Suffice it to say that significant up-front effort should be put into protocol development to assure that the data collected are of high quality, are well-understood, and support desired metric extraction.

EXPOSURE ASSESSMENT IN THE REAL WORLD

The more plain and satisfying our state appears, the more we may know that we are living in an unreal world. For the real world is not satisfying.
—G.K. Chesterton (1906)

Hypothetical mechanisms that attempt to explain observed biological effects of exposure to EMF can be tested in a laboratory setting. Commercial exposure systems are available which permit accurately controlled exposures of cell cultures (in vitro) and animals (in vivo). When necessary, active cancellation of external sources can be utilized over the entire ELF range, thus isolating experiments from the vagaries of real-world magnetic fields.

In the real world, all bets are off. Fields are not uniformly distributed. There is no control over the relative orientation of the DC and AC fields. Waveforms may not be sinusoidal. Sources turn on and off during acquisition. Transients seem to come from nowhere. Significantly, the pristine conditions required to initiate certain hypothetical biological processes may be difficult to find. When conducting exposure assessment in support of epidemiology, one must recognize and take into account the unpleasantries of real-world EMF environments. Data-acquisition protocols must be robust enough to permit meaningful measurements to be made in less-than-ideal settings.

A Real-World Example

Exposure assessment performed in the Finnish garment industry[1] illustrates the complexity that may be encountered in a real-world situation. This is in contrast to the appliance measurements, discussed later, that are mostly performed in a laboratory. Measurements very similar to those listed in Table 3 were performed in garment factories in Finland.

Acquisition of magnetic field data can be performed by referencing either to the position of the field source, such as a sewing machine motor, or to the position of the operator, in this case a seamstress. Both can be of value for the extraction of biomechanism-based metrics. If a sensor is physically attached to the seamstress, then the actual fields she experiences while performing her work can be recorded, and metrics tied to her personal exposure can be estimated. If, on the other hand, the complete volume in which the seamstress works is carefully mapped relative to the sewing machine motor, meaningful bioeffects metrics can still be extracted. This is most effectively achieved by extracting metrics based on a model of the seamstress' body placed in the three-dimensional field map. Both techniques were used in collecting and analyzing the Finnish garment industry data.

---

[1] Hansen, N.H., L.M. Gillette, B.W. Wilson. EMF exposure assessment in the Finnish garment industry: Evaluation of proposed EMF exposure metrics (in preparation).

It was assumed that the seamstress would remain relatively motionless while performing work at a sewing machine. Therefore, instead of strapping a sensor to the seamstress while she worked, a sensor was clamped to a stand and located at the approximate position of the seamstress' sternum. This measurement was not representative of exposure for seamstresses who moved from one machine to another while performing their work (Fig. 1). However, this approach minimized impact on worker productivity while we were performing measurements. Using this setup, ELF spot measurements, 200-second ELF operator exposure data, and high-frequency dB/dt measurements were performed. In addition, average workday exposures were determined for several workers who wore EMDEX II meters while performing their normally assigned tasks.

Two typical operator exposure waveforms are shown in Figure 2. An AC induction motor (Fig. 2A) runs continuously while the seamstress engages and disengages a manual clutch with a foot treadle. The seamstress is exposed to a relatively large, nearly constant AC field throughout her work shift. Somewhat less common is the electronically controlled DC motor (Fig. 2B), which has a much lower back-

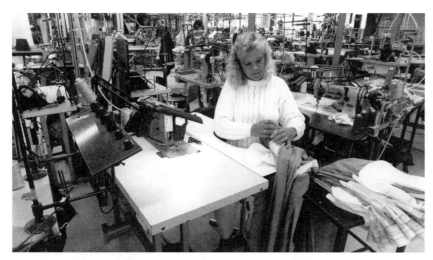

FIG. 1. A seamstress at a sewing workstation. It is common for one worker to alternate between multiple machines to perform various tasks.

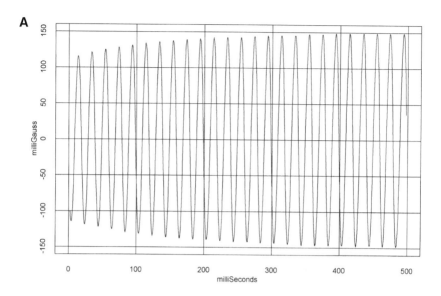

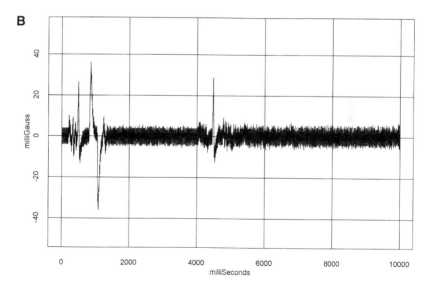

FIG. 2. (A) One-half second of operator exposure flux-density data for an AC induction sewing machine motor. The increase in amplitude corresponds to the beginning of the sewing operation. (B) Ten seconds of operator exposure flux-density data for an electronically controlled sewing machine motor. Low-frequency transients riding on low-level, 50-Hz AC correspond to running the motor for short bursts.

ground AC sinusoidal field, with significant low-frequency transients appearing when the motor is actually turning.

Exposure waveforms such as these can be interpreted in terms of coherence and transients by use of the metrics defined previously; namely, percent time in coherence ($\%t_{coh}$) and signal-to-noise of the maximum transient (S/N_{trans}). Metrics were extracted and are shown in Table 4 for the sewing machine motors featured in Figure 2. Two widely used metrics, $B_{AC,RMS}$ and RoC, are shown for comparison.

For the electronically controlled DC motor (C in Table 4), the 50-Hz sinusoid is interrupted by the actuation of the motor, resulting in a low $\%t_{coh}$ value. These low-frequency transients are quite small compared to the sinusoidal amplitude of motor B, an AC induction motor. With respect to the seamstress, motor B had a signal-to-noise value exceeding unity. The relatively constant sinusoidal fields of motor A resulted in a higher $\%t_{coh}$ value. The dB/dt transient (Fig. 3) resulting from a switch closure in a thermal appliqué heater is at too high a frequency to affect these bioeffects metrics.

The number of motors studied was too small to investigate possible correlation between the different metrics; hence, we cannot ascertain the suitability of the common, more easily extracted metrics ($B_{AC,RMS}$, RoC) as surrogates for the biomechanism-based metrics. It is apparent, however, that a very constant AC waveform would tend to result in low values of RoC and high values of $\%t_{coh}$. It is not obvious that exist-

TABLE 4
Metrics Extracted for Operator Exposure Flux-Density Data

ID	Motor type	$B_{AC,RMS}$ (mG)	RoC (MG/sec)	$\%t_{coh}$	S/N_{trans}
A	AC induction	3.242	0.004	58%	0.464
B	AC induction	110.527	0.208	31%	1.038
C	Electronically controlled DC	24.563	0.287	11%	0.262

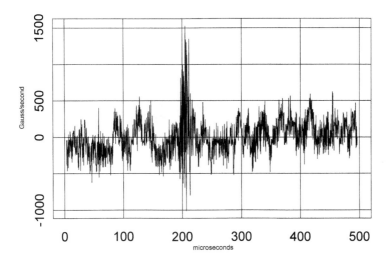

FIG. 3. One-half millisecond of high-frequency dB/dt waveform. The large transient corresponds to a switch closure in a thermal appliqué heater.

ing measures based on periodically sampled $B_{AC,RMS}$ would be adequate surrogates for S/N_{trans}.

Existing metrics have even less relevance to the question of resonance. Figure 4 is a resonance contour map showing a seamstress seated at a sewing machine. The IPR theory requires certain levels of static flux density to set cyclotron resonances at harmonics of the utility frequency (in this case, 50 Hz). As can be seen in the figure, lines of constant static flux density (B_{DC}) corresponding to harmonics of the resonance of the lithium ion (see Eq. 6c) intersect the seamstress' body. For resonance to occur, the AC field must be parallel to the DC field, with magnitudes that cause an increase in probability according to Equation 7. It would be remarkable indeed if a periodic sampling meter happened to be located at the points in the seamstress' body that satisfied these conditions. It is difficult to envision how any approach other than detailed mapping of the AC and DC fields in the operator space could yield meaningful resonance metrics when one considers the complex geometries of magnetic fields warped by ferro-

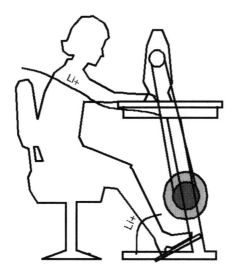

Fig. 4. Lines of constant static flux density (B_{DC}) corresponding to harmonics of the cyclotron resonance for the Li^+ ion.

magnetic objects. This is a dramatic illustration of the difficulties encountered outside of the controlled laboratory environment.

Table 5 shows $\% V_{res}$ extracted for several ions having potential biological significance. Large pieces of ferromagnetic material in the sewing machines and peripheral objects create significant gradients in the Earth's magnetic field. Hence, resonances for several ions are possible within a relatively small area.

A Second Look at Laboratory Measurements

Work done previously (Gauger 1984) has characterized appliances and other electrical equipment for their exposure potential. Narrow-band, 60-Hz AC RMS flux density versus distance was measured. Efforts are now under way (Hansen et al. 1996) to perform more detailed measurements of appliances that will permit the extraction of metrics having relevance to bioelectromagnetics research. Table 6 contains metrics extracted for a set of six appliances and serves to illustrate the potential problems of performing meaningful measurements in the labora-

TABLE 5
Percent Body-in-Resonance Metric for Four Sewing Machines and 12 Ions[a]

ID	S⁶⁻	Li⁺	Mn⁷⁺	S⁴⁻	Cr⁶⁺	Mn⁶⁺	Mg²⁺	Mn⁴⁺	Cr³⁺	Mn³⁺	Fe³⁺	Ca²⁺
A	10%	92%	26%	7%	1%	3%	17%	91%	1%	3%	2%	1%
D	35%	68%	43%	43%	9%	4%	29%	78%	1%	0%	0%	0%
E	13%	45%	25%	7%	7%	0%	58%	62%	0%	0%	0%	0%
F	63%	90%	85%	73%	40%	8%	3%	90%	0%	5%	0%	0%

[a] Resonance conditions were not satisfied for other ions evaluated.

tory. The actual waveform acquisitions were performed at the approximate position of the operator's sternum during normal usage.

The controlled environment available in the laboratory can simplify measurements, but it can also result in metric values that have little relevance to real-world situations. Note the remarkably high $\%t_{coh}$ values in Table 6. These data resulted from placing the sensor in a stationary stand while acquiring flux-density information. This, of course, was not typical of appliance operators, who would normally be moving about. To assure that the extracted metrics are representative of real-world situations, we now involve a live subject in our measurements. The sensor is strapped to the subject, who performs normal work.

Also lacking from the laboratory are environmental factors such as background noise and location-specific variability. Typically, surrounding furniture, building structures, and other ferrous material containing objects are not simulated in the laboratory. Thus, the extraction of resonance metrics is difficult. However, in the laboratory

TABLE 6
Preliminary Results for Six Appliances

Appliance	$B_{AC,RMS}$ (mG)	dB/dt_{PK} (mG/sec)	RoC (mG/sec)	S/N_{trans}	$\%t_{coh}$
Can opener	274.7	21.4	0.132	0.101	82%
Computer monitor	265.9	10.8	0.019	0.029	99%
Electric drill	250.4	2.8	0.004	0.011	99%
Hair clippers	497.3	62.5	0.349	2.377	100%
Microwave oven	263.4	10.9	0.019	0.068	99%
Space heater	229.3	2.3	0.002	0.005	100%

we are able to study ferrous objects to determine their impact on both AC and static fields. Although such research helps predict the effect such objects will have in a real-world environment, there is no substitute for making measurements at real locations.

Figure 5 shows a resonance map for Li^+ made in a secretarial office. The static field levels present inside an office are determined by local geomagnetic field intensity, shielding effects of the building frame, perturbations in the field due to nearby ferromagnetic objects such as table legs, and local sources of static field such as permanent magnets in motors. Replicating this combination of factors in the laboratory would have been very difficult indeed.

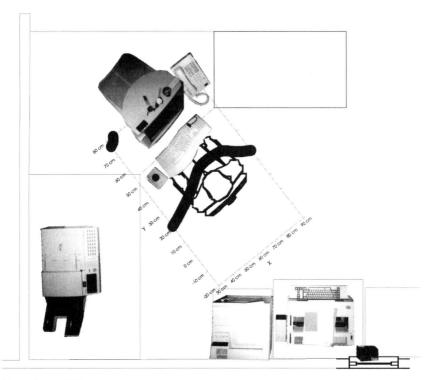

Elevation = 100cm.

FIG. 5. A secretarial office, viewed from above, showing contours ($\pm 10\%$) of constant flux density corresponding to resonances of Li^+.

Suggestions for Study Design

The design of data-acquisition protocols for exposure assessment studies should take into account the metrics discussed previously. We began this chapter by posing two questions:

1. What constitutes *dose* in bioelectromagnetics?

2. How can a useful definition of *dose* be factored into practical exposure assessment studies?

We essentially evaded the first question by stating that our definition of dose is imprecise because no causal mechanisms have been verified. Nevertheless, we can define several dose metrics representative of the various bioeffects mechanism theories currently being tested. This being the case, we can address the second question by factoring these metrics into the data-acquisition protocols designed for exposure assessment studies. By improving the linkage between theoretical laboratory research and measurements made in the field, the question of what causes EMF bioeffects will be better addressed.

Cost is a major concern for large studies. In most cases, the detailed field characterization described in this chapter would be far too expensive. The actual value of collecting volumes of characterization data will depend, to a large degree, on the types of sources involved, their location, and the actual objectives of the study. The variability of requirements from one study to another is so great that only very general suggestions can be made here:

1. Clearly determine which hypotheses will be tested in the study. If testing the hypothesis that nighttime exposure to AC fields from alarm clocks suppresses the production of melatonin, then it is probably adequate to periodically sample AC RMS flux density. If, however, one wants to test one or more bioeffects mechanism theories, then data must be collected that will support extraction of the relevant metrics.

2. Look for surrogates for expensive measurements. For testing theories related to coherence and transients, it may be possible to perform detailed measures on a small subset of sources to determine a surrogate measure. For the sewing machine example, motor brand and model may be well-correlated to coherence and transient metrics. With brand and model as a surrogate metric, a

record could be kept of each seamstress' equipment usage to see when there is a correlation between the type of motor used and an observed health effect. Of course, this would be effective only if each seamstress predominantly used only one type of machine.

3. Perform at least a limited number of on-site surveys. To test theories that depend on field geometries, such as IPR, there may be no substitute for detailed in-the-field measurements. Even when there is no interest in testing bioeffects theories, a few detailed measurements should be performed to see what the periodic sampling meter is hiding.

4. Take great care in developing data-acquisition and metric-extraction protocols. Make sure it is clearly understood which theories can and cannot be tested given the type of data acquisition that is to be performed.

SUMMARY

Our understanding of dose in bioelectromagnetics is limited by our imprecise knowledge about the causal mechanisms behind EMF biological effects. By developing useful metrics that reflect the various bioeffects theories, we are in a better position to test these theories. We reviewed metrics defined for three theories: coherence, transients, and IPR. Testing will be enhanced if studies are designed with adequate data-acquisition protocols that support the extraction of relevant dose metrics.

ACKNOWLEDGMENTS

This work was supported by the U.S. Department of Energy through the EMF RAPID Program under contract AC06-76RL0 1830. The digitized human cadaver data used in the resonance metric calculations was provided by The Visible Human Project™, National Library of Medicine, Bethesda, Maryland.

REFERENCES

Adair, R.K. 1991. Constraints on biological effects of weak extremely-low-frequency electromagnetic fields. *Physiol. Rev.* A43:1039–1048.

Adair, R.K. 1992. Criticism of Lednev's mechanism for the influence of weak magnetic fields on biological systems. *Bioelectromagnetics* 13:231–235.

Blackman, C.F., S.G. Benane, D.E. House, J.R. Rabinowitz, W.T. Joines. 1984. A role for the magnetic component in the field-induced efflux of calcium ions from brain tissue. In: Abstracts of the Sixth Annual Meeting of The Bioelectromagnetics Society, Atlanta, Georgia, Abstract Sa-4.

Blackman, C.F., S.G. Benane, D.E. House, J.P. Blanchard. 1996. Independent replication of the 12 mG magnetic field effect on melatonin and MCF-7 cells in vitro. In: Abstracts of the 18th Annual Bioelectromagnetics Society Meeting, June 9–14, Victoria, B.C., Canada, #A-1-2, pp. 1–2.

Blanchard, J.P., C.F. Blackman. 1994. Clarification and application of an ion parametric resonance model for magnetic field interactions with biological systems. *Bioelectromagnetics* 15:217–238.

Chesterton, G.K. 1906. *Dickens and America.* Quoted in *The Columbia Dictionary of Quotations*, Columbia University Press, 1993.

Foster, K.R., H.P. Schwan. 1989. Dielectric properties of tissues and biological materials: A critical review. *CRC Crit. Rev. Biomed. Eng.* 17(1):25–104.

Gauger, J.R. 1984. *Household Appliance Magnetic Field Survey.* Technical Report E06549-3, Chicago: IIT Research Institute.

Halle, B. 1988. On the cyclotron resonance mechanism for magnetic field effect on transmembrane ion conductivity. *Bioelectromagnetics* 9:381–385.

Hansen, N.H., B.W. Wilson. 1995. Measurement methods and metric extraction algorithms in support of EMF bio-effects mechanism hypothesis evaluation. In: Abstracts of the Annual Review of Research on Biological Effects of Electric and Magnetic Fields from the Generation, Delivery, and Use of Electricity, November 12–16, Palm Springs, California, Abstract P-51, p. 107. Frederick, Maryland: W/L Associates, Ltd.

Hansen, N.H., B.W. Wilson, W.R. Canada. 1996. Bio-effects mechanism based exposure assessment of appliances in the home and workplace. In: Abstracts of the 18th Annual Bioelectromagnetics Society Meeting, June 9–14, Victoria, B.C., Canada, Abstract P-14, p. 202.

Lednev, V.V. 1991. Possible mechanism for the influence of weak magnetic fields on biological systems. *Bioelectromagnetics* 12:71–75.

Lee, G.M., M.B. Yost, R.R. Neutra, D.D. Hristova, T. Tarshis, R. Hiatt, A.R. Leonard. 1992. Descriptive assessment of 24-hour personal exposure to 60-Hz magnetic fields using a rate-of-change metric. In: Abstracts of the First World Congress for Electricity and Magnetism in Biology and Medicine, Lake Buena Vista, Florida, June 14–19, Abstract J-3.

Liboff, A.R. 1985. Cyclotron resonance in membrane transport. In: *Interactions Between Electromagnetic Fields and Cells*, A Chiabrera, C. Nicolini, H.P. Schwan, eds., pp. 281–296. London: Plenum Publishing Corp.

Liburdy, R.P., T.R. Sloma, R. Sokolic, P. Yaswen. 1993. ELF magnetic fields, breast cancer, and melatonin: 60 Hz fields block melatonin's oncostatic action on ER$^+$ breast cancer cell proliferation. *J. Pineal Res.* 14:89–97.

Litovitz, T.A., D. Krause, J.M. Mullins. 1991. Effect of coherence time of the applied magnetic field on ornithine decarboxylase activity. *Biochem. Biophys. Res. Commun.* 178:862–865.

Litovitz, T.A., D. Krause, C.J. Montrose, J.M. Mullins. 1994a. Temporally incoherent magnetic fields mitigate the response of biological systems to temporally coherent magnetic fields. *Bioelectromagnetics* 15:399–409.

Litovitz, T.A., C.J. Montrose, P. Doinov, K.M. Brown, M. Barber. 1994b. Superimposing spatially coherent electromagnetic noise inhibits field-induced abnormalities in developing chick embryos. *Bioelectromagnetics* 15:105–113.

McLeod, B.R., S.D. Smith, K.E. Cooksey, A.R. Liboff. 1987. Ion cyclotron resonance frequencies enhance Ca^{2+} mobility in diatoms. *J. Bioelectr.* 6:1–12.

Podgoretskii, M.I. 1960. On the modulation and beats in quantum transitions. Preprint p-491. United International Institute for Nuclear Research, Dubna.

Podgoretskii, M.I., O.A. Khrustalev. 1964. Interference effects in quantum transitions. *Soviet Phys. Uspekhi* 6:682–700.

Sandweiss, J. 1990. On the cyclotron resonance model of ion transport. *Bioelectromagnetics* 11:203–205.

Sastre, A., R. Kavet, J.L. Guttman, J.C. Weaver. Residential magnetic field transients induce transmembrane voltages that may exceed thermal noise. *Bioelectromagnetics* (in press).

Smith, S.D., B.R. McLeod, A.R. Liboff, K.E. Cooksey. 1987. Calcium cyclotron resonance and diatom motility. *Bioelectromagnetics* R:215–227.

Wachtel, H., R. Pearson, K. Ebi. 1996. Rental status and wire code are risk factors for childhood cancer. In: Abstracts of the 18th Annual Bioelectromagnetics Society Meeting, June 9–14, Victoria, B.C., Canada, Abstract A-2-3, p. 6.

PART II
Issues in
Field Perception

6 Magnetoreception in Terrestrial Vertebrates: Implications for Possible Mechanisms of EMF Interaction with Biological Systems

JOHN B. PHILLIPS
MARK E. DEUTSCHLANDER
Department of Biology, Indiana University,
Bloomington, Indiana

CONTENTS

INTRODUCTION
THEORETICAL MODELS OF MAGNETORECEPTION
    Radical Pair-Based Mechanisms (photoreceptor models)
    Magnetite-Based Mechanisms
    Comparison of Radical Pair- and Magnetite-Based
        Magnetoreception Mechanisms
USES OF THE GEOMAGNETIC FIELD IN ANIMALS
    Magnetic Compass Orientation
    Magnetic Navigation
    A Magnetic Zeitgeber for Entrainment of Circadian Rhythms?
LOCALIZATION OF RECEPTORS AND FUNCTIONAL
   PROPERTIES OF MAGNETORECEPTION MECHANISMS:
   PHYSIOLOGICAL EVIDENCE
    Pineal Interactions with Earth-Strength Magnetic Fields

(continued)

CONTENTS (continued)

Evidence for a Visually Based Magnetic Compass
The Trigeminal System
LOCALIZATION OF RECEPTORS AND FUNCTIONAL PROPERTIES
  OF MAGNETORECEPTION MECHANISMS: BEHAVIORAL EVIDENCE
    Wavelength-Dependent Effects of Light on Magnetic Compass
      Orientation
    Magnetite-Based Magnetoreception and
      Magnetic Navigation
SUMMARY: IMPLICATIONS FOR EMF RESEARCH

INTRODUCTION

Neurophysiological and behavioral studies of geomagnetic field sensitivity ("magnetoreception") in terrestrial animals are beginning to elucidate biophysical mechanisms of interaction between biological systems and the geomagnetic field (Beason and Semm 1987; Beason et al. 1995; Phillips and Borland 1992a–c; Semm et al. 1984; Demaine and Semm 1985; Semm and Beason 1990; Wiltschko et al. 1993, 1994; Wiltschko and Wiltschko 1995b). The findings of these studies are relevant in three ways to investigators interested in biological effects of manmade electric and magnetic fields (EMF). First, two biophysical mechanisms are currently being investigated by researchers interested in both magnetoreception and EMF effects—mechanisms involving radical pair reactions (Brocklehurst and McLauchlan 1996; Canfield et al. 1994, 1995; Grissom 1995; McLauchlan 1992; Schulten 1982; Schulten and Windemuth 1986; Scaiano et al. 1994; Walleczek 1994) and mechanisms involving particles of biogenic magnetite (Edmonds 1996; Kirschvink and Gould 1981; Kirschvink et al. 1985; Yorke 1979). Magnetoreception studies that provide evidence for a radical pair-based mechanism (possibly involving specialized photoreceptors) and/or a magnetite-based mechanism lend credibility to the results of

EMF studies that implicate these two mechanisms as possible sites of interaction of EMF with biological systems.

The two remaining areas of overlap between magnetoreception and EMF studies relate directly to the focus of this book: the effects of EMF on the circadian rhythm of melatonin levels in rodents and, possibly, humans. Animal experiments involving extremely low frequency (ELF) EMF and single, abrupt EMF changes suggest that the pineal gland, a neuroendocrine end organ of the visual system, may be directly involved in mediating the neuroendocrine changes in melatonin (and other downstream hormones) associated with EMF exposure (Welker et al. 1983; Olcese et al. 1985; Wilson et al. 1989, 1990; Reiter 1992, 1993; Wilson 1994; Yellon 1994; Kato et al. 1993, 1994a, b; also see chapters in Part III, Section 3, in this volume). Some researchers have suggested that this effect may be mediated by a direct interaction of EMF with retinal photoreceptors (Olcese et al. 1985, 1988a, b; Reuss and Olcese 1986; Olcese and Reuss 1986; Olcese 1990). Studies of geomagnetic sensitivity in a variety of animals implicate photoreceptors as at least one primary site of interaction with the Earth's magnetic field (Phillips and Borland 1992a, b, 1994; Semm et al. 1984; Wiltschko et al. 1993; Wiltschko and Wiltschko 1995a, b). These findings suggest that there may be a direct functional connection between geomagnetic sensitivity and the in vivo EMF effects on melatonin.

Finally, studies of magnetoreception in animals have provided evidence for an extremely high level of sensitivity to variation in the intensity and/or inclination of the geomagnetic field. Evidence for responses to changes in an Earth-strength field as little as 100 nT (approximately 0.2% change), and possibly lower, has been obtained in both behavioral and neurophysiological studies (Rodda 1984b; Keeton et al. 1974; Larkin and Keeton 1976; Kowalski et al. 1988; Wagner 1983; Semm and Beason 1990). There is growing evidence that in some vertebrates these high levels of sensitivity may be mediated by a specialized magnetoreception system involved in deriving "map" (geographic position) information from natural spatial variation in the geomagnetic field. Such a system would be sensitive enough to detect the regular, daily temporal variation in the geomagnetic field. And, indeed, bicoordinate navigation by terrestrial vertebrates, in which the use of "magnetic map" information has been implicated, appears to be influenced by natural temporal variation in the geomagnetic field (Keeton et al. 1974; Kowalski et al. 1988; Larkin and Keeton 1976; Rodda 1984b). These findings point to the need for a reconsideration of an idea that is currently given little credibility; i.e., that natural temporal variation in the geomagnetic field may serve as a Zeitgeber ("time giver") for the entrainment of circadian rhythms (Bliss and Heppner 1976; Brown and Chow 1976; Brown and Scow 1978; Welker et al. 1983).

This chapter attempts to present a coherent picture of the possible uses and functional characteristics of magnetoreception in terrestrial vertebrates in order to provide the basis for discussion of common questions that have arisen in both the magnetoreception and EMF literatures. For instance, one crucial question is whether some of the effects of EMF (e.g., effects on melatonin in rodents) are mediated by a sensory system(s) specialized for detection of the geomagnetic field or, instead, result from "nonspecific" effects on biological processes that are not involved in geomagnetic field detection. Of these two alternatives, the former is by far the most accessible to critical tests.

The advantage of studying an effect mediated by a specific sensory channel is that a sensory mechanism will have been "optimized" by natural selection to respond to a specific range of stimuli and function in specific behavioral contexts. This characteristic makes it possible to generate reasonable *a priori* assumptions about the functional properties of the sensory mechanism, and about the correspondence between the functional properties of behavioral and neurophysiological responses to specific types of stimuli. For example, magnetic compass orientation must be mediated by a magnetoreception system that is sensitive to, and is likely to be optimized for detection of, the directional properties of a magnetic field that approximates the intensity of the geomagnetic field. Moreover, the directional sensitivity of this system must be represented in the neural channels that carry information to the central nervous system. Finally, if the directional response of the underlying magnetoreception mechanism is altered by exposure to a particular experimental condition (e.g., a particular wavelength of light or frequency of EMF), this experimental treatment should produce a similar or related effect on the *direction* of magnetic compass orientation in the animal. These characteristics make it possible to define a range of stimuli and stimulus parameters that should affect the sensory system (and to confirm these predictions using complementary behavioral and neurophysiological approaches). This "functional signature" can then be used to determine whether the underlying sensory system is likely to mediate responses to other types of stimuli [e.g., power-frequency (60-Hz) EMF]. Thus, if particular types of stimuli or experimental treatments (e.g., pulse remagnetization, exposure to particular wavelengths of light or frequencies of EMF; discussed herein) are found to uniquely affect a particular type of sensory mechanism, these experimental treatments can be used to carry out critical tests of the involvement of the same or similar sensory mechanism(s) in mediating other physiological responses (e.g., neuroendocrine responses to EMF).

This chapter will focus on the correspondence between the results of behavioral and neurophysiological studies of the magnetoreception mechanism(s) involved in spatial orientation by terrestrial vertebrates. We will first introduce two of the proposed mechanisms for geomagnetic transduction in terrestrial vertebrates. Then we will discuss aspects of spatial orientation behavior in which sensitivity to the Earth's magnetic field is thought to play a role, and the functional requirements/constraints that these "behavioral contexts" place on the underlying sensory mechanism(s). Finally, we will summarize behavioral and neurophysiological evidence concerning the functional properties of the underlying mechanism(s). In particular, we will examine evidence suggesting that there are two distinct magnetoreception mechanisms in terrestrial vertebrates that are specialized to respond to different components of the magnetic field, and both of which may be present in the same organism. Throughout this discussion, we will consider whether one or both of these magnetoreception mechanisms, or similar biophysical process(es), are involved in mediating possible health-related neuroendocrine effects of EMF on biological systems, as well as the implications such an involvement would have for the design of experiments to identify the critical stimulus parameters that potentially trigger adverse effects on biological systems. Our hope is that this chapter will help stimulate a convergence of interests among researchers working in applied areas to investigate potential health effects of EMF and researchers working on basic questions concerning the sensory mechanism(s) of geomagnetic field detection in terrestrial organisms.

THEORETICAL MODELS OF MAGNETORECEPTION

Radical Pair-Based Mechanisms (photoreceptor models)

Interest in the possibility that specialized photoreceptors might be involved in obtaining directional ("compass") information from the geomagnetic field was triggered by a theoretical model proposed by Leask (1977). While Leask's "optical-pumping" model was important in stimulating much of the early qualitative work on the visual system's involvement in magnetoreception, there now is general consensus that the requirements necessary for the optical-pumping mechanism to operate are not met in biological systems (e.g., the requirement of an internal source of energy in the radio frequency range). Currently, the most plausible model to implicate specialized photoreceptors in magnetoreception is the "radical pair" model proposed by Schulten (Schulten 1982; Schulten and Windemuth 1986). Schulten's model invokes a reaction belonging to the general family of photo-induced electron transfer reactions. Most molecules have a singlet ground state; i.e., the spins of paired electrons are antiparallel, so that the resulting magnetic moments cancel out and the net magnetic moment of the molecule is equal to zero. Absorption of a photon of light, however, may cause the molecule (A) to accept an electron from a neighboring donor molecule (D), resulting in a radical pair ($^1A^*$ + $^1D \oslash {}^2A^-$ + $^2D^+$). This interaction results in both members of the radical pair having a net magnetic moment from the spin of the unpaired electron, which tends to be strongly influenced by the magnetic moments resulting from the nuclear spins (hyperfine interactions), causing the electron's magnetic moment to precess around the net nuclear magnetic moment. An external magnetic field adds to the nuclear magnetic moment, and causes the electron to precess around the resultant (nuclear + external) magnetic field vector with a frequency in the radio frequency (RF) range (i.e., the Zeeman interaction).

If the unpaired electrons associated with the members of the radical pair retain their antiparallel spin alignments, transfer of an electron from molecule A back to molecule D will result in both members of the pair returning to a singlet ground state. However, because the unpaired electrons associated with the two radicals are not constrained by sharing an orbital with another electron, one of the electrons may "flip" so that the two electrons are in parallel spin alignments. In this case, transfer of an electron from A back to D will yield a triplet excited state in which the excited electron and the remaining unpaired electron in the ground state have parallel spin alignments, so that the magnetic moments of the two electrons sum together. A molecule in a triplet excited state exhibits distinctly different properties from the same molecule in a singlet excited state. For example, the singlet excited state of rhodopsin may be more efficient than the triplet excited state at initiating the visual cascade that triggers a change in the membrane potential of a photoreceptor.

The presence of a static external field can increase the probability that one of the unpaired electrons in the radical pair will flip, so that back transfer of an electron will result in a triplet, rather than a singlet, excited state. Moreover, a particular alignment of the magnetic field may create an energy relationship between one of the triplet substates and the singlet state that is favorable for so-called intersystem crossing. In an ordered array of molecules, therefore, the triplet state yield (and, thus, the efficiency of subsequent biochemical reactions in which the excited molecule participates) may exhibit a dependence on the alignment of the external field.

The effect of a static magnetic field on the triplet state yield from this type of radical pair reaction can exhibit a complex dependence on a variety of factors, including the intensity and alignment of the external static field, the characteristics of the molecule involved (e.g., the strength of the hyperfine interactions), the spatial and temporal characteristics of the interaction between the two radicals (e.g., "cage lifetime"), and the presence and characteristics (frequency, intensity, alignment, etc.) of any external AC fields (see Schulten 1982; Schulten and Windemuth 1986; Canfield et al. 1994, 1995). As a consequence, the range of external magnetic field intensities that can appreciably affect triplet yield varies widely in different radical pair systems, but tends to have lower limits of magnetic field intensity that are 1–2 orders of magnitude higher than the intensity of the geomagnetic field (~ 0.05 mT) (Grissom 1995). Nevertheless, some radical pair systems may be sensitive to an Earth-strength magnetic field (Schulten 1982; Schulten and Windemuth 1986; Grissom 1995; Brocklehurst and McLauchlan 1996). Moreover, if the radical pair reaction takes place in the membrane surrounding a superparamagnetic (SPM) magnetite particle, it would be exposed to a stronger local field whose alignment would "track" that of the geomagnetic field (J. Kirschvink, personal communication). It is primarily an empirical question, therefore, whether a radical pair mechanism is used by animals for detection of the geomagnetic field and/or whether such mechanisms play a role in other physiological effects of static fields or EMF on biological systems (Brocklehurst and McLauchlan 1996).

In general, a biological process that involves a radical pair mechanism may be sensitive to the axis (but not polarity) of an Earth-strength magnetic field (Schulten 1982). It is unlikely to be sensitive to small changes (changes of less than 10% or so) in magnetic field intensity. A magnetoreception system mediated by a radical pair mechanism, therefore, is apt to serve as an "axial" compass (like that observed in birds; Wiltschko and Wiltschko 1972, 1988), rather than an intensity detector. An important difference between a magnetic compass that utilizes a radical pair-based mechanism and a biochemical pathway involving a radical pair reaction that exhibits nonspecific effects of EMF or static fields is that the design of the magnetic compass is likely to have been optimized by natural selection to respond to the directional properties of the magnetic field. Therefore, the population of molecules that interact with the magnetic field is apt to occur in a highly ordered, presumably membrane-bound, array to maximize the directional sensitivity of the receptor. Moreover, the local molecular environment is likely to have been modified to optimize the relative geometry and spacing of the radical pair, and to shield the system from competing effects or thermal buffeting. Finally, a radical pair-based magnetic compass would have to be interfaced with a neural processing system capable of extracting directional information from the complex, three-dimensional patterns likely to be generated by this type of mechanism due to the radial and axial symmetry of the response (Schulten and Windemuth 1986; J. Canfield, personal communication).

Although, in principle, a radical pair-based magnetoreception mechanism might be located anywhere in the body, there are a number of reasons why this type of mechanism is apt to occur in a specialized photoreceptor. First, if a radical pair-based magnetoreception system requires photoexcitation for the initial formation of the radical pair, location in a photoreceptor would be advantageous, because it would provide access to an abundant supply of photons (Schulten 1982; Schulten and Windemuth 1986). Second, the highly ordered membrane environment present in the outer segments of rods and/or cones would be well-suited for detecting the directional effects of the geomagnetic field on ordered arrays of molecules (Schulten 1982; Schulten and Windemuth 1986). Finally, in some photoreceptors a high degree of order extends to the geometry of adjacent light-absorbing molecules. For example, the retinula 1–6 cells in the compound eye of flies contain two light-absorbing pigments—a photopigment maximally sensitive to blue-green light (450–500 nm) and a "sensitizing" pigment maximally sensitive to ultraviolet light (340–370 nm) that transfers energy to the photopigment (Kirschfeld et al. 1977). Both peaks of spectral sensitivity exhibit a dependence on the E-vector of plane-polarized light, but are maximally sensitive to different E-vector alignments (Horridge and Mimura 1975). This suggests not only that the molecules are in an ordered array with respect to the microvilli that make up the light-sensitive rhabdome of the photoreceptor, but also that the relative geometry of the two molecules is fixed.

Schulten's (1982) proposal that a radical pair-based mechanism might affect the efficiency of visual transduction suggests that animals might be able to perceive the geomagnetic field as a visual pattern superimposed on its surroundings, or to detect the magnetic field by means of a separate parallel pathway that is not involved in processing other visual stimuli. Interest in the possible involvement of the visual system in magnetoreception has led to a number of studies investigating the dependence of behavioral and neurophysiological responses to directional properties of the magnetic field on the presence and/or wavelength of light (e.g., Semm et al. 1984; Semm and Demaine 1986; Phillips and Borland 1992a, b; Phillips and Sayeed 1993; Lohmann and Lohmann 1993; Wiltschko et al. 1993; Wiltschko and Wiltschko 1995b; Munro et al. in press; and see pages 143 and 147). However, the presence or absence of light dependence or light sensi-

tivity alone does not provide sufficient evidence either to implicate or
to rule out a radical pair mechanism. If the initial formation of the radical pair requires photoexcitation, a magnetoreception mechanism
based on a radical pair reaction should exhibit light dependence.
However, if the radical pair is formed as an intermediate in a biochemical reaction that does not require photoexcitation (Canfield et al.
1994, 1995; Grissom 1995), the magnetoreception mechanism may not
require light or be associated with the visual system in any way.

It is also possible, at least in theory, for a biochemical source of high-
energy quanta [e.g., similar to the biochemical pathways involved in
bioluminescence (Hastings 1983; McCapra 1990)] to substitute for
environmental light under certain conditions, resulting in an otherwise light-dependent radical pair mechanism that could function in
the absence of environmental light. Moreover, a radical pair mechanism that is *not* light-dependent also might have become associated
with the visual system (e.g., downstream in the visual cascade, or in
secondary visual neurons) because of the well-developed spatial-pro-
cessing capabilities of the visual system . If so, an effect of the presence
and/or wavelength of light could arise as a consequence of this association, rather than being a property of the radical pair mechanism itself.
Finally, a photoreceptor-based mechanism that involves particles of
magnetite is also possible (Edmonds 1996; see next section). Thus, evidence which suggests that a particular response to magnetic stimuli is
affected by the presence or absence of light must be interpreted with
care, and can only be taken as compelling evidence for or against the
involvement of a radical pair mechanism when additional evidence is
obtained (see Table 1).

Magnetite-Based Mechanisms

Two size classes of magnetite particles are potentially useful for detection of the Earth's magnetic field (Kirschvink and Gould 1981;
Kirschvink and Walker 1985). Large, single-domain (SD) particles have
a magnetic moment that is constrained by shape anisotropy to lie
along the long axis of the particle in either of two opposite directions.
In smaller SPM particles, the magnetic moment is not constrained by
the particle's structure and can wander freely without rotation of the
particle, aligning itself in an Earth-strength field with a time constant

TABLE 1
Properties of Magnetoreception Mechanism

Sensitivity to	Magnetite	Radical pair
Polarity of static magnetic field	No: neither SPM particles nor freely rotating SD particles (Edmonds 1996; Kirschvink and Gould 1991; Kirschvink and Walker 1985). Yes: SD particles unable to rotate freely with respect to surrounding tissue (Kirschvink and Gould 1991; Kirschvink and Walker 1985), but polarity may be "discarded" by subsequent neural processing.	No (Schulten 1982; Schulten and Windemuth 1986).
Small changes in static field intensity	Sensitivity as low as 1–10 nT possible by averaging across large ($>10^{6-7}$) population of SD particles (Yorke 1979, 1981; Kirschvink and Walker 1985).	Unlikely below 1,000–10,000 nT (Schulten 1982; Schulten and Windemuth 1986).
ELF EMF (<100 Hz)	Arrays of SD particles potentially sensitive to 60-Hz EMF down to a few hundred nT, and possibly lower (Kirschvink et al. 1993).	Unknown.
High-frequency EMF (>1 MHz)	Broadly tuned in the 0.5–10 GHZ range. Effects may require low frequency modulation (Kirschvink 1996).	Possible frequency-specific effects; for example, in 1- to 5-MHz range (Canfield et al. 1994, 1995). No information available on lower limits of sensitivity, but likely to vary widely in different radical pair systems.

continued

TABLE 1 (continued)
Properties of Magnetoreception Mechanism

Sensitivity to	Magnetite	Radical pair
Light	Yes or No. Interaction of magnetite with static field independent of light. However, light dependence may arise secondarily due to properties of transduction and/ or neural processing mechanisms (e.g., Kirschvink 1996, Edmonds 1996).	Yes or No. Depends on variety factors including whether initial formation of radical pair requires photoexcitation and/ or properties of neural processing mechanism (Grissom1995; Schulten 1982, Schulten and Windemuth 1986; Canfield et al. 1994, 1995).
Pulse remagnetization	No: SPM particles, or freely rotating SD particles. Yes: SD particles fixed with respect to surrounding tissue (Kalmijn and Blakemore 1978).	No.

Shading indicates properties likely to be uniquely associated with one of the two mechanisms (and thus, useful in distinguishing between the two).

varying from seconds to days. Deposits of magnetic material, in some cases identified as SD or SPM particles of magnetite, have now been found in a variety of higher animals that exhibit magnetic sensitivity (reviewed in Kirschvink et al. 1985).

A magnetite-based receptor could respond to the direction and/or intensity of the magnetic field (Kirschvink and Walker 1985) by coupling SD or SPM particles to a suitable transduction mechanism (e.g., hair cells or stretch receptors) that causes a change in membrane conductance (Kirschvink et al. 1993). Another ingenious suggestion for a magnetite-based magnetoreceptor stems from the observation that the strong, local magnetic fields associated with a magnetite particle can align certain types of pigment molecules that are nearby in solution. If the magnetic moments of a three-dimensional array of SD magnetite particles track the external field, the alignment of a solution of pigment molecules surrounding the particles and, therefore, the light-transmission properties of the pigment molecules may depend on magnetic field alignment (Edmonds 1996). If an organelle containing the magnetite particles and pigment solution were located in the path of incoming light (e.g., carotenoid pigments contained in oil droplets found in the inner segments of some vertebrate photoreceptors), this change in the transmission of light would cause a modulation of light intensity reaching the visual pigment. The result would be a light-dependent, photoreceptor-based magnetoreceptor mediated by a magnetite-based mechanism.

Receptors utilizing particles of biogenic magnetite could, in theory, mediate either axial or polar responses to the magnetic field (Kirschvink and Gould 1981; Kirschvink and Walker 1985; Edmonds 1996). In general, axial sensitivity (sensitivity to the axis, but not the polarity, of the magnetic field) would be exhibited by magnetite-based receptors in which the magnetic moments of individual particles were free to rotate with respect to the surrounding tissue and to "track" the alignment of an external, Earth-strength magnetic field. As a consequence, the net magnetic moment produced by individual particles, or arrays of particles, would change in alignment relative to the animal's body (1) as the animal changes its body alignment relative to an external field, or (2) as the alignment of an external field changes relative to the animal's body. Polar sensitivity (sensitivity to the polarity of the magnetic field) would be exhibited by magnetite-based receptors in which the particles' magnetic moments were at least partially constrained (not free to rotate) with respect to the surrounding tissue. If the receptor mechanism involves SD particles of magnetite that are spaced far enough apart that they do not interact, polar sensitivity would arise if the individual particles are constrained by the surrounding tissue. A magnetite-based receptor would also exhibit polar sensitivity if SD or SPM particles are arranged in linear arrays ("chains") in which the spacing between adjacent particles is small enough that the strength of the interactions between the particles is greater than the strength of the interactions of individual particles with the external field. The interactions between adjacent particles in this type of linear array would constrain the particles' magnetic moments to align (in one of two opposite directions) with the long axis of the chain.

Comparison of Radical Pair- and Magnetite-Based Magnetoreception Mechanisms

Although much of the effort to distinguish between radical pair- and magnetite-based mechanisms, including experiments carried out by our laboratory (see pp. 147–153), has been focused on the effects of light on behavioral and neurophysiological responses to magnetic stimuli (e.g., Semm et al. 1984; Semm and Demaine 1986; Phillips and Borland 1992a–c, 1994; Lohmann and Lohmann 1993; Wiltschko et al. 1993), it is incorrect to assume that a radical pair-based magnetoreception mechanism would necessarily require light or that a magnetite-based magnetoreception mechanism would necessarily be non-light-dependent. Properties that are potentially more useful in distinguishing between these two types of mechanisms include (1) sensitivity to the polarity of the magnetic field, (2) sensitivity to small changes in static field intensity, (3) sensitivity to RF EMF, and (4) sensitivity to pulse remagnetization (see pp. 156–157). Table 1 summarizes a number of these properties and refers the reader to the relevant references. Properties that are likely to be uniquely associated with one of the two mechanisms (and thus, that should be useful in distinguishing between the two) are shaded in Table 1.

USES OF THE GEOMAGNETIC FIELD IN ANIMALS

Magnetic Compass Orientation

The best-documented role of the geomagnetic field in spatial orientation is as a source of directional compass information. Indeed, this is the only capacity in which the use of the geomagnetic field by animals has been unequivocally demonstrated. Behavioral and/or neurophysiological evidence for directional magnetic field sensitivity has been obtained for more than 40 species, including representatives of all major groups of jawed vertebrates and a variety of invertebrates (see Wiltschko and Wiltschko 1995a for review). Evidence for magnetic field sensitivity, however, is by no means unequivocal in every case for which data have been presented. At this juncture, there are only a handful of experimental systems for which successful replication by different laboratories (or even by the same laboratory) has demonstrated that the evidence for magnetic field sensitivity is reproducible (see Wiltschko and Wiltschko 1995a). Despite potential concerns about some of the reports of magnetic field sensitivity, the existence of this sensory capability in animals is not in doubt. Indeed, even the most conservative reading of the available literature suggests that sensitivity to the direction of the geomagnetic field is widespread among animals.

Magnetic Navigation

In contrast to the use of magnetic compass information, the possibility that some terrestrial organisms may derive geographic position ("map") information from spatial gradients in one or more parameters of the magnetic field remains controversial (e.g., Lednor 1982; Walcott 1991). A number of studies that provide support for the possibility of a "magnetic map" have been completed over the last 2–3 years. Because some of these studies have only recently been published, or have yet to be submitted for publication, we will discuss these findings and their implications in some detail.

A gradient map, such as the proposed magnetic map, requires an animal to learn the alignment and, possibly, the steepness of one or more environmental gradients in the vicinity of its home range or territory, and to extrapolate the gradients beyond its area of familiarity. A comparison of the value of such a map factor at an unfamiliar site to the home value would provide information about the animal's position along the gradient in relationship to home. Nonparallel gradients of two different factors would allow bicoordinate position-fixing ("true navigation") (Wallraff 1991; Phillips 1996). Depending on the sensory apparatus, an organism possessing a map based on the geomagnetic field could theoretically utilize a gradient of inclination, horizontal intensity, vertical intensity, or total intensity to derive one of the map parameters.

Recent interest in the magnetic map hypothesis was triggered by studies showing that the initial homeward orientation of homing pigeons (*Columba livia*) may be influenced by natural temporal variation and, possibly, by spatial anomalies (irregularities) in the geomagnetic field (Keeton et al. 1974; Larkin and Keeton 1976; Walcott 1978; Kiepenheuer 1982, 1986; Wagner 1983; Kowalski et al. 1988; Lednor and Walcott 1988; but see Walcott 1991). Spatial variation in the intensity of the geomagnetic field averages 3–5 nT/km in the north temperate zone. However, localized spatial irregularities in the geomagnetic field can produce gradients that are stronger or weaker by an order of magnitude or more, and can differ markedly in direction from the global alignment of the field. The magnitude of normal, daily, temporal variation in the geomagnetic field varies with latitude, but averages 20–30 nT at mid-northern and southern latitudes. Magnetic storms resulting from solar activity can result in daily fluctuations of up to an order of magnitude or so greater (Fig. 1). One measure of the deviations from the regular daily pattern of temporal variation are the K indices, which have been used by researchers to look for correlations between disturbance of the geomagnetic field and variation in orientation responses (Keeton et al. 1974; Larkin and Keeton 1976; Rodda 1984b; Kowalski et al. 1988).

Because normal geographic gradients in the magnetic field are extremely weak, spatial irregularities and temporal fluctuations in the magnetic field can have a significant effect on local values of geomagnetic field parameters. Therefore, under some conditions spatial irregularities and temporal fluctuations should produce large errors in estimates of the home direction in orientation derived from a magnetic map. Indeed, the threshold for effects of naturally occurring temporal and spatial variation in the magnetic field on homing may be as low as 10 nT (Rodda 1984b; Keeton et al. 1974; Larkin and Keeton 1976; Kowalski et al. 1988; Wagner 1983). This extremely high level of sensitivity would be needed for a map sense that was able to resolve differences in geographic position of as little as 1–2 km. However, such variation would be too weak to affect a magnetic compass (Wiltschko 1972).

It is tempting to compare the high level of sensitivity necessary to detect geographic variation in the magnetic field with that exhibited by the electroreception system of elasmobranch fish, which can detect the weak electrical fields induced in a marine environment by movement through the geomagnetic field (Kalmijn 1981, 1982). The detection problem, however, is fundamentally different. The electroreception system of elasmobranch fish is able to detect electrical fields on

Daily Variation in Total Intensity

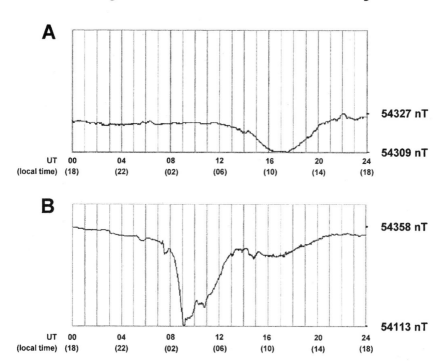

FIG. 1. Natural temporal variation in the total intensity of the geomagnetic field. (A) On a magnetically "quiet" day, temporal variation is largely confined to the daylight hours, and exhibits a fairly regular pattern that varies predictably with time of year. (B) During a magnetic storm, the regular daily pattern of temporal variation can be disrupted by large, abrupt changes in the magnetic field that may be several times the magnitude of normal daily variation. (Data obtained from USGS/NGIC 1990.)

the order of nV/cm by directly comparing the charge distribution on opposite sides of the body. By comparison, spatial variation in the geomagnetic field is superimposed on a background field that is approximately 10,000 times larger (e.g., the gradient of total intensity averages around 5 nT/km out of a total of approximately 50,000 nT). Moreover, the difference in magnetic total intensity across the head or body of a small vertebrate (1–10 cm in width) would be approximately

0.000001% to 0.0000001% of the background field. It would be impossible, therefore, for a terrestrial animal to sense the direction of the magnetic gradient by sampling at a single location. Geographic gradients in the magnetic field could only be sensed by taking "point" samples at a series of well-separated locations in a known spatial relationship to one another. Consistent with this method of sampling is the observation that species exhibiting map-based homing (true navigation) go through an early developmental stage during which they rely on "vector" navigation and/or path integration to keep track of geographic position (Perdeck 1958; Rodda and Phillips 1992). Map-based homing is only exhibited by older, more experienced individuals that presumably have had an opportunity to sample the relevant geophysical parameters (e.g., magnetic field parameters such as inclination and/or total intensity) over a relatively large area.

The difficulty inherent in detecting the extremely weak geographic gradients in the magnetic field is compounded by several factors in addition to spatial irregularities and temporal variation. Even when the local gradients of magnetic field parameters such as total intensity and inclination are extremely regular, it may be difficult for an animal to make fine-scale determinations of geographic position. Potential sources of error include the temperature sensitivity of the underlying magnetoreception system (Yorke 1979), and microscale irregularities at or near ground level. To date, no attempt has been made to quantify the magnitude of error that would be introduced by these sources; however, such sources of error would be especially problematic for ectothermic organisms that move relatively slowly at ground level (e.g., most amphibians and reptiles). Nevertheless, studies of amphibians and reptiles (like those of birds) have provided evidence that is consistent with an ability to derive map information from the geomagnetic field.

Rodda (1984a, b, 1985) obtained evidence that yearling American alligators (*Alligator mississippiensis*) use a route-based mechanism (i.e., path integration), rather than a bicoordinate map, to derive the geographic position information necessary for homing. In contrast, alligators in their second year or older appeared to rely on site-based information, suggesting that they use a true bicoordinate map. Rodda (1984b) found a correlation between "errors" in the direction of homeward orientation exhibited by older alligators and natural temporal variation in the inclination and/or horizontal intensity of the geomagnetic field. In contrast, yearlings showed no effect of temporal variation in the magnetic field. Because both age groups had access to the same sources of compass information, Rodda's findings are consistent with the possibility that the temporal variation in the geomagnetic field may have been affecting a magnetic map. If so, these data suggest that alligators may be sensitive to changes in magnetic inclination of as little as 0.01–0.02°. A change in inclination of 0.01° would result from the addition of a field of approximately 10 nT aligned perpendicularly to the geomagnetic field.

For an animal, such as the alligator, that during its first few years of life moves relatively short distances (< 5–10 km), natural temporal variation in the geomagnetic field could introduce large errors in map information derived from the geomagnetic field. Rodda's (1984b) findings suggest strategies that may be used by alligators to minimize the errors introduced by temporal variation. The home direction selected by older alligators in Rodda's study appeared to reflect the difference between the magnetic field value measured just prior to capture (or averaged over the entire night before capture) and the value measured the following night at the time of release. Errors in estimates of relative geographic position caused by temporal variation in the magnetic field would be reduced by minimizing the time interval between measurements taken at the two locations and/or by taking readings at night when the magnetic field is relatively stable (Rodda 1984b). Evidence from homing pigeons is also consistent with the possibility that a comparison of magnetic parameters measured immediately before and after displacement may play a role in the map component of homing under some circumstances (Papi et al. 1983).

Additional support for the use of the geomagnetic field to derive geographic position has come from studies of hatchling sea turtles. Lohmann and Lohmann (1994, 1996) found that when hatchling loggerhead sea turtles (collected from nests on their natal beaches) were exposed to values of magnetic inclination, or intensity, that would normally be encountered at the extremes of their range, the turtles shifted the direction of magnetic compass orientation to a new heading that might help prevent them from being displaced beyond their normal range by ocean currents. These data do not suggest that hatchling sea turtles have a bicoordinate map, which presumably would require a knowledge of the geographic variation in the magnetic field built up through experience during long-distance movements. Rather, Lohmann and Lohmann (1994, 1996) suggest that the response of hatchling sea turtles to the magnetic field changes may represent an innate "recognition" mechanism that helps prevent young turtles from straying beyond the boundaries of their normal range into regions where conditions (e.g., water temperatures) are not favorable for survival. If this interpretation is correct, the geomagnetic field provides hatchling sea turtles with a rudimentary sense of geographic position. Furthermore, Lohmann and Lohmann (1994) observed a significant difference in the direction of orientation exhibited by hatchling sea turtles exposed to inclinations of 58° (the local inclination on the natal beach) and 60°, indicating that the turtles can resolve a 2° change in inclination. This difference corresponds to the change in inclination that would be produced by the addition of a field of approximately 2,000 nT aligned perpendicularly to the ambient field.

Further experimental evidence for the use of geographic position information derived from the magnetic field has come from recent studies of a migratory bird, the silvereye (*Zosterops lateralis*) (Fischer et al. in preparation[1]). Adult silvereyes were captured on their breeding grounds in Tasmania off the southern coast of Australia before the fall migration and then transported to Armidale, New South Wales, approximately halfway to the northern boundary of the population's winter range on the eastern coast of Australia. They were divided into two groups and held indoors in the ambient magnetic field until they exhibited migratory activity. When tested indoors in the ambient magnetic field of Armidale, the two groups of silvereyes exhibited seasonally appropriate, northeasterly orientation as demonstrated previously in this species (Wiltschko et al. 1993, 1994). One group was subsequently exposed to a 12% (approximately 6,000 nT) decrease in the

---

[1] Fischer, J.H., U. Munro, J.B. Phillips. Use of a geomagnetic "map" by a migratory bird. (Manuscript in preparation.)

vertical intensity of the magnetic field resulting in values of magnetic inclination, vertical intensity, and total intensity comparable to those that occur in the vicinity of the northern boundary of the population's winter range ("simulated northern displacement"). The second group was exposed to a 12% increase in vertical intensity resulting in values of the three magnetic field parameters comparable to those normally experienced near the beginning of their fall migration from Tasmania ("simulated southern displacement"). Both experimental manipulations produced changes in total magnetic field intensity (approximately 9–10%) below values that have been shown to affect the magnetic compass in another migratory bird, the European robin (*Erithacus rubecola*) (Wiltschko 1972).

Silvereyes exposed to the simulated southern displacement continued to show a seasonally appropriate migratory orientation to the north-northeast that was stronger than in the control condition, although this difference was not statistically significant. In contrast, the responses of birds exposed to the simulated northern displacement were randomly distributed (they failed to exhibit a consistent direction of orientation, as might be expected in the final stages of migration), and differed significantly from the control condition. These findings are consistent with the possibility that silvereyes use magnetic inclination and/or intensity to derive one coordinate of a bicoordinate map. However, the data do not rule out an alternative explanation, which is that silvereyes fly in a fixed northeasterly compass direction during the fall migration until they encounter specific values of magnetic inclination and/or intensity associated with the northern boundary of the population's winter range. This second alternative is similar to the "range boundary" hypothesis suggested by Lohmann and Lohmann (1994) to explain effects of changes in magnetic inclination on the orientation of young sea turtles.

To date, the response of silvereyes to changes in vertical intensity smaller than 12% (and the corresponding changes in total intensity and inclination) has not been investigated. If silvereyes are using the magnetic field to delineate the boundary of the population's range, a relatively low level of sensitivity might suffice. For example, an ability to detect differences in the magnetic field of 1–2% (i.e., a change of 500–1000 nT in vertical intensity, and/or a corresponding change in inclination or total intensity) would allow silvereyes to resolve differ-ences in north-south position with a resolution of roughly 100–200 km. In contrast, if silvereyes are using the magnetic field as a source of map information that allows individual birds to return to specific summer or winter territories, they would need a much higher level of sensitiv-ity. For example, a magnetic map sense accurate to within 10 km or so would require an ability to detect differences in vertical (or total) intensity on the order of 50 nT and/or differences in inclination of approximately 0.05°. Further experiments to determine the threshold of the silvereyes' response, and to identify the specific magnetic field parameter or parameters to which they are responding, would clearly be of considerable interest.

Preliminary data from a study of the homing orientation of eastern red-spotted newts (*Notophthalmus viridescens*) are also consistent with the possibility that a magnetic field parameter may be involved in map-based homing. Initial results suggest that changes in magnetic inclination of approximately 2° have a significant effect on the direc-tion of homing orientation, but have no effect on shoreward magnetic compass orientation, which does not require map information (J. Fischer, J.B. Phillips, and S.C. Borland, research in progress). The magnetic field manipulation was produced by introducing an artificial field of approximately 2,000 nT aligned in the vertical plane roughly perpendicular to the geomagnetic field so that the total magnetic field intensity remained unchanged. If replicable, these results would be consistent with the possibility that magnetic inclination is used to derive one coordinate of the navigational map. It must be kept in mind, however, that in order for newts to derive useful information about geographic position within their normal range of movement (< 5 km), they would have to detect differences in magnetic inclina-tion that are 100–1000 times smaller than the manipulations used in these experiments (0.02–0.002° depending on the steepness of the local gradient) and/or corresponding differences in the vertical or horizon-tal intensity (both of which are affected by the change in inclination). Moreover, since magnetic inclination is measured relative to gravity, a gravitational reference system with a comparable level of sensitivity would be required.

A Magnetic Zeitgeber for Entrainment of Circadian Rhythms?

An idea suggested many years ago (Bliss and Heppner 1976; Brown and Chow 1976; Brown and Scow 1978; Welker et al. 1983) that is currently given little credibility, is that the regular daily pattern of temporal variation in the geomagnetic field may provide a Zeitgeber, or timing cue, that plays a role in the entrainment of circadian rhythms. Temporal variation tends to be relatively high during the day (at least 20–30 nT, often higher); whereas at night the geomagnetic field tends to be relatively stable (see Fig. 1) (Skiles 1985). Theoretically, if an organism could perceive the temporal fluctuations in one or more of the parameters of the geomagnetic field, these fluctuations could supplement, or take the place of, the photoperiod for entrainment of circadian rhythms (e.g., for an animal that spends part of the day in a burrow where it is not exposed to the light–dark cycle). It is not surprising, therefore, that the current concern about possible EMF effects on circadian production of melatonin has led to a resurgence of interest in the possibility of a magnetic Zeitgeber.

Several reasons provide impetus for further study of the possibility of a magnetic Zeitgeber. First, sensory apparatus that would be necessary to detect the daily pattern of temporal variation in the geomagnetic field should be *identical in all important respects* to that required to detect the natural spatial variation in the geomagnetic field during short-distance (< 5 km) movements (for which there is growing evidence; see previous discussion). The second reason to examine the possibility of a magnetic Zeitgeber is the growing evidence for a magnetoreception system, possibly involving particles of magnetite, that may exhibit the requisite level of sensitivity (Semm and Beason 1990; Table 2, and see p. 144). Detection of both temporal and spatial variation in the geomagnetic field would require (1) sensitivity in the range of 10 nT or less and (2) an ability to compare the values of a specific magnetic field parameter(s) taken at widely separated points in time and/or space. Thus, a conclusive demonstration of the use of the magnetic field to derive map or geographic position information for short distance movements would provide *prima facie* evidence for the high level of sensitivity that would be necessary to detect natural temporal variation in the magnetic field. Indeed, evidence for effects of natural temporal variation on the direction of homing orientation

TABLE 2

Absolute Levels of Sensitivity to Magnetic Stimuli:
Neurophysiological and Behavioral Studies

Study	Type of response	Sensitivity
Beason and Semm 1987; Semm and Beason 1990	Recordings from the ophthalmic branch of trigeminal nerve and trigeminal nucleus in adult bobolinks	Responses of individual units down to 100–200 nT. (See page 144.) Entire system might be at least an order of magnitude more sensitive (i.e., ~ 5–10 nT).
Keeton et al. 1974; Larkin and Keeton 1976; Kowalski et al. 1988	Effects of natural temporal variation in geomagnetic field on orientation of homing pigeons	Correlations consistent with sensitivity to variation in geomagnetic field of < 100 nT.
Kiepenheuer 1982, 1986; Wagner 1983	Initial orientation of homing pigeons at natural magnetic anomalies	Disruption of initial orientation at strong magnetic anomalies could be due to variation in the geomagnetic field or in some other geophysical parameter (e.g., gravity). If effects of weak magnetic anomalies are due to variation in geomagnetic field, then responses are consistent with sensitivity to variation of < 100 nT.
Rodda 1984b	Effects of natural temporal variation in geomagnetic field on homing orientation of American alligators	Correlations consistent with effects of ~0.01–0.02° change in inclination (equivalent to ~10–20 nT field applied perpendicular to the geomagnetic field; see text)

continued

TABLE 2 (continued)

Absolute Levels of Sensitivity to Magnetic Stimuli: Neurophysiological and Behavioral Studies

Study	Type of response	Sensitivity
Lohmann and Lohmann 1994, 1996	Change in direction of magnetic compass orientation by hatchling sea turtles	Response to 2° change in inclination in one experimental treatment (equivalent to ~2000 nT field applied perpendicular to the geomagnetic field; see text), and to a 9000-nT change in total intensity
Fisher et al. (in preparation)[1]	Effects of experimental manipulation of static magnetic field on migratory orientation of adult silvereyes	Response to ~6,000 nT changes in vertical intensity (corresponding to "map" displacements of ~1200 km); smaller changes not tested. Use of a magnetic map potentially would require much higher sensitivity (e.g., map resolution of 100 km would require sensitivity to changes of approximately 500 nT; greater resolution would require higher sensitivity).
Fischer, Phillips, and Borland (unpublished data)	Effects of experimental manipulation of magnetic inclination on the homing orientation of eastern newts	Response to 2° change in inclination (equivalent to ~2000-nT field applied perpendicular to the geomagnetic field); smaller changes in inclination not yet tested. Magnetic map that would provide useful information within newt's normal range of movement (< 5 km) would require sensitivity to inclination changes of 0.02–0.002° (i.e., equivalent to field of ~2–20 nT perpendicular to geomagnetic field).

[1] Fisher, J.H., U. Munro, J.B. Phillips. Use of a geomagnetic "map" by a migratory bird. (Manuscript in preparation).

(Rodda 1984b; Keeton et al. 1974; Larkin and Keeton 1976; Kowalski et al. 1988; Wagner 1983; and see pp. 125–129) suggests that at least some terrestrial vertebrates are capable of detecting natural temporal variation in the geomagnetic field.

LOCALIZATION OF RECEPTORS AND FUNCTIONAL PROPERTIES OF MAGNETORECEPTION MECHANISMS: PHYSIOLOGICAL EVIDENCE

Pineal Interactions with Earth-Strength Magnetic Fields

Semm et al. (1980) were the first to provide physiological evidence suggesting that the visual system and the pineal gland might be involved in magnetoreception. In particular, they found that single units in the pineal gland of the guinea pig (*Cavia aperea*) were sensitive to an abrupt rotation of the vertical component of the magnetic field. Similar experiments carried out on pigeons, bobolinks (*Dolichonyx oryzivorus*), and rats (*Rattus norvigicus*) (Semm et al. 1982; Semm 1983; Beason and Semm 1987; Reuss et al. 1983) showed that, in addition to changes in the vertical component of the magnetic field, pineal cells also respond to abrupt changes in the horizontal component of the magnetic field. Such abrupt changes in the magnetic field, however, can induce relatively large electrical currents within an organism (see Reiter and Richardson 1992), so that the pineal cells in these experiments may have been responding to the induced electrical artifacts and not to the magnetic field per se. Therefore, studies using abrupt EMF changes do not provide unequivocal evidence for geomagnetic sensitivity.

In order to minimize electrical artifacts and provide better evidence for magnetic field sensitivity, a gradual change in the magnetic field must be used to elicit a response. Gradual changes in the horizontal component of the magnetic field have been shown to affect the spontaneous firing rate of pineal cells in birds (Demaine and Semm 1985), suggesting that at least in birds, pineal cells are sensitive to Earth-strength magnetic fields rather than, or in addition to, electrical currents that are induced in the tissue when abruptly changing magnetic stimuli are used (Semm et al. 1982; Beason and Semm 1987).

Biochemical changes in the pineal [e.g., changes in nocturnal melatonin and serotonin-N-acetyltransferase (NAT)] also have been used in attempts to demonstrate geomagnetic field sensitivity in both rodents and birds (see Table 3). As in some of the electrophysiological studies

TABLE 3

Summary of Subjects, Stimuli, and Results from Studies Investigating Biochemical Changes Associated with Static Earth-Strength Magnetic Field Manipulations[1]

Study	Subject(s)	Stimulus type: 1.Type of change 2. Rate of change 3. Total exposure time	Findings
Welker et al. 1983	Sprague-Dawley rat (*Rattus norvegicus*)	1. Inversion of horizontal component and changes in inclination of 5°–15° 2. Abrupt 3. 15 minutes–2 hours	Nighttime exposure to change in the field resulted in depression of pineal NAT (serotonin N-acetyltransferase) and melatonin, and serum melatonin.
Olcese et al. 1985	Sprague-Dawley rat	1. 50° rotation in horizontal component 2. Abrupt 3. 30 minutes	Pineal NAT and melatonin were inhibited only in intact animals. No effect seen in blinded animals.
Reuss and Olcese 1986	Sprague-Dawley rat	1. 50° rotation in horizontal component 2. Abrupt 3. 30 minutes	Pineal NAT and HIOMT (hydroxyindole-O-methyltransferase) were inhibited under red light. No effect seen in darkness.

[1]All stimuli exposures were at night unless otherwise indicated.

continued

TABLE 3 (continued)

Summary of Subjects, Stimuli, and Results from Studies Investigating Biochemical Changes Associated with Static Earth-Strength Magnetic Field Manipulations

Study	Subject(s)	Stimulus type: 1. Type of change 2. Rate of change 3. Total exposure time	Findings
Olcese and Reuss 1986	Sprague-Dawley (albino) rat, Long-Evans (hypopig-mented) hooded rat, Golden hamster (*Mesocricetus auratus*)	1. 50° rotation in horizontal component 2. Abrupt 3. 30 minutes	Both types of rat exhibited decrease in pineal melatonin. No effect seen in hamster pineal melatonin.
Khoory 1987	Wistar rat	1. Reduction of magnetic field to 0.0025 mT 2. Abrupt 3. 30 minutes	No effect on pineal NAT or melatonin.
Olcese et al. 1988b	Sprague-Dawley rat (normal and light-induced photoreceptor degenerates)	1. 50° rotation in horizontal component 2. Abrupt 3. 30 minutes	Normal rats exhibited reduced levels of retinal dopamine and norepinephrine, but no effect on retinal NAT. No effects in photoreceptor-degenerate animals.
Rudolph et al. 1988	Wistar-Fullinsdorf rat	1. Inversion of horizontal component 2. Abrupt 3. 60 minutes	Decrease in pineal cyclic adenosine monophosphate (cAMP).

continued

TABLE 3 (continued)

Summary of Subjects, Stimuli, and Results from Studies Investigating Biochemical Changes Associated with Static Earth-Strength Magnetic Field Manipulations

Study	Subject(s)	Stimulus type: 1.Type of change 2. Rate of change 3. Total exposure time	Findings
Stehle et al. 1988	Mongolian gerbil (*Meriones unguiculatus*; both pigmented and albino) and Sprague-Dawley rat	1. 60° rotation of horizontal component 2. Abrupt 3. 30 minutes	All subjects except pigmented gerbils exhibited deceases in pineal NAT and melatonin.
Olcese and Hurlbut 1989	Sprague-Dawley rat, Richardson's ground squirrel (*Spermophilus richardsonii*), Golden hamster	1. 72° clockwise rotation of horizontal component 2. Abrupt 3. 30 minutes, daytime exposure	Reduced levels of retinal dopamine in rat and squirrel, increased levels of retinal dopamine in hamster.
Olcese 1990	Sprague-Dawley rat (albino) and ACI rat (fully pigmented)	1. Rotation of horizontal component 2. Abrupt 3. 30 minutes	Decrease in pineal NAT in albino rats, but not in ACI rats.
	RCS rat (inherited retinal dystrophy) and Rdy rat (genetic controls)	1. Rotation of horizontal component 2. Abrupt 3. 30 minutes	Decrease in retinal dopamine in normal rats (Rdy), but not in RCS, retinal-degenerate rats.

continued

TABLE 3 (continued)

Summary of Subjects, Stimuli, and Results from Studies Investigating Biochemical Changes Associated with Static Earth-Strength Magnetic Field Manipulations

Study	Subject(s)	Stimulus type: 1. Type of change 2. Rate of change 3. Total exposure time	Findings
Lerchl et al. 1990	Sprague-Dawley rat, AMES mouse (*Mus musculus*)	1. Inversion of the horizontal component 2. Abrupt 3. On/off at 5-minute intervals for 1 hour	In mice: increased levels of pineal 5 HT (serotonin). In rats: increased 5 HT and 5 HIAA (5-hydroxyindole acetic acid); decreased pineal NAT; no effect on serum or pineal melatonin.
Lerchl et al. 1991	Sprague-Dawley rat	1. Inversion of the horizontal component 2. Pulsed and gradual (i.e., 1 second) 3. On/off at 1-minute intervals for 1 hour	Increased pineal 5HT and 5HIAA level, and decreased levels of pineal NAT and melatonin only in pulsed-field exposures.
Schneider et al. 1994a	Pied flycatcher (*Ficedula hypoleuca*)	1. Change in horizontal direction and/or intensity 2. Abrupt 3. 5 × 30-minute exposures	Decreased serum melatonin with combined change in intensity and direction, not with only change in intensity or direction.

(Semm et al. 1982; Semm 1983; Beason and Semm 1987; Reuss et al. 1983), however, most of these studies have used a single, abrupt change in an Earth-strength field as the stimulus, increasing the likelihood that the observed effects were due to induced electrical currents, not to the magnetic field (Lerchl et al. 1991; Reiter and Richardson 1992). While sensitivity to induced electrical currents may provide little, if any, information about the mechanism(s) of magnetoreception in terrestrial organisms, such sensitivity provides a possible explanation for the reported effects of ELF EMF on pineal function (e.g., Kato et al. 1993, 1994a, b; Yellon 1994). Whereas a quick inversion of the magnetic field would produce a single, large, induced electrical current in tissue, ELF EMF would produce a much smaller electrical current that would be repeated with every oscillation of the field. Therefore, the results of studies using an abrupt change in an Earth-strength field may help elucidate the mechanism of ELF EMF effects on melatonin and pineal function (for review, see Olcese 1990), and so we will briefly review the findings here.

Welker et al. (1983) first demonstrated that a single exposure to an abrupt rotation of the horizontal component of the magnetic field during the night resulted in depression of pineal melatonin and NAT levels in rats held under red light. Effects of the magnetic field inversion, however, were eliminated by transection of the optic nerve (Olcese et al. 1985) and by the absence of the red light (Reuss and Olcese 1986). These results indicate that both an intact retina and optic nerve are required for the observed effects on rat pineal, suggesting that retinal photoreceptors may be the site of biological interaction for the abrupt field change. Such effects on the retina could subsequently effect the pineal via the retinohypothalamic-pineal pathway.

Olcese et al. (1988b) found that during the night, abrupt deflection of the horizontal component of the magnetic field caused a reduction in dopamine and norepinephrine levels in the rat retina. Retinal effects were absent in rats in which the outer segments of the photoreceptors had degenerated as a consequence of 8 weeks of exposure to constant light (Olcese et al. 1988b), and in rats with inherited retinal dystrophy (Olcese 1990). These data provide direct support for a photoreceptor-based mechanism for biochemical responses to abrupt field changes in the retina of mammals.

In birds, melatonin responses to EMF changes (Schneider et al. 1994a) may not require retinal photoreceptors. Demaine and Semm (1985) demonstrated magnetic sensitivity in pineal cells that was independent of retinal input. Unlike the mammalian pineal, the avian pineal is intrinsically photosensitive (Semm and Demaine 1983). One class of avian pinealocytes resembles rudimentary photoreceptors and contains a photoreceptive opsin protein (Okano et al. 1994). The pineal data from birds, therefore, are consistent with a photoreceptor-based mechanism for EMF effects. Furthermore, Demaine and Semm (1985) used a gradual change in the magnetic field to elicit pineal cell responses. As a consequence, the responses they observed were unlikely to be due to electrical artifacts and, therefore, are consistent with a photoreceptor-based magnetoreception mechanism.

The evidence for an effect of magnetic stimuli on melatonin concentration in the pineal (apparently mediated by photoreceptors) and the dependence of this effect on the phase of the light–dark cycle have caused some investigators to suggest that natural variation in the geomagnetic field may play some role circadian rhythms of rodents and birds (for example Olcese et al. 1988a; Welker et al. 1983). At this point, however, induced electrical currents caused by the abrupt changes in the magnetic field used in many of the experiments cannot be ruled out, and, in some cases, appear to be the most likely explanation for the observed effects (Lerchl et al. 1990; Reiter and Richardson 1992). Lerchl et al. (1991) compared pineal responses in rodents exposed to a repeated, "pulsed" (abrupt on/off), magnetic stimulus versus a repeated, gradual (1 second ramped field change) stimulus. Pineal biochemical responses were exhibited only in animals exposed to the pulsed stimuli, suggesting that induced currents were responsible for the pineal effects caused by repeated magnetic field changes. Whether their results can explain the pineal responses reported by Welker et al. (1983) and others (Olcese et al. 1985; Reuss and Olcese 1986; Olcese and Reuss 1986; Rudolph et al. 1988; Stehle et al. 1988; Olcese 1990) is unclear, because several different exposure conditions were used in these studies; e.g., repeated versus single magnetic field changes and varying magnitudes of horizontal deflection (see Table 3 for specific details of these studies).

Regardless of whether the effects of abrupt EMF changes on pineal function in rodents are mediated by a sensory mechanism specialized for detection of the geomagnetic field, or instead, are mediated by induced electrical currents on a system not involved in magnetoreception, the site of EMF interaction appears to be the retinal photoreceptors (Olcese et al. 1985, 1988b; Reuss and Olcese 1986; Olcese 1990). Neurophysiological recordings using gradual field changes to study pineal/magnetic field interactions in pigeons suggest that, at least in birds, magnetic field effects may be mediated by a photoreceptor-based magnetoreception mechanism (Demaine and Semm 1985). These neurophysiological data also are consistent with the possibility that natural magnetic stimuli may play some role in circadian periodicity in birds (Demaine and Semm 1985; Schneider et al. 1994a, b). Furthermore, the similarity of the pineal response (i.e., reduction of nocturnal melatonin) in the studies of birds using gradual magnetic field changes to that observed in studies of rodents using abrupt field changes and ELF EMF suggests that gradual, abrupt, and ELF field effects may be mediated by a common mechanism (possibly photoreceptor-based magnetoreceptors located in the retina and/or pineal) that may be sensitive to both magnetic and induced electric stimuli.

Evidence for a Visually Based Magnetic Compass

In addition to the study of the pineal by Demaine and Semm (1985), several experiments have been performed using gradual rotation of the magnetic field to characterize the physiological correlates of geomagnetic sensitivity in the avian visual system. Semm and colleagues (Semm et al. 1984; Semm and Demaine 1986) performed electrophysiological studies showing responses to very slow (90-second) rotations of an Earth-strength magnetic field in a number of centers in the pigeon brain that receive visual input [e.g., the lateral and superior vestibular nuclei, the nucleus of the basal optic root (nBOR), the optic tectum, etc.]. Single units in the nBOR were selectively responsive over a small range of alignments of the magnetic field, suggesting that nBOR encodes information about the direction of the magnetic field and, therefore, may be part of the magnetic compass of birds. Furthermore, the responses of the brain nuclei to magnetic field rotations were shown to be dependent on input from the retina and on the presence of light. Magnetic field responses exhibited by nBOR units appeared to be influenced by the wavelength of light, showing peak sensitivities around 500 or 580 nm (Semm and Demaine 1986).

The Trigeminal System

Physiological evidence for a nonvisually based magnetoreception system has come from recordings in the nervous system of a migratory bird, the bobolink. Units from the ophthalmic branch of the trigeminal nerve respond to changes in the rotation of the vertical or horizontal component of the Earth's magnetic field as well as to changes in intensity of as little as 50–200 nT (Beason and Semm 1987; Semm and Beason 1990; P. Semm personal communication). Magnetic stimuli used in these experiments included rectangular pulses, sinusoidally oscillating fields, and a slowly moving bar magnet; therefore, electrically induced artifacts were not likely to be responsible for all these effects. The trigeminal nerve innervates the ethmoidal region, where particles of single-domain magnetite have been found in bobolinks (Beason and Nichols 1984; Beason 1989) and a variety of other vertebrates (Kirschvink et al. 1985). The absolute sensitivity of the trigeminal nerve responses, as well as the anatomical proximity of the nerve to tissue containing magnetite, suggest that magnetite may be the transducer in this system.

Interestingly, light-dependent responses to magnetic stimuli also have been recorded in the optic tectum and pineal of the bobolink, suggesting the existence of two independent magnetoreception systems in the same organism (Beason and Semm 1987). These findings are consistent with behavioral evidence for the presence of two magnetoreception systems in terrestrial vertebrates (see next section).

There has been some concern about the validity of the central nervous system recordings, because the responses to magnetic stimuli are observed in some preparations but not in others (Semm personal communication). However, the case for a photoreceptor-based magnetic compass and a magnetite-based/trigeminal system in vertebrates is strengthened by the results of independent behavioral studies presented in the next section.

LOCALIZATION AND FUNCTIONAL PROPERTIES OF MAGNETORECEPTION MECHANISMS: BEHAVIORAL EVIDENCE

Behavioral responses to Earth-strength magnetic fields have been characterized primarily on the basis of four properties: (1) sensitivity to the polarity of the magnetic field (e.g., Wiltschko and Wiltschko 1972, 1988; Beason 1989; Arendse 1978; Phillips 1986b; Burda et al. 1990; Light et al. 1993); (2) dependence on the presence of light (e.g., Arendse 1978; Phillips and Borland 1992b; Lohmann and Lohmann 1993); (3) dependence on the wavelength of light (Phillips and Borland 1992a; Phillips and Sayeed 1993; Wiltschko et al. 1993; Wiltschko and Wiltschko 1995b; Beason and Phillips, unpublished data); and (4) sensitivity to pulse remagnetization (Wiltschko et al. 1994; Beason et al. 1995; Munro et al. in press). Most "compass" responses exhibited by terrestrial vertebrates are independent of the polarity of the magnetic field (i.e., exhibit axial sensitivity) and are dependent on, or sensitive to, light (see Wiltschko and Wiltschko 1995a). Animals which exhibit axial sensitivity to the geomagnetic field rely on the inclination, or dip angle, of the magnetic field to distinguish between the two ends of the magnetic axis; i.e., poleward versus equatorward (Wiltschko and Wiltschko 1972, 1988). Several lines of behavioral evidence suggest that axial compass responses are mediated by a light-dependent, possibly photoreceptor-based, magnetoreception mechanism (see next section).

Several compass responses, however, provide interesting exceptions to the general pattern. For example, Light et al. (1993) found that hatchling sea turtles exhibited an axial magnetic compass response, while in a closely related species, Lohmann and Lohmann (1993) found that hatchlings continued to respond to changes in magnetic field alignment after several minutes in total darkness. These findings are compatible with either a radical pair mechanism that does not require photoexcitation for generation of the radical pair (or that can substitute a biochemical source of energy when light is not available) or with a magnetite-based mechanism in which the magnetic moments of SPM or SD particles are free to rotate with respect to the surrounding tissue (see Table 1). Additional research will be necessary to distinguish between these (and other) alternative explanations for the sea turtle's magnetic compass response.

Newts exhibiting the compass component of homing also appear to be an exception. The newt's homing response exhibits polar sensitivity (Phillips 1986b), but also is influenced by the wavelength of light (Phillips and Borland 1994). We have speculated that these properties arise from an interaction between a light-dependent magnetic compass and a non-light-dependent magnetic intensity, or inclination, detector that is involved in deriving map information from the geomagnetic field (Phillips and Borland 1994; and see next section).

The last exception has been observed in the only mammal for which the functional characteristics of a behavioral response to the magnetic field have been characterized—the African mole rat (*Cryptomys hottentotus*). Burda et al. (1990) provided family groups of the African mole rat with uniformly dispersed nesting material in a visually symmetrical, circular arena, and found that they spontaneously built nests in a particular direction relative to the magnetic field. This response was sensitive to the polarity of the magnetic field and persisted in total darkness (see Wiltschko and Wiltschko 1995a). These findings suggest that a magnetite-based magnetoreception mechanism mediates the mole rats' nest-building, directional preference (see Table 1). It is unclear, however, whether the apparently innate directional preference evident in the nest-building response of African mole rats should be classified as a compass response in the same sense as the shoreward orientation of newts (see next section). It is certainly possible that the mole rats are primarily using the geomagnetic field as a source of compass information. For example, nest position or alignment in this species could function as a directional reference that is used when leaving the nest (e.g., for foraging or "tunnel digging"). Alternatively, however, the alignment of the nest might make it easier for mole rats to maintain a particular body alignment relative to the magnetic field that facilitates measurements of spatial or temporal variation in a particular parameter of the magnetic field (e.g., inclination or intensity; Phillips and Borland 1994). Thus, while it may turn out that the same form of orientation behavior (e.g., compass orientation) may be mediated by different magnetoreception mechanisms in different species, it is also possible that the involvement of different magnetoreception mechanisms (e.g., magnetite-based versus photoreceptor-based mechanisms) may indicate that the two behaviors, although superficially similar, serve different functions. In order to further address some of the questions concerning the functional properties and behavioral context(s) of magnetic orientation in rodents, we are conducting experiments to characterize the magnetic nest-building response of the Siberian hamster (*Phodopus sungorus*) (Deutschlander et al. 1996).

Wavelength-Dependent Effects of Light on Magnetic Compass Orientation

To date, the results of experiments investigating the influence of changes in the wavelength of light on magnetic compass orientation have been published for four species. In the eastern red spotted newt (Phillips and Borland 1992a) and the fruit fly (*Drosophila melanogaster*) (Phillips and Sayeed 1993), changes in the wavelength of light were found to produce a 90° shift in the direction of magnetic compass orientation. Newts that had been trained to an artificial shore in an outdoor tank under full-spectrum light and were tested under violet or blue (400- or 450-nm) light exhibited shoreward magnetic compass orientation that was indistinguishable from that obtained under full-spectrum light (Fig. 2A). In contrast, newts that were tested under green, yellow, or orange (500-, 550-, or 600-nm) light exhibited orientation that was shifted by 90° from the orientation of full-spectrum controls (Fig. 2B). Fruit flies have also been found to exhibit a 90° difference in the direction of magnetic compass orientation when tested under two different wavelengths of light (365 nm and 500 nm). These wavelengths were chosen because they preferentially excite two spectral mechanisms found in the most abundant class of photoreceptors (the retinula 1–6 cells) in the compound eye (Phillips and Sayeed 1993).

Unlike newts and fruit flies, two species of migratory birds (the silvereye and the European robin) (Wiltschko et al. 1993; Wiltschko and Wiltschko 1995a, b), were found to orient in a seasonally appropriate migratory direction relative to the magnetic field under full-spectrum, blue (443-nm; silvereyes only), and yellow (571-nm) light. Under longer wavelengths of light (588 nm and 633 nm), however, their bearings were randomly distributed with respect to the magnetic field (Wiltschko et al. 1993; Wiltschko and Wiltschko 1995a, b). In contrast, newts were able to orient with respect to the magnetic field at wavelengths from 400–600 nm (with the exception of 475 nm; see p. 151),

Shoreward Compass Orientation

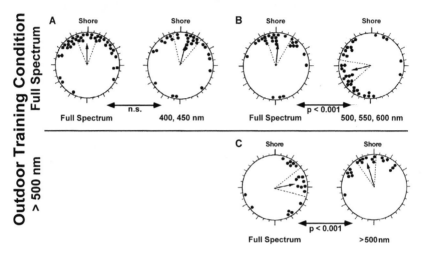

Testing Condition

FIG. 2. Wavelength-dependent effects of light on the shoreward magnetic compass response of newts (modified from Phillips and Borland 1992a). Each pair of distributions shows data from newts tested in the same experiments under full-spectrum light (left distribution) or under wavelengths from a specific region of the spectrum (right distribution). A brief summary of experimental methods is provided (below). (A and B) Shoreward magnetic compass orientation of newts trained under natural skylight. (A) Controls tested under full-spectrum light were oriented towards shore. Newts tested under 400- and 450-nm light also oriented towards shore, and were indistinguishable from controls. (B) Full-spectrum controls were oriented towards shore. Newts tested under 500-, 550- and 600-nm light oriented approximately 90° counterclockwise of shore, and differed significantly from full-spectrum controls ($p < 0.001$, Watson U^2 test, Batschelet 1981). (C) Shoreward magnetic compass orientation of newts trained under long-wavelength light. After training under long-wavelength (> 500-nm) light, newts tested under full-spectrum light oriented approximately 90° clockwise of shore. Newts tested under wavelengths > 500 nm were oriented in the shoreward magnetic direction. The two distributions were significantly different ($p < 0.001$, Watson U^2 test).

Methods. Groups of newts were trained in water-filled, outdoor tanks with an artificial shore at one end, and then released individually at the center of a visually symmetric, dry indoor arena. Directional responses were measured at a radius of 20 cm from the center of the arena. Each data point is the magnetic bearing of

caption continued on facing page

but were randomly distributed when tested under wavelengths in the near-infrared (> 715-nm; Phillips and Borland 1992b) range. Given the long-wavelength shift in the newt's shoreward response, the absence of a wavelength-dependent shift in magnetic compass orientation of migratory birds is intriguing. However, these data do not rule out similar underlying biophysical mechanisms in newts and birds. Like fruit flies, most birds have a population of ultraviolet-sensitive photoreceptors with a peak of sensitivity around 370 nm (Chen et al. 1984). Thus, further tests are needed to determine if birds exhibit a 90° difference in the direction of magnetic compass orientation under ultraviolet and visible light, similar to that observed in fruit flies (Phillips and Sayeed 1993).

Because the shoreward magnetic compass response of newts is learned, Phillips and Borland (1992a) were able to carry out control experiments designed to distinguish a direct effect of long-wavelength light on the magnetic compass from a nonspecific effect on the newts' behavior. In initial experiments, newts that were trained outdoors under full-spectrum light exhibited a 90°, counterclockwise shift in the direction of magnetic compass orientation when tested under long-wavelength (500 nm) light (Fig. 2B). We reasoned that if this 90° shift was due to a direct effect on the newts' magnetic compass, then newts *trained under long-wavelength light* should learn a direction of orienta-

---

an individual newt. Individual newts were tested only once, in one of four magnetic field alignments (i.e., magnetic north at north, east, south, or west; Phillips 1986a), and the magnetic bearings were pooled relative to the direction towards shore in the training tank. As a consequence of the use of the four symmetrical magnetic field alignments, the pooled distribution retained only the component of orientation that was a consistent magnetic response. Arrows at the center of distributions indicate significant mean vector bearings; lengths of arrows are proportional to the mean vector lengths 'r' (radius of circle corresponds to r = 1). Dashed lines indicate the 95% confidence interval for the mean vector bearing. Discrete wavelengths of light were produced using broad-band interference filters (40 ± 2 nm bandwidth) and adjusted to equal quantal flux. In tests where newts were trained under long-wavelength light, the outdoor tanks were enclosed in sheets of a yellow gel filter (Lee Filters #101), which transmitted less than 1% of light at wavelengths below 490 nm and less than 0.1% at wavelengths below 470 nm. For testing under long-wavelength light in (C), a filter made of the same yellow gel material was placed in the light path to the indoor arena.

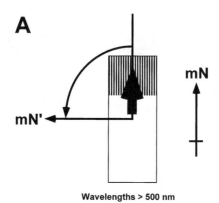

Wavelengths > 500 nm

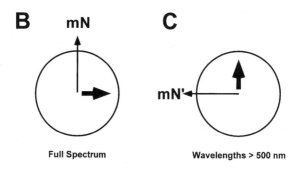

Full Spectrum   **Wavelengths > 500 nm**

FIG. 3. Predicted orientation of newts after training under long-wavelength light if the wavelength-dependent 90°-shift is due to a direct effect of light on the underlying magnetoreception mechanism. (A) Schematic of one of the outdoor training tanks aligned with artificial shore toward magnetic north. If long-wavelength light (i.e., wavelengths > 500 nm) causes the newts' perceived magnetic north (mN') to be rotated 90° counterclockwise from true magnetic north (mN), then the direction of shore will appear to the newts to be toward magnetic east. (B) When subsequently tested in the indoor arena *under full-spectrum light*, directional information obtained from the magnetic field will be rotated 90° clockwise from what the newts experienced during training. Orientation in the shoreward direction learned during training under long-wavelength light will cause the newts to orient 90° *clockwise* of the actual shoreward direction. (C) In contrast, when tested *under long-wavelength light*, the magnetic field will appear to be rotated 90° counterclockwise of its actual direction, as it appeared in training [see (A)]. As a consequence, the direction of shore learned during training under long-wavelength light will correspond to the actual direction of shore relative to the magnetic field, resulting in unshifted orientation.

tion relative to the magnetic field that is shifted 90° *clockwise* of true shore direction (Fig. 3A). Therefore, when newts trained under long-wavelength light are *tested under full-spectrum light*, their orientation relative to the magnetic field should be shifted 90° clockwise of the true shore direction (Fig. 3B). In contrast, newts trained *and* tested under long-wavelength light should orient in the correct shoreward direction (Fig. 3C). As shown in Figure 2C, the orientation of newts trained under long-wavelength light was consistent with these predictions, providing strong evidence that light has a direct effect on the underlying magnetoreception mechanism.

Figure 4 presents a simple model that was proposed to explain the wavelength-dependent, 90° shift in the magnetic compass orientation of newts (Phillips and Borland 1992a). According to this model, the magnetic field alters the efficiency of phototransduction involving two spectral mechanisms that have antagonistic effects on the response of the magnetoreceptor, resulting in complementary bimodal patterns (Figs. 4A, C). The "complimentary bimodal pattern" model was tested by observing the shoreward compass response of newts under 475-nm light, which is intermediate between the spectral regions that produced normal ($\leq$450 nm) and shifted (500 nm) orientation. Light at wavelengths around 475 nm should excite the two spectral mechanisms more or less equally, and cause the two complementary patterns to cancel each other out (Fig. 4B). As predicted, newts tested under 475-nm light were randomly distributed with respect to the magnetic field (Phillips and Borland 1992a).

If the two spectral mechanisms that contribute to the newt's magnetic compass are similar in absolute sensitivity, broad-band light present under natural conditions also would be expected to degrade or eliminate the newt's ability to obtain compass information from the magnetic field due to similar activation of the two spectral mechanisms. Controls tested under full-spectrum light, however, exhibited magnetic compass orientation that is indistinguishable from newts tested under 400- and 450-nm light (Fig. 2A). These findings indicate that full-spectrum light is primarily exciting the short-wavelength mechanism. Therefore, newts appear to avoid the problem of equal excitation of the two spectral mechanisms by reducing the relative sen-

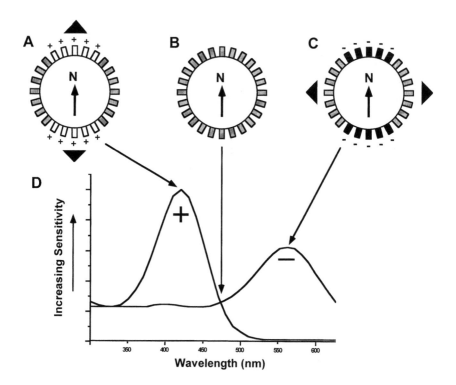

FIG. 4. A hypothetical magnetoreception system consisting of a circular array of receptors (small rectangles). (A) Under short-wavelength light, receptors aligned within a certain angle of either end of the magnetic axis exhibit an increase in response (light-colored rectangles) relative to receptors in alignments that are not affected by the magnetic field (shaded rectangles). Arrowheads at the edge of the circular array indicate the axis that will appear to have the highest level of response. (B) Under an intermediate wavelength of light ($\sim$ 475 nm) that activates the two spectral mechanisms [see (D)] more-or-less equally, the response of the receptors is independent of magnetic field alignment (shaded rectangles). (C) Under long-wavelength light, receptors in alignments that are affected by the magnetic field exhibit a decrease in response (dark rectangles) relative to receptors in alignments that are unaffected by the magnetic field (shaded rectangles). The axes with the highest level of response (indicated by arrows) differ by 90° in (A) and (C). (D) Absorption spectra of two hypothetical spectral mechanisms proposed to mediate the newt's light-dependent magnetic compass response showing the lower sensitivity of the long-wavelength spectral mechanism (see text), as well as the equal absorption of the two mechanisms at wavelengths $\sim$ 475 nm. Note that this hypothesis does not predict the direction along the magnetic axis that will be interpreted as magnetic north (see Phillips and Borland 1992a).

sitivity of the long-wavelength spectral mechanism (Fig. 4D; and Phillips and Borland 1992a).

Because a reduction in the sensitivity of one of the two spectral mechanisms appears to be necessary for the newt's magnetic compass to operate under natural (i.e., broad-band) lighting conditions, it is surprising that natural selection has not completely eliminated one of the two spectral mechanisms. For example, if the wavelength dependence of the newt's magnetic compass response were a consequence of antagonistic long-wavelength and short-wavelength inputs onto a second-order cell, it seems likely that natural selection would have eliminated one of these two inputs, resulting in an achromatic visual pathway in which directional information from the magnetic field was unaffected by the spectral content of light. Evidence that this has not occurred (Fig. 2) suggests that the two spectral mechanisms (1) may not act independently, (2) may be essential components of the biophysical process responsible for magnetic field detection and, therefore, (3) may be present in the same cell. Our working hypothesis, therefore, is that the wavelength dependence of the newt's magnetic compass response arises at the level of individual receptor cells (e.g., a single class of photoreceptor that contains two spectral mechanisms).

Our interest in whether the wavelength-dependent, 90° shift in the magnetic compass response of newts is an intrinsic property of the primary receptors stems in part from the discovery of unusual photoreceptors in the pineal complex (parietal eye) of lizards (Solessio and Engbretson 1993). The spectral properties of these parietal eye photoreceptors closely resemble the spectral properties predicted to underlie the magnetic compass response of newts (Phillips and Borland 1992a). Solessio and Engbretson obtained recordings from isolated parietal eye photoreceptors that demonstrated the presence of two spectral mechanisms, one absorbing at short wavelengths ($lambda_{max}$ = 440 nm), which causes a hyperpolarization of the cell membrane, and a second absorbing at long wavelengths ($lambda_{max}$ = 495 nm), which causes a depolarization of the cell membrane. Thus, unlike typical vertebrate photoreceptors, the parietal eye photoreceptors have two spectral mechanisms in the same cell which have antagonist effects on the response of the cell. Similar photoreceptors are thought to be present in the frontal organ, an outgrowth of the pineal complex, found in some amphibians (Eldred and Nolte 1978). Currently, we are conducting behavioral experiments to see if the spectral mechanisms that mediate the light-dependent magnetic compass response in the newt are located in the pineal complex (M.E. Deutschlander, J.B. Phillips, and S.C. Borland, research in progress).

Solessio and Engbretson (1993) suggest that the parietal eye photoreceptors of lizards might play a role in the entrainment of circadian rhythms. Their model of the photoreceptor's response to daily changes in the intensity and spectral composition of natural skylight indicates that the parietal eye receptor should exhibit sharp response peaks at dawn and dusk and, thus, would be well-suited to signal the transitions between the photophase and scotophase. If we find that pineal photoreceptors, similar to those reported by Solessio and Engbretson (1993), are involved in the magnetic compass response of newts, these data would suggest that there may be a common element (the same class of photoreceptor) responsible for light-dependent entrainment of circadian rhythms, and for light-dependent detection of the directional properties of the geomagnetic field (supporting the conclusions of Semm et al. 1980, 1982; Semm 1983; Semm and Demaine 1986). If confirmed, this would still leave open the question of whether magnetic field sensitivity is a fortuitous byproduct of a specialized receptor mechanism responsible for delineating the light–dark phases of the photocycle, or alternatively, whether the magnetic field is directly involved in the entrainment of circadian rhythms.[2]

---

[2] A photoreceptor-based magnetoreception system (e.g., one involving a radical pair mechanism) (Schulten 1982; Schulten and Windemuth 1986) is unlikely to be sensitive enough to detect the natural temporal variation in the geomagnetic field (see discussion on pp. 118, 124, and Table 1). We have argued elsewhere, however, that the accuracy necessary to measure the *spatial* variation in the geomagnetic field may require a "hybrid" system that uses an input from the light-dependent magnetic compass to position a non-light-sensitive, presumably magnetite-based, magnetic inclination or intensity detector in a fixed alignment relative to the magnetic field (Phillips and Borland 1994; and see next section). If a similar system is involved in detecting the daily pattern of *temporal* variation in the geomagnetic field, a stimulus that affected *either* the light-dependent magnetic compass or the non-light-sensitive, possibly magnetite-based, detector would be likely to alter the temporal information derived from the magnetic field.

Magnetite-Based Magnetoreception and Magnetic Navigation

Initial evidence that some vertebrates may have two distinct magnetoreception systems was obtained in a study comparing the effects of inverting the vertical component of the magnetic field on the shoreward compass orientation and homing orientation of newts (Phillips 1986b). Newts that were homing (which requires map as well as compass information) were found to be sensitive to the horizontal polarity of the magnetic field ("polar" sensitivity). In contrast, newts exhibiting shoreward compass orientation (which requires only compass information) responded only to the axis of the magnetic field ("axial" sensitivity) and used inclination or dip angle to distinguish between the two ends of the magnetic axis.

As discussed previously, an axial magnetic compass response, like the shoreward magnetic compass orientation of newts, could be mediated by either a photoreceptor-based magnetoreception mechanism or by a magnetite-based magnetoreception mechanism (i.e., one in which the magnetic moments of SD or SPM particles are free to rotate with respect to the surrounding tissue). In contrast, a polar magnetic compass response, like the homing orientation of newts, could be mediated by a magnetite-based mechanism (i.e., one in which the magnetic moments are at least partially constrained with respect to the surrounding tissue). Polar sensitivity, however, is inconsistent with the expected properties of a photoreceptor-based mechanism (Table 1). Surprisingly, more recent studies have demonstrated that homing orientation in newts, like shoreward compass orientation, is altered under long-wavelength light (Phillips and Borland 1994). In contrast to the 90° shift in shoreward compass orientation observed under long-wavelength light (Fig. 2), newts tested in 550- and 600-nm light in the homing experiments were randomly distributed with respect to the magnetic field.

The properties of the magnetic response of homing newts are consistent with a "hybrid" system that receives inputs from both the light-dependent compass and from a non-light-sensitive magnetic intensity/inclination detector (Phillips and Borland 1994). Specifically, the light-dependent magnetic compass may be used to position the intensity/inclination detector in a specific horizontal alignment relative to the magnetic field in order to obtain the precise measurements necessary to derive map information. The involvement of a magnetite-based intensity detector could account for the polar sensitivity of the newts' homing response, while an input from a light-dependent magnetic compass could account for the wavelength-dependent effects of light on the response. Moreover, the interaction of these two inputs could produce additional properties that are not characteristic of either magnetoreception mechanism; e.g., random orientation under long-wavelength light (Phillips and Borland 1994).

Experiments using pulse remagnetization are consistent with the possibility that a magnetite-based magnetoreceptor also may be used by migratory birds to obtain map information from the geomagnetic field. The magnetic orientation of experienced, adult migratory birds (silvereyes, bobolinks, and European robins) is influenced by prior treatment with a single brief magnetic pulse that has an intensity greater than the coercivity of SD particles of magnetite (Wiltschko et al. 1994; Beason et al. 1995; Wiltschko and Wiltschko 1995b). This treatment causes SD particles in which the magnetic moment is aligned antiparallel to the pulse to be remagnetized in the opposite direction (Kalmijn and Blakemore 1978). In the bobolink, the effect of pulse remagnetization on the direction of magnetic orientation was found to differ with the alignment of the pulse relative to the bird's head (Beason et al. 1995), as would be expected if the magnetite particles were not free to rotate with respect to the surrounding tissue. Furthermore, in silvereyes, an effect of pulse remagnetization was only observed in older, experienced birds (Wiltschko et al. 1994), which are thought to rely on magnetic map information to determine the direction of migration (Perdeck 1958). The identical treatment was found to have no effect on the magnetic orientation of young, inexperienced birds captured before their first migration (Munro et al. in press), which do not rely on map information (Perdeck 1958). This difference in the responses of young and old birds to pulse remagnetization is consistent with an effect on a magnetite-based, magnetoreception mechanism that is involved in deriving map information from the geomagnetic field. The age-dependent effects of pulse remagnetization treatment are also important because they suggest that the effect of pulse remagnetization is not likely to be due to an electrical artifact induced by the rapid magnetic pulse; such an artifact would likely be similar in young and old birds due to their similar body size and morphology.

Two additional lines of evidence suggest that pulse remagnetization does not affect a magnetic compass. Young silvereyes that are not affected by pulse remagnetization (Munro et al. in press) nevertheless exhibit the same wavelength-dependent effects of light on magnetic compass orientation[3] as those exhibited by older, experienced silvereyes (Wiltschko et al. 1993). These findings suggest that the young birds are utilizing the same light-dependent magnetic compass as adults. Secondly, Beason and Semm (1996) have obtained evidence that if the trigeminal nerve is blocked with a local anesthetic, the behavioral response of experienced adult bobolinks to pulse remagnetization is eliminated. As in previous experiments (Beason et al. 1995), pulse remagnetization caused a shift in the direction of migratory orientation of birds that did not have the trigeminal nerve blocked. When the ophthalmic branch of the trigeminal nerve was subsequently blocked, however, the birds returned to the seasonally appropriate migratory direction just as in the control condition. These data suggest that the magnetic compass was unaffected by the trigeminal nerve block; blocking the nerve did not cause random orientation in the absence of celestial light cues, as would be expected if the birds were unable to use their magnetic compass. These experiments suggest that pulse remagnetization affects some component of the bird's navigational system other than the compass (e.g., the map). Furthermore, these findings are consistent with the previous suggestion that magnetic responses recorded in the trigeminal nerve are mediated by a magnetite-based receptor that plays a specialized role in the map component of homing (Beason and Semm 1987; Semm and Beason 1990; and see p. 144).

A magnetic-based magnetoreceptor that is involved in the map component of homing may have a limited operating range (i.e., a so-called "sensory window"). For example, the neural mechanisms that process the output of such a receptor may filter out unusually large

---

[3] Munro, U., J.B. Phillips, W. Wiltschko. Importance of light and magnetite in the magnetic orientation of migratory birds. (Manuscript in preparation.)

fluctuations in the magnetic field caused by magnetic storms (Fig. 1). The possibility that detection of geomagnetic spatial variation by animals may be limited to a relatively narrow sensory window seems plausible in light of the fact that in both manmade and biological detector systems, high levels of sensitivity are typically achieved at the expense of operating range.

A sensory window also may exist in the temporal domain. Both the normal daily pattern of temporal variation in the geomagnetic field and the variation resulting from changes in geographic position (map location) involve gradual changes in one or more magnetic parameters (intensity, inclination, etc.). In contrast, magnetic disturbance associated with solar flares and sunspot activity often involve rapid and erratic fluctuations in the magnetic field (Fig. 1). Such disturbances would make spatial or temporal information derived from the magnetic field unreliable. A magnetoreception system that is used to derive spatial (map) and/or temporal information from the geomagnetic field, therefore, is likely to incorporate mechanisms to "low-pass filter" the response, making the system relatively insensitive to rapid changes in the magnetic field. Therefore, if terrestrial organisms have a specialized magnetoreception system to detect the naturally occurring spatial and/or temporal variation in the geomagnetic field, this system is likely to be sensitive to extremely small (10–100 nT) changes in magnetic total intensity (or comparable changes in one or more other magnetic field parameters). The system may filter out, or saturate in response to, large (> 100 nT), rapid fluctuations in the magnetic field which, under natural conditions, are associated with magnetic storms. Thus, large changes in an Earth-strength magnetic field may be no more effective, or may even be less effective, than small changes in eliciting a response that is mediated by this type of magnetoreception system. This should be especially true for terrestrial organisms that move relatively short distances and, therefore, would never experience large spatial variation in the geomagnetic field.

SUMMARY: IMPLICATIONS FOR EMF RESEARCH

Sensitivity to the Earth's magnetic field is widespread in terrestrial organisms. Both behavioral and neurophysiological evidence suggests that there may be two magnetoreception mechanisms present in some vertebrates, one system functioning as a magnetic compass and the other providing geomagnetic-based map information. Evidence from amphibians and birds suggest that the magnetic compass mechanism is light-sensitive, based in the visual system, and may involve a specialized photoreceptor. Currently under way in our lab are studies that will help to determine whether a specialized class of photoreceptors found in the pineal complex of amphibians and reptiles (Eldred and Nolte 1978; Solessio and Engbretson 1993) represents a common element in light-dependent detection of the Earth's magnetic field and light-dependent entrainment of circadian rhythms. If a similar photoreceptor-based magnetoreception mechanism is present in rodents, it would be a possible site of interaction between EMF and the pineal/melatonin system. Since the pineal is not intrinsically light-sensitive in rodents, this mechanism would presumably have to reside in the retina, and could affect the pineal via the retinohypothalamic-pineal pathway. Indeed, pineal responses to abruptly changing, Earth-strength magnetic stimuli in rodents appear to depend on both the presence of light (Reuss and Olcese 1986) and intact photoreceptors in the retina (Olcese et al. 1985, 1988b). Whether these are effects mediated by a magnetoreception system or are effects of the magnetic field manipulation on a "nonspecialized system" (e.g., induced effects on the electric fields of the eye) is unclear at this time. However, the similarity of the effect of abrupt changes in an Earth-strength magnetic field and ELF EMF on rodent pineal physiology (i.e., a decrease in nocturnal melatonin levels) suggests that there is a common biological response to these two types of stimuli. In other words, the evidence that abrupt, Earth-strength magnetic field manipulations alter pineal physiology due to an interaction with retinal photoreceptors (Reuss and Olcese 1986; Olcese et al. 1985, 1988b) implicates a retinal source for ELF EMF pineal responses in mammals. This retinal hypothesis for ELF EMF effects in rodents has predictable properties (dependence on the absence/presence of light, the wavelength of light, and an intact visual system) and is clearly testable, but does not explicitly suggest a biophysical mechanism for ELF EMF interaction (see Table 1).

If a light-dependent magnetoreception system involving a radical-pair mechanism, like that proposed by Schulten (1982), is responsible for the observed effects of Earth-strength magnetic fields on rodent pineal physiology, it is unlikely that such a mechanism would be sensitive to weak (< 10% of the geomagnetic field) ELF EMF stimuli. On the other hand, the sensitivity of this type of mechanism to high-frequency EMF has not been adequately addressed (Table 1). Preliminary observations in our laboratory suggest that light-dependent magnetic compass responses in some animals may be sensitive to low-level, broad-band EMF in the radio frequency (RF) range, and that failure to control for this factor may be a major cause of variability in behavioral and neurophysiological responses to magnetic stimuli. Computers, power supplies, light sources, and other electronic devices can radiate RF through coil systems that are used to produce magnetic and ELF EMF stimuli. In addition, levels of RF may change depending on a variety of factors, including changes in grounding configuration (e.g., whether the coil system is disconnected from ground when a magnetic or ELF EMF stimulus is turned off). Moreover, rapidly changing or "pulsed" magnetic stimuli which have been found to be effective in eliciting changes in pineal function and melatonin levels in rodents (Lerchl et al. 1990, 1991; Olcese and Reuss 1986; Olcese et al. 1985, 1988a, b; Reiter 1992; Welker et al. 1983) tend to have more high-frequency components than more slowly varying stimuli, and the switches used to produce these stimuli may introduce additional high-frequency transients. Careful controls are needed to determine whether the presence of low-level RF "noise" is responsible for some of the observed effects that have been attributed to abruptly changing magnetic stimuli and ELF EMF, and/or whether RF "noise" is responsible for the difficulty of replicating some of these effects. On the positive side, experiments involving controlled RF stimuli may provide a productive avenue to investigate the involvement of a radical pair (or related) mechanism in mediating responses to magnetic and EMF stimuli (Table 1).

The presence of a second, possibly magnetite-based, mechanism of magnetoreception in terrestrial vertebrates provides another potential site of EMF interaction. The available evidence concerning this second mechanism suggests that it is a magnetic intensity (or inclination) detector that is not light sensitive, and, at least in some animals, may play a specialized role in deriving map information from the geomagnetic field. Behavioral and neurophysiological evidence suggest this magnetite-based system may have an extremely high level of sensitivity (Rodda 1984b; Keeton et al. 1974; Larkin and Keeton 1976; Kowalski et al. 1988; Wagner 1983; Semm and Beason 1990), possibly being able to detect changes of a few tens of nT in the geomagnetic field. The high gain that would be necessary to achieve this putative level of sensitivity and the characteristics of naturally occurring stimuli suggest that this system may be adapted to respond to a restricted range of stimulus parameters in both the intensity and frequency domains. As a consequence, the response of this system to artificial magnetic stimuli and, potentially, to EMF would be unlikely to exhibit a linear intensity/response relationship. Thus, only the component of a temporally varying stimuli that falls within narrow intensity and frequency windows may be an effective stimuli for this type of system. Studies carried out to date, which point to the existence of magnetite-based magnetoreception mechanisms, however, have provided relatively little information about (1) the specific parameter(s) of the magnetic field to which this type of magnetoreception system is sensitive (e.g., inclination or total intensity); (2) the range of values of the parameter(s) to which this magnetoreception system is capable of responding; and (3) the physical conditions required for such a system to operate. Therefore, if the animals used in studies on EMF possess a magnetite-based magnetoreception system, the absence of effect(s) of certain types of EMF stimuli on these animal models must be interpreted with care.

Studies of animal homing responses suggest that natural magnetic variation associated with solar flares and sunspot activity (typically < 100 nT) may effect the homing abilities of animals such as the American alligator (Rodda 1984b) and the pigeon (Keeton et al. 1974; Larkin and Keeton 1976; Kowalski et al. 1988). These findings, in conjunction with the high level of magnetic sensitivity reported in the trigeminal system (Semm and Beason 1990), point to the need to reevaluate the the possibility that temporal variation in the geomagnetic field can provide a Zeitgeber for circadian rhythms in some organisms (Bliss and Heppner 1976; Brown and Chow 1976; Brown and Scow 1978; Welker et al. 1983). Investigation of this possibility will require an even greater emphasis on the use of stimulus parameters that fall within the intensity and frequency ranges of naturally occurring geomagnetic stimuli, standardization of pre-exposure conditions, and elimination of other Zeitgebers (e.g., light–dark cycles, feeding schedules, social stimuli, etc.).

Several investigators have argued that evidence for the visual system's involvement in responses to Earth-strength magnetic field manipulations indicates the existence of a visually based (possibly radical pair-mediated) geomagnetic Zeitgeber (e.g., Olcese et al. 1985; Reuss and Olcese 1986). At present, it seems unlikely that a magnetoreceptor based on a radical pair mechanism would be able to detect naturally occurring temporal or spatial variations in the geomagnetic field. In contrast, a magnetite-based magnetoreceptor, at least in theory, could provide the necessary sensitivity (Yorke 1979; Kirschvink and Walker 1985). Phillips and Borland (1994) have suggested one way in which a magnetite-based receptor might be functionally linked to a photoreceptor-based magnetoreception mechanism to facilitate precise, reproducible magnetic measurements that would be needed for a magnetic map or Zeitgeber. Whether or not Earth-strength magnetic effects observed in rodents (e.g., Olcese et al. 1985; Welker et al. 1983) are mediated by such a "hybrid" magnetoreception mechanism may be a profitable avenue for future research.

The issues addressed in this chapter are by no means inconsequential for investigators interested in possible effects of EMF on animal models. An investigator may fail to demonstrate EMF effects, or incorrectly interpret such effects (e.g., EMF effects that exhibit nonlinear dose–response properties), if the appropriate stimulus parameters, physical conditions, and (possibly) behavioral contexts are not taken into account. Clearly, some basis for selecting particular combinations of stimulus parameters, exposure conditions, and behavioral contexts is needed. The results of ongoing behavioral studies of the geomagnetic field's role in the spatial orientation behavior of animals may provide a starting point for such considerations. Furthermore, our current knowledge of the functional properties of magnetoreception in terrestrial vertebrates has reached a point where it should be possible to determine if similar mechanisms mediate EMF effects in animal models. At the very least, such experiments would help to narrow the range of possible mechanisms of EMF interaction with biological systems.

REFERENCES

Arendse, M.C. 1978. Magnetic field detection is distinct from light detection in the invertebrates *Tenebrio* and *Talitrus*. *Nature* 274:358–362.

Batschelet, E. 1981. *Circular Statistics in Biology*. New York: Academic Press.

Beason, R.C. 1989. Use of an inclination compass during migratory orientation by the bobolink (*Dolichonyx oryzivorus*). *Ethology* 81:291–299.

Beason, R.C., J.E. Nichols. 1984. Magnetic orientation and magnetically sensitive material in a transequatorial migratory bird. *Nature* 309:151–153.

Beason, R.C., P. Semm. 1987. Magnetic responses of the trigeminal nerve system of the bobolink (*Dolichonyx oryzivorus*). *Neurosci. Lett.* 80:229–234.

Beason, R.C., P. Semm. 1996. Does the avian ophthalmic nerve carry magnetic navigational information? *J. Exp. Biol.* 199:1241–1244.

Beason, R.C., N. Dussourd, M.E. Deutschlander. 1995. Behavioral evidence for the use of magnetic material in magnetoreception by a migratory bird. *J. Exp. Biol.* 198:141–146.

Bliss, V.L., F.H. Heppner. 1976. Circadian activity rhythm influenced by near zero magnetic field. *Nature* 261:411–412.

Brocklehurst, B., K.A. McLauchlan. 1996. Free radical mechanism for the effects of environmental electromagnetic fields on biological systems. *Int. J. Radiat. Biol.* 69:3–24.

Brown, F.A., C.S. Chow. 1976. Uniform daily rotations and biological rhythms and clocks in hamsters. *Physiol. Zool.* 49:263–285.

Brown, F.A., K.M. Scow. 1978. Magnetic induction in a circadian cycle in hamsters. *J. Interdiscp. Cycle Res.* 9:137–145.

Burda, H., S. Marhold, T. Westenberger, R. Wiltschko, W. Wiltschko. 1990. Magnetic compass orientation in the subterranean rodent *Cryptomys hottentotus*. *Experientia* 46:528–530.

Canfield, J.M., R.L. Belford, P.G. Debrunner, K.J. Schulten. 1994. A perturbation theory treatment of oscillating magnetic fields in the radical pair mechanism. *Chem. Phys.* 182:1–18.

Canfield, J.M., R.L. Belford, P.G. Debrunner, K.J. Schulten. 1995. A perturbation theory treatment of oscillating magnetic fields in the radical pair mechanism using the Liouville equation. *Chem. Phys.* 195:59–69.

Chen, D.-M., J.S. Collins, T.H. Goldsmith. 1984. The ultraviolet receptor in bird retinas. *Science* 285:337–340.

Demaine, C., P. Semm. 1985. The avian pineal as an independent magnetic sensor. *Neurosci. Lett.* 62:119–122.

Deutschlander M.E., J.B. Phillips, S.C. Borland, L.E. Anderson, B.W. Wilson. 1996. Are *in vivo* effects of EMF in mammals mediated by a sensory system specialized for detection of the geomagnetic field?: The case for geomagnetic sensitivity in the rodent, *Phodopus sungorus*. In: Abstracts of the 18th Annual Bioelectromagnetic Society Meeting, British Columbia, June 9–14, p. 262. Frederick, Maryland: Bioelectromagnetics Society

Edmonds, D.T. 1996. A sensitive optically detected magnetic compass for animals. *Proc. Royal Soc. London B.* 263:295–298.

Eldred, W.D., J. Nolte. 1978. Pineal photoreceptors: Evidence for a vertebrate visual pigment with two physiologically active states. *Vision Res.* 18:29–32.

Grissom, C.B. 1995. Magnetic field effects in biology: A survey of possible mechanisms with emphasis on radical-pair recombination. *Chem. Rev.* 95:3–24.

Hastings, J.W. 1983. Biological diversity, chemical mechanisms and the evolutionary origins of bioluminescent systems. *J. Mol. Evol.* 19:309–321.

Horridge, G.A., K. Mimura. 1975. Fly photoreceptors. I. Physical separation of two visual pigments in *Calliphora* retinula cells 1–6. *Proc. Royal Soc. London B* 190:211–224.

Kalmijn, A. 1981. Biophysics of geomagnetic field detection. *IEEE Trans. Biomed. Eng.* 17:1113–1124.

Kalmijn, A. 1982. Electric and magnetic detection in elasmobranch fishes. *Science* 218:916–918.

Kalmijn, A.J., R.P. Blakemore, 1978. The magnetic behavior of mud bacteria. In: *Animal Migration, Navigation and Homing*, K. Schmidt-Koenig and W.T. Keeton, eds., pp 354–355. New York: Springer-Verlag.

Kato, M., K. Honma, T. Shigemitsu, Y. Shiga. 1993. Effects of exposure to a circularly polarized 50-Hz magnetic field on plasma and pineal melatonin levels in rats. *Bioelectromagnetics* 14:97–106.

Kato, M., K. Honma, T. Shigemitsu, Y. Shiga. 1994a. Circularly polarized 50-Hz magnetic field exposure reduces pineal gland and blood melatonin concentrations in Long-Evans rats. *Neurosci. Lett* 166:59–62.

Kato, M., K. Honma, T. Shigemitsu, Y. Shiga. 1994b. Recovery of nocturnal melatonin concentration takes place within one week following cessation of 50-Hz circularly polarized magnetic field exposure for six weeks. *Bioelectromagnetics* 15:489–492.

Keeton, W.T., T.S. Larkin, D.M. Windsor. 1974. Normal fluctuations in the Earth's magnetic field influence pigeon orientation. *J. Comp. Physiol.* 95:95–103.

Khoory, R. 1987. Compensation of the natural magnetic field does not alter N-acetyltransferase activity and melatonin content of the rat pineal gland. *Neurosci. Lett.* 76:215–220.

Kiepenheuer, J. 1982. The effect of magnetic anomalies on the homing behavior of pigeons: an attempt to analyze the possible factors involved. In: *Avian Navigation*, F. Papi, H. Wallraff, eds., pp. 120–128. Berlin: Springer-Verlag.

Kiepenheuer, J. 1986. A further analysis of the orientation behavior of homing pigeons released within magnetic anomalies. In: *Biophysical Effects of Steady Magnetic Fields*, G. Maret, N. Boccara, J. Kiepenheuer, eds., pp. 148–153. Berlin: Springer-Verlag.

Kirschfeld, K., N. Franceschin, B. Minke. 1977. Evidence for a sensitizing pigment in fly photoreceptors. *Nature* 269:386–390.

Kirschvink, J.L. 1996. A possible mechanism for coupling nonthermal levels of radiation to biological systems. *Bioelectromagnetics* 17:242–245.

Kirschvink, J.L., J.L. Gould. 1981. Biogenic magnetite as a basis for magnetic field detection in animals. *Biosystems* 13:181–201.

Kirschvink, J.L., M.M. Walker. 1985. Particle-size considerations for magnetite-based magnetoreceptors. In: *Magnetite Biomineralization and Magnetoreception in Organisms: A New Biomagnetism*, J.L. Kirschvink, D.S. Jones, B.J. MacFadden, eds., pp. 243-254. New York: Plenum Press.

Kirschvink, J.L., D.S. Jones, B.J. MacFadden, eds. 1985. *Magnetite Bio-mineralization and Magnetoreception in Organisms: A New Bio-magnetism.* New York: Plenum Press.

Kirschvink, J.L., J.D. Ricci, M.H. Nesson, S.J. Kirschvink. 1993. *Magnetite-Based Magnetoreceptors in Animals: Structural, Behavioral, and Biophysical Studies.* Technical Report TR-102008, Palo Alto, California: Electric Power Research Institute (EPRI).

Kowalski, U., R. Wiltschko, E. Fuller. 1988. Normal fluctuations of the geomagnetic field may affect initial orientation of pigeons. *J. Comp. Physiol. A* 163: 593-600.

Larkin, T., W.T. Keeton. 1976. Bar magnets mask the effect of normal magnetic disturbances on pigeon orientation. *J. Comp. Physiol.* 110:227–231.

Leask, M.J.M. 1977. A physicochemical mechanism for magnetic field detection by migrating birds and homing pigeons. *Nature* 267:144–145.

Lednor, A.J. 1982. Magnetic navigation in pigeons: Possibilities and problems. In: *Avian Navigation,* F. Papi, H.G. Wallraff, eds., pp. 109-119. Berlin: Springer-Verlag.

Lednor, A.J., C. Walcott. 1988. Orientation of homing pigeons at magnetic anomalies. *Behav. Ecol. Sociobiol.* 22:3–8.

Lerchl, A., K.O. Nonaka, K.-A. Stokkan, R.J. Reiter. 1990. Marked rapid alterations in nocturnal pineal serotonin metabolism in mice and rats exposed to weak intermittent magnetic fields. *Biochem. Biophys. Res. Commun.* 169:102–108.

Lerchl, A., K.O. Nonaka, R.J. Reiter. 1991. Pineal gland "magnetosensitivity" to static fields is a consequence of induced electrical currents (eddy currents). *J. Pineal Res.* 10:109–116.

Light, P., M. Salmon, K.J. Lohmann. 1993. Geomagnetic orientation of loggerhead sea turtles: Evidence for an inclination compass. *J. Exp. Biol.* 182:1–10.

Lohmann, K.J., C.M. Lohmann. 1993. A light-independent magnetic compass in the leatherback sea turtle. *Biol. Bull.(Woods Hole)* 185:149–151.

Lohmann, K.J., C.M. Lohmann. 1994. Detection of magnetic inclination angle by sea turtles: A possible mechanism for determining latitude. *J. Exp. Biol.* 194:23–32.

Lohmann, K.J., C.M. Lohmann. 1996. Detection of magnetic field intensity by sea turtles. *Nature* 380:59–61.

Mai, J.K., P. Semm. 1990. Pattern of brain glucose utilization following magnetic stimulation. *J. Hirnforsch.* 31:331–336.

McCapra, F. 1990. The chemistry of bioluminescence: Origins and mechanism. In: *Light and Life in the Sea*, P.J. Herring, A.K. Cambell, L. Maddock, eds., pp. 265-278. New York: Cambridge University Press.

McLauchlan, K. 1992. Are environmental magnetic fields dangerous? *Phys. World* 5:41–45.

Munro, U., J.A. Munro, J.B. Phillips, W. Wiltschko. Evidence for a magnetite-based navigational "map" in birds. *Naturwissenschaften* (in press).

Okano, T., T. Yoshizawa, Y. Fukada. 1994. Pinopsin is a chicken pineal photoreceptive molecule. *Nature* 372:94–97.

Olcese, J. 1990. The neurobiology of magnetic field detection in rodents. *Prog. Neurobiol.* 35:325–330.

Olcese, J., E. Hurlbut. 1989. Comparative studies on the retinal dopamine response to altered magnetic fields in rodents. *Brain Res.* 498:145–148.

Olcese, J., S. Reuss. 1986. Magnetic field effects on pineal gland melatonin synthesis: Comparative studies of albino and pigmented rodents. *Brain Res.* 369:365–368.

Olcese, J., S. Reuss, L. Vollrath. 1985. Evidence for the involvement of the visual system in mediating magnetic field effects on pineal melatonin synthesis in the rat. *Brain Res.* 333:382–384.

Olcese, J., S. Reuss, P. Semm 1988a. Geomagnetic field detection in rodents. *Life Sci.* 42:605–613.

Olcese, J., S. Reuss, J. Stehle, S. Steinlechner, L. Vollrath. 1988b. Responses of the mammalian retina to experimental alteration of the ambient magnetic field. *Brain Res.* 448:325–330.

Papi, F. E. Meschini, N.E. Baldaccini. 1983. Homing behavior of pigeons released after having been placed in an alternating magnetic field. *Comp. Biochem. Physiol.* 76A:673–682.

Perdeck, A.C. 1958. Two types of orientation on migrating *Sturnus vulgaris* and *Fringilla coelebs* as revealed by displacement experiments. *Ardea* 46:1–37.

Phillips, J.B. 1986a. Magnetic compass orientation in the Eastern red-spotted newt (*Notophthalmus viridescens*). *J. Comp. Physiol.* 158:103–109.

Phillips, J.B. 1986b. Two magnetoreception pathways in a migratory salamander. *Science* 233:765–767.

Phillips, J.B. 1996. Magnetic navigation. *J. Theoret. Biol.* 180:309–319.

Phillips, J.B., S.C. Borland. 1992a. Behavioral evidence for the use of a light-dependent magnetoreception mechanism by a vertebrate. *Nature* 359:142–144.

Phillips, J.B., S.C. Borland 1992b. Magnetic compass orientation is eliminated under near-infrared light in the eastern red-spotted newt *Notophthalmus viridescens*. *Anim. Behav.* 44:796–797.

Phillips, J.B., S.C. Borland. 1992c. Wavelength-specific effects of light on magnetic compass orientation of the eastern red-spotted newt *Notophthalmus viridescens*. *Ethol. Ecol. & Evol.* 4:33–42.

Phillips, J.B., S.C. Borland. 1994. Use of a specialized magnetoreception system for homing. *J. Exp. Biol.* 188:275–291.

Phillips, J.B., O. Sayeed. 1993. Wavelength-dependent effects of light on magnetic compass orientation in *Drosophila melanogaster*. *J. Comp. Physiol.* 172:303–308.

Phillips, J.B., K. Adler, S.C. Borland. 1995. True navigation by an amphibian. *Anim. Behav.* 50:855–858.

Reiter, R.J. 1992. Alterations of the circadian melatonin rhythm by the electromagnetic spectrum: A study in environmental toxicology. *Regul. Toxicol. Pharmacol.* 15:226–244.

Reiter, R.J. 1993. Electric and magnetic fields and melatonin production. *Biomed. & Pharmacother.* 47:439–444.

Reiter, R.J., B.A. Richardson. 1992. Magnetic field effects on pineal indoleamine metabolism and possible biological consequences. *FASEB J.* 6:2283–2287.

Reuss, S., J. Olcese. 1986. Magnetic field effects on rat pineal gland: Role of retinal activation by light. *Neurosci. Lett.* 64:97–101.

Reuss, S., P. Semm, L. Vollrath. 1983. Different types of magnetically sensitive cells in the rat pineal gland. *Neurosci. Lett.* 40:23–26.

Reuss, S., J. Olcese, L. Vollrath, M. Skalej, M. Meves. 1985. Lack of an effect of NMR-strength magnetic fields on rat pineal melatonin synthesis. *IRCS Med. Sci.* 13:471.

Rodda, G.H. 1984a. Homeward paths of displaced juvenile alligators as determined by radiotelemetry. *Behav. Ecol. Sociobiol.* 14:241–246.

Rodda, G.H. 1984b. The orientation and navigation of juvenile alligators: Evidence of magnetic sensitivity. *J. Comp. Physiol.* 154:649–658.

Rodda, G.H. 1985. Navigation in juvenile alligators. *Z. Tierpsychol.* 68:65–77.

Rodda, G.H., J.B. Phillips. 1992. Navigational systems develop along similar lines in amphibians, reptiles and birds. *Ethol. Ecol. & Evol.* 4:43–51.

Rudolph, K., A. Wirz-Justice, K. Krauchi, H. Feer. 1988. Static magnetic fields decrease nocturnal pineal cAMP in the rat. *Brain Res.* 446:159–160.

Scaiano, J.C., F.L. Cozens, J. McLean. 1994. Model for the rationalization of magnetic field effects *in vivo*: Application of the radical-pair mechanism to biological systems. *Photochem. Photobiol.* 59:585–589.

Schneider, T., H. Thalau, P. Semm. 1994a. Effects of light or different Earth-strength magnetic fields on the nocturnal melatonin concentration in a migratory bird. *Neurosci. Lett.* 168:73–75.

Schneider, T., H. Thalau, P. Semm, W. Wiltschko. 1994b. Melatonin is crucial for the migratory orientation of Pied Flycatchers (*Ficedula hypoleuca* pallas). *J. Exp. Biol.* 194:255–262.

Schulten, K. 1982. Magnetic field effects in chemistry and biology. *Adv. Solid State Phys.* 22:61–83.

Schulten, K., A. Windemuth. 1986. Model for a physiological magnetic compass. In: *Biophysical Effects of Steady Magnetic Fields*, G. Maret, ed. pp. 99-106. Berlin: Springer-Verlag.

Semm, P. 1983. Neurobiological investigations on the magnetic sensitivity of the pineal gland in rodents and pigeons. *J. Comp. Biochem. Physiol.* 76:683–689.

Semm, P., C. Beason. 1990. Responses to small magnetic variations by the trigeminal system of the bobolink. *Brain Res. Bull.* 25:735–740.

Semm, P., C. Demaine. 1983. Electrical responses to direct and indirect photic stimulation of the pineal gland of the pigeon. *J. Neural Transm.* 58:281–289.

Semm, P., C. Demaine. 1986. Neurophysiological properties of magnetic cells in the pigeon's visual system. *J. Comp. Physiol.* 159:619–625.

Semm, P., T. Schneider, L. Vollrath. 1980. Effects of an Earth-strength magnetic field on electrical activity of pineal cells. *Nature* 288:607–608.

Semm, P. T. Schneider, L. Vollrath, W. Wiltschko. 1982. Magnetic sensitivity in pineal cells in pigeons. In: *Avian Navigation*, F. Papi, H. Wallraff, eds., pp. 329–337. Berlin: Springer-Verlag.

Semm, P., D. Nohr, C. Demaine, W. Wiltschko. 1984. Neural basis of the magnetic compass: Interactions of visual, magnetic and vestibular inputs in the pigeon's brain. *J. Comp. Physiol.* 155:283–288.

Skiles, D.D. 1985. The geomagnetic field: Its nature, history, and biological relevance. In: *Magnetite Biomineralization and Magnetoreception in Organisms: A New Biomagnetism*, J.L. Kirschvink, D.S. Jones, B.J. MacFadden, eds., pp. 43-102. New York: Plenum Press.

Solessio, E., G. Engbretson. 1993. Antagonistic chromatic mechanisms in photoreceptors of the parietal eye of lizards. *Nature* 364:442–445.

Stehle, J., S. Reuss, H. Schroeder, M. Henschel, L. Vollrath. 1988. Magnetic field effects on pineal N-acetyltransferase activity and melatonin content in the gerbil—Role of pigmentation and sex. *Physiol. Behav.* 44:91–94.

USGS/NGIC. 1990. USGS/NGIC Geomagnetic Observatory Data 1990 (CD-ROM). United States Geological Survey, National Geomagnetic Information Center, Denver, Colorado.

Wagner, G. 1983. Natural geomagnetic anomalies and homing in pigeons. *Comp. Biochem. Physiol.* 76A:691–700.

Walcott, C. 1978. Anomalies in the earth's magnetic field increase the scatter of pigeon's vanishing bearings. In: *Animal Migration, Navigation and Homing*, K. Schmidt-Koenig, W.T. Keeton, eds., pp. 143–151. Berlin: Springer-Verlag.

Walcott, C. 1991. Magnetic maps in pigeons. In: *Orientation in Birds*, P. Berthold, ed., pp. 38–51. Basel: Birkhauser.

Walleczek, J. 1994. Immune cell interactions with extremely low frequency magnetic fields: Experimental verification and free radical mechanisms. In: *On the Nature of Electromagnetic Field Interactions with Biological Systems*, A.H. Frey, ed., pp. 167–180. Austin, Texas: R.G. Landes Co.

Wallraff, H.G. 1991. Conceptual approaches to avian navigation systems. In: *Orientation in Birds*, P. Berthold, ed., pp. 128–165. Basel: Birkhauser.

Welker, H.A., P. Semm, R.P. Willig, J.C. Commentz, W. Wiltschko, L. Vollrath. 1983. Effects of an artificial magnetic field on serotonin N-acetyltransferase activity and melatonin content in the rat pineal gland. *Exp. Brain Res.* 50:426–432.

Wilson, B.W. 1994. Neuroendocrine responses to electric and magnetic fields. In: *Biological Effects of Electric and Magnetic Fields*, D.O. Carpenter, S. Ayrapetyan, eds., pp. 287–313. New York: Academic Press.

Wilson, B.W., R.G. Stevens, L.E. Anderson 1989. Neuroendocrine mediated effects of electromagnetic-field exposure: Possible role of the pineal gland. *Life Sci.* 45:1319–1332.

Wilson, B.W., R.G. Stevens, L.E. Anderson, eds. 1990. *Extremely Low Frequency Electromagnetic Fields: The Question of Cancer*. Columbus, Ohio: Battelle Press.

Wiltschko, W. 1972. The influence of magnetic total intensity and inclination on the directions chosen by migrating European Robins. In: *Animal Orientation and Navigation*, S.R. Galler, K. Schmidt-Koenig, G.J. Jacobs, R.E. Belleville, eds., pp. 569–578. Washington, D.C.: NASA SP-262, U.S. Government Printing Office.

Wiltschko, W., R. Wiltschko. 1972. Magnetic compass of European robins. *Science* 176:62–64.

Wiltschko, W., R. Wiltschko. 1988. Magnetic orientation in birds. *Curr. Ornithol.* 5:67–121.

Wiltschko, R., W. Wiltschko, eds. 1995a. *Magnetic orientation in animals (Zoophysiology v. 33)*. Berlin: Springer-Verlag.

Wiltschko, W., R. Wiltschko. 1995b. Migratory orientation of European robins is affected by the wavelength of light as well as by a magnetic pulse. *J. Comp. Physiol. A* 177:363–369.

Wiltschko, W., U. Munro, H. Ford, R. Wiltschko. 1993. Red light disrupts magnetic orientation of migratory birds. *Nature* 364:525–527.

Wiltschko, W., U. Munro, R.C. Beason, H. Ford, R. Wiltschko. 1994. A magnetic pulse leads to a temporary deflection in the orientation of migratory birds. *Experientia* 50:697–700.

Yellon, S.M. 1994. Acute 60-Hz magnetic field exposure effects on the melatonin rhythm in the pineal gland and circulation of the adult Djungarian hamster. *J. Pineal Res.* 16:136–144.

Yorke, E.D. 1979. A possible magnetic transducer in birds. *J. Theoret. Biol.* 77:101–105.

Yorke, E.D. 1981. Sensitivity of pigeons to small magnetic field variations. *J. Theor. Biol.* 89:533–537.

7 Action of Melatonin on Magnetic Field Inhibition of Nerve-Growth-Factor-Induced Neurite Outgrowth in PC-12 Cells

CARL F. BLACKMAN
SHAWNEE G. BENANE
DENNIS E. HOUSE
National Health and Environmental Effects Research Laboratory, U.S. Environmental Protection Agency, Research Triangle Park, North Carolina

CONTENTS

INTRODUCTION
MATERIALS AND METHODS
   Exposure System
   Growth, Preparation, and Exposure of Cells
   Assay Procedures and Data Presentation
   Statistical Analyses
RESULTS
DISCUSSION AND CONCLUSIONS
ACKNOWLEDGMENTS
REFERENCES

INTRODUCTION

Exposure of PC-12 cell clones to 50-Hz magnetic fields for a 22-hour period has been shown to alter the relative number of cells or cell clusters exhibiting neurite outgrowth (Blackman et al. 1993a, b). For the parental cell line, PC-12, which was primed with nerve growth factor (NGF) before testing, inhibition of neurite outgrowth occurred in a field-strength-dependent manner between 6 and 10 μT root mean square (RMS; 60 and 100 mG RMS). These results occurred from a direct interaction of 50-Hz magnetic fields with the cells, and were not dependent on the induced electric field, according to standard criteria (Misakian and Kaune 1990). Further, this assay system has been used extensively to demonstrate consistency between the biological response and the predictions of the ion parametric resonance (IPR) model (Blanchard and Blackman 1994), under parallel AC/DC magnetic field exposure (Blackman et al. 1994, 1995b, c).

Subsequent tests, reported in this chapter, show that melatonin modulates magnetic field effects on neurite outgrowth in PC-12. Melatonin is an important hormone whose nocturnal pulsatile influence may affect virtually every cell in the body. In addition to its influence on ultradian rhythms, melatonin has oncostatic properties (Tamarkin et al. 1981; Narita and Kudo 1985; Hill and Blask 1988; Leone et al. 1988; Kereni et al. 1990; Dogliotti et al. 1990; Blask 1993; Blask et al. 1991; Cos et al. 1991; Gonzalez et al. 1991; Lissoni et al. 1991), and recently has been shown to be a potent free radical scavenger (Reiter et al. 1994; Tan et al. 1993a, b, 1994). We previously investigated the potential influence of melatonin on membrane-based cell responses and reported its influence on modulation of intercellular communication through gap junctions (Ubeda et al. 1995b), and on neurite outgrowth from PC-12D cells stimulated with magnetic fields (Ubeda et al. 1996). The relationship of these findings to the present will be discussed briefly later in this chapter.

MATERIALS AND METHODS

Exposure System

The exposure system included two coils constructed in the Helmholtz configuration [two 1000-turn, 20-cm-diameter coils of enameled wire, aligned coaxially 10 cm apart and oriented to produce a vertical magnetic field (Blackman et al. 1993a)]. Since both coils were energized, sinusoidal magnetic fields of uniform flux density were generated coaxially on the center line between the coils in a region where the samples were placed. Because of the many turns of wire in the coil, only 2.95 mA produced the flux density examined in this study. The Helmholtz-coil exposure system and a Co-Netic™ metal magnetic field shield (Magnetic Shield Corp., Bensenville, Illinois) were housed in a 5% CO_2 incubator (Forma, Marietta, Ohio, model 3156) maintained at 37°C. We placed the coil system in the upper two-thirds of the incubator space on a specially constructed plastic shelf, with the control samples housed in a tube-configured Co-Netic™ shield positioned near the bottom of the incubator space, with the long axis fore and aft to allow air circulation and to facilitate positioning the dishes (for more details, see Blackman et al. 1993a). The ambient static and 60-Hz magnetic fields within the exposure chamber were measured using a Bartington MAG-03 fluxgate magnetometer (GMW, Redwood City, California) (Table 1). The 50-Hz AC magnetic field was produced by a function generator and an ammeter, connected in series with the coils. The shielded control cells were not exposed to the 50-Hz magnetic field because it was oriented perpendicularly to the axis of the shield.

TABLE 1
Ambient Magnetic Field Conditions[a]

Frequency	Location	Axis[b] x	y	z	Mean	Angle
60 Hz	Coil[c]	0.21	0.32	0.32	0.50	39°
	Shield	0.010	0.015	0.017	0.025	43°
DC	Coil[c]	6	18	37	42	58°
	Shield	4	1	3	5	37°

[a] Flux density in μT. These values are representative for the exposure volume.
[b] In horizontal plane, x denotes axis front-to-back; y, left-to-right. The vertical axis is denoted by z.
[c] In the coil exposure volume.

A frequency meter verified the setting on the function generator. All generating and monitoring equipment was located remotely from the incubator. Upon energization, the current was manually ramped up to the desired value over 1 to 2 seconds to minimize induction of transient electric fields in the dishes.

The flux density of the 50-Hz magnetic field used in these experiments was measured with a calibrated Gaussmeter (model 640, F.W. Bell, Orlando, Florida) and Hall effect probe within the CO_2 incubator at locations inside the coils occupied by the dishes. By performing this measurement within the exposure system, the reported value reflects the influence of the inner walls of the incubator, whose proximity to the coils reduced the actual flux density by ~20% from calculated values for free space. This reduction in flux density was found to be uniform over the region occupied by the cells in each dish.

Growth, Preparation, and Exposure of Cells

PC-12 cells were obtained from the Tissue Culture Facility at the University of North Carolina at Chapel Hill. The cells were grown on six-well, collagen-coated plates, in a 5% CO_2 incubator at 37°C, using RPMI 1640 medium (Gibco, Gaithersburg, Maryland, #320-1875)—supplemented with 10% horse serum and 5% fetal calf serum—and 100 units/ml each of penicillin and streptomycin. NGF (50 ng/ml, Sigma #6009, Sigma Chemical, St. Louis, Missouri) was added to the plates every other day for 6 days. On day 7, the cells were washed to remove remaining NGF, then the cells were removed from the plates and stored at –80°C in 1-ml volumes of 8×10^5 cells/ml. For experimental treatments, the primed cells were thawed and diluted so that 5-ml volumes, at 2×10^4 cells/ml, could be plated on collagen-coated, 35-mm dishes. For details of these procedures, see Blackman et al. (1993b, 1994).

In the first experiment, 11 dishes were plated with cells, 5 ng/ml of NGF was added to 10 of them, and melatonin (Sigma Chemical, #M-5250) was added to 8 of those 10 dishes in decade concentration steps from 10^{-12} to 10^{-5} M. Two dishes without melatonin, one with and one without NGF, served as controls. The other dish with NGF but without melatonin served as a comparison to those with melatonin added. After

22 hours of incubation without imposed magnetic fields, the cells in each dish were assayed. This experiment was conducted three times.

In the second experiment, eight dishes were plated with cells, 5 ng/ml of NGF was added to seven of those dishes, and five of the seven dishes received different concentrations of melatonin. In one part of the experiment, the melatonin concentrations were 10^{-12}, 10^{-11}, 10^{-10}, 10^{-9}, and 10^{-8} M; in the other, 10^{-9}, 10^{-8}, 10^{-7}, 10^{-6}, and 10^{-5} M. Six of the dishes containing NGF, five containing melatonin and one without, were placed in the magnetic field exposure system. In addition, one dish with NGF and one without were placed in the same incubator but inside a tube composed of Co-Netic™ metal. This shield reduced the flux density of the 50-Hz magnetic field generated by the exposure system to less than 1%, thereby creating the sham exposure for two sets of controls: one with and one without NGF. These controls were not exposed to either magnetic fields or melatonin.

Each magnetic field exposure was for 22 hours to a 50-Hz, vertically oriented, uniform magnetic field at a flux density of 23 μT RMS (230 mG RMS) in an ambient DC magnetic field flux density of 37 μT vertical and 19 μT horizontal. Each concentration series of melatonin was run three independent times.

Assay Procedures and Data Presentation

We used standard procedures for assaying the relative changes in neurite outgrowth of the PC-12 cells in our tests (Greene and Tischler 1976; Greene 1977; Rukenstein and Greene 1983; Blackman et al. 1993b, 1995b, c). The cells were examined by light microscopy in a blinded fashion in pseudo randomized areas located in the center of each dish ($\leq$ 0.3-cm radius). The neurite outgrowth assays were performed by scoring the percentage of individual cells and cell clumps (also called "cells" here) either with a neurite length greater than the cell body, or with neurites containing either a branch or a growth cone (these last two categories accounted for approximately 5% of the total cells scored positive). All cells were counted within each microscope field, and at least 100 cells were assayed in each dish. The number of cells with neurites divided by the total number of cells examined gave the percent cells with neurites.

Controls shielded from magnetic field exposure were included in all assays and used to normalize each result. The response of the treated cells was normalized to the range of response observed for cells without magnetic field exposure, with the minimum of the range established by cells with no NGF (designated the background level of neurite outgrowth) and the maximum of the range established by cells with 5 ng/ml of NGF (Blackman et al. 1995b, c). This calculation gave a normalized neurite outgrowth (NNO) response that could be compared between various treatments. Since the absolute maximal neurite outgrowth production possible for PC-12 cells is larger than that produced by 5 ng/ml of NGF, it is theoretically possible that an NNO cell response could be greater than 100% (see Rukenstein and Greene 1983).

Statistical Analyses

Statistical analyses were performed on the degree of effects of melatonin on NNO in magnetic field-exposed PC-12 cells. First, an analysis of variance with replication and melatonin concentrations as variables was performed separately for each of the two melatonin ranges to determine if melatonin had a significant influence. Second, a Dunnett's test was performed comparing all melatonin values in each range to their control which was under identical magnetic field conditions to examine the cell response at each melatonin concentration.

RESULTS

In the absence of magnetic fields, the neurite outgrowth response of PC-12 cells with 5 ng/ml NGF was observed to be unaffected by a range of melatonin concentrations from 10^{-12}–10^{-5} M (Fig. 1). However, in both series of experiments with different concentrations of melatonin (10^{-12}–10^{-8} and 10^{-9}–10^{-5} M), melatonin modulated the inhibition of neurite outgrowth caused by the magnetic field (Fig. 2). In the melatonin range between 10^{-12} and 10^{-8} M, concentrations of 10^{-10}, 10^{-9}, and 10^{-8} M caused a statistically significant amelioration in the inhibition of neurite outgrowth produced by the magnetic field. In the melatonin range between 10^{-9} and 10^{-5} M, concentrations of 10^{-9}, 10^{-8}, and 10^{-7} M melatonin ameliorated the field action, whereas 10^{-6} and 10^{-5} M

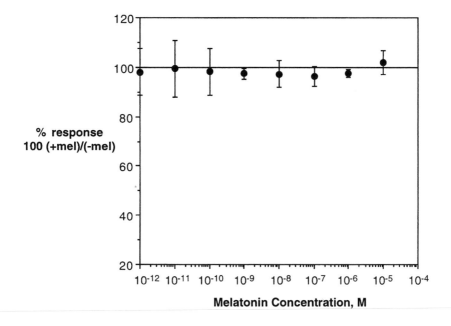

FIG. 1. Neurite outgrowth stimulated by 5 ng/mL NGF in PC-12 cells: Comparison of cell responses with melatonin (+mel) and without melatonin (−mel). Symbols represent the mean ± 2 SE of three runs.

melatonin enhanced the field inhibition of neurite outgrowth. The cell responses at 10^{-9} and 10^{-8} M melatonin were comparable between series, as shown in Figure 2.

DISCUSSION AND CONCLUSIONS

This study examined whether melatonin could affect membrane-related signaling processes in nervous system-derived cells in the presence or absence of magnetic fields. NGF-stimulated neurite outgrowth in PC-12 cells was selected because it represents a fundamental signaling process in nervous system development, and because we have previously shown that magnetic fields can directly influence that process (Blackman et al. 1993b). If melatonin can be shown to exert a

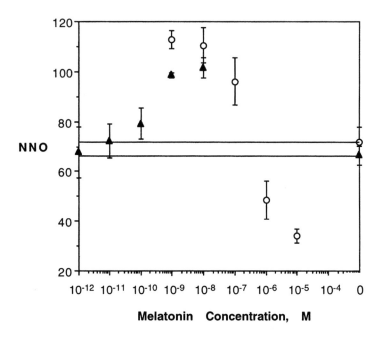

FIG. 2. Influence of 23-μT, 50-Hz magnetic fields on neurite outgrowth stimulated by 5 ng/mL NGF in PC-12 cells: Comparison of normalized neurite outgrowth with and without melatonin present. Symbols represent the mean ± 2 SE of three runs. Two ranges of melatonin were tested: closed triangles are from cells treated with melatonin concentrations between 10^{-12} and 10^{-8} M; open circles, between 10^{-9} and 10^{-5} M. Data at zero melatonin level show reduction in cell response compared to no magnetic field exposure, which is 100 (see text for details).

modulating influence on neurite outgrowth when the cells are stimulated either with NGF or with NGF and magnetic fields, this may indicate another action of melatonin in addition to its oncostatic properties (Tamarkin et al. 1981; Narita and Kudo 1985; Hill and Blask 1988; Leone et al. 1988; Kereni et al. 1990; Dogliotti et al. 1990; Blask 1993; Blask et al. 1991; Cos et al. 1991; Gonzalez et al. 1991; Lissoni et al. 1991) and free radical-scavenging potential (Reiter et al. 1994; Tan et al. 1993a, b, 1994), and thus provide another means for probing aspects of melatonin's mechanism(s) of action.

The results of this study demonstrate that melatonin alone, without an imposed magnetic field, does not influence the NGF stimulation of neurite outgrowth in PC-12 cells when melatonin is present in decade concentration steps from 10^{-12} to 10^{-5} M. This range covers the physiological ($\sim 10^{-10}$–10^{-9} M) and pharmacological ($\sim 10^{-6}$–10^{-5} M) concentration regions. In contrast, when a 50-Hz magnetic field of 23 μT was present, the cell neurite outgrowth response was altered by this concentration range of melatonin in a biphasic manner. The physiological concentration region of melatonin ameliorated the magnetic field-induced inhibition of neurite outgrowth, whereas the pharmacological concentration region enhanced the field-induced inhibition. Thus, melatonin is demonstrated to modulate the action of a signaling agent, NGF, in PC-12 cells when melatonin and NGF are applied in the presence of a 50-Hz magnetic field. While the underlying basis for this phenomenon is not apparent, it represents an intriguing relationship between two seemingly unrelated effects.

We have also studied neurite outgrowth in the PC-12D subline of PC-12 cells. The PC-12D line, in contrast to the parental line, does not need to be primed with NGF before becoming responsive to NGF in this 22-hour assay. PC-12D cells respond to a 50-Hz magnetic field by producing neurites in the *absence* of NGF stimulation (Blackman et al. 1993a). Recently, Ubeda et al. (1996) demonstrated that melatonin at 10^{-10} M prevented the magnetic field induction of neurite outgrowth in this subline. Although magnetic fields induced a different response in PC-12 and in PC-12D cell lines, the action of physiological levels of melatonin in both cell lines is to counter the action of the magnetic field. This consistency of action reinforces the premise that melatonin influences the interaction of nervous system-derived cells with magnetic fields, and helps refine the search for the specific mechanism(s) of action.

Melatonin also has been shown to alter another membrane-based signaling mechanism—the movement of ions and small molecules between cells via gap junction communication. Inhibition of gap junction communication has been implicated in the processes that lead to reduced growth control in cells, and thus to tumor development. Ubeda et al. (1995b) showed that a physiological level of melatonin (10^{-10} M) enhanced gap junction communication between normal

C3H10T½ cells in culture, whereas this melatonin-enhanced communication was eliminated by 30-minute exposure to 1.6-mT, 50-Hz magnetic fields (Ubeda et al. 1995a). Some chemicals associated with chlorination disinfection of drinking water, and known to cause tumors in rodents, have been shown to inhibit gap junction communication (Benane et al. 1996), and physiological levels of melatonin have been demonstrated to partially reverse that inhibition for a subgroup of those chemicals (Blackman et al. 1995a).

The results of the present study demonstrated that melatonin affects membrane-related signaling processes in nervous system-derived cells in the presence of 50-Hz magnetic fields. Furthermore, physiological and pharmacological concentrations of melatonin had opposing influences. The development of models to explain the complicated interactions of melatonin in biological systems, alone and in concert with magnetic fields, may provide useful tools from which to utilize melatonin in a therapeutic context.

ACKNOWLEDGMENTS

We wish to thank J.P. Blanchard, J.A. Elder, and A.M. Richard for helpful suggestions during the preparation of this manuscript. The research described in this article has been reviewed by the National Health and Environmental Effects Research Laboratory, U.S. Environmental Protection Agency, and is approved for publication. Approval does not signify that the contents necessarily reflect the views and policies of the Agency, nor does mention of trade names or commercial products constitute endorsement or recommendation for use.

The work described here was supported in part by interagency agreements with the U.S. Department of Energy, Office of Energy Management, IAG# DE-AI01-89CE34024 and DE-AI01-94CE34007.

REFERENCES

Benane, S.G., C.F. Blackman, D.E. House. 1996. Effect of perchloroethylene and its metabolites on intercellular communication in clone 9 rat liver cells. *J. Toxicol. Environ. Health* 48:427–438.

Blackman, C.F., S.G. Benane, D.E. House, M.M. Pollock. 1993a. Action of 50-Hz magnetic fields on neurite outgrowth in pheochromocytoma cells. *Bioelectromagnetics* 14:273–286.

Blackman, C.F., S.G. Benane, D.E. House. 1993b. Evidence for direct effect of magnetic fields on neurite outgrowth. *FASEB J.* 7:801–806.

Blackman, C.F., J.P. Blanchard, S.G. Benane, D.E. House. 1994. Empirical test of an ion parametric resonance model for magnetic field interactions with PC-12 cells. *Bioelectromagnetics* 15:239–260.

Blackman, C.F., S.G. Benane, D.E. House. 1995a. Action of perchloroethylene and metabolites on intercellular communication is modulated by melatonin. In: Abstracts of the Annual Meeting of the American Society for Cell Biology, December 9–13, 1995, Washington, DC, #1104, p. 190a.

Blackman, C.F., J.P. Blanchard, S.G. Benane, D.E. House. 1995b. An alternate assay for measuring IPR model validity. In: Abstracts of the Annual Review of Research on Biological Effects of Electric and Magnetic Fields from the Generation, Delivery, and Use of Electricity, November 12–16, Palm Springs, California, #A-5, p. 4.

Blackman, C.F., J.P. Blanchard, S.G. Benane, D.E. House. 1995c. The ion parametric resonance model predicts magnetic field parameters that affect nerve cells. *FASEB J.* 9:547–551.

Blanchard, J.P., C.F. Blackman. 1994. Clarification and application of an ion parametric resonance model for magnetic field interactions with biological systems. *Bioelectromagnetics* 15:217–238.

Blask, D.E. 1993. Melatonin in oncology. In: *Melatonin. Biosynthesis, Physiological Effects, and Clinical Applications*, H.-S. Yu and R.J. Reiter, eds., pp. 448–475. Boca Raton, Florida: CRC Press.

Blask, D.E., D.B. Pelletier, S.M. Hill, A. Lemus-Wilson, D.S. Grosso, S.T. Wilson, M.E. Wise. 1991. Pineal melatonin inhibition of tumor promotion in the N-nitroso-N-methylurea of mammary carcinogenesis: Potential involvement of antiestrogenic mechanisms in vivo. *J. Cancer Res. Clin. Oncol.* 117:526–532.

Cos, S., D.E. Blask, A. Lemus-Wilson, A.B. Hill. 1991. Effects of melatonin on the cell cycle kinetics and estrogen-rescue of MCF-7 human breast cancer in culture. *J. Pineal Res.* 10:36–42.

Dogliotti, L., A. Berruti, T. Buniva, M. Torta, A. Bottini, M. Tampellini, M. Terzolo, R. Faggiuolo, A. Angeli. 1990. Melatonin and human cancer. *J. Steroid Biochem. Mol. Biol.* 37:983–987.

Gonzalez, R., A. Sanchez, J.A. Ferguson, C. Balmer, C. Daniel, A. Cohen, W.A. Robinson. 1991. Melatonin therapy of advanced human malignant melanoma. *Melanoma Res.* 1:237–243.

Greene, L.A. 1977. A quantitative bioassay for nerve growth factor (NGF) activity employing a clonal pheochromocytoma cell line. *Brain Res.* 133:350–353.

Greene, L.A., A.S. Tischler. 1976. Establishment of a noradrenergic clonal line of rat adrenal pheochromocytoma cells which respond to nerve growth factor. *Proc. Natl. Acad. Sci.* (USA) 73:2424–2428.

Hill, S.M., D.E. Blask. 1988. Effects of the pineal hormone on the proliferation and morphological characteristics of human breast cancer cells (MCF-7) in culture. *Cancer Res.* 48:6121–6126.

Kereni, N.A., E. Padula, G.M. Feuer. 1990. Oncostatic effects of the pineal gland. *Drug Metabol. Drug Interact.* 8:313–319.

Leone, A.M., R.E. Silman, B.T. Hill, R.D.H. Wheland, S.A. Shellard. 1988. Growth inhibitory effects of melatonin and its metabolites against ovarian tumor cell lines in vitro. In: *The Pineal Gland and Cancer*, D. Gupta, A. Attanasio, and R.J. Reiter, eds., pp. 273–281. London: Brain Research Promotion.

Lissoni, P., S. Barni, G. Cattaneo, G. Tancini, G. Esposti, D. Esposti, F. Fraschini. 1991. Clinical results with the pineal hormone melatonin in advanced cancer resistant to standard antitumor therapies. *Oncology* 48:448–450.

Misakian, M., W.T. Kaune. 1990. Optimal experimental design for in vitro studies with ELF magnetic fields. *Bioelectromagnetics* 11:251–255.

Narita, T., H. Kudo. 1985. Effect of melatonin on B16 melanoma growth in athymic mice. *Cancer Res.* 45:4175–4177.

Reiter, R.J., D.-X. Tan, B. Poeggeler, A. Menendez-Pelaez, L.-D. Chen, S. Saarela. 1994. Melatonin as a free radical scavenger: Implications for aging and age-related processes. *Ann. N.Y. Acad. Sci.* 719:1–12.

Rukenstein, A., L.A. Greene. 1983. The quantitative bioassay of nerve growth factor: Use of frozen "primed" PC12 pheochromocytoma cells. *Brain Res.* 263:177–180.

Tamarkin, L., M. Cohen, D. Roselle, C. Reichter, M. Lippman, B. Chabner. 1981. Melatonin inhibition and pinealectomy enhancement of 7-12-dimethylbenz(a)-anthracene-induced mammary tumors in rat. *Cancer Res.* 41:4432–4436.

Tan, D.-X., L.-D. Chen, B. Poeggeler, L.C. Manchester, R.J. Reiter. 1993a. Melatonin: A potent, endogenous hydroxyl radical scavenger. *Endocr. J.* 1:57–60.

Tan, D.-X., B. Poeggeler, R.J. Reiter, L.-D. Chen, S. Chen, L.C. Manchester, L.R. Barlow-Walden. 1993b. The pineal hormone melatonin inhibits DNA-adduct formation induced by the chemical carcinogen safrole in vivo. *Cancer Lett.* 70:65–71.

Tan, D.-X., R.J. Reiter, L.-D. Chen, B. Poeggeler, L.C. Manchester, L.R. Barlow-Walden. 1994. Both physiological and pharmacological levels of melatonin reduce DNA adduct formation induced by the carcinogen safrole. *Carcinogenesis* 15:215–218.

Ubeda A., M.A. Trillo, D.E. House, C.F. Blackman. 1995a. A 50-Hz magnetic field blocks melatonin-induced enhancement of junctional transfer in normal C3H10T½ cells. *Carcinogenesis* 16(12):2945–2949.

Ubeda, A., M.A. Trillo, D.E. House, C.F. Blackman. 1995b. Melatonin enhances junctional transfer in normal C3H10T½ cells. *Cancer Lett.* 91:241–245.

Ubeda, A., M.A. Trillo, D.E. House, C.F. Blackman. 1996. Melatonin prevents magnetic field-induced neurite outgrowth in a subline of pheochromocytoma cells, PC-12D. *Bioelectrochem. Bioenerg.* 39:77–81.

PART III
Circumstantial Case

SECTION 1
Melatonin Effects on Breast Cancer

8 Systemic, Cellular, and Molecular Aspects of Melatonin Action on Experimental Breast Carcinogenesis

David E. Blask

Laboratory of Experimental Neuroendocrinology/
Oncology, Bassett Research Institute,
Cooperstown, New York

Contents

Introduction
Melatonin and Experimental Cancer In Vivo
Effects of Surgical and "Physiological" Pinealectomy on
Carcinogen-Induced Mammary Carcinogenesis in Rats
Influence of Treatment Protocol and Environmental Factors
Initiation Versus Promotion and the Influence of
Pinealectomy and/or Constant Light
Potential Mechanisms of Melatonin Action on the
Initiation of Carcinogen-Induced Mammary Tumors In Vivo
Melatonin and Experimental Cancer In Vitro:
Human Breast Cancer Cell Growth Studies
Cellular and Molecular Mechanisms of Melatonin
Action on Human Breast Cancer Cells
Cellular Aspects Involving Esradiol, Prolactin,
and Other Growth Factors

(continued)

CONTENTS (continued)

Melatonin Binding Sites in Murine and
    Human Breast Cancer
Melatonin Modulation of Nonmelatonin, Hormone-
    Receptor Expression in Human Breast Cancer Cells
Melatonin Control of Transcriptional Events
Melatonin Interaction with Redox Mechanisms:
    Reduced Glutathione and Nitric Oxide
Melatonin's Effects on Calcium Homeostasis
CONCLUSIONS
REFERENCES

INTRODUCTION

The incidence of and mortality from breast cancer, the second leading cause of cancer deaths in women in industrialized countries, are increasing worldwide (Davis et al. 1990). As the most common and serious malignancy of the reproductive tract in American women, breast cancer represents 31% of all cancers in women; one in eight women can expect to develop the disease over her lifetime (Parker et al. 1996). At the time of clinical diagnosis of metastatic disease, about 60% of breast cancers are found to be estrogen receptor positive (ER^+). Major progress has been made in the endocrine treatment of ER^+ breast cancer, particularly with nonsteroidal anti-estrogen tamoxifen. Nevertheless, one-third to one-half of women who develop breast cancer will die of metastatic disease (Jordan and Murphy 1991; Jordan 1994). In spite of great strides in our understanding of breast cancer biology, virtually nothing is known about the etiology and/or evolution of this disease (Donegan and Spratt 1988).

Breast cancer cells not only respond directly to a variety of mitogenic hormones including estrogen, progesterone, and prolactin, but their growth is also modulated by paracrine, autocrine, and intracrine growth factors such as insulin-like growth factor (IGF-1) and transforming growth factor (TGF) α and β (Friess et al. 1993). Ultimately, breast cancer cellular homeostasis may depend on a dynamic balance between these stimulatory and inhibitory growth factors as well as hormones of neuroendocrine origin. Some of the neurohormones potentially important in the regulation of breast cancer growth include peptide hormones such as gonadotropin-releasing hormone and somatostatin (Schally et al. 1984).

The emergence of melatonin as yet another important neuroendocrine regulator of neoplastic growth has provoked a new phase of pineal gland research into the basic mechanisms of melatonin action at the systemic, cellular, and molecular levels. A number of experimental neoplasms have been studied with respect to the ability of melatonin and its analogues to influence cancer growth both in vivo and in vitro. These neoplasms encompass tumors of the breast, prostate, uterus, cervix, ovary, pituitary, skin, neural tissue, lung, liver, colon, and connective tissue (Blask 1984, 1990, 1993; Blask and Hill 1988). In vivo investigations almost exclusively have employed animal models of human tumor growth, while in vitro studies have been directed primarily toward human cancer cells; transformed and nontransformed murine cell lines have been used to a lesser extent. The nature of the neoplastic growth response to melatonin in vivo and in vitro depends to a large extent on a variety of experimental factors, including dose, timing and duration of treatment, route of administration, photoperiod, and culture conditions. Although much less is known about melatonin's effects on the initiation of malignant transformation, under most circumstances to date, melatonin has been found to inhibit tumor growth in vivo and in vitro, prompting its designation as an oncostatic compound (Blask 1984, 1993; Blask and Hill 1988). However, there are instances when melatonin either stimulates or has no effect on tumorigenesis depending on the time of day it is administered, suggesting that it may ultimately function as a "chrono-oncomodulatory" neurohormone (Blask 1993).

Because this volume focuses on the potential role of magnetic fields as an etiological agent in the genesis of both experimental and clinical breast cancer, the following discussion will focus on experimental findings related to melatonin's regulatory influence on breast cancer. This chapter will provide the reader with background information that will complement subsequent chapters on magnetic field enhancement of breast carcinogenesis via mechanisms ostensibly involving inhibition of melatonin secretion from the pineal gland (Beniashvili et al. 1991; Löscher et al. 1993, 1994), as well as via the antagonism of its oncostatic action at the level of the breast cancer cell (Liburdy et al. 1993; Liburdy 1994; Blask et al. 1993). Additionally, this chapter will present new research findings relating to melatonin's mechanism(s) of action on breast cancer growth at the cellular and molecular levels, thus forming a conceptual framework with which the reader may consider potential mechanisms of magnetic field interference with melatonin's oncostatic action.

MELATONIN AND EXPERIMENTAL BREAST CANCER IN VIVO

Effects of Surgical and "Physiological" Pinealectomy on Carcinogen-Induced Mammary Carcinogenesis in Rats

Of initial interest to investigators seeking a possible relationship of melatonin to breast cancer was whether the endogenous, nocturnal melatonin signal itself serves as an important physiological regulatory signal in the control of breast carcinogenesis. This question was initially addressed by investigators (Aubert et al. 1980; Tamarkin et al. 1981) who surgically pinealectomized female rats several weeks before administration of the chemical carcinogen 7,12-dimethylbenz(a)anthracene [DMBA; an initiator of primarily prolactin-sensitive mammary adenocarcinomas (Welsch 1985)], and then compared tumor incidence, as well as latency to tumor onset, with that in pineal-intact cohorts. Although an initial study reported a lack of effect of pinealectomy on DMBA-induced mammary tumorigenesis (Aubert et al. 1980), subsequent studies clearly demonstrated that pinealectomy enhanced or promoted development of mammary tumors in DMBA-treated rats maintained on diurnal lighting (light:dark 12:12 or 10:14) as compared with pineal-intact controls (Tamarkin et al. 1981; Kothari et al. 1984; Shah et al. 1984). We later confirmed this finding (Blask et al. 1991b) in the N-nitroso-N-methylurea (NMU) model of mammary cancer, which is sensitive to the direct growth-promoting effects of both prolactin and estradiol (E_2) (Welsch 1985) (Fig. 1). Therefore, these studies provide compelling evidence that the nocturnal melatonin signal is yet

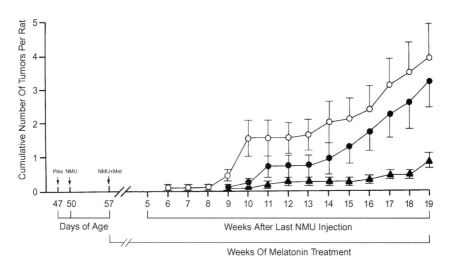

FIG. 1. Effects of either daily afternoon injections (1600–1800 hours) of vehicle (●) or melatonin (500 μg; (▲), or of pinealectomy ("Pinx") (○) during the early and late promotion phases of NMU-induced mammary tumorigenesis on the mean (± SE) cumulative number of palpable mammary tumors per rat. Melatonin versus vehicle control, p < 0.05. (Reprinted from Blask et al. 1991a with permission from Plenum Publishing Corp.)

another important component of a complex array of growth-regulatory hormones and factors implicated in breast carcinogenesis.

Experiments using constant light exposure as a method of "physiological" pinealectomy have been employed as an alternative strategy for demonstrating the enhancing effect of reduced melatonin on tumorigenesis. Like pinealectomy, constant light exposure negates the expression of the nocturnal melatonin signal and in turn promotes DMBA-induced mammary tumorigenesis (Kothari et al. 1984; Shah et al. 1984). Although it is tempting to ascribe enhanced mammary tumorigenesis in both pinealectomized and constant light-exposed animals to the lack of a nightly melatonin surge, it is important to note that these two manipulations are not exactly equivalent in the outcomes they produce. For example, while the circadian melatonin signal is eliminated in both pinealectomized and constant light-exposed animals, the activity rhythm—which is still entrained to the photoperiod (it occurs every 24 hours) in pinealectomized rats—initially free-runs in constant light-exposed rats with a periodicity of about 25.1 hours (Cassone 1992). However, more prolonged exposure to constant lighting conditions (several weeks to months) culminates in complete suppression of circadian rhythmicity and its replacement by ultradian rhythms (period < 20 hours) (Depres-Brummer et al. 1995). Additionally, constant light-exposed female rats enter into constant estrus (Fiske 1941; Lawton and Schwartz 1967) while estrous cycles remain normal in pinealectomized animals (Moore and Rapport 1971; Reiter 1980). Furthermore, prolactin levels are consistently elevated in constant light-exposed animals (Vaticon et al. 1980) but not in pinealectomized rats (Relkin et al. 1972; Blask et al. 1991b). Clearly, not all of the effect of constant light in promoting DMBA-induced mammary tumorigenesis may necessarily be due purely to the elimination of the endogenous melatonin rhythm. Thus, a critical issue left to resolve is whether differences in the expression of circadian rhythmicity, irrespective of or in addition to the suppression of the melatonin signal, may account for differences in tumorigenesis.

Influence of Treatment Protocol and Environmental Factors

Several studies show a marked and consistent suppressive effect of melatonin, at doses ranging from 25 μg–1 mg and injected daily for 7–335 days, on either transplantable (Anisimov et al. 1973; Karmali et al. 1978), spontaneous (Wrba et al. 1986; Subramanian and Kothari 1991a), or carcinogen-induced mammary cancer in either female mice or rats (Aubert et al. 1980; Tamarkin et al. 1981; Shah et al. 1984; Blask 1984; Blask et al. 1986, 1991b). Clearly, the DMBA and NMU models of chemically initiated mammary carcinogenesis have provided the most comprehensive picture of the oncostatic effects of melatonin in vivo (Blask 1993). Although the earliest report of melatonin's action on DMBA-induced tumors revealed that morning injections resulted in a stimulatory effect of this indoleamine (Hamilton 1969), subsequent DMBA investigations demonstrated that daily, late-afternoon injections of melatonin inhibited mammary tumorigenesis. These findings suggest that these tumors exhibit a diurnal rhythm of sensitivity to melatonin (Blask 1993). In fact, a diurnal rhythm of sensitivity to the oncostatic effect of melatonin is apparent in the NMU tumor model.

Melatonin injected only during the late afternoon, 2 hours before lights off, was effective in inhibiting tumorigenesis while morning injections, a few hours after lights on, had no impact on tumor development (Blask et al. 1990, 1991a, 1992).

The oral administration of melatonin via drinking water also is quite effective in suppressing DMBA-induced mammary cancer growth (Kothari 1987; Kothari and Subramanian 1992), indicating that melatonin retains its oncostatic properties following absorption from the gastrointestinal tract and first-pass metabolism by the liver. Interestingly, DMBA itself reduces the circulating levels of melatonin presumably via an action on melatonin's pineal production. In this way, some of DMBA's carcinogenic action may result in part from its ability to suppress nightly pineal melatonin output (Bartsch et al. 1990).

Some studies have shown that alterations in environmental factors such as nutritional intake or photoperiodic exposure significantly influence the tumorigenic response to melatonin in rats with DMBA-induced mammary cancers. For example, in rats placed on a modest regimen of caloric restriction (i.e., 30%), melatonin is much more efficacious in suppressing tumorigenesis than in animals fed ad libitum (Blask 1984; Blask et al. 1986). With respect to photoperiod, the anticarcinogenic effect of melatonin appears to be enhanced in rats maintained on constant light as compared with animals maintained on short photoperiod (Shah et al. 1984; Kothari 1987).

Initiation Versus Promotion and the Influence of Pinealectomy and/or Constant Light

In most of the early studies using the DMBA model, melatonin treatment encompassed both the initiation and promotion (tumors already established) phases of carcinogenesis, making it virtually impossible to determine whether the inhibitory action of melatonin was on tumor initiation, promotion, or both (Blask 1993). In the first study restricting melatonin administration to the promotion phase of DMBA-induced mammary tumorigenesis, late-afternoon melatonin injections (200 μg) administered only twice a week decreased both the size and number of mammary tumors (Aubert et al. 1980).

More recently, melatonin's influence on the initiation-versus-promotion phases of carcinogenesis was examined in animals that were either pinealectomized or maintained on constant light (Subramanian and Kothari 1991b). In the initiation experiments, either intact or pinealectomized female rats maintained on either constant light or short photoperiod (light:dark 10:14) were administered vehicle or melatonin (200 μg) through drinking water for 1 week before and 1 week following DMBA treatment at 55 days of age. Melatonin substantially diminished tumor incidence in pineal-intact rats maintained on either constant light or short photoperiod. However, in pinealectomized animals, melatonin was completely ineffective in suppressing tumor development in rats on either photoperiodic regimen. The promotion study was similar to the initiation study with the exception that melatonin treatment was delayed until 1 week following DMBA administration but continued thereafter for a total of 7 months. Interestingly, when restricted to the promotion phase, melatonin therapy was equally effective in suppressing tumorigenesis in either intact, pinealectomized, and/or constant light-exposed animals. Although no effect of melatonin on final tumor number was evident under any experimental condition, melatonin did delay the latency to onset of tumor appearance in all situations. These results suggest that an intact pineal gland and presumably its endogenous melatonin rhythm are required for exogenous melatonin's oncostatic effect on tumor initiation, but not promotion, in this model system. An earlier study reported similar results of pinealectomy on the tumor response to melatonin administration encompassing both the initiation and promotion phases of carcinogenesis (Tamarkin et al. 1981). Although we previously found a suppressive effect of melatonin restricted to the promotion phase in this model system (Blask 1984; Blask et al. 1986), we have not observed melatonin inhibition of tumor initiation (Blask, unpublished results).

In the NMU model system, we also have addressed the initiation-versus-promotion issue and determined that daily, late-afternoon melatonin injections (500 μg/day) restricted to the initiation phase of NMU-induced mammary tumorigenesis failed to inhibit tumor development (Blask et al. 1991b); however, when restricted to the promotion phase, melatonin was effective in suppressing tumorigenesis (Fig. 1). The antipromotion effect of melatonin in this model system is further substantiated by the ability of melatonin to completely block E_2-

induced regrowth of NMU tumors that had regressed in response to ovariectomy (Blask et al. 1991b). As alluded to earlier, melatonin therapy administered in the morning a few hours after lights on is completely ineffective in inhibiting NMU-induced mammary tumorigenesis (Blask et al. 1990, 1991a, 1992). Interestingly, pinealectomy (lack of a melatonin signal?) makes these tumors responsive to the antipromotion effects of melatonin therapy administered in the morning; however, late-afternoon melatonin treatment still appears to be more effective than late-morning melatonin in suppressing tumorigenesis in pinealectomized rats (Blask et al. 1990, 1991a). Taken together, these results suggest that there is diurnal rhythm of mammary tumor sensitivity to exogenous melatonin during the promotion phase that is dependent on the endogenous melatonin signal (Blask 1994).

Potential Mechanisms of Melatonin Action on the Initiation of Carcinogen-Induced Mammary Tumors In Vivo

A variety of factors may explain why some investigators have been able to inhibit initiation of DMBA-induced mammary carcinogenesis while we failed to affect tumor initiation in either the DMBA or NMU models. For example, in the DMBA system, we administer the carcinogen intravenously and melatonin by subcutaneous injection (Blask et al. 1986); others typically administer DMBA via the intragastric route and melatonin orally via drinking water (Kothari 1987; Kothari and Subramanian 1992), therefore subjecting these compounds to first-pass metabolism by the liver. Thus, melatonin might inhibit tumor initiation by limiting the absorption of DMBA or by decreasing its activation and increasing its detoxification by phase-I (cytochromes b_5 and P450) and phase-II (glutathione S-transferase; GST) xenobiotic metabolizing enzymes in the liver (Kothari and Subramanian 1992).

Melatonin administration in drinking water (200 μg/day) recently has been reported to not only raise total glutathione (GSH) levels but the levels of other important enzymes of the glutamyl cycle, such as GST in the mammary gland and liver tissues in female rats treated with DMBA (Kothari and Subramanian 1992). It has been proposed that melatonin's inhibition of the initiation step of DMBA-induced mammary carcinogenesis may be brought about in part by an increased detoxification of DMBA by elevated GSH and GST levels. Additionally, a melatonin-induced inhibition of phase-I enzymes also may lead to decreased activation of DMBA (Kothari and Subramanian 1992).

Another mechanism by which melatonin might inhibit carcinogen-initiated mammary carcinogenesis is its ability to inhibit carcinogen-induced DNA adduct formation, as has been demonstrated in the liver (Reiter et al. 1994; Tan et al. 1994). Since the ultimate epoxide derivative of DMBA forms DNA adducts in mammary epithelial cells (DiGiovanni and Juchau 1980), it is conceivable that melatonin may block the formation of these adducts as a result of its own intrinsic antioxidant properties and/or through the stimulation of GSH and GST (Reiter et al. 1994; Tan et al. 1994; Kothari and Subramanian 1992). However, if such a mechanism was operating, we would expect inhibition of tumor initiation in both our DMBA and NMU studies, because NMU also forms adducts with DNA (Kumar et al. 1990). Perhaps in our studies, any effect of melatonin on liver metabolism of DMBA was limited by the parenteral route of administration of both substances. Unlike DMBA, which is metabolically activated in the liver and mammary gland to its ultimate carcinogenic form, 3,4-dihydro-diol-1, 2-epoxide (DiGiovanni and Juchau 1980), NMU directly alkylates DNA and activates H-*ras* and K-*ras* oncogenes (Kumar et al. 1990). Because NMU does not require metabolic activation to cause malignant transformation, melatonin might not have an impact on the direct initiation of carcinogenesis by this nitrosamine.

Another potential anti-initiation mechanism of mammary tumorigenesis by melatonin may involve melatonin-induced alterations in the structure and proliferative capacity of the normal mammary ductal system, suggesting that it may act as a differentiating agent. For example, melatonin treatment of female rats or mice results in a decrease in the number of terminal end and alveolar buds, as well as a decrease in the amount of mammary gland DNA synthesis that may create a more "differentiated" ductal system, which might then render the mammary epithelium refractory to the effects of a carcinogen such as DMBA (Shah et al. 1984; Kothari 1988; Subramanian and Kothari 1991a). Studies in vitro suggest that pharmacological doses of melatonin could act directly on mammary tissue to maintain the differentiated state (Sanchez-Barceló et al. 1990). Furthermore, physiological concentrations of melatonin may induce a "partially differentiated" phenotype in MCF-7 human breast cancer cells in vitro (Crespo et al. 1994).

Other evidence suggests that melatonin suppression of circulating prolactin, E_2, and IGF-1 levels (Tamarkin et al. 1981; Shah et al. 1984; Subramanian and Kothari 1991a; Scaglione et al. 1992), as well as the expression of epidermal growth factor receptors and c-*erb2* oncoprotein (Scaglione et al. 1992), may be responsible for inhibiting murine mammary tumorigenesis in vivo, because these hormones and growth factors are endogenous promoters of mammary cancer (Freiss et al. 1993). However, we have never observed a melatonin-induced decrease in either prolactin or E_2 levels in rats with either DMBA- or NMU-induced tumors (Blask et al. 1986, 1991b). Rather, it appears more likely that melatonin may act directly at the level of breast cancer cells to inhibit the mitogenic actions of E_2, prolactin, and other growth factors (Hill et al. 1992; Cos and Blask 1994; Lemus-Wilson et al. 1995). Moreover, melatonin may stimulate immune mechanisms to slow or halt breast cancer growth once it is initiated (Maestroni and Conti 1993). The potential cellular and molecular mechanisms by which melatonin inhibits mammary tumorigenesis during the growth-promotion phase are addressed in greater detail in subsequent sections of this chapter.

MELATONIN AND EXPERIMENTAL BREAST CANCER IN VITRO: HUMAN BREAST CANCER CELL GROWTH STUDIES

The demonstration that melatonin inhibits the growth of monolayer cultures of ER^+ human breast cancer cells (MCF-7) supplemented with 10% fetal bovine serum (FBS) in vitro established for the first time that physiologically relevant levels of this neurohormone have a direct oncostatic effect on breast cancer cells, while higher or lower concentrations exert little or no influence (Hill and Blask 1988) (Fig. 2). These findings formed the basis of a model system of human breast cancer growth with which to probe the cellular and molecular mechanisms of melatonin's oncostatic action; this system will be discussed later in this chapter (see p. 213).

Melatonin not only inhibits the proliferation of monolayer cultures of MCF-7 cells but also cells cultured in an anchorage-independent system as well (Cos and Blask 1990). However, the bell-shaped,

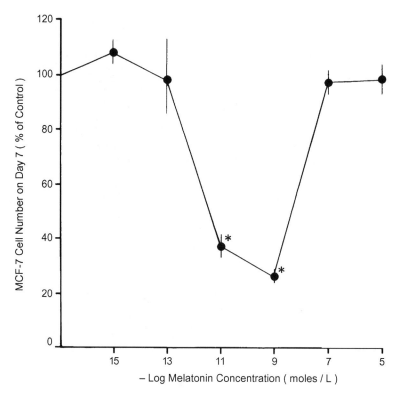

FIG. 2. Bell-shaped dose–response of MCF-7 cell proliferation in monolayer culture to the effects of increasing concentrations of melatonin. Each point is the mean ($\pm$ SE) percentage of inhibition of cell growth as a percentage of the growth of vehicle-treated controls (100%) following 7 days of culture in Dulbecco's Modified Eagle's Medium (DMEM) containing 10% FBS. Asterisk indicates $p < 0.01$ versus controls and other melatonin doses. (Reprinted from Hill and Blask 1988 with permission from the American Association for Cancer Research.)

dose–response curve characteristic of melatonin action on monolayer cultures changes to a linear dose–response relationship in soft agar culture (Fig. 3). Additionally, as the amount of FBS is reduced in the medium, MCF-7 cells lose their responsiveness to melatonin until they are totally refractory in serum-free, chemically defined medium (Blask and Hill 1986; Hill 1986; Hill and Blask 1986). In fact, we have found

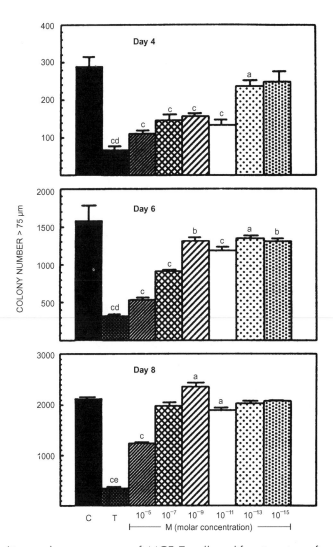

FIG. 3. Linear dose–response of MCF-7 cell proliferation in soft agar suspension culture to the effects of different concentrations of melatonin during an 8-day culture period in DMEM containing 10% FBS. Data are expressed as the mean (± SE) colony number per plate. Designations of a, b, or c indicates $p < 0.05$ compared to controls (C) ; d or e indicates $p < 0.05$ tamoxifen (T)-treated versus all melatonin (M)-treated groups. (Reprinted from Cos and Blask 1990 with permission from Elsevier Science Ireland, Ltd.)

that MCF-7 cell sensitivity to melatonin can vary dramatically from robust to little or no response with different batches of FBS obtained from different, or even the same, commercial sources (unpublished results). In addition to serum factors, different growth rates of MCF-7 cells, as determined by different initial plating densities, have a profound impact on the responsiveness of these cells to melatonin. For example, physiological melatonin is more effective in inhibiting the growth of fast-growing (short doubling time) MCF-7 cells initally plated at high density than slower-growing cells (long doubling time) initally plated at low density (Cos and Sanchez-Barceló 1995). Moreover, the "circadian-like" presentation of physiological levels of melatonin to MCF-7 cells is more effective in inhibiting cell growth than continuous exposure (Cos and Sanchez-Barceló 1994). These findings emphasize the importance of culture conditions, particularly serum components and plating density-determined growth rates, in setting the level of MCF-7 cell sensitivity to melatonin inhibition.

Characteristic changes in the ultrastructural morphology of MCF-7 cells occur in response to continuous exposure to melatonin. These changes include reduced numbers of surface microvilli, cytoplasmic and ribosomal shedding, disruption of mitochondrial cristae, vesiculation of smooth endoplasmic reticulum, and increased numbers of autophagic vacuoles (Hill and Blask 1988). This morphological picture has been confirmed and extended by Crespo et al. (1994), who concluded that such a profile of ultrastructural features suggests that these cells are undergoing a transition to a more differentiated phenotype in the presence of melatonin. Melatonin exerts its antiproliferative and apparent differentiating action by delaying the progression of cells from G_1/G_0 to the S-phase of the cell cycle (Cos et al. 1991) (Fig. 4). Other studies using partially synchronized MCF-7 cells suggest that they are most susceptible to inhibition by melatonin during the S-phase of the cell cycle (Cos et al. 1993).

Because MCF-7 cells represent metastatic breast cancer cells, Cos and Sanchez-Barceló (1996) examined whether physiological melatonin would inhibit the invasiveness of these cells measured in Falcon cell culture membrane inserts coated with an extract of basement membrane components (Matrigel™; Collaborative Biomedical Products, Bedford, MA). They found that melatonin not only reduced

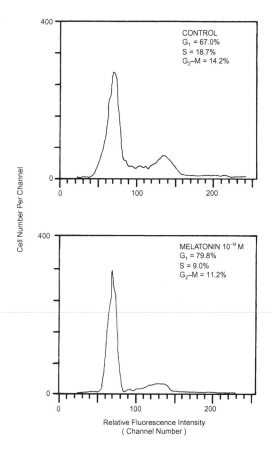

FIG. 4. DNA histograms of cell cycle phase distributions of vehicle-treated (upper panel) or melatonin-treated (lower panel) MCF-7 breast cancer cells after 5 days of monolayer culture in DMEM containing 10% FBS. Phase distributions were determined by flow cytometry of cells stained with propidium iodide. (Reprinted from Cos et al. 1991 with permission from Munksgaard International Publishers, Ltd., Copenhagen.)

the ability of MCF-7 cells to attach to and traverse the basement membrane, it also counteracted the ability of E_2 to stimulate cell adhesion and invasiveness. Pretreatment of the cells with melatonin induced the same inhibitory effect on unstimulated and E_2-stimulated attachment and invasion. Melatonin also reduced the chemotactic response of MCF-7 cells toward the extracellular matrix molecule fibronectin.

These important results indicate that physiological melatonin inhibits both the proliferation and invasiveness of MCF-7 cells in vitro. The decreased invasiveness of these cells may be due to a reduction in cell attachment, cell motility, and/or the production of matrix degradative enzymes (Cos and Sanchez-Barceló 1996).

Melatonin's direct inhibitory effect on MCF-7 cell growth in culture has now been replicated by a number of other independent laboratories. While the majority of these investigators reported an inhibitory effect of physiological melatonin (de Launoit et al. 1990; L'Hermite-Baleriaux et al. 1990; Liburdy et al. 1993; Cos and Sanchez-Barceló 1994, 1995; Crespo et al. 1994; Furuya et al. 1994; Blackman et al. 1996), the remaining researchers detected either a cytotoxic or cytostatic effect of melatonin only at pharmacological levels (Shellard et al. 1989; Bartsch et al. 1992). Interestingly, one group who initially reported an oncostatic effect of melatonin on MCF-7 cell growth (L'Hermite-Baleriaux et al. 1990) subsequently reported no effect (L'Hermite-Baleriaux and de Launoit 1992). When closely examined, the latter study revealed a variety of culture conditions that were different from ours; most notably, the length of incubation, which was 12 days in the study by L'Hermite-Baleriaux and de Launoit (1992) versus 5–7 days in our system (Blask and Hill 1986; Hill and Blask 1988; Cos et al. 1991; Hill et al. 1992). Another difference was that they used MCF-7 cells that were apparently hypersensitive to E_2, because they achieved a twofold increase in MCF-7 cell growth with E_2 in 10% FBS in which cell growth, in our hands, is already maximally stimulated. This difference suggests that they either used a batch serum that was low in E_2 or inadvertently tested an MCF-7 subline that was already biased toward growth-stimulatory effects from endogenous estrogens in their FBS, thus overshadowing any growth inhibition by melatonin. In this regard, MCF-7 cells from different laboratories have been shown to vary widely in basal and E_2-stimulated growth rates, in responses to inhibition by the anti-estrogen tamoxifen, and in ER and progesterone receptor content (Osborne et al. 1987). It is conceivable that similar variations in responsiveness to melatonin could exist among MCF-7 cell sublines from different laboratories, particularly under different culture conditions.

Cellular and Molecular Mechanisms of Melatonin Action on Human Breast Cancer Cells

Cellular Aspects Involving Estradiol, Prolactin, and Other Growth Factors

The first clue that the estrogen-growth response pathway is crucial for melatonin's oncostatic effect on MCF-7 human breast cancer cell growth in vitro was the demonstration that neither physiological nor pharmacological concentrations had an inhibitory effect on the growth of ER⁻ human breast cancer cell lines (Hill et al. 1992). Melatonin's ability to block E_2-stimulated MCF-7 cell growth as well as E_2-induced rescue of tamoxifen-inhibited cells further attests to the importance of the estrogen-growth response system as a component of the mechanisms mediating melatonin's oncostatic action in vitro (Cos et al. 1991; Hill et al. 1992). Interestingly, E_2 is also capable of rescuing MCF-7 cells from melatonin-induced growth arrest (Cos et al. 1991), and essentially reverses the differentiating effect of melatonin on these cells (Crespo et al. 1994).

As alluded to previously, in addition to estrogens, the hormonal regulation of breast cancer growth encompasses a complex array of other estrogen-inducible endocrine, paracrine, and autocrine substances, including prolactin, EGF, or TGFα, IGF-1, and cathepsin D (Freiss et al. 1993). In serum-free, chemically defined medium, melatonin inhibits the release of several proteins synthesized by MCF-7 cells, including an E_2-inducible 52 kD glycoprotein which may correspond to the autocrine growth stimulator cathepsin-D (Hill 1986; Blask and Hill 1988). Additionally, melatonin not only increases the levels of inhibitory growth factor activity (TGFβ?) in medium conditioned by MCF-7 cells (Cos and Blask 1994), it also inhibits the capacity of E_2-induced growth factor activity (Cos and Blask 1994), prolactin (Lemus-Wilson et al. 1995), and EGF itself (Cos and Blask 1994) to stimulate MCF-7 cell growth. In the case of inhibiting prolactin-stimulated MCF-7 cell growth, melatonin exhibits the same basic bell-shaped, dose–response curve as it does in the presence of 10% FBS (Lemus-Wilson et al. 1995) (Fig. 5). Taken together, these results indicate that melatonin exerts its oncostatic effect in vitro by modulating the secretion and/or action of E_2-inducible endocrine, paracrine, or autocrine growth factors.

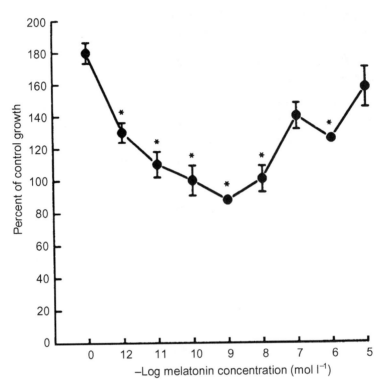

FIG. 5. Bell-shaped dose–response of MCF-7 cell proliferation, stimulated by human prolactin (20 ng/mL), to increasing concentrations of melatonin following 3 days of monolayer culture in DMEM containing 5%, charcoal-stripped FBS. Each point represents the mean (± SE) percent of the control growth rate (100%) in response to human prolactin alone (without melatonin). Asterisk indicates $p < 0.05$ melatonin + prolactin versus prolactin alone. (From Lemus-Wilson et al. 1995 from Macmillian Press, Ltd., United Kingdom.)

Melatonin Binding Sites in Murine and Human Breast Cancer

We originally reported 2-[^{125}I]iodomelatonin (2-IMLT) binding sites in mammary cancers generated by the chemical carcinogen NMU in adult, female Sprague-Dawley rats. Crude membrane fractions of NMU-induced mammary tumors demonstrated highly specific 2-IMLT binding that increased linearly with increasing tissue concentrations (Blask et al. 1990; Burns et al. 1990). The binding of 2-IMLT to these tumor membranes was characterized by a relatively low binding affinity (K_D = 9.6 nM) and moderate capacity (B_{max} = 67.8 fmole/mg protein), and the rank order of potency of a number of melatonin analogs for competition with 2-IMLT binding indicated a melatoninergic process. However, because the binding was of relatively low affinity, it is unlikely that it represents binding to the recently cloned MLT_{1a} or MLT_{1b} membrane receptors that are of much higher affinity (K_D 20–160 pM; Reppert and Weaver 1995). In spite of these 2-IMLT binding sites in NMU-induced tumors, we still don't know whether they actually mediate the oncostatic signal provided by either exogenous or endogenous melatonin in rats with NMU-induced tumors. Nevertheless, if these binding sites are indeed involved in transmitting melatonin's oncostatic message in vivo, then their low-affinity state may explain why pharmacological levels of exogenous melatonin (20 μg) are required to inhibit the growth of carcinogen-induced mammary tumors (Stankov et al. 1991).

As mentioned previously, the administration of melatonin either orally or by injection has been shown to inhibit the development of spontaneous adenocarcinomas in female mice (Wrba et al. 1986; Subramanian and Kothari 1991a). Furthermore, melatonin suppresses the normal development of the mammary parenchyma in mice (Sanchez-Barceló et al. 1990). While melatonin binding sites have not been reported to exist in mouse mammary tumors, 2-IMLT binding sites were recently characterized in crude membrane preparations of mammary glands from normal female BALB/c mice (Recio et al. 1994). These binding sites appeared to exhibit a diurnal rhythm in binding affinity and receptor number such that the highest-affinity binding and lowest receptor number occurred during the light phase 4 hours before lights off, while the lowest-affinity binding and highest receptor number occurred during the dark phase 3 hours before lights on. However, whether these represent authentic melatonin receptors remains problematic, because compounds such as hydroxyindoles and dopaminergic agents bind with higher affinity to 2-IMLT binding sites than either melatonin or 6-chloromelatonin in competition experiments. Nevertheless, the relatively low affinity of these binding sites

(K_D = 1–3 nM) also might explain why large doses of melatonin are required to inhibit spontaneous mammary carcinogenesis in mice.

Limited work has been done with respect to identifying 2-IMLT binding sites in human breast cancer tissue. The results of one small study (Stankov et al. 1991) revealed that some ER^+ breast cancers were also positive while some ER^- tumors were negative for 2-IMLT binding. In the remaining tumors in which ER status was unknown, half were positive while the other half were negative for 2-IMLT binding. These results are interesting in light of the fact that the ER^+ human breast cancer cell line MCF-7 is very weakly positive (≈ 0.7 fmoles/mg protein) for 2-IMLT binding in both membrane and nuclear fractions (Stankov et al. 1991), and exhibits low-level expression of transcripts for the cloned, membrane-bound melatonin receptor (Mel_{1a}) (Reppert and Weaver 1995) that are only detectable with reverse transcription–polymerase chain reaction technology (S. Hill, personal communication). Thus, it appears doubtful at this juncture that authentic, high-affinity, membrane-bound melatonin receptors play a significant role in mediating the direct oncostatic effects of melatonin on breast cancer cell growth.

MELATONIN MODULATION OF NONMELATONIN, HORMONE-RECEPTOR EXPRESSION IN HUMAN BREAST CANCER CELLS

Melatonin regulation of heterologous receptors such as the ER in human breast cancer cells was first examined by Danforth et al. (1983), who found that physiological concentrations of melatonin augmented both cytoplasmic and nuclear estrogen binding activity in MCF-7 cells within 40 minutes of exposure; the increase persisted for 5 hours. While the binding affinity was unaffected by melatonin, receptor number increased by approximately 80% over controls, indicating an up-regulatory action of melatonin on MCF-7 cells.

Since the Danforth et al. report, Molis and colleagues (1993) performed extensive studies on melatonin's ability to modulate ER expression in MCF-7 cells, and documented effects of physiological melatonin on ER expression in MCF-7 cells that contradict the initial work of Danforth et al. (1983). In the Molis et al. study, over a period of 6–48 hours of continuous incubation of MCF-7 cells with melatonin (1 nM) in steroid-depleted medium, ER number progressively decreased—with the maximum inhibition occurring after 24 hours of incubation—while binding affinity was unaffected (Fig. 6). Melatonin also caused a dose- and time-dependent reduction in levels of immunoreactive ER, with maximal suppression occurring with 1 nM melatonin following 12 hours of incubation (Fig. 6). Surprisingly, pharmacological concentrations of melatonin induced a 50% rise in immunoreactive ER levels following 48 hours of incubation. Melatonin's down-regulation of the ER apparently results from an indirect mechanism involving transcriptional regulation (see next section) rather than direct binding to the hormone-binding domain of the ER. The reason for the discrepancy between the Danforth et al. (1983) and Molis et al. (1993) studies may be due to different culture conditions and/or sublines of MCF-7 cells (Osborne et al. 1987).

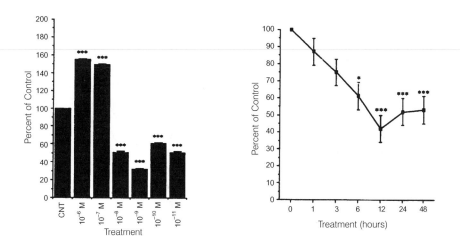

FIG. 6. Dose–response (left panel) and time-course (right panel) effects of melatonin on ER protein expression in MCF-7 human breast cancer cells cultured 48 hours in phenol red-free DMEM supplemented with 5%, charcoal-stripped FBS. Western blot analysis of total cellular protein was performed by resolving the protein by SDS-PAGE followed by immunoblotting with the H222 monoclonal antibody to the human ER. Autoradiograms from Western blot analyses were quantified by scanning densitometry and results were presented as percent of control (100%). Single asterisk indicates $p < 0.05$; triple asterisk, $p < 0.001$ versus controls. (Reprinted from Molis et al. 1993 with permission from the *International Journal of Oncology.*)

MELATONIN CONTROL OF TRANSCRIPTIONAL EVENTS

Extending their work on melatonin modulation of the expression of ER protein in MCF-7 cells, Molis et al. (1994) examined whether melatonin's suppression of ER expression is exerted at the transcriptional level. Like its effect on ER protein expression, 1 nM melatonin substantially reduced the steady-state levels of ER mRNA by 44% as early as 3 hours of culture, and by 76% as late as 48 hours of culture in MCF-7 cells incubated in 10% FBS (Fig. 7). In fact, the bell-shaped, dose–response signature of melatonin's inhibition of cell proliferation (Hill and Blask 1988; Lemus-Wilson et al. 1995) (Figs. 2 and 5) also characterized melatonin's action on ER mRNA expression (Fig. 8). Nuclear run-on experiments revealed that melatonin's inhibitory action on ER mRNA expression was due to the suppression of the transcription of the ER gene. Apparently, this regulation was independent of both new protein synthesis as well as a direct interaction of melatonin with the ER and subsequent feedback on its own expression. Furthermore, they found that melatonin did not affect the stability of the ER transcript. Although it is not clear by what mechanism(s) melatonin suppresses ER gene transcription in human breast cancer cells, Molis et al. (1994) propose that melatonin's extremely lipophilic nature may allow it to diffuse into the nucleus to directly bind with promoter sequences and inhibit ER gene transcription. Additional possibilities suggested by this group include melatonin binding to and sequestration of key transcriptional regulatory factors, or the induction of critical negative regulatory transcription factors perhaps via an interaction with a nuclear melatonin binding protein.

Melatonin also modulates the expression of c-*fos* and c-*myc* (Molis et al. 1995), immediate early genes important in E_2-induced proliferation of MCF-7 cells in culture (Wilding et al. 1988). For example, the proto-oncogene product of c-*fos* is a transcription factor that is a key target of signal transduction in processes such as cell proliferation (van der Burg et al. 1990). While melatonin induces a sustained elevation in the steady-state concentrations of c-*myc* mRNA within 3 hours, it causes a transient initial rise in c-*fos* mRNA followed by precipitous decrease. In the case of other estrogen-inducible proteins, melatonin stimulates, also within a few hours, the expression of steady-state levels of pS2 mRNA, as well as an initial rise followed by a drop in TGFα mRNA; in

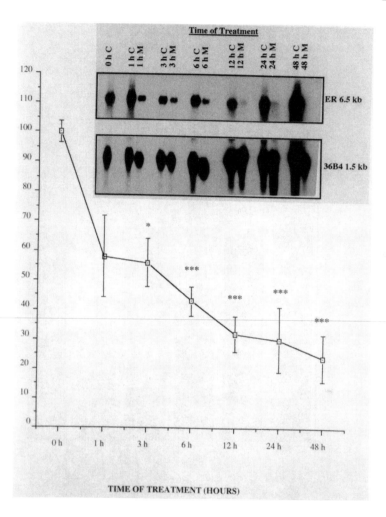

FIG. 7. Time course of MCF-7 cell steady-state ER mRNA expression in response to melatonin (10^{-9} M) following 48 hours of culture in DMEM supplemented with 10% FBS. Control cells were incubated with vehicle. Northern blots were probed with a ^{32}P-labeled, 2.1-kb human ER cDNA and a 0.2-kb, 36B4 cDNA to monitor loading. Autoradiograms from Northern blot analyses were quantifed by scanning densitometry and normalization with 36B4 mRNA. Each point represents the mean ($\pm$ SE) ER mRNA level as a percent of the control (100%). Asterisk indicates $p < 0.05$; triple asterisk, $p < 0.001$ versus control. (Reprinted from Molis et al. 1994 with permission from The Endocrine Society, Bethesda, Maryland.)

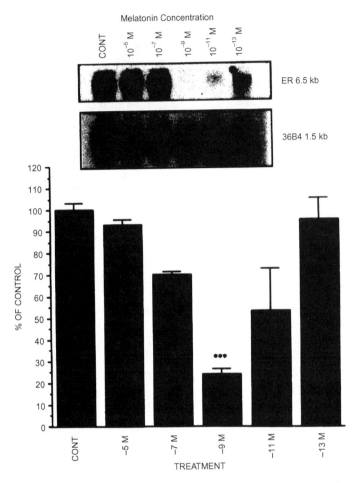

FIG. 8.   Dose–response of MCF-7 cell steady-state ER mRNA levels to various concentrations of melatonin following 48 hours of culture in DMEM supplemented with 10% FBS. Consult the legend for Fig. 7 for additional details. Triple asterisk indicates p (0.001 versus control. (Reprinted from Molis et al. 1994 with permission from The Endocrine Society, Bethesda, Maryland.)

contrast, levels of progesterone receptor mRNA steadily fall in MCF-7 cells following their exposure to physiological melatonin. Melatonin also significantly stimulates the expression of the mRNA for TGFβ, an important inhibitory autocrine growth factor (Freiss et al. 1993) that may account for the increased inhibitory growth-factor activity we observe in conditioned medium from the melatonin-treated MCF-7 cells mentioned previously (Cos and Blask 1994). Molis et al. (1995) infer from these results that mechanisms more rapid than down-regulation of ER are important in melatonin's modulation of their expression, while longer-term modulation of these transcripts may be strongly influenced by melatonin's down-regulation of ER expression.

Melatonin Interaction with Redox Mechanisms: Reduced Glutathione and Nitric Oxide

Elevated intracellular concentrations of reactive oxygen species and free radicals can create a pro-oxidant state within cells with the potential not only to lead to cancer initiation but promotion/progression as well (Ceruti 1985). As the most ubiquitous nonprotein thiol produced by mammalian cells, reduced glutathione (GSH) is among the most potent and crucial antioxidant molecule in the intracellular compartment, providing it with a reducing environment. GSH is synthesized via the glutamyl cycle from its constituent amino acids in two consecutive enzymatic steps involving the rate-limiting enzyme γ-glutamyl-cysteine synthetase and GSH synthetase (Meister 1991). We have taken advantage of a highly specific inhibitor of GSH synthesis—L-buthionine sulfoximine (L-BSO), which blocks the rate-limiting step of GSH synthesis and depletes cells of their GSH content (Meister 1991)—to determine whether GSH is involved in the mechanism of melatonin's direct inhibitory effect on MCF-7 human breast cancer cell growth in culture.

The simultaneous and continuous incubation of MCF-7 cells with melatonin (1 nM) and L-BSO (1–10 μM) resulted in a complete blockade of melatonin's oncostatic effect on cell growth, indicating that the depletion of GSH somehow renders these cells incapable of responding to melatonin (Blask and Wilson 1994; Blask et al. 1994). Similar results have been reported for the cytotoxic effect of the diterpene drug taxol in this same cell line (Leibmann et al. 1993). That the depletion of GSH rather than an interaction with L-BSO with melatonin was responsible for eliminating melatonin's oncostatic effect is substantiated by the ability of GSH added back to the cultures to restore melatonin's ability to inhibit cell proliferation in the presence of L-

BSO. Therefore, the oncostatic action of melatonin in MCF-7 cells appears to depend on the presence of adequate, perhaps threshold levels of intracellular GSH. In fact, melatonin itself raises GSH levels in MCF-7 cells, an effect that is completely blocked by L-BSO (Blask and Wilson 1994; Blask et al. 1994). This melatonin-induced increase in the GSH content of breast cancer cells is consistent with the report of Subramanian and Kothari (1992), alluded to previously, showing that melatonin treatment increases the GSH levels in normal or DMBA-transformed mammary tissue in female rats. That melatonin itself may actually be interacting with GSH to produce its oncostatic action in MCF-7 cells via a free radical-scavenging mechanism is suggested by recent data demonstrating a synergistic effect of melatonin and GSH in suppressing free radical formation (Poeggeler et al. 1995).

Nitric oxide (NO) has emerged as an extremely important intracellular signal-transduction molecule (Moncada and Higgs 1993). Not only does NO function in a variety of physiological processes, it also acts as either a free radical or antioxidant species (Stamler et al. 1992). This fascinating molecule has been shown to exert a cytostatic, antiproliferative effect on melanoma (Maragos et al. 1993) and breast cancer (Lepoivre et al. 1989), presumably via an inhibition of ribonucleotide reductase, the rate-limiting step in DNA synthesis (Bitonti et al. 1994). The redox state of the intracellular environment can determine specific redox forms of NO which, in turn, may target specific cellular processes such as DNA synthesis and elicit a particular biological response such as cytostasis (Girard and Potier 1993). Because melatonin may alter the redox state of breast cancer cells in conjunction with GSH (Blask and Wilson 1994; Blask et al. 1994; Poeggeler et al. 1995), we wanted to determine whether NO is involved in the mechanism(s) mediating the oncostatic effect of melatonin on MCF-7 cells in vitro.

We approached this question by blocking the synthesis of NO and determining what effect this manipulation had on the antiproliferative action of melatonin in MCF-7 cells. The synthesis of NO can be inhibited by N-monomethyl-L-arginine (NMMA), a potent inhibitor of both the inducible (i) and constitutive (c) forms of NO synthase (NOS), the rate-limiting enzyme in the synthesis of NO from L-arginine and molecular O_2 (Moncada and Higgs 1993). It was recently shown that MCF-7 cells express both iNOS and cNOS activities at low levels, resulting in the production of low ambient levels of NO as well (Bani et al. 1995). In the presence of NMMA, melatonin fails to inhibit MCF-7 cell growth in culture (Fig. 9). This finding suggests that melatonin may stimulate NO production in these cells, as has recently been shown for the pep-

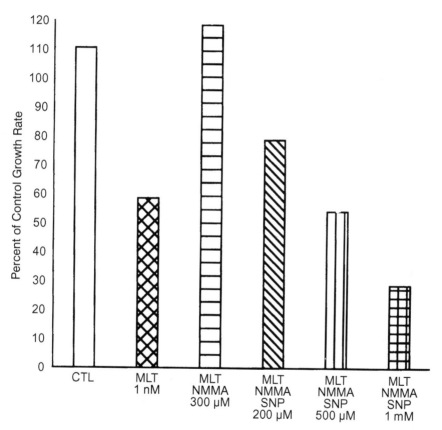

FIG. 9. Effects of the NOS synthesis blocker N-monomethyl-L-arginine (NMMA) (300 μM) and the NO donor sodium nitroprusside (SNP) (200 μM–1 mM) on melatonin (MLT) (1 nM) inhibition of MCF-7 cell proliferation following 5 days of monolayer culture in DMEM supplemented with 10% FBS. Control (CTL) cells were incubated with vehicle. Data represent the mean percent of the control growth rate (100%). Standard errors are less than 5% of each mean. MLT versus CTL or MLT + NMMA, $p < 0.05$; MLT + NMMA + SNP (all concentrations) versus MLT + NMMA or CTL, $p < 0.05$.

tide hormone relaxin (Bani et al. 1995). This conclusion is provisionally supported by a recent report that physiologically relevant levels of melatonin stimulate NO production in human monocytes (Morrey et al. 1994). When increasing concentrations of sodium nitroprusside (an NO donor) are added to the cell cultures containing melatonin plus NMMA, melatonin's inhibition of cell growth is restored in a dose-dependent manner (Blask and Wilson 1994; Blask et al. 1994), providing further evidence for a melatonin-stimulating effect on NO production in MCF-7 cells. These results also suggest that NO is involved in mediating melatonin's direct, oncostatic action on human breast cancer cells perhaps through an interaction with GSH. Thus, entrance of melatonin into MCF-7 cells to maintain elevated GSH levels may create the appropriate intracellular redox state for the formation of a redox form of NO that inhibits ribonucleotide reductase, and thus DNA synthesis. It may be that melatonin in the intracellular compartment might act as part of a coupling or "molecular switch" mechanism for GSH and NO, perhaps via calcium/calmodulin (Ca^{2+}/CaM), which regulates cNOS (Moncada and Higgs 1993) to inhibit cell proliferation.

Melatonin's Effects on Calcium Homeostasis

Calcium exerts an important mitogenic effect on cancer cell growth, including the proliferation of MCF-7 human breast cancer cells (Banyard and Tellam 1985; Simpson and Arnold 1986). In fact, peptide growth factors as well as estrogen cause an increase in intracellular Ca^{2+} levels presumably by stimulating the influx of Ca^{2+} into cells (Moolenaar et al. 1984; Morley et al. 1992). Calcium/calmodulin, which may be an ER-binding protein (Castoria et al. 1988), also plays an important role not only in the proliferation of normal cells but in the growth of neoplastic cells, presumably by effects on intracellular processes including cell cycle progression and cytoskeletal integrity. For example, agents that increase Ca^{2+}/CaM levels and disrupt cytoskeletal integrity stimulate cell proliferation, whereas the opposite effects are manifested with Ca^{2+}/CaM antagonists (Rasmussen and Means 1987). Melatonin's influence on Ca^{2+} metabolism includes its (1) binding to Ca^{2+}/CaM (Benitez-King and Anton-Tay 1993), (2) action as a Ca^{2+}/CaM antagonist (Benitez-King et al. 1994), (3) ability to modulate Ca^{2+}/CaM levels (Benitez-King et al. 1994), and (4) capacity to act as a blocker of voltage-sensitive Ca^{2+} channels (Vaněček 1995).

In view of the pivotal role played by Ca^{2+} in neoplastic cell proliferation, we tested whether physiological melatonin would inhibit Ca^{2+}-dependent MCF-7 cell growth, as well as whether such an inhibition would be GSH-dependent. MCF-7 cells were incubated in either normal Ca^{2+}-containing Dulbecco's Modified Eagle's Medium (DMEM; Gibco, BRL Products, Gaithersburg, MD) or in Ca^{2+}-free DMEM in the presence or absence of melatonin (1 nM) or $CaCl_2$ (1.2, 1.4, or 2.6 mM). Although Ca^{2+}-free DMEM was used, the serum (10% FBS) in the medium contributed a small amount of Ca^{2+}, resulting in a final concentration in each plate of approximately 0.09 mM as opposed to the 1.4-mM concentration found in regular DMEM. Following 5 days of incubation with no medium changes, MCF-7 cell growth in the Ca^{2+}-free medium was half that of control MCF-7 cells grown in normal DMEM, while the addition of $CaCl_2$ to Ca^{2+}-free cultures resulted in a dose-related increase in cell growth. This result confirmed that MCF-7 cell proliferation is, in part, Ca^{2+}-dependent (Simpson and Arnold 1986). However, when melatonin was added to cells cultured in Ca^{2+}-free DMEM replenished with $CaCl_2$, the growth-stimulatory effect of Ca^{2+} was totally blocked. In fact, cell growth in these treatment groups was actually about 34% lower than in the Ca^{2+}-free control cultures (Blask, unpublished results). Furthermore, melatonin was ineffective in suppressing MCF-7 cell growth as well as inducing any further increase in intracellular levels of GSH in Ca^{2+}-free medium. However, when Ca^{2+} levels were increased through the addition of $CaCl_2$ to Ca^{2+}-free medium, melatonin's antiproliferative effect, as well as its ability to increase intracellular stores of GSH, were restored; this effect was blocked by L-BSO (Fig. 10).

Taken together, these results indicate that physiological melatonin blocks Ca^{2+}-induced growth signaling perhaps by blocking the influx of Ca^{2+} via L-type, voltage-sensitive Ca^{2+} channels, and/or by having other effects on Ca^{2+} metabolism such as altering Ca^{2+}/CaM levels or intracellular Ca^{2+} stores in these cells. Thus, it appears that melatonin's oncostatic action on MCF-7 cell growth in vitro may be a GSH-, NO-, and Ca^{2+}-dependent process that perhaps requires a coupling between these growth signal-transduction pathways, with melatonin acting as a

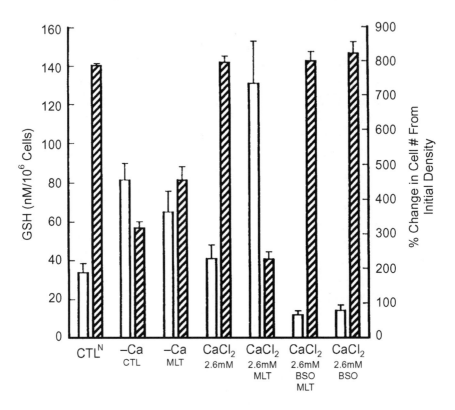

FIG. 10. The growth (hatched bars) and total (reduced + oxidized) GSH levels (open bars) of monolayer cultures of MCF-7 cells treated with either vehicle (CTL), melatonin (MLT) (1 nM), $CaCl_2$ (2.6 mM), MLT + $CaCl^2$, MLT + buthionine sulfoximine (BSO) (10 μM) + $CaCl_2$, or BSO + $CaCl_2$ for a 5-day culture period in Ca^{2+}-free DMEM supplemented with 10% FBS. Data represent the mean ($\pm$ SE) GSH levels or percent change in cell number from the initial plating density. N = DMEM with calcium, -Ca = DMEM without calcium. CTL (-Ca) versus CTL^N, $p < 0.05$; $CaCl_2$ versus CTL (-Ca), $p < 0.05$; MLT + $CaCl_2$ versus $CaCl_2$, $p < 0.05$.

these growth signal-transduction pathways, with melatonin acting as a molecular switch.

Conclusions

Although exogenous administration of melatonin in vivo at a particular time of day (i.e., late afternoon) inhibits tumor growth during the promotion phase of experimental mammary carcinogenesis, it is clearly the oncostatic action of the endogenous, nocturnal melatonin signal that is most relevant to the question regarding influence of electric and magnetic fields on breast cancer (Stevens 1987, 1993). Stevens' (Stevens et al. 1992) original hypothesis held that magnetic fields promote mammary cancer growth either by eliminating or attenuating the oncostatic melatonin signal generated by the pineal gland. Subsequently, the hypothesis was extended to include a magnetic field blockade or attenuation of physiological melatonin's oncostatic action at the level of the breast cancer cell (Liburdy et al. 1993; Blask et al. 1993). As will be evident from subsequent chapters by Löscher and Liburdy (Chapters 20–22), there is some experimental evidence to support both of these aspects of the Stevens hypothesis. Certainly, the pinealectomy and constant-light studies cited in this chapter indicate that eliminating the endogenous nocturnal melatonin signal enhances carcinogen-induced mammary tumorigenesis in female rats. Perhaps even more intriguing is the idea that magnetic fields may have a direct "desensitizing" effect on the human breast cancer cell response to the oncostatic action of physiologically relevant levels of melatonin (Liburdy et al. 1993; Blask et al. 1993; Blackman et al. 1996). If, in fact, magnetic fields interact with melatonin at the cellular and/or molecular levels in cancer cells, then a variety of target sites—ranging from membrane receptors and signal-transduction pathways to nuclear transcriptional events (Table 1)—may be susceptible to magnetic field interdiction of the oncostatic melatonin signal. Hopefully, the foregoing discussion has illuminated some of the possible mechanism(s) by which magnetic fields may attenuate the direct oncostatic action of melatonin on breast cancer growth, and will lead to the design of new experiments addressing the putative link between magnetic fields, melatonin, and breast carcinogenesis.

TABLE 1
Summary of Possible Melatonin Actions on Breast Cancer Growth-Related Cellular and Molecular Mechanisms Encompassing Signal Reception, Signal Transduction, and Nuclear Events

Melatonin Action via Signal Reception
Estrogen receptor expression
Epidermal growth factor expression
Estradiol, prolactin, epidermal growth factor growth signals
Melatonin receptor expression (?)

Melatonin Action via Signal Transduction
cyclic AMP (?)
Glutathione
Nitric oxide
Calcium

Melatonin Action via Nuclear Events
Estrogen receptor mRNA expression
Progesterone receptor expression
Transforming growth factors (α and β) mRNA expression
c-*myc* mRNA expression
c-*fos* mRNA expression
pS2 mRNA expression
c-*erb*2 oncoprotein expression

REFERENCES

Anisimov, V.N., V.G. Morozov, V.K. Kbvavinson, V.M. Dilman. 1973. Correlations of anti-tumour activity of pineal and hypothalamic extract, melatonin and sygethin in mouse transplantable mammary tumours. *Vopr. Onkol.* 19:99–101.

Aubert, C., P. Janiaud, J. Lecalvez. 1980. Effect of pinealectomy and melatonin on mammary tumour growth in Sprague-Dawley rats under conditions of lighting. *J. Neural Transm.* 47:121–130.

Bani, D., E. Masini, M.G. Bello, M. Bigazzi, T.B. Sacchi. 1995. Relaxin activates the L-arginine–nitric oxide pathway in human breast cancer cells. *Cancer Res.* 55:5272–5275.

Banyard, M.R.C., R.L. Tellam. 1985. The free cytoplasmic calcium concentration of tumorigenic and non-tumorigenic human somatic cell hybrids. *Br. J. Cancer* 51:761–766.

Bartsch, C., H. Bartsch, T.H. Lippert, D. Gupta. 1990. Effect of the mammary carcinogen 7,12-dimethylbenz(a)anthracene on pineal melatonin biosynthesis, secretion, and peripheral metabolism. *Neuroendocrinology* 52:538–544.

Bartsch, H., C. Bartsch, W.E. Simon, B. Flehmig, I. Ebels, T.H. Lippert. 1992. Antitumor activity of the pineal gland: Effect of unidentified substances versus the effect of melatonin. *Oncology* 49:27–30.

Beniashvili, D.S., V.G. Bilanishvili, M.Z. Menabde. 1991. Low-frequency electromagnetic radiation enhances the induction of rat mammary tumors by nitrosomethyl urea. *Cancer Lett.* 61:75–79.

Benitez-King, G., F. Anton-Tay. 1993. Calmodulin mediates melatonin cytoskeletal effects. *Experientia* 49:635–641.

Benitez-King, G., L. Huerto-Delgadillo, L. Samano-Coronel, F. Anton-Tay. 1994. Melatonin effects on cell growth and calmodulin synthesis in MDCK and N1E-115 cells. In: *Advanced in Pineal Research, Vol. 7*, G.J.M. Maestroni, A. Conti, R.J. Reiter, eds., pp. 57–61. London: John Libbey.

Bitonti, A.J., J.A. Dumont, T.L. Bush, E.A. Cashmain, D.E. Cross-Doersen, P.S. Wright, D.P. Matthews, J.R. McCarthy, D.A. Kaplan. 1994. Regression of human breast tumor xenografts in response to (E)-2'-deoxy-2'-(fluoromethylene) cytidine, an inhibitor of ribonucleoside diphosphate reductase. *Cancer Res.* 54:1485–1490.

Blackman, C.F., S.G. Benane, D.E. House, J.P. Blanchard. 1996. Independent replication of the 12 mG magnetic field effect on melatonin and MCF-7 cells in vitro. In: Abstracts of the 18th Annual Bioelectromagnetics Society Meeting, June 9–14, 1996, Victoria, B.C., Canada, #A-1-2, pp. 1–2.

Blask, D.E. 1984. The pineal: An oncostatic gland? In: *The Pineal Gland*, R.J. Reiter, ed., pp. 253–284. New York: Raven Press.

Blask, D.E. 1990. The emerging role of the pineal gland and melatonin in oncogenesis. In: *Extremely Low Frequency Electromagnetic Fields:*

The Question of Cancer, B.W. Wilson, R.G. Stevens, L.E. Anderson, eds., pp. 319–335. Columbus, Ohio: Battelle Press.

Blask, D.E. 1993. Melatonin in oncology. In: *Melatonin. Biosynthesis, Physiological Effects, and Clinical Applications*, H.-S. Yu and R.J. Reiter, eds., pp. 448–475. Boca Raton, Florida: CRC Press.

Blask, D.E. 1994. Neuroendocrine aspects of circadian pharmacodynamics. In: *Circadian Cancer Therapy*, W.J.M. Hrushesky, ed., pp. 39-54. Boca Raton, Florida: CRC Press.

Blask, D.E., S.M. Hill. 1986. Effects of melatonin on cancer: Studies on MCF-7 human breast cancer cells in culture. *J. Neural Transm.* Suppl. 21:433–449.

Blask, D.E., S.M. Hill. 1988. Melatonin and cancer: Basic and clinical perspectives. In: *Melatonin—Clinical Perspectives*, A. Miles, D.R.S. Philbrick, C. Thompson, eds., pp. 128–173. New York: Oxford University Press.

Blask, D.E., S.T. Wilson. 1994. Melatonin and oncostatic signal transduction: Evidence for a novel mechanism involving glutathione and nitric oxide. In: *Advances in Pineal Research, Vol. 8*, M. Moller, P. Pevét, eds., pp. 465–471. London: John Libbey.

Blask, D.E., S.M. Hill, K.M. Orstead, J.S. Massa. 1986. Inhibitory effects of the pineal hormone melatonin and underfeeding during the promotional phase of 7,12-dimethylbenzanthracene (DMBA)-induced mammary tumorigenesis. *J. Neural Transm.* 67:125–138.

Blask, D.E., S. Cos, S.M. Hill, D.M. Burns, A. Lemus-Wilson, D.B. Pelletier, L. Liaw, A. Hill. 1990. Breast cancer: A target site for the oncostatic actions of pineal hormones. In: *Advances in Pineal Research, Vol. 4*, R.J. Reiter, A. Lukaszyk, eds., pp. 267–274. London: John Libbey.

Blask, D.E., S. Cos, S.M. Hill, D.M. Burns, A. Lemus-Wilson, D.S. Grosso. 1991a. Melatonin action on oncogenesis. In: *Role of Melatonin and Pineal Peptides in Neuroimmunomodulation*, F. Fraschini, R.J. Reiter, eds., pp. 233–240. New York: Plenum Press.

Blask, D.E., D.B. Pelletier, S.M. Hill, A. Lemus-Wilson, D.S. Grosso, S.T. Wilson, M.E. Wise. 1991b. Pineal melatonin inhibition of tumor promotion in the N-nitroso-N-methylurea of mammary carcinogenesis: Potential involvement of antiestrogenic mechanisms in vivo. *J. Cancer Res. Clin. Oncol.* 117:526–532.

Blask, D.E., S.T. Wilson, S. Cos, A.M. Lemus-Wilson, L. Liaw. 1992. Pineal and circadian influence on the inhibitory growth response of experimental breast cancer to melatonin. *Endocr. Soc.* Abst. 1025:308.

Blask, D.E., S.T. Wilson, J.D. Saffer, M.A. Wilson, L.E. Anderson, B.W. Wilson. 1993. Culture conditions influence the effects of weak magnetic fields on the growth-response of MCF-7 human breast cancer cells to melatonin *in vitro*. In: Abstracts of the Annual Review of Research on Biological Effects of Electric and Magnetic Fields from the Generation, Delivery, and Use of Electricity, Savannah, Georgia, October 31–November 4, Abstract P-45, p. 65. Frederick, Maryland: W/L Associates, Ltd.

Blask, D.E., S.T. Wilson, A.M. Lemus-Wilson. 1994. The oncostatic and oncomodulatory role of the pineal gland and melatonin. In: *Advances in Pineal Research, Vol. 7*, G.J.M. Maestroni, A. Conti, R.J. Reiter, eds., pp. 235–241. London: John Libbey.

Burns, D.M., S. Cos Corral, D. Blask. 1990. Demonstration and partial characterization of 2-iodomelatonin binding sites in experimental mammary cancer. *Endocr. Soc.* Abst. 151:62.

Cassone, V.M. 1992. The pineal gland influences rat circadian activity rhythms in constant light. *J. Biol. Rhythms*, 7:27–40.

Castoria, G., A. Migliaccio, E. Nola, F. Auricchio. 1988. In vitro interaction of estradiol receptor with Ca^{2+}-calmodulin. *Mol. Endocrinol.* 2:167–174.

Ceruti, P.A. 1985. Prooxidant states and tumor promotion. *Science* 227:375–381.

Cos, S., D.E. Blask. 1990. Effects of the pineal hormone melatonin in the anchorage-independent growth of human breast cancer cells (MCF-7) in a clonogenic culture system. *Cancer Lett.* 50:115–119.

Cos, S., D.E. Blask. 1994. Melatonin modulates growth factor activity in MCF-7 human breast cancer cells. *J. Pineal Res.* 17:25–32.

Cos, S., E.J. Sanchez-Barceló. 1994. Differences between pulsatile or continuous exposure to melatonin in MCF-7 human breast cancer cell proliferation. *Cancer Lett.* 85:105–109.

Cos, S., E.J. Sanchez-Barceló. 1995. Melatonin inhibition of MCF-7 human breast-cancer cells growth: Influence of cell proliferation rate. *Cancer Lett.* 93:207–212.

Cos, S., E.J. Sanchez-Barceló. 1996. Melatonin reduces the invasion capacity of MCF-7 human breast cancer cells. In vitro studies. In: Abstracts of the 7th Colloquium of the European Pineal Society, Sitges, Spain, March 28–31, p. 75.

Cos, S., D.E. Blask, A. Lemus-Wilson, A.B. Hill. 1991. Effects of melatonin on the cell cycle kinetics and estrogen-rescue of MCF-7 human breast cancer in culture. *J. Pineal Res.* 10:36–42.

Cos, S., F. Fernandez, E.J. Sanchez-Barceló. 1993. Influence of cell cycle phase on melatonin inhibitory action in MCF-7 cells. In: Abstracts of the 6th Colloquium of the European Pineal Society, Copenhagen, Denmark, July 23–27, E26.

Crespo, D., C. Fernandez-Viadero, R. Verduga, V. Overjero, S. Cos. 1994. Interaction between melatonin and estradiol on morphological and morphometric features of MCF-7 human breast cancer cells. *J. Pineal Res.* 16(4):215–222.

Danforth, D.N., L. Tamarkin, M. Lippman. 1983. Melatonin increases estrogen receptor binding activity of human breast cancer cells. *Nature* 305:323–325.

Davis, D.E., D. Hoel, J. Fox, A. Lopez. 1990. International trends in cancer mortality in France, West Germany, Italy, Japan, England and Wales, and the USA. *Lancet* 336:474–481.

de Launoit, J.L. Pasteels, M. L'Hermite, M. L'Hermite-Baleriaux. 1990. In vitro effect of melatonin on cell cycle kinetics of mammary cancer cell lines. *Endocr. Soc.* Abst. 140:59.

Deprés-Brummer, P., F. Levi, G. Metzger, Y. Touitou. 1995. Light-induced suppression of the rat circadian system. *Am. J. Physiol.* 268:R1111–R1116.

DiGiovanni, J., M.R. Juchau. 1980. Biotransformation and bioactivation of 7,12-dimethylbenz(a)anthracene (7,12-DMBA). *Drug Metab. Rev.* 11:61–101.

Donegan, W.L., S.S. Spratt, eds. 1988. *Cancer of the Breast,* Philadelphia: Saunders.

Fiske, V.M. 1941. Effect of light on sexual maturation, estrous cycles, and anterior pituitary of the rat. *Endocrinology,* 29:187–196.

Freiss, G., C. Pretois, F. Vignon. 1993. Control of breast cancer cell growth by steroids and growth factors: Interactions and mechanisms. *Breast Cancer Res. Treat.* 27:57–68.

Furuya, Y., K. Yamaoto, N. Kohno, Y.S. Ku, Y. Saitoh. 1994. 5-fluo-rouracil attenuates an oncostatic effect of melatonin on estrogen-sensitive human breast cancer (MCF-7). *Cancer Lett.* 81:95–98.

Girard, P., P. Potier. 1993. NO, thiols and disulfides. *FEBS Lett.* 320:7–8.

Hamilton, T. 1969. Influence of environmental light and melatonin upon mammary tumour induction. *Br. J. Surg.* 56:764–766.

Hill, S.M. 1986. *Antiproliferative Effect of the Pineal Hormone Melatonin on Human Breast Cancer Cells In Vitro.* Doctoral Dissertation, University of Arizona, Tucson.

Hill, S.M., D.E. Blask. 1986. Melatonin inhibition of MCF-7 breast cancer cell proliferation: Influence of serum factors, prolactin and estradiol. *Endocr. Soc. Abst.* 863:246.

Hill, S.M., D.E. Blask. 1988. Effects of the pineal hormone on the proliferation and morphological characteristics of human breast cancer cells (MCF-7) in culture. *Cancer Res.* 48:6121–6126.

Hill, S.M., L.L. Spriggs, M.A. Simon, H. Muraoka, D.E. Blask. 1992. The growth inhibitory action of melatonin on human breast cancer cells is linked to the estrogen response system. *Cancer Lett.* 64:249–256.

Jordan, V.C. 1994. Molecular mechanisms of antiestrogen action in breast cancer. *Breast Cancer Res. Treat.* 31:41–52.

Jordan, V.C., C.S. Murphy. 1991. Endocrine pharmacology of anti-estrogens as antitumor agents. *Endocr. Rev.* 11:578–610.

Karmali, R.A., D.F. Horrobin, T. Ghayur. 1978. Role of the pineal gland in the aetiology and treatment of breast cancer. *Lancet* 2:1002.

Kothari, L. 1987. Influence of chronic melatonin on 9,10-dimethyl-1,2-benzanthracene (DMBA)-induced mammary tumorigenesis. *Oncology* 44:64–66.

Kothari, L. 1988. Effect of melatonin on the mammary gland morphology, DNA synthesis, hormone profiles and incidence of mammary cancer in rats. In: *The Pineal Gland and Cancer*, D. Gupta, A. Attanasio, R.J. Reiter, eds., pp. 210–219. London: Brain Research Promotion.

Kothari, L., A. Subramanian. 1992. A possible modulatory influence of melatonin on representative phase I and phase II drug metabolizing enzymes in 9,10-dimethyl-1,2-benzanthracene induced rat mammary tumorigenesis. *Anti-Cancer Drugs* 3:623–628.

Kothari, L., P.N. Shah, M.C. Mhatre. 1984. Pineal ablation in varying photoperiods and the incidence of 9,10-dimethylbenzanthracene-induced mammary cancer in rats. *Cancer Lett.* 22:99–102.

Kumar, R., S. Sukumar, M. Barbacid. 1990. Activation of *ras* oncogenes preceding the onset of neoplasia. *Science* 248:1101–1104.

Lawton, I., N.B. Schwartz. 1967. Pituitary-ovarian function in rats exposed to constant light. A chronological study. *Endocrinology* 81:497–508.

Leibmann, J.E., S.M. Hahn, J.A. Cook, C. Lipshultz, J.B. Mitchell, D.C. Kaufman. 1993. Glutathione depletion by L-buthionine sulfoximine antagonizes taxol cytotoxicity. *Cancer Res.* 53:2066–2070.

Lemus-Wilson, A., P.A. Kelly, D.E. Blask. 1995. Melatonin blocks the stimulatory effects of prolactin on human breast cancer cell growth in culture. *Br. J. Cancer* 72: 72:1435–1440.

Lepoivre, M., H. Boudbid, J.F. Petit. 1989. Antiproliferative activity of gamma-interferon combined with lipopolysaccharide on murine adenocarcinoma: Dependence on an L-arginine metabolism with production of nitrite and citrulline. *Cancer Res.* 49:1970–1976.

L'Hermite-Baleriaux, M., Y. de Launoit. 1992. Is melatonin really an in vitro inhibition of human breast cancer cell proliferation? *In Vitro Cell. & Devel. Biol.* 28A:583–584.

L'Hermite-Baleriaux, M., M. L'Hermite, J.L. Pasteels, Y. de Launoit. 1990. Effect of melatonin on the proliferation of human mammary cancer cells in culture. *Eur. Pineal Study Group* 161.

Liburdy, R.P. 1994. Cellular interactions with electromagnetic fields: Experimental evidence for field effects on signal transduction and cell proliferation. In: *On the Nature of Electromagnetic Field Interactions*, A.H.Frey, ed, pp. 99–125. Austin, Texas: R.G. Landes Co..

Liburdy, R.P., T.R. Sloma, R. Sokolic, P. Yaswen. 1993. ELF magnetic fields, breast cancer, and melatonin: 60 Hz fields block melatonin's oncostatic action on ER$^+$ breast cancer cell proliferation. *J. Pineal Res.* 14:89–97.

Löscher, W., M. Mevissen, W. Lehmacher, A. Stamm. 1993. Tumor promotion in a breast cancer model by exposure to a weak alternating magnetic field. *Cancer Lett.* 71:75–81.

Löscher, W., U. Wahnschaffe, M. Mevissen, A. Lerchl, A. Stamm. 1994. Effects of weak alternating magnetic fields on nocturnal melatonin production and mammary carcinogenesis in rats. *Oncology* 51:288–295.

Maestroni, G.J.M., A. Conti. 1993. Melatonin in relation to the immune system. In: *Melatonin. Biosynthesis, Physiological Effects, and Clinical Applications*, H.-S. Yu and R.J. Reiter, eds., pp. 289–309. Boca Raton, Florida:CRC Press.

Maragos, C.M., J.M. Wang, J.A. Hrabie, J.J. Oppenheim, L.K. Keefer. 1993. Nitric oxide/nucleophile complexes inhibit the in vitro proliferation of A375 melanoma cells via nitric oxide release. *Cancer Res.* 53:564–568.

Meister, A. 1991. Glutathione deficiency produced by inhibition of its synthesis, and its reversal: Applications in research and therapy. *Pharmacol. & Ther.* 51:155–194.

Molis, T., M.R. Walters, S.M. Hill. 1993. Melatonin modulation of estrogen receptor expression in MCF-7 human breast cancer cells. *Int. J. Oncol.* 3:687–694.

Molis, T.M., L.L. Spriggs, S.M. Hill. 1994. Modulation of estrogen receptor mRNA expression by melatonin in MCF-7 human breast cancer cells. *Mol. Endocrinol.* 8:1681–1690.

Molis, T.M., L.L. Spriggs, Y. Jupiter, S.M. Hill. 1995. Melatonin modulation of estrogen-regulated proteins, growth factors, and proto-oncogenes in human breast cancer. *J. Pineal Res.* 18(2):93–103.

Moncada, S., A. Higgs. 1993. The L-arginine-nitric oxide pathway. *New Engl. J. Med.* 329:2002–2012.

Moolenaar, W.H., L.G.J. Tertoolen, S.W. de Laat. 1992. Growth factors immediately raise cytoplasmic free Ca^{2+} in human fibroblasts. *J. Biol. Chem.* 259:8066–8069.

Moore, R.Y., R.L. Rapport. 1971. Pineal and gonadal function in the rat following cervical sympathectomy. *Neuroendocrinology* 7:361–374.

Morley, P., J.F. Whitfield, B.C. Vanderhyden, B.K. Tsan, J.L. Schwartz. 1992. A new, non-genomic estrogen action: The rapid release of intracellular calcium. *Endocrinology* 131:1305–1312.

Morrey, K.M., J.A. McLachlan, C.D. Serkin, O. Bakouche. 1994. Activation of human monocytes by the pineal hormone melatonin. *J. Immunol.* 153:2671–2680.

Osborne, C.K., K. Hobbs, J.M. Trent. 1987. Biological differences among MCF-7 human breast cancer cell lines from different laboratories. *Breast Cancer Res. Treat.* 9:111–121.

Parker, S.L., T. Tong, S. Bolden, P.A. Wingo. 1996. Cancer Statistics 1996. *CA Cancer J. Clin.* 65:5–27.

Poeggeler, B., R.J. Reiter, R. Hardeland, E. Sewerynck, D. Melchiorri, L.R. Barlow-Walden. 1995. Melatonin, a mediator of electron transfer and repair reactions, acts synergistically with the chain-breaking antioxidants ascorbate, trolox, and glutathione. *Neuroendocrinol. Lett.* 19:87–92.

Rasmussen, C.D., A.R. Means. 1987. Calmodulin is involved in regulation of cell proliferation. *EMBO J.* 6:3961–3968.

Recio, J., M.D. Mediavilla, D.P. Cardinali, E.J. Sanchez-Barceló. 1994. Pharmacological profile and diurnal rhythmicity of 2-[^{125}I]-iodomelatonin binding sites in murine mammary tissue. *J. Pineal Res.* 16:10–17.

Reiter, R.J. 1980. The pineal and its hormones in the control of reproduction in mammals. *Endocrin. Rev.* 1:109–131.

Reiter, R.J., D.-X. Tan, B. Poeggeler, L.-D. Chen, A. Menendez-Pelaez. 1994. Melatonin, free radicals and cancer initiation. In: *Advances in Pineal Research, Vol. 7*, G.J.M. Maestroni, A. Conti, R.J. Reiter, eds., pp. 211–228. London: John Libbey

Relkin, R., M. Adachi, S.A. Kahan. 1972. Effects of pinealectomy and constant light and darkness on prolactin levels in the pituitary and plasma and on pituitary ultrastructure of the rat. *J. Endocrinol.* 54:263–268.

Reppert, S.M., D.R. Weaver. 1995. Melatonin madness. *Cell* 83:1059–1062.

Sanchez-Barceló, E.J., M.D. Mediavilla, H.A. Tucker. 1990. Influence of melatonin on mammary gland growth: In vivo and in vitro studies. *Proc. Soc. Exp. Biol. Med.* 194:103–107.

Scaglione, F., G. Dermartini, V. Lucini, S. Capsoni, D. Esposti. 1992. Melatonin and DMBA induced tumors: Action on growth factors. *Endocr. Soc. Abst.* 1028:308.

Schally, A.V., A.M. Comaru-Schally, T.W. Redding. 1984. Antitumor effects of analogs of hypothalamic hormones in endocrine dependent cancers. *Proc. Soc. Exp. Biol. Med.* 175:259–281.

Shah, P.N., M.C. Mhatre, L.S. Kothari. 1984. Effect of melatonin on mammary carcinogenesis in intact and pinealectomized rats in varying photoperiods. *Cancer Res.* 44:3403–3407.

Shellard, S.A., R.D.H. Whelan, B.T. Hill. 1989. Growth inhibitory and cytotoxic effects of melatonin and its metabolites on human tumour cell lines in vitro. *Br. J. Cancer* 60:288–290.

Simpson, R.V., A.J. Arnold. 1986. Calcium antagonizes 1,25-dihydroxyvitamin D_3 inhibition of breast cancer cell proliferation. *Endocrinology* 119:2284–2289.

Stamler, J.S., D.J. Singel, J. Loscalzo. 1992. Biochemistry of nitric oxide and its redox-activated forms. *Science* 258:1898–1902.

Stankov, B., V. Lucini, F. Scaglione, B. Cozzi, M. Righi, G. Canti, G. Dermantini, F. Fraschini. 1991. 2-[^{125}I]iodomelatonin binding in normal and neoplastic tissues. In: *Role of Melatonin and Pineal Peptides in Neuroimmunomodulation*, F. Fraschini, R.J. Reiter, eds., pp. 117–125. New York: Plenum Press.

Stevens, R.G. 1987. Electric power use and breast cancer: A hypothesis. *Am. J. Epidemiol.* 125:556–561.

Stevens, R.G. 1993. Breast cancer and electric power. *Biomed. & Pharmacother.* 47:435–438.

Stevens, R.G., S. Davis, D.B. Thomas, L.E. Anderson, B.W. Wilson. 1992. Electric power, pineal function, and the risk of breast cancer. *FASEB J.* 6:853–660.

Subramanian, A., L. Kothari, L. 1991a. Melatonin, a suppressor of spontaneous murine mammary tumors. *J. Pineal Res.* 10:136–140.

Subramanian, A., L. Kothari, L. 1991b. Suppressive effect by melatonin on different phases of 9,10-dimethyl-1,2-benzanthracene (DMBA)-induced rat mammary gland carcinogenesis. *Anti-Cancer Drugs* 2:297–303.

Tamarkin, L., M. Cohen, D. Roselle, C. Reichter, M. Lippman, B. Chabner. 1981. Melatonin inhibition and pinealectomy enhancement of 7-12-dimethylbenz(a)-anthracene-induced mammary tumors in rat. *Cancer Res.* 41:4432–4436.

Tamarkin, L., D. Danforth, A. Lichter, E. De Moss, M. Cohen, B.Chabner, M. Lippman. 1983. Decreased nocturnal plasma melatonin peak in patients with estrogen receptor positive breast cancer. *Science* 216:1003–1005.

Tan, D.-X., R.J. Reiter, L.-D. Chen, B. Poeggeler, L.C. Manchester, L.R. Barlow-Walden. 1994. Both physiological and pharmacological levels of melatonin reduce DNA adduct formation induced by the carcinogen safrole. *Carcinogenesis* 15:215–218.

van der Burg, B., R.P. de Groot, L. Isbrucker, W. Kruijer, S.W. de Latt. 1990. Stimulation of TPA-responsive element activity by a cooperative action of insulin and estrogen in human breast cancer cells. *Mol. Endocrinol.* 4:1720–1726.

Vaněček, J. 1995. Melatonin inhibits increase of intracellular calcium and cyclic AMP in neonatal rat pituitary via independent pathways. *Mol. Cell. Endocr.* 107:149–153.

Vaticon, M.D., C. Fernandez-Galaz, A. Esquinfino, A. Tejero, E. Aguilar. 1980. Effects of constant light on prolactin secretion in adult female rats. *Horm. Res.* 12:277–288.

Welsch, C.W. 1985. Host factors affecting the growth of carcinogen-induced rat mammary carcinomas: A review and tribute to Charles Brenton Huggins. *Cancer Res.* 45:3415–3443.

Wilding, G., M.E. Lippman, E.P. Gelmann. 1988. Effects of steroid hormones and peptide growth factors on protooncogene c-*fos* expression in human breast cancer cells. *Cancer Res.* 48:802–805.

Wrba, H., F. Halberg, A. Dutter. 1986. Melatonin circadian-stage-dependently delays breast tumor development in mice injected daily for several months. *Chronobiol.* 13:123–126.

PART III
Circumstantial Case

SECTION 2
Light Effects on Melatonin

9 Light and Melatonin in Humans

LENNART WETTERBERG
Karolinska Institute, Stockholm

CONTENTS

INTRODUCTION
MELATONIN PRODUCTION INFLUENCED BY LIGHT
  AND DARKNESS
MELATONIN AND MOOD DISORDERS
    Melatonin Monitors the Internal Body Rhythms in Humans
    Diurnal Rhythm Disturbances and Depression
    Seasonal Variations and Depression
FACTORS INFLUENCING MELATONIN PRODUCTION
MELATONIN IN MENTAL DISORDERS
THE LOW-MELATONIN SYNDROME
MELATONIN, CORTISOL, AND MONOAMINE OXIDASE
  IN PLATELETS AS MARKERS FOR DEPRESSION—
  A MULTIDIMENSIONAL ANALYSIS
MELATONIN AND LIGHT TREATMENT IN DEPRESSION
    Outcome of 10 Days of Light Treatment in Depression
GENERAL EFFECTS OF LIGHT ON MELATONIN
MELATONIN RECEPTORS IDENTIFIED
MELATONIN SEPARATES SUBGROUPS OF INDIVIDUALS WITH
  "ELECTRIC HYPERSENSITIVITY"
MELATONIN AS A POTENTIAL THERAPEUTIC AGENT
REFERENCES

233

INTRODUCTION

Melatonin production in the pineal gland of mammals follows a free-running endogenous rhythm with a period approximating 24 hours. This endogenous rhythm is synchronized to the light–dark cycle by light suppression of pineal melatonin synthesis acting though the suprachiasmatic nucleus (Klein et al. 1991). As a result, in the adult, melatonin is produced at night and its synthesis is suppressed during the day. The duration of daylight and darkness varies both with season and latitude, and these variables, in turn, affect the supply of food. The duration of darkness also regulates the duration of melatonin production in some species, particularly seasonal breeders; by acting as a gonadal repressor, melatonin serves to coordinate the time of birth with available food supply, and thereby enhances survival (Reiter 1991).

Already at the beginning of the 20th century, Simpsom and Galbraith (1906) observed that variations in body temperature (lower temperature at night), are influenced by the light–dark cycle. In the 1950s, Pittendrigh (1954) demonstrated that an inner biological clock governed temperature control. Suprachiasmatic nuclei of the hypothalamus in the midbrain serve as regulators of endogenous rhythms. Suprachiasmatic nuclei cells have been transplanted from one strain of hamsters with a short diurnal rhythm to another strain, with the result that the shorter rhythm from the host strain was transferred to the recipient (Ralph et al. 1990). Further investigations point to the importance of light for synchronizing circadian rhythms in general (Pittendrigh 1954, 1979).

MELATONIN PRODUCTION INFLUENCED BY LIGHT AND DARKNESS

Both light and darkness affect pineal melatonin production (Wetterberg 1978). Formation of melatonin from the pineal gland is rhythmically regulated by alterations in light/darkness that affect noradrenaline concentrations through nerve pathways from the retina to the hypothalamus and suprachiasmatic nuclei, via the thoracic spinal cord and upper cervical ganglion to the pineal gland. The nerve endings release noradrenaline at the β-adrenergic receptors, which stimulates the transformation of ATP to cyclic AMP (cAMP) and thereby increases protein synthesis in the pineal gland. The activity of two enzymes, serotonin N-acetyl transferase (NAT) and hydroxyindole-O-methyl transferase (HIOMT), increases in darkness and makes possible the synthesis of melatonin from serotonin. Melatonin is immediately secreted from the pineal gland into the blood. Blood levels of melatonin reach their highest values during the night at about 0200 hours. During daytime and with exposure to bright light at night, melatonin formation decreases.

MELATONIN AND MOOD DISORDERS

Melatonin Monitors Internal Body Rhythms in Humans

Melatonin has been studied in depressive disorders since Wetterberg et al. (1979) reported a patient with higher cortisol levels during depression than during recovery, and with a concomitant decrease in the nocturnal serum melatonin level from 0.12 nmol/L to 0.06 nmol/L. Also in this patient, the peak level of melatonin occurred earlier (midnight) during the depressive episode than during recovery (0400 hours). The potential use of melatonin as a biological marker in depression was obvious. Not only is melatonin dependent on both noradrenergic and serotonergic transmissions for its regulation, it also seems to be related to the hypothalamic-pituitary-adrenal (HPA) axis, which is affected in depressive states [elevated nocturnal cortisol levels and early escape in the dexamethasone suppression test (DST)]. In adult patients with depression, a coupling between the rhythms of secretion of melatonin and of cortisol (adrenal cortical hormone), as well as possible rhythm disturbances of these two hormones, were reported by Wetterberg et al. (1979).

Additionally, melatonin is useful in indicating the phase and amplitude of the biological clock mechanism. The variation in melatonin concentrations over a 24-hour period allows scientists to study the hypothesis of free-running rhythm failure in subtypes of depression, and to test the phase-advance theory of affective illness introduced by Halberg (1968). Free-running rhythm refers to the genetically determined internal rhythm, which each healthy individual may display when isolated from all external time cues. Normally, the internal body rhythm is synchronized with the external clock; i.e., the light–dark cycle arising from the sun–earth rotation. A free-running rhythm may be longer or shorter than 24 hours; this is the basis for the term circadian, meaning nearly 24 hours. Phase advance refers to a behavioral or hormonal rhythm with an appearance earlier than its normal circadian pattern. The phase-advance theory of manic-depressive illness hypothesizes a pathological, phase-advanced free-running rhythm, which is based on internal (e.g., body-temperature rhythm versus sleep–wake cycle) and external (e.g., body-temperature rhythm versus light–dark cycle) desynchronization of physiological functions. The phase-advance theory was evaluated by Kripke (1983), who proposed that depression may be the result of an internal desynchronization of circadian oscillators, with the strong oscillator being phase advanced in relation to a weak oscillator. The internal rhythm also could be phase delayed, as has been proposed to be the case in seasonal affective disorder, or "winter depression" (Lewy et al. 1987; Sack and Lewy 1988).

Temporal external desynchronization such as in jet lag can occur in some individuals during flights over time zones. Rapid time-zone changes may even precipitate mood disorders in predisposed persons, as Jauhar and Weller (1982) showed in a study at Heathrow Airport in London. Healy (1987) has convincingly argued for a "circadian rhythm dysfunction in affective disorders" linking "rhythm and blues." It is obvious that as a rhythm-regulating factor and a marker for rhythm disturbances, melatonin offers a valuable tool in research on mood disorders.

Diurnal Rhythm Disturbances and Depression

A disturbed diurnal rhythm—which could include sleep and appetite disturbances, early-morning awakening, difficulty in concentration, and body-temperature variations—is a common symptom in depression. Sleep deprivation is a treatment mode for depression that has been investigated during recent decades. Complete 40-hour sleep deprivation has been evaluated (Roy-Byrne et al. 1984), as well as partial sleep deprivation (Schilgen and Tolle 1980) and rapid eye movement (REM) sleep deprivation (Vogel et al. 1980). These therapies have shown significant improvement in the symptoms of depression on a short-term basis. Sleep deprivation, however, has not been compared to placebo. Also, there have been difficulties in assessing whether the sleep deprivation effect is truly antidepressant or merely symptomatic.

Hypothetically, sleep deprivation operates by a chronobiological mechanism irrespective of whether the effect is antidepressant or symptomatic. This hypothesis is supported by the observation of changes in body-temperature rhythm during this treatment (Pflug et al. 1981).

Acute exposure to light at night reduces the nocturnal decline of core body temperature and inhibits the secretion of melatonin. Results show that the elevation of core body temperature induced by nocturnal exposure to bright light can be reversed completely by circumventing the decline of serum melatonin levels with concurrent oral administration of melatonin. That melatonin acts as the mediator of the effect of light on core body temperature provides a rationale for the use of oral melatonin as an aid in the re-entrainment of body-temperature rhythm in desynchronized conditions (Cagnacci et al. 1993).

Seasonal Variations and Depression

Seasonal variations in the incidence of depression and suicide in mood disorders are well-documented (Eastwood and Peacocke 1976; Eastwood and Stiasny 1978; Rosenthal et al. 1983). Circannual rhythms in pineal function in animals have been reported over the last two decades (Griffiths et al. 1979; Illnerová and Vaněček 1980). Seasonal variation in pineal gland weights in human autopsy material has been described (Wetterberg 1978). Seasonal variations in melatonin production measured in 24-hour serum levels and in urine have been shown at least on some latitudes (Arendt et al. 1977; Wetterberg et al. 1981; Wirz-Justice and Arendt 1979). Based on these reports, it is probable that some forms of depression could be biochemically linked to a disturbance in melatonin production, secretion, or function. The close relationship between the pituitary, adrenal, thyroid, and gonadal systems and the pineal gland, and especially melatonin, may be reflected in corresponding neuropsychoendocrine dysfunctions of clinical importance. Serum and plasma melatonin determinations may thus be of interest in different disease states and diagnostic subgroups.

Factors Influencing Melatonin Production

It is clear that factors other than psychiatric diagnoses are of importance for melatonin levels. It has been reported that bright light (Lewy et al. 1980; Wetterberg 1978), age (Attanasio et al. 1985; Iguchi et al. 1982; Nair et al. 1986; Sharma et al. 1989; Thomas and Miles 1989; Waldhauser and Waldhauser 1988, review; Wetterberg 1979), body weight (Arendt et al. 1982; Ferrier et al. 1982), body height (Beck-Friis et al. 1984), use of glasses (Erikson et al. 1983), use of drugs (e.g., β-adrenergic receptor blocking agents: Beck-Friis et al. 1983; Hanssen et al. 1977; Moore et al. 1979; chlorpromazine: Smith et al. 1979; antide-pressant drugs: for review see Checkley and Palazidou 1988), and genetic variation (Wetterberg et al. 1983) are among factors that, to dif-ferent degrees and under various circumstances, may influence mela-tonin levels in humans.

In addition, melatonin antiserum may react with platicizers such as dimethyl phthalate, which may be found in various plastic materials and as an ingredient of insect-repellent formulations (Wetterberg et al. 1984). When sampling tissues, it is important to avoid platicizers in the collection tubes and pipettes. Furthermore, the platicizers may inter-fere with melatonin function and affect various mechanisms that depend on intact melatonin receptors, as has recently been discussed in relation to environmental hazards of different plastic material.

The issue of age and melatonin has been addressed separately in a comparative study between healthy controls and two groups of patients, one with depression and one with alcoholism (Wetterberg et al. 1992). Two normal control populations, separated by 8,000 miles and 24 degrees of latitude, had similar mean values for overnight uri-nary melatonin concentrations. These values were significantly higher than 6-month values for depressed subjects and abstinent alcoholic subjects, while means for the two clinical populations were similar. Age and urinary melatonin concentrations in the control and clinical populations were inversely related, but the slopes of the linear regres-sion equations were 10 times steeper for the control groups than for the clinical populations. Differences in age and sex distribution accounted for some of the disparities, although controls still differed from the clinical populations, even after sex and age were factored out. The disparate slopes for age and melatonin concentrations may con-tribute to some of the conflicting findings of studies comparing popu-lations of different ages. The total melatonin content in the samples from alcoholic subjects, but not the depressed subjects, was lower than that for controls. The difference in melatonin concentration between controls and patients was not accounted for by difference in duration of urinary collection period, hours of sleep, or body weight.

Defining the influence of season and latitude on melatonin production has become important in interpreting the growing literature on melatonin in health and disease. These factors are potential variables and conceivably could contribute to the resolution of contradictory findings. A recent worldwide study on nighttime melatonin production provided a unique opportunity to examine for geographic and seasonal effects on normative nighttime urinary melatonin concentration (Wetterberg et al. 1993). In this study, monthly melatonin concentrations were obtained on normal subjects of varying ethnicity living in widely different climatic, dietary, social, and geographic circumstances. The study was carried out at 19 centers in 14 countries distributed on 5 continents at latitudes from 31,01° south to 69,40° north. The mean serum melatonin concentration for 321 individuals, (age 39 ± 9 years) from the 19 centers in the worldwide study was 274 ± 120 pmol/L, with a similar individual distribution at all sites (Wetterberg et al. 1993).

MELATONIN IN MENTAL DISORDERS

Current views on the use of melatonin as a tool in the diagnosis of mental disorders were reviewed by Miles et al. (1988). Other extensive overviews concerning melatonin and its physiological functions are found in three monographs: by Yu and Reiter (1993), by Wetterberg (1993), and by Arendt (1995).

Specific findings relating serum melatonin to clinical variables in patients with mood disorders have been reported by Wetterberg et al. (1981), Beck-Friis (1983), and Beck-Friis et al. (1984, 1985a, b). The conclusions in these studies were based on the examination of 87 individuals, including acutely ill patients with major depression according to the Research Diagnostic Criteria (RDC) of Spitzer et al. (1978), patients in clinical remission, and healthy control subjects. Brown et al. (1987), using the Hamilton factor scores (Rhoades and Overall 1983), reported correlation between the clinical symptoms of depressed mood ($r = -0.43$, $p < 0.04$), reality disturbance ($r = -0.41$, $p < 0.04$), and a decrease of nocturnal serum melatonin, but no correlation for symptom clusters of somatization, diurnal variation, agitation/anxiety, weight loss, or cognitive or vegetative factors. The symptom clusters of depressed mood also included motor retardation, inability to work, suicide items, indications of reality disturbance, symptoms of guilt feelings, depersonalization, and paranoid symptoms such as suspiciousness, referential thinking, and delusions. In summary, nighttime melatonin levels may vary in different groups of depressed patients. Several studies have, however, found samples of patients with low nighttime levels of melatonin.

THE LOW-MELATONIN SYNDROME

The clinical finding of a subgroup of depression with "low-melatonin syndrome" was introduced by our research team (Beck-Friis 1983). The study included 31 acutely depressed inpatients diagnosed with major depressive illness according to RDC (Spitzer et al. 1978) and 33 healthy control subjects. Seventeen of the depressed patients had early escape of DST (serum cortisol not suppressed by dexamethasone) and 15 had a normal DST. Twenty-six of these patients were restudied 1 month to 1 year later while in a state of partial or complete remission. Clinical ratings were made with the Comprehensive Psychopathological Rating Scale (CPRS) (Åsberg et al. 1978).

When the depressed patients were divided into those with an abnormal response to the DST (DST+) and those with a normal response (DST-), a statistical difference was found. Melatonin (MT) max in the DST+ depressed patients (n = 17) was 0.19 ± 0.03 nmol/L; in the DST- group (n = 15) it was 0.30 ± 0.03 nmol/L. The statistical analysis of the hypothesis of equal MT max between the DST+, DST-, and control groups showed a significant difference in MT max between the groups (p = 0.004). When the depressed patients (n = 26) were restudied in clinical remission, the MT max levels did not change significantly (0.24 ± 0.03 nmol/L in relapse; 0.23 ± 0.04 nmol/L in remission). The same was true for the DST+ and DST- groups. In the DST+ group, the cortisol levels and response in the DST normalized. This difference in melatonin and cortisol levels between relapse and remission led us to test the possibility of melatonin as a trait marker for certain types of depressions. Therefore, we further studied the clinical features of these patients (Beck-Friis et al. 1985b).

Patients with no reported diurnal variation of depressive symptoms (n = 7) had significantly lower MT max levels (0.15 ± 0.05 nmol/L) than patients with reported diurnal variation (n = 25; 0.26 ± 0.03 nmol/L, p = 0.047). Patients with no more than three registered depressive periods in the summer (June–August) (n = 12) had significantly lower mean MT max levels (0.17 ± 0.04 nmol/L) than patients with three or less corresponding periods (n = 20). When the number of months with registered depressions was divided by the number of registered depressive episodes, patients in the DST+ group had a significantly higher quotient (7.4 ± 1.0 nmol/L) than patients in the DST- group (4.1 ± 0.2 nmol/L, p = 0.01), indicating that patients with abnormal DST had longer depressive episodes. A trend toward higher frequency of patients with more than three registered depressive periods during the summer was found in the DST+ group compared to the DST- group (p = 0.08). Eight of 12 (67%) of the patients in the DST- group, but only 3 of 16 (19%) of the patients in the DST+ group reported an increase of depressive symptoms during the spring (p = 0.02). Patients in the DST+ group seemed to have their depressive episodes more equally distributed during the year, in contrast to the patients in the DST- group, who tended to have their depressive episodes more frequently in spring and autumn (Beck-Friis et al. 1985b).

It was suggested that the following features constitute a low-melatonin syndrome: low nocturnal melatonin levels, an abnormal DST, a disturbed 24-hour rhythm of cortisol, and, as the main clinical feature, a less pronounced daily and annual cyclic variation in depressive symptomatology. Clinically, this means that the depression is more or less unlinked to the influence of external temporal cues. In this study, there was a correlation between low nocturnal melatonin levels and the symptoms of lassitude, sadness, and inability to feel, as reported on the CPRS clinical rating. Also, there was a correlation between low melatonin levels and cluster of conative and emotional retardation symptoms. Findings by Brown et al. (1987) also support the correlation between low melatonin levels and depressed mood and/or retardation symptoms. The different studies about depression and low melatonin have previously been reviewed in detail by Wetterberg et al. (1990).

In summary, all but three studies have shown low melatonin in depressed patients: Jimerson et al. (1977), Stewart and Halbreich (1989), and Thompson et al. (1988). Jimerson et al. used a bioassay, which has not been used in other studies. The patients were diagnosed as moderately to severely depressed, but no clinical ratings were shown. No difference was observed in the nocturnal melatonin rhythm between patients and control subjects during 1 or 2 baseline days, a sleep-deprivation day, and a recovery day. The number of patients in the study by Thompson et al. (1990) [n = 9 (5 females)] does not seem sufficient, especially when testing patients according to their DST status. Furthermore, the selection and diagnoses of patients in this study seem mixed. Six patients were drug-free for at least 1 year, and three were chronically depressed patients admitted for assessment for prefrontal lobotomy and who had been drug-free for at least 6 weeks. Thus, the selection of the patients in this study differs from the selection of the patients in the Stockholm study (Beck-Friis 1983; Wetterberg et al. 1981). Patients with various mixtures of depression were included in the study by Stewart and Halbreich (1989). The authors mention that the high levels of daytime melatonin suggest a nonspecificity of the assay. In our opinion, these three studies do not convincingly refute the association between low melatonin and some types of depressive disorders.

The relation between low melatonin levels and disturbances in the HPA axis has been supported in many studies but not all, and therefore needs further evaluation. Steiner and Brown (1985) and Brown et al. (1985) found melatonin levels to be decreased in depressed patients, but found no association between low melatonin levels and suppression in the DST. Boyce (1985) found no clear association between melatonin secretion and the HPA axis. Lang and Sizonenko (1988) recently reviewed the literature on reported possible interactions between adrenal and pineal functions in mammals, and found that no definite conclusions on this issue can be made as yet; however, they suggested a possible age-dependent relationship. Demisch et al. (1988) suggested in a study of dexamethasone administration in healthy subjects that dexamethasone affects nocturnal production of melatonin by means of mechanisms within the pineal gland. Kennedy et al. (1989) reported on melatonin and cortisol levels in 33 female subjects of comparable age with eating disorders. They found significantly higher nocturnal levels of plasma cortisol in the patients compared with the control subjects; however, when patients were divided according to depression status, those with concurrent major depression had significantly lower nocturnal melatonin melatonin values than the nondepressed groups. The depressed patients in this study also had a significantly lower ratio of melatonin to cortisol.

When looking at the relationship between low-melatonin syndrome and the diagnosis of melancholia in DSM-III-R (American Psychiatric Association 1987), the rigidity of the diagnostic criteria should be taken into consideration. Rigidity of the criteria may explain the lack of a correlation between low melatonin and melancholia in some studies. In DSM-III-R, the diagnosis of major depressive disorder with melancholic features is made by including criteria such as early-morning awakening and symptoms that are worse in the morning. However, Rafaelsen and Mellerup (1978) showed that the diurnal symptom variation disappeared during the most severe states of melancholia, but reappeared when the patients had started responding to treatment. Thus, the diurnal rhythm disturbances in melancholia are dynamic, not static.

Furthermore, in a Swedish study by von Knorring et al. (1977), early awakening and increased dysphoric mood in the early morning were not specific for "depressive syndrome" but were typically also seen in other diagnostic groups; e.g., in those with anxiety disorders and neurotic depressions. Rhythmic variations of melancholic symptoms therefore seem to relate more closely to health than to the most severe state of melancholia. In a chronobiological sense, health can be defined as the individual's maintained ability to make rhythms well-functioning; i.e., to adapt external and internal biological rhythms. Melatonin and a normal pineal function seem to be involved in this adaptation. In depressed patients, therefore, low melatonin levels hypothetically may impair this adaptation with a subsequent locked rhythmic capacity manifested in persistence of dysphoric mood and prolonged depressive episodes. The finding of our study that patients with low-melatonin syndrome could have longer depressive periods than patients with higher melatonin levels also may indicate that the low-melatonin patient group received inadequate therapy.

Melatonin levels could serve as a marker for noradrenergic tone in the brain. If low melatonin concentrations reflect a deficiency of noradrenaline at receptor sites, the possibility that the low-melatonin syndrome might respond to noradrenergic antidepressive pharmacotherapy should be tested. A dysfunction in the serotonergic system could theoretically also lead to a low-melatonin syndrome. The diagnostic categories in DSM-IV (American Psychiatric Association 1994), with specifiers for melancholic features, atypical features, and seasonal pattern, allow for symptomatic classifications of major depressive disorders and will be helpful in the further diagnostics using several biological markers, one of which is melatonin. On the functional level, low-melatonin syndrome in depression may be interpreted as a loss of rhythm amplitude, which could be a sign of dysfunction between the pineal gland and the suprachiasmatic nuclei in the hypothalamus (Klein et al. 1991).

The low nocturnal melatonin levels in these depressed patients is likely genetically determined (Wetterberg et al. 1983). The recent findings by Reppert et al. (1996) of melatonin receptors in the "biological clock" are in line with such a hypothesis. A new frontier in the knowledge about melatonin recently opened up when Reppert's group reported on two specific types of melatonin receptors, cloned and localized to specific areas on the human genome. Melatonin1a (Mel_{1a}) receptors are mapped to chromosome 4q35.1 and may be involved in genetically based circadian and neuroendocrine disorders (Slaugenhaupt et al. 1995). The Melatonin1b (Mel_{1b}) receptors, which are localized to chromosome 11q21-22 (Reppert et al. 1995), may mediate the action of melatonin on the retinal level and participate in some of the atypical mood disorders responding to light treatment.

The genetically predisposed pineal rhythm function and the melatonin levels may be influenced by environmental factors in critical periods of life; e.g., impaired parent–child relationship, early psychic traumas, or other stressful factors in the first few years of life, when the fundamentals of self-esteem and self-respect are laid down. Psychological injuries and traumas during such critical periods, hypothetically, could influence the ground for self-esteem according to the concepts of the narcissistic development formulated by Kohut (1971) and Kernberg (1975), and also could influence the soma (e.g., the endocrine system). Such a hypothesis is supported by the findings of Yuwiler (1985), who reported that steroid treatment in newborn rats reduced normal catecholamine-induced increase in pineal NAT activity, indicating that stress in the neonatal period can alter pineal function. These animal studies support some of the psychoanalytic theories about the relationship between stress exposure and psychic trauma in early childhood and adult psychopathology. Breier et al. (1988) recently reported a significant correlation between early parental loss, development of adult psychopathology, and endocrine changes in the HPA axis with elevated levels of cortisol and adrenocorticotropic hormone (ACTH). In the aforementioned study by Beck-Friis et al. (1985b), depressed adult patients but not the healthy subjects who lost one parent before the age of 17, whether by death or divorce, had very low levels of nocturnal melatonin and differed from patients with no reported parental loss. If this hypothesis holds true, many individuals in western societies who live in a single-parent household may be at risk for melatonin deficiency and the subsequent potential health risks.

The question arises whether low melatonin is a state or trait marker for depression (Miles and Thomas 1988; Sack and Lewy 1988). Relating melatonin and pineal function to the "rhythm-generating system," low melatonin in depressive states—as expressed in the low-melatonin syndrome—can be seen as a trait marker for the clinical time course of the depressive state. However, in other subtypes of mood disorders not related to melatonin—e.g., in patients with bipolar disorders and, hypothetically, especially in patients with rapid cycling (DSM-IV) (i.e., patients with rapid and sudden mood swings)—changes in the melatonin secretion amplitude also may be state-dependent.

MELATONIN, CORTISOL, AND MONOAMINE OXIDASE IN PLATELETS AS MARKERS FOR DEPRESSION—A MULTIDIMENSIONAL ANALYSIS

New diagnostic trends emphasize the importance of reliable biological markers to differentiate subtypes of depressive disorders. This differentiation will enable clinicians to choose the appropriate therapy for the individual patient and/or to better predict the patient's response to different biological therapies such as pharmacotherapy, light therapy, or electroconvulsive therapy.

Multidimensional analysis of several biological factors may reveal hidden subgroups, as has recently been demonstrated in a study of depressed patients where monoamine oxidase (MAO) and cortisol were examined together with melatonin (Wahlund et al. 1995). In the follow-up study, a total number of 28 acutely ill inpatients fulfilling the RDC of major affective disorder were investigated and compared to 20 apparently healthy subjects. The patients were followed for 10 years and the diagnoses evaluated according to the ICD classification. ICD-296 includes 296B, 296D, 296E, and 296X; i.e., unipolar affective psychosis, bipolar affective psychosis with melancholia, bipolar affective psychosis mixed form, and nonspecific affective psychosis, respectively. ICD-300 represents 300E; i.e., neurotic depression. Platelet MAO activity was assayed as well as serum melatonin and cortisol at the beginning of the study. The DST also was performed with the oral administration of 1 mg dexamethasone at 2200 hours and serum samples drawn at 0800, 1600, and 2200 hours the following day. Maximum post-DST cortisol level (Cpdx) were used for calculation. Discrimination of subgroups of depressed patients and separation of controls from patients were evaluated using biochemical variables with exploratory data analysis, principle component analysis, and discriminant analysis.

The multivariate data analysis was performed in several steps: The total sample was analyzed in three dimensions by means of rotating the three standardized and scaled biochemical variables in a 3-D computer program. The data set consisted of two main nonspherical clusters. In order to visualize the 3-D findings, principle component analysis and multidimensional scaling were performed. The principle component analysis was performed on melatonin, platelet MAO activity, and maximum Cpdx; the two first standardized principle components captured 83% of total variance.

The results showed that Cpdx was a powerful dicriminator between patients with affective psychosis and patients with neurotic depression. Using all three variables (platelet MAO activity, peak nocturnal melatonin, and Cpdx), it was possible to separate ICD categories 296 and 300 with a higher accuracy of 90% sensitivity and 89% specificity. Thus, the two clinical subgroups of depressed patients showed diverse patterns in the three variables compared to controls, indicating a biological difference between the clinical groups. Melatonin may thus be combined with other biological markers to improve the diagnostic power of different clinical subgroups. The use of melatonin in combination with such markers may prove useful in predicting a prognosis, as well as in choosing the right treatment for the individual patient with different subtypes of major depression.

MELATONIN AND LIGHT TREATMENT IN DEPRESSION

Although its mechanism of action remains to be explained, light therapy appears to be a safe and useful treatment for patients with depression (Avery et al. 1990; James et al. 1985; Kjellman et al. 1993; Kripke et al. 1992; Lewy et al. 1982; Rosenthal et al. 1984; Sack et al. 1990; Terman et al. 1989; Wirz-Justice et al. 1993; Thalén et al. 1995a). We recently have reported that depressed patients with nonseasonal pattern have less efficient treatment outcome compared to depressed patients with a seasonal pattern (Kjellman et al. 1993; Thalén et al. 1995a, b). Ninety patients with a major depressive disorder were classified according to seasonal or nonseasonal pattern. They were clinically evaluated before and after light treatment in the morning or in the evening. The results of this study suggest a specific nonplacebo effect of light treatment in depressed patients with seasonal pattern. For the present report, we have been using matched groups of patients with seasonal or nonseasonal depression receiving light treatment either in the morning or in the evening.

The amplitude and the circadian phase hypotheses of light treatment in depression were tested using melatonin as a marker of circadian rhythm. According to the amplitude hypothesis, the amount of melatonin produced will increase by light treatment due to increase in β-adrenergic receptor activity. We also tested the hypothesis about the relationship between timing of light and therapeutic outcome to elucidate which one—morning or evening light—was most effective. Some researchers maintain that timing of light is not critical (James et al. 1985) whereas others have reported that bright light is more effective in the treatment of depression when light is administered in the morning (Lewy et al. 1985, 1987). The authors consider that most patients with seasonal depression have a phase delay of their biological rhythm, mainly revealed by the delayed sleep–wake cycle and verified by the dim-light melatonin onset (Lewy et al. 1987).

The phase position of the nightly serum melatonin profile was established before light treatment in depressed patients. The timing of the treatment was given without previous knowledge about the internal circadian phase position in the individual patient. If the phase-shift hypothesis of depression is correct, patients with a phase-delayed sleep–wake cycle and delayed internal rhythms manifested by a delayed melatonin phase position should accordingly benefit from morning light, not by light treatment in the evening. Patients with a phase-advanced sleep–wake cycle and advanced internal rhythms manifested by an advanced melatonin phase should, according to the same hypothesis, benefit from evening light, not by light treatment in the morning.

To explore the relationship of melatonin as an internal amplitude and rhythm marker, we studied depressed patients with either seasonal or nonseasonal patterns and addressed the following questions:

1. Is there a difference in melatonin amplitude and phase position between depressed patients with seasonal and nonseasonal pattern before as well as after light treatment, and when treatment is given in the morning or in the evening?

2. Will the melatonin phase position predict a preferential treatment response to morning or evening light?

3. Is a low circadian amplitude of melatonin related to less favorable therapeutic response?

4. Is the degree of suppression and the rebound of serum melatonin by light exposure at night (2200–2300 hours) correlated to the therapeutic outcome of light treatment?

The light treatment was applied in a room with white ceiling, walls, and floor. The reflection from 24 fluorescent tubes in the ceiling gave indirect light with a luminance of 350 candela/m^2, giving an approximate illuminance of 1500 lux 0.8 m above the floor. The patients were clad in white clothes to minimize light absorption and to give maximal reflection (Thalén et al. 1995c).

The light source was full-spectrum light with one of two different light temperatures: 4000 kelvin (kelvin A, n = 13) and 6500 kelvin

(kelvin B, n = 50), with no significant subgroup differences in assignment. The time of light treatment was either 0600–0800 hours (morning light) or 1800–2000 hours (evening light) for 10 consecutive days. A
light test to measure degree of suppression of serum melatonin concentration and a possible rebound of serum melatonin was performed
with bright light between 2200–2300 hours using the light tubes of 6500
kelvin with a luminance of 350 candela/m^2 as the light source. The light
test was performed with the same light source as during the light treatment. The serum samples were analyzed for melatonin by the radioimmunoassay method of Wetterberg et al. (1978). The lower limit of
detection was 0.01 nmol/L. The intra-assay coefficient of variation for
samples 0.1–0.15 nmol/L was 12.3%; for > 0.15 nmol/L, 7.4%; and for
< 0.10 nmol/L, 28% (n = 100). The interassay coefficient of variation for
serum melatonin levels > 0.15 nmol/L was 4.8% (n = 60). For each
individual the area under the profile time curve (AUC; an index of
melatonin production) for melatonin was calculated by means of the
trapezoidal rule. Because the time points are not equidistant, AUC is a
more consistent estimate of the average hormone level than the arith-
metic mean value. AUC was highly correlated to the maximum nightly
value of the melatonin profile (before treatment: r = 0.95, p < 0.001;
after treatment: r = 0.96, p < 0.001) (Thalén et al. 1995c).

Melatonin phase position estimated as the "time center of gravity"
before light treatment was not significantly related to a month of treatment, diagnosis, or time of light treatment, and there were no factor
interactions. After 10 days of light treatment, patients treated with
morning light significantly advanced their phase and patients treated
with evening light significantly delayed their phase, p < 0.001.
Patients treated with light in the morning had significantly later time
center of gravity than patients treated with evening light.

Outcome of 10 Days of Light Treatment in Depression

Clinical ratings: After 10 days of light treatment, the patients with seasonal pattern improved significantly more than nonseasonal patients
[Hamilton Depression Rating Scale (HDRS; Hamilton 1967) relative
changes p < 0.001]. The mean relative improvement in HDRS was
more than 50% in the 42 patients with a seasonal pattern and less than
21% in the 21 patients with a nonseasonal pattern. There was no sig-

nificant interaction between diagnosis and time of light treatment, nor were there any significant differences in improvement between patients with or without antidepressant medication and patients treated in the morning or in the evening.

Serum melatonin production expressed as AUC was significantly negatively correlated to age [- 0.039 (pmol/L) x (hours/year); p < 0.02]. The patients selected for morning light treatment were significantly younger than those selected for evening light treatment (morning: 46 ± 2; evening: 55 ± 2 years; p < 0.002). The age of the patients was not significantly correlated to the absolute or relative clinical improvement according to the clinical ratings in HDRS. An analysis of regression between the variables of age and melatonin AUC showed no significant differences between patients with a seasonal and nonseasonal pattern. The melatonin amplitude was significantly decreased by light when both patient groups were combined (Thalén et al. 1995c).

There are some specific questions that could be answered about possible differential effect of light on serum melatonin between depressed patients with and without seasonal pattern. There was no difference in melatonin amplitude between patients with seasonal and nonseasonal pattern, neither before nor after light treatment, nor when treatment was given in the morning or in the evening. The melatonin phase position did not predict a preferential treatment response to morning or evening light. A low circadian amplitude of melatonin did not correlate to less favourable therapeutic response. The degree of light suppression or rebound of serum melatonin in relation to light exposure at night from 2200–2300 hours was not significantly related to the therapeutic outcome of light treatment.

GENERAL EFFECTS OF LIGHT ON MELATONIN

There are some interesting results related to the questions about the general effects of bright light on serum melatonin amplitude and phase position. The amplitude hypothesis, formulated as an increase in the β-adrenergic receptor activity at the pinealocytes, would result in an increase in melatonin formation. In the whole group of depressive patients, light treatment instead caused a significant lowered secretion of melatonin.

Salinas et al. (1992) also found that bright light of 3000 lux lowered melatonin but dim light of 300 lux gave a rebound of melatonin. Our finding of lowered melatonin following light treatment argues against the amplitude hypothesis stating that an increase in melatonin following light treatment should indicate an increase in receptor sensitivity related to the melatonin rhythm-generating system. Because we now find an overall significant decrease in melatonin amplitude even in patients with clinical improvement in the depressive symptoms, we may test the further hypothesis that light treatment has similar effects on central neurotransmitter activities such as the serotonin-specific re-uptake inhibitor fluoxetine, which also decreases melatonin levels (Childs et al. 1995) in contrast to fluvoxamine and tricyclic antidepressants (Skene et al. 1994).

Light is likely to act via the retinal-hypothalamic-pineal pathway and lower melatonin levels by effects on the pinealocytes. Continuing the reasoning that the therapeutic effect of light is similar to fluoxetine, light may decrease β-adrenergic function. Fluoxetine alone did not produce β-adrenoreceptor down-regulation, but significantly reduced cAMP accumulation after 2 weeks of treatment (Baron et al. 1988). Melatonin also might be lowered by stimulation of alpha$_2$ adrenoreceptor agonist (Palazidou et al. 1989). Furthermore, light treatment may change receptor sensitivity at the hypothalamic level. There is some evidence in seasonally depressed patients of dysregulation in serotonergic neurotransmission that normalizes following light treatment (Jacobsen et al. 1994). The suprachiasmatic nucleus mediates the reduction in melatonin produced by acute exposure to light at night; this action may be modulated by serotonergic receptor activity (Thompson et al. 1990). It is possible that light treatment down-regulates the suprachiasmatic nuclei output and, as a consequence, the production of melatonin. The findings of similarities between light treatment and the effects of fluoxetine but not of other serotonin-specific re-uptake inhibitors may be a useful discovery in the further elucidation of the antidepressant effects of light treatment.

The effects of light on melatonin have been studied by Terman et al. (1988) and Lewy et al. (1985), both groups reporting phase-advancing effects of morning light in patients with seasonal depression. Lewy and coworkers reported that the changes of melatonin phase were of therapeutic importance, relating a phase advancement of the melatonin rise in the evening after treatment to a better clinical effect (Lewy et al. 1985, 1987).

Lemmer et al. (1994) showed a significant phase advance in the circadian rhythm of melatonin when bright light was given to young healthy individuals in the morning, but not when given in the evening. The two-oscillators hypothesis indicates a different regulatory mechanism for melatonin onset in the evening and for melatonin offset in the morning. It appears that in both animals and humans, the evening melatonin production onset does not necessarily phase shift in parallel with the morning offset (Illnerová et al. 1993). The findings of Lemmer et al. (1994) that healthy individuals do not shift their melatonin phase when light is given in the evening but depressed patients phase shift when light is given either in the evening or in the morning would indicate a disturbance or instability of the evening melatonin onset oscillator in depression. Rao et al. (1992), on the other hand, found no significant effects of morning light treatment on melatonin rhythms in nonseasonal depressive patients. Winton and coworkers found in depressed patients that the clinical effect of light treatment was dissociated from the effect on the nightly melatonin rhythm (Winton et al. 1989). The same research group also found a normal circadian rhythm of melatonin in patients with seasonal affective disorder (Checkley et al. 1993). An interesting finding was a difference in cerebral blood flow between depressed patients and controls in response to artificial light, pointing to the possibility of a general lowered cerebral metabolism in depression that might be normalized by light treatment (Murphy et al. 1993). This hypothesis needs to be tested in further studies. Wirz-Justice et al. (1993) found that morning and evening light were equally effective as antidepressant but did not determine a more exact change of circadian phase position, because serum melatonin was estimated from the excretion of a urinary melatonin metabolite.

The interest in light-regulation of the pineal hormone melatonin as a serotonin-related neurotransmitter has received new momentum since it has been shown that a single pulse of light is capable of inducing the circadian phase-dependent gene expression in neurons (Takahashi 1993). A genetic predisposition for high responsiveness to light may occur in patients with seasonal depression (Nurnberger 1988). The biological correlate to this responsiveness may involve melatonin production, which has been shown to be under genetic control (Wetterberg et al. 1983).

MELATONIN RECEPTORS IDENTIFIED

The altered gene expression induced by light and its effect on melatonin production may account for a specific effect that may mediate the antidepressant effect of phototherapy. Melatonin also regulates seasonal reproductive function and modulates several circadian rhythms in many mammals. The recent cloning and characterization of a high-affinity receptor for melatonin from the human is the next step in the identification of one of the hypothetical vulnerability factors of seasonal depression (Reppert et al. 1996). The receptor genes encode several proteins that are members of a group within the G-protein coupled receptor family. In situ hybridization studies of melatonin receptor mRNA in mammals reveal signals in the hypophysial tissue and the hypothalamic suprachiasmatic nucleus. The high-affinity melatonin receptor is likely to mediate the circadian actions of melatonin in humans.

Only complete results with more patients followed for longer periods and taking the response of several other hormones into account are useful for determining the possible predictive value of the different melatonin measures. The recent discoveries about melatonin receptors will give new momentum to the studies of melatonin amplitude and phase position during light treatment in depressed patients to elucidate interaction with other possible biological correlates.

MELATONIN SEPARATES SUBGROUPS OF INDIVIDUALS WITH "ELECTRIC HYPERSENSITIVITY"

In a pilot study of 354 office workers in four Swedish companies, nightly urinary melatonin excretion was analyzed. Of the 354 individuals, 92 were identified as suffering from "hypersensitivity to electricity" (Wadman et al. 1996). The 92 self-reported cases were subdivided into four groups based on their reported symptoms. The 92 cases and the 262 controls did not differ in their mean nightly urinary melatonin excretion. However, one subgroup with "skin symptoms" showed lower melatonin compared to an other group with "many symptoms" of the "electric hypersensitivity" syndrome. The results suggest that different symptom groups of patients with this syndrome may have some relationship with melatonin levels. Further studies are called for to identify possible subgroups with low melatonin, which might benefit from melatonin substitution.

MELATONIN AS A POTENTIAL THERAPEUTIC AGENT

Should there be individuals identified with very low melatonin, the pineal hormone is now available for treatment. However, clinical trials are needed. In 1995, melatonin appeared in the health stores in the United States, and the claims are that the hormone cures everything from cancer and aging to insomnia and jet lag. The open sale to the public caused a shortage of melatonin on the market (Bonn 1996). In some countries, melatonin is available only by doctor's prescription, or not at all until proper toxicological studies and double-blind controlled investigations of its effect and side effects have been elucidated. There are persons who suffer from melatonin deficiency; e.g., following removal of the pineal gland. Melatonin supplementation has been successfully used in some persons who lack their own production (Petterborg et al. 1991). Melatonin also may correct rhythm disturbances; e.g., in blind children with non-24-hour sleep–wake cycle (Palm et al. 1991). Melatonin is thus a potent rhythm regulatory hormone and is in many countries classified and regulated as a medication.

The recent findings of at least two distinct melatonin receptors, Mel_{1a} and Mel_{1b}, hypothetically signaling different biological messages [e.g., one regulating the sleep–wake cycle and one the reproductive functions (Reppert et al. 1996)], will be helpful in the further search of the proper medical application of melatonin. As a further result of the receptor research, specific melatonin agonists and antagonist are now being developed. These pharmacological tools will be helpful in the further elucidation of the physiological and pharmacological effects of melatonin. There is clear evidence that melatonin is useful when correctly timed in certain types of human rhythm disorders leading to sleep problems. There is, however, insufficient scientific evidence for any other therapeutic use of melatonin in humans as yet, and there is no information on its possible harmful long-term side effects.

REFERENCES

American Psychiatric Association. 1987. *Diagnostic and Statistical Manual of Mental Disorders*, 3rd Edition, Revised. American Psychiatric Association: Washington, DC.

American Psychiatric Association. 1994. *Diagnostic and Statistical Manual of Mental Disorders*, 4th Edition, Revised. American Psychiatric Association: Washington, DC.

Arendt, J. 1995. *Melatonin and the Mammalian Pineal Gland*. London: Chapman and Hall.

Arendt J., A. Wirz-Justice, J. Bradtke. 1977. Annual rhythm of serum melatonin in man. *Neurosci. Lett.* 7:327–330.

Arendt, J., S. Hampton, J. English, P. Kwasowski, V. Marks. 1982. 24-hour profiles of melatonin, cortisol, insulin, C-peptide and GIP following a meal and subsequent fasting. *Clin. Endocrinol.* 16:89–95.

Åsberg, M., S.A. Montgomery, C. Perris, D. Schalling, G. Sedvall. 1978. A comprehensive psychopathological rating scale. *Acta Psychiatr. Scand.* (Suppl) 271:5–27.

Attanasio, A., P. Borrelli, D. Gupta. 1985. Circadian rhythms in serum melatonin from infancy to adolescence. *J. Clin. Endocrinol. & Metab.* 61:388–390.

Avery, D.H., A. Khan, S.R. Dager, G.B. Cox, D.L. Dunner. 1990. Bright light treatment of winter depression: Morning versus evening light. *Acta Psychiatr. Scand.* 82:335–338.

Baron, B.M., A.M. Ogden, B.W. Siegel, J. Stegeman, R.C. Ursillo, M.W. Dudley. 1988. Rapid down regulation of beta-adrenergic adrenoreceptors by co-administration of desimipramine and fluoxetine. *Eur. J. Pharmacol.* 154:125–134.

Beck-Friis, J. 1983. *Melatonin in Depressive Disorders—A Methodological and Clinical Study of the Pineal-Hypothalamic-Pituitary-Adrenal Cortex System*. Academic thesis, Karolinska Institute, Stockholm, Sweden.

Beck-Friis, J., T. Hanssen, B.F. Kjellman. 1983. Serum melatonin and cortisol in human subjects after the administration of dexamethasone and propranolol. *Psychopharmacol. Bull.* 19:646–648.

Beck-Friis, J., D. von Rosen, B.F. Kjellman, J.G. Ljunggren, L. Wetterberg. 1984. Melatonin in relation to body measures, sex, age, season and the use of drugs in patients with major affective disorders and healthy subjects. *Psychoneuroendocrinology* 9:261–277.

Beck-Friis, J., J.G. Ljunggren, M. Thorén, D. von Rosen, B.F. Kjellman, L. Wetterberg. 1985a. Melatonin, cortisol and ACTH in patients with major depressive disorders and healthy humans with special reference to the outcome of the dexamethasone suppression test. *Psychoneuroendocrinology* 10:173–186.

Beck-Friis, J., B.F. Kjellman, B. Aperia, F. Undén, D. von Rosen, J.G. Ljunggren, L. Wetterberg. 1985b. Serum melatonin in relation to clinical variables in patients with major depressive disorders and hypothesis of a low melatonin syndrome. *Acta Psychiatr. Scand.* 71:319–330.

Bonn, D. 1996. Melatonin's multifarious marvels: Miracle or myth? *Lancet* 347:184.

Boyce, P.M. 1985. 6-Sulphatoxymelatonin in melancholia. *Am. J. Psychiatry* 142:125–127.

Breier, A., J.R. Kelsoe, P.D. Kirwin, S.A. Beller, O.M. Wolkowitz, D. Pickar. 1988. Early parental loss and development of adult psychopathology. *Arch. Gen. Psychiatry* 45:987–993.

Brown, R.P., J.H. Kocsis, S. Caroff, J. Amsterdam, A. Winokur, P.E. Stokes, A. Frazer. 1985. Differences in nocturnal melatonin secretion between melancholic depressed patients and control subjects. *Am. J. Psychiatry* 142:811–816.

Brown, R.P., J.H. Kocsis, S. Caroff, J. Amsterdam, A. Winokur, P. Stokes, A. Frazer. 1987. Depressed mood and reality disturbance correlate with decreased nocturnal melatonin in depressed patients. *Acta Psychiatr. Scand.* 76:272–275.

Cagnacci, A., R. Soldani, S.S.C. Yen. 1993. The effect of light on core body temperature is mediated by melatonin in women. *J. Clin. Endocrinol. & Metab.* 76:1036.

Checkley, S.A., E. Palazidou. 1988. Melatonin and antidepressant drugs: Clinical pharmacology. In: *Melatonin: Clinical Perspectives*, A.

Miles, D.R.S. Philbrick, S. Thompson, eds., pp. 190–204. New York: Oxford University Press.

Checkley, S.A., D.G. Murphy, M. Abbas, M. Marks, F. Winton, E. Palazidou, D.M. Murphy, C. Franey, J. Arendt. 1993. Melatonin rhythms in seasonal affective disorder. *Br. J. Psychiatry* 163:332–337

Childs, P.A., I. Rodin, N.J. Martin, N.H.P. Allen, L. Plaskett, P.J. Smythe, C. Thompson. 1995. Effects of fluoxetine on melatonin in patients with seasonal affective disorder and matched controls. *Br. J. Psychiatry* 166:196–198.

Demisch, L., K. Demisch, T. Nickelsen. 1988. Influence of dexamethasone on nocturnal melatonin production in healthy adult subjects. *J. Pineal Res.* 5:317–322.

Eastwood, M.R., J. Peacocke. 1976. Seasonal pattern of suicide, depression and electroconvulsive therapy. *Br. J. Psychiatry* 129:472–475.

Eastwood, M.R., S. Stiasny. 1978. Psychiatric disorder, hospital admission and season. *Arch. Gen. Psychiatry* 35:769–771.

Erikson, C., R. Küller, L. Wetterberg. 1983. Nonvisual effects of light. *Neuroendocrinol. Lett.* 5:412.

Ferrier, I.N., J. Arendt, E.C. Johnstone. 1982. Reduced nocturnal melatonin secretion in chronic schizophrenia: Relationship to body weight. *Clin. Endocrinol.* 17:181–187.

Griffiths, D., R.F.A. Seamark, M.M. Bryden. 1979. Summer and winter cycles in plasma melatonin levels in the elephant seal. *Aust. J. Biol. Sci.* 32:581–586.

Halberg, F. 1968. Physiologic considerations underlying rhythmometry, with special reference to emotional illness. In: Abstracts of the Symposium Bel-Air III, Geneva, Masson et Cie, p. 73.

Hamilton, M. 1967. Development of a rating scale for primary depressive illness. *Br. J. Clin. Psychol.* 6:278–296.

Hanssen, T., T. Heyden, I. Sundberg, L Wetterberg. 1977. Effect of propranolol on serum melatonin. *Lancet* 2:309.

Healy, D. 1987. Rhythm and blues: Neurochemical, neuropharmacological and neuropsychological implications of a hypothesis of a circadian rhythm dysfunction in affective disorders (review). *Psychopharmacology* 93:271–285.

Iguchi, H., K.I. Kato, H. Ibayashi. 1982. Age-dependent reduction in serum melatonin concentrations in healthy human subjects. *J. Clin. Endocrinol. & Metab.* 55:27–29.

Illnerová, H., J. Vaněček. 1980. Pineal rhythm in N-acetyltransferase activity in rats under different artificial photoperiods and natural daylight in the course of a year. *Neuroendocrinology* 31:321–326.

Illnerová, H., L. Samkova, M. Buresova. 1993. Light entrainment of rat and human circadian melatonin rhythms. In: *Light and Biological Rhythms in Man*, L. Wetterberg, ed., pp. 161–171. New York: Pergamon Press.

Jacobsen, F.M., E.A. Muller, N.E. Rosenthal, S. Rogers, J.L. Hill, D.L. Murphy. 1994. Behavioral responses to intravenous meta-chlorophenylpiperazine in patients with seasonal affective disorder and control subjects before and after phototherapy. *Psychiatry Res.* 52:181–197.

James, S. P., T.A. Wehr, D.A. Sack, B.L. Parry, N.E. Rosenthal. 1985. Treatment of seasonal affective disorder with light in the evening. *Br. J. Psychiatry* 147:424–428.

Jauhar, P., M.P.I. Weller. 1982. Psychiatric morbidity and time zone changes: A study from Heathrow Airport. *Br. J. Psychiatry* 140:231–235.

Jimerson, D.C., H.J. Lynch, R.M. Post, R.J. Wurtman, W.E. Bunney Jr. 1977. Urinary melatonin rhythms during sleep deprivation in depressed patients and normals. *Life Sci.* 20:1501–1508.

Kennedy, S.H., P.E. Garfinkel, V. Parienti, D. Costa, B.M. Brown. 1989. Changes in melatonin levels but not cortisol levels are associated with depression in patients with eating disorders. *Arch. Gen. Psychiatry* 46:73–78.

Kernberg, O. 1975. *Borderline Conditions and Pathological Narcissism.* New York: Jason Aronson.

Kjellman, B.F., B.-E. Thalén, L. Wetterberg. 1993. Light treatment of depressive states: Swedish experiences at latitude 59° North. In: *Light and Biological Rhythms in Man*, L. Wetterberg, ed., pp. 351–370. New York: Pergamon Press.

Klein, D.C., R.Y. Moore, S.M. Reppert, eds. 1991. *Suprachiasmatic Nucleus: The Mind's Clock.* Oxford Press: New York.

Kohut, H. 1971. *The Analysis of the Self.* New York: International Universities Press.

Kripke, D.F. 1983. Phase-advance theories for affective illness. In: *Circadian Rhythms in Psychiatry*, T.A. Wehr, F.K. Goodwin, eds., pp. 41–69. Pacific Grove, California: Boxwood Press.

Kripke, D.F., D.J. Mullaney, M.R. Klauber, S.C. Risch, J.C. Gillin. 1992. Controlled trial of bright light for nonseasonal major depressive disorders. *Biol. Psychiatry* 31:119–134.

Lang, U., P.C. Sizonenko. 1988. Melatonin and human adrenocortical function. In: *Melatonin: Clinical Perspectives*, A. Miles, D.R.S. Philbrick, C. Thompson, pp. 79–91. New York: Oxford University Press.

Lemmer, B., T. Brühl, K. Witte, B. Pflug, W. Köhler, Y. Touitou. 1994. Effects of bright light on circadian patterns of cyclic adenosine monophosphate, melatonin and cortisol in healthy subjects. *Eur. J. Endocrinol.* 130:472–477.

Lewy, A.J., T.A. Wehr, F.K. Goodwin, D.A. Newsome, S.P. Markey. 1980. Light suppresses melatonin secretion in humans. *Science* 210:1267–1269.

Lewy, A.J., K.A. Herbert, N.E. Rosenthal, T.A. Wehr. 1982. Bright artificial light. Treatment of a manic depressive patient with a seasonal mood cycle. *Am. J. Psychiatry* 139:1496–1498.

Lewy, A.J., R.L. Sack, C.M. Singer. 1985. Bright light, melatonin and biological rhythms: Implications for the affective disorders. *Psychopharmacol. Bull.* 21:368–372.

Lewy, A.J., R.L. Sack, S. Miller, T.M. Hoban. 1987. Antidepressant and circadian phase-shifting effects of light. *Science* 235–354.

Miles, A., D.R. Thomas. 1988. Melatonin and laboratory medicine. In: *Melatonin: Clinical Perspectives*, A. Miles, D.R.S. Philbrick, S. Thompson, eds., pp. 253–279. New York: Oxford University Press.

Miles, A, D.R.S. Philbrick, C. Thompson, eds. 1988. *Melatonin: Clinical Perspectives.* New York: Oxford University Press.

Moore, D.C., L. Paunier, P.C. Sizonenko. 1979. Effects of adrenergic stimulation and blockade on melatonin secretion in the human. In: *The Pineal Gland of the Vertebrates Including Man*, J. Ariens Kappers, P. Pevét, eds., pp. 517–521. Amsterdam: Elsevier North-Holland.

Murphy D.G., D.M. Murphy, M. Abbas, E. Palazidou, C. Binnie, J. Arendt, D. Campos-Costa, S.A. Checkley. 1993. Seasonal affective disorder: Response to light as measured by electroencephalogram, melatonin suppression, and cerebral blood flow. *Br. J. Psychiatry* 163:327–337.

Nair, N.V.P., N. Hariharasubramanian, C. Pilapil, I. Isaac, J.X. Thavundayil. 1986. Plasma melatonin—An index of brain aging in humans. *Biol. Psychiatry* 21:141–150.

Nurnberger, J.I., W. Berritini, L. Tamarkin, J. Hamovit, J. Norton, E. Gershon. 1988. Supersensitivity to melatonin suppression by light in young people at high risk for affective disorder. *Neuropsychopharmacology* 1:217–223.

Palazidou, E., A. Papadopoulos, A. Sitsen, S. Sthal, S. Checkley. 1989. An alpha₂ adrenoreceptor anatagonist, Org 3770, enhances nocturnal melatonin secretion in man. *Psychopharmacology* 97:115–117.

Palm, L., G. Blennow, L. Wetterberg. 1991. Correction of non-24-hour sleep/wake cycle by melatonin in a blind retarded boy. *Ann. Neurol.* 29(3)336–39.

Petterborg, L.J., B.E. Thalén, B. Kjellman, L. Wetterberg. 1991. Effect of melatonin replacement on serum hormone rhythms in a patient lacking endogenous melatonin. *Brain Res. Bull.* 27:181–85.

Pflug, B., A. Johnsson, A.T. Ekse. 1981. Manic-depressive states and daily temperature. Some circadian studies. *Acta Psychiatr. Scand.* 63:277.

Pittendrigh, C.S. 1954. On temperature independence in the clock–system controlling emergence in *Drosophila*. *Proc. Natl. Acad. Sci. USA* 40:1018.

Pittendrigh, C.S. 1979. Some functional aspects of circadian pacemakers. In: *Biological Rhythms and Their Central Mechanism*, M. Suda, Hayaishi, H. Nakagawa, eds., p. 3. Amsterdam: Elsevier/North-Holland Biomedical Press.

Rafaelsen, O.J., E.T. Mellerup. 1978. Circadian rhythms in depressive disorders. In: *Depressive Disorders*, F.K. Stuttgart, ed., pp. 409–417. Stuttgart: Schattauer.

Ralph, M.R., R.G. Foster, F.C. Davis, M. Menaker. 1990. Transplanted suprachiasmatic nucleus determines circadian period. *Science* 247:975.

Rao M.L., B. Muller-Oerlinghausen, A. Mackert, B. Sterbel, R.D. Stieglitz, H.P. Volz. 1992. Blood serotonin, serum, melatonin and light therapy in healthy subjects and in patients with nonseasonal depression. *Acta Psychiatr. Scand.* 86:127–132.

Reiter, R.J. 1991. Pineal gland: Interface between the photoperiodic environment and the endocrine system. *Trends Endocrinol. Metab.* 1:13–19.

Reppert, S.M., C. Godson, C.D. Mahle, D.R. Weaver, S.A. Slaugenhaupt, J.F. Gusella. 1995. Molecular characterization of a second melatonin receptor expressed in human retina and brain: The Mel_{1b} melatonin receptor. *Proc. Natl. Acad. Sci. USA* 92:8734–8738.

Reppert, S.M., D.R. Weaver, C. Godson. 1996. Melatonin receptors step into the light: Cloning and classification of subtypes. *Trends Pharmacol. Sci.* 17:100–102.

Rhoades, H.M., J.E. Overall. 1983. The Hamilton Depression Scale: Factor scoring and profile classification. *Psychopharmacol. Bull.* 19:91–96.

Rosenthal, N.E., D.A. Sack, T.A. Wehr. 1983. Seasonal variation in affective disorders. In: *Circadian Rhythms in Psychiatry*, T.A. Wehr, F.K. Goodwin, eds., pp. 185–201. Pacific Grove, California: Boxwood Press.

Rosenthal, N.E., D.A. Sack, J.C. Gillin, A.J. Lewy, F.K. Goodwin, Y. Davenport, P.S. Mueller, D.A. Newsome, T.A. Wehr. 1984. Seasonal affective disorder: A description of the syndrome and preliminary findings with light therapy. *Arch. Gen. Psychiatry* 41:72–80.

Roy-Byrne, P.P., T.W. Uhde, R.M. Post. 1984. Antidepressant effects of one night's sleep deprivation: Clinical and theoretical implications. In: *Neurobiology of Mood Disorders*, R.M. Post, J.C. Ballenger, eds., p. 817. Baltimore: Williams & Wilkins.

Sack, R.L., A.J. Lewy. 1988. Melatonin and major affective disorders. In: *Melatonin: Clinical Perspectives*, A. Miles, D.R.S. Philbrick, C. Thompson, pp. 205–227. New York: Oxford University Press.

Sack, R.L., A.J. Lewy, D.M. White, C.M. Singer, M.J. Fireman, R. Vandiver. 1990. Morning vs. evening light treatment for winter depression. *Arch. Gen. Psychiatry* 47:343–351.

Salinas, E.O., C.M. Hakim-Kreis, M.L. Piketty, R.M. Dardennes, C.Z. Musa. 1992. Hypersecretion of melatonin following diurnal exposure to bright light in seasonal affective disorder: Preliminary results. *Biol. Psychiatry* 32:387–398.

Schilgen, B., R. Tolle. 1980. Partial sleep deprivation as therapy for depression. *Arch. Gen. Psychiatry* 37:267.

Sharma, M., J. Palacios-Bois, G. Schwartz G, H. Iskandar, M. Thakur, R. Quirion, N.P. Nair. 1989. Circadian rhythms of melatonin and cortisol in aging. *Biol. Psychiatry* 25:305–319.

Simpsom, S., J.J. Galbraith. 1906. Observations on the normal temperature of the monkey and its diurnal ariation, and on the effect of changes in the daily routine on the variation. *Trans. R. Soc. Edinb.* 45:5.

Skene, D.J., C.J. Bojkowski, J. Arendt. 1994. Comparision of the effects of acute fluoxamine and desipramine administration on melatonin and cortisol production in humans. *Br. J. Clin. Pharmacol.* 37:181–186.

Slagenhaupt, S.A., A.L. Roca, C.B. Liebert, M.R. Altherr, J.F. Gusella, S.M. Reppert. 1995. Mapping of the gene for the Mel$_{1a}$-melatonin receptor to human chromosome 4 (*MTNR1A*) and mouse chromosome 8 (*Mtnr1a*). *Genomics* 27:355–357.

Smith, J.A., J.L. Barnes, T.J. Mee. 1979. The effect of neuroleptic drugs on serum and cerebrospinal fluid melatonin concentration in psychiatric subjects. *J. Pharm. Pharmacol.* 31:246–248.

Spitzer, R.L., J. Endicott, E. Robins. 1978. Research Diagnostic Criteria: Rationale and reliability. *Arch. Gen Psychiatry* 35:773–782.

Steiner, M., G.M. Brown. 1985. Melatonin–cortisol ratio and the dexamethasone suppression test in newly admitted psychiatry inpatients. In: *The Pineal Gland: Endocrine Aspects* (Advances in the Biosciences, Vol. 53), G.M. Brown, S.D. Wainwright, eds., pp. 347–353. Oxford: Pergamon Press.

Stewart, J.W., U. Halbreich. 1989. Plasma melatonin levels in depressed patients before and after treatment with antidepressant medication. *Biol. Psychiatry* 25:33–38.

Takahashi, J.S. 1993. Biological rhythms: From gene expression to behavior. In: *Light and Biological Rhythms in Man*, L. Wetterberg, ed., pp. 3–20. New York: Pergamon Press.

Terman, M., J.S. Terman, F.M. Quitkin, T.B. Cooper, E.S. Lo, J.M. Gorman, J.N. Stewart, P.J. McGrath. 1988. Response of melatonin cycle to phototherapy for seasonal affective disorder. *J. Neural. Transm.* 72:147–165.

Terman, M., Terman, J.S., F.M. Quitkin, P.J. McGrath, J.W. Stewart, B. Rafferty. 1989. Light therapy for seasonal affective disorder. A review of efficacy. *Neuropsychopharmacology* 2:1–22.

Thalén, B.-E., B.F. Kjellman, L. Mørkrid, R. Wibom, L. Wetterberg. 1995a. Light treatment in seasonal and nonseasonal depression. *Acta Psychiatr. Scand.* 91:352–360.

Thalén, B.-E., B.F. Kjellman, L. Mørkrid, L. Wetterberg. 1995b. Seasonal and nonseasonal depression: A comparison of clinical characteristics in Swedish patients. *Eur. Arch. Psychiatry Clin. Neurosci.* 245:101–108.

Thalén, B.-E., B.F. Kjellman, L. Mørkrid, L. Wetterberg. 1995c. Melatonin in light treatment in seasonal and nonseasonal depression. *Acta Psychiatr. Scand.* 92:274–284.

Thomas, D.R., A. Miles. 1989. Melatonin secretion and age. *Biol. Psychiatry* 25:364–367.

Thompson, C., C. Franey, J. Arendt, S.A. Checkley. 1988. A comparison of melatonin secretion in normal subjects and depressed patients. *Br. J. Psychiatry* 152:260–266.

Thompson, C., D. Stinson, A. Smith. 1990. Seasonal affective disorder and season-dependent abnormalities of melatonin depression by light. *Lancet* 336:703–706.

Vogel, G.W., F. Vogel, R.S. McAbee, A.J. Thurmond. 1980. Improvement of depression by REM sleep deprivation. New findings and a theory. *Arch. Gen. Psychiatry* 37:247.

von Knorring, L., C. Perris, E. Strandman. 1977. Diurnal variation in intensity of symptoms in patients of different diagnostic groups. *Arch. Psychiatr. Nervenkr.* 244:295–312.

Wadman, C., Ö. Medhage, U. Bergqvist, G. Linder, R. Wibom, B. Knave, L. Wetterberg. 1996. Differences in melatonin between "electric hypersensistive" and healthy individuals—A case–control study. Reported at the IOCH Congress.

Wahlund, B., J. Sääf, L. Wetterberg. 1995. Classification of patients with affective disorders using platelet monoamine oxidase activity, serum melatonin and post dexamethasone cortisol. *Acta Psychiatr. Scand.* 91:313–321.

Waldhauser, F., M. Waldhauser. 1988. Melatonin and aging. In: *Melatonin: Clinical Perspectives*, A. Miles, D.R.S. Philbrick, S. Thompson, eds., pp. 174–189. New York: Oxford University Press.

Wetterberg, L. 1978. Melatonin in humans: Physiological and clinical studies. *J. Neural Transm.* (Suppl) 13:289–310.

Wetterberg, L. 1979. Clinical importance of melatonin. *Prog. Brain Res.* 52:539–547.

Wetterberg, L. 1993. *Light and Biological Rhythms in Man*. New York: Pergamon Press.

Wetterberg, L., O. Eriksson, Y. Friberg, B. Vangbo. 1978. A simplified radioimmunoassay for melatonin and its application to biological fluids: Preliminary observation on the half–life of plasma melatonin in man. *Clin. Chem. Acta* 86:169–177.

Wetterberg, L., J. Beck-Friis, B. Aperia, U. Petterson. 1979. Melatonin/ cortisol ratio in depression. *Lancet* 2:1361.

Wetterberg, L., B. Aperia, J. Beck-Friis, B.F. Kjellman, J.G. Ljunggren, U. Petterson, Å Sjölin, A. Tham, F. Undén. 1981. Pineal-hypothalamic-pituitary function in patients with depressive illness. In: *Steroid Hormone Regulation of the Brain*, K. Fuxe, J.A. Gustafsson, L. Wetterberg, eds., pp. 397–403. Oxford: Pergamon Press.

Wetterberg, L., L. Iselius, J. Lindsten. 1983. Genetic regulation of mela-tonin excretion in urine. *Clin. Genet.* 24:403–406.

Wetterberg, L, J. Sääf, B. Norén, E. Waldenlind, Y. Friberg. 1984. Interference with the radioimmunoassay of melatonin by dimethyl phtalate. *J. Steroid Biochem.* 20:63.

Wetterberg, L., J. Beck-Friis, B.F. Kjellman. 1990. Melatonin as a marker for a subgroup of depression in adults. In: *Biological Rhythms, Mood Disorders, Light Therapy, and the Pineal Gland*, M. Shafii, S.L. Shafii, eds., pp. 69–95. Washington, DC: American Psychiatric Press.

Wetterberg, L., B. Aperia, D.A. Gorelick, H.E. Gwirtzman, M.T. McGuire, E.A. Serefetinides, A. Yuwiler. 1992. Age, alcoholism and depression are associated with low levels of urinary melatonin. *J. Psychiatr. Neurosci.* 17:215–224.

Wetterberg, L., G. Eberhard, L. von Knorring, M.A. Kohan, E. Ylipää, W. Rutz, T. Bratlid, V. Lacoste, C. Thompson, H. Yoneda, N.E. Rosenthal, M. McGuire, A. Polleri, M. Freedman, D.J. Morton, J. Redman, J.D. Bergiannaki, C. Shapiro, A. Yuwiler. 1993. Chapter 19:

The influence of age, sex, height, weight, urine volume and latitude on melatonin concentrations in urine. In: *Light and Biological Rhythms in Man*, L. Wetterberg, ed., pp. 275–286. New York: Pergamon Press.

Winton, F., T. Corn, L.W. Huson, C. Franey, J. Arendt, S. Checkley. 1989. Effects of light treatment upon mood and melatonin in patients with seasonal affective disorders. *Psychol. Med.* 19:585–590.

Wirz-Justice, A., J. Arendt. 1979. Diurnal, menstrual cycle and seasonal indole rhythms in man and their modification in affective disorders. In: *Biological Psychiatry Today*, J. Obiols, C. Ballús, E. Gonzáles Monclús, et al., eds., pp. 294–302. Amsterdam: Elsevier North-Holland.

Wirz-Justice, A., P. Graw, K. Kräuchi, B. Gisin, A. Jochum, J. Arendt, H.-U. Fisch, C. Buddeberg, W. Plödinger. 1993. Light therapy in seasonal affective disorder is independent of time of day or circadian phase. *Arch. Gen. Psychiatry* 50:929–937.

Yu, H.-S., R.J. Reiter. 1993. *Melatonin, Biosynthesis, Physiological Effects, and Clinical Applications*. Boca Raton, Florida: CRC Press.

Yuwiler, A. 1985. Neonatal steroid treatment reduces catecholamine-induced increases in pineal serotonin *N*-acetyltransferase activity. *J. Neurochem.* 44:1185–1193.

10 Signal Transduction of Light for Melatonin Regulation in Humans

GEORGE C. BRAINARD
Department of Neurology, Jefferson Medical College,
Thomas Jefferson University, Philadelphia, Pennsylvania

CONTENTS

INTRODUCTION
PARADOXICAL EFFECTS OF LIGHT INTENSITY ON
    MELATONIN CONTROL
THE LIGHT-INDUCED MELATONIN SUPPRESSION
    RESPONSE IN HUMANS
THE ROLE OF OCULAR PHYSIOLOGY IN MELATONIN
    REGULATION
RESOLVING THE PARADOXICAL LIGHT INTENSITY EFFECTS
    ON MELATONIN
THE ROLE OF LIGHT WAVELENGTH IN MELATONIN
    REGULATION
CONCLUSION
ACKNOWLEDGMENTS
REFERENCES

INTRODUCTION

Light is essential to life on Earth. In terms of human life, light can be a potent force for healing and biological change. Over the past 15 years, there has been extensive documentation that human health can be powerfully influenced by light entering the eyes. In addition to supporting vision, light detected by the eyes is a potent stimulus for controlling the circadian and neuroendocrine systems (Aschoff 1981; Wurtman et al. 1985; Wetterberg 1993; Lam in press). The potency of light in regulating human physiology has led researchers and clinicians to explore the therapeutic capacity of light. Increasingly, published data indicate that light may be used to alleviate the depressed mind, resolve sleep disruption, normalize eating problems, quiet mood swings, ameliorate menstrual dysfunction, and stabilize the disrupted rhythms of shift workers and jet travelers (Wurtman et al. 1985; Rosenthal and Blehar 1989; Wetterberg 1993; Lam in press).

This book seeks to explain why breast cancer incidence markedly rises as countries industrialize. A key aim of this text is to explore a hypothesis that may account for the marked breast cancer in modern societies. Stated simply, this hypothesis contends that members of industrialized societies have two novel elements in their environments which may increase their susceptibility to cancer: increased exposure to electric and magnetic fields (EMF), and increased exposure to light during the night (Stevens et al. 1992). This hypothesis is predicated on three sets of observations:

1. Melatonin can be suppressed by light during the night in many species, including humans.
2. Melatonin can be suppressed by exposure to EMF in rodent studies.
3. Melatonin can suppress mammary tumorigenesis in animals.

The principal focus of this chapter is the regulation of human melatonin by light. It is important to note that more than 50 years of studies on the effects of light on the pineal gland in diverse animal species preceded the more recent experiments on the human pineal gland and melatonin (Kitay and Altschule 1954; Aschoff 1981; Binkley 1988). It also must be emphasized that light has many biological effects in animals and humans beyond the regulation of melatonin; for example, to the broader circadian and neuroendocrine systems, as mentioned previously (Aschoff 1981; Wurtman et al. 1985; Wetterberg 1993). Considering the broader capacity of light to influence human physiology and health, the hypothesis at the core of this book may be too restrictive in examining melatonin as the central factor linking environmental light and EMF to the rising incidence of breast cancer. Nevertheless, the melatonin hypothesis is bound to be useful in guiding both experimental and epidemiological investigations.

PARADOXICAL EFFECTS OF LIGHT INTENSITY ON MELATONIN CONTROL

To understand the role of light intensity in regulating melatonin in healthy human subjects, it is useful to begin by considering an apparent paradox. Specifically, two separate experiments were done within the same laboratory, by the same team of investigators, following a similarly structured protocol. As illustrated in Figure 1, the results from these two studies are in complete contradiction. Data from the first experiment clearly demonstrated that exposure to light at 100 lux induced a full suppression of high nocturnal levels of plasma melatonin in normal subjects (Gaddy et al. 1993). Data from the second experiment, however, clearly showed that exposure to 100 lux did not suppress nocturnal melatonin in normal volunteers (Brainard et al. 1994a). How should these results be interpreted? Is one set of data wrong and the other right? Was one of the experiments conducted incorrectly? Are the suppressive effects of light on melatonin not repeatable?

On closer examination, the two studies portrayed in Figure 1 have a remarkable number of similarities. In both experiments: (1) nearly equivalent numbers of healthy subjects from the Philadelphia metropolitan area were studied, (2) the mean ages of the subjects were identical (24 years), (3) the light exposure was broad-band white light at 100 lux, (4) all plasma samples were collected by antecubital venipuncture, (5) exposure time began at 0200 hours and lasted at least 1 hour, (6) the radioimmunoassay technique (Rollag and Nieswender 1976) for quantifying plasma melatonin was the same, (7) the senior investigators were the same, and (8) the data reduction and statistical testing were

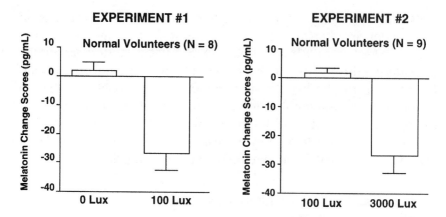

FIG. 1. This illustration of studies on the effect of 100 lux on melatonin portrays an apparent paradox. The two graphs show two separate experiments done by the same research team in the same laboratory. The data from Experiment 1 clearly indicate that exposure of healthy subjects to 100 lux induced a full suppression of nocturnal melatonin (Gaddy et al. 1993). The data from Experiment 2, however, just as clearly show that exposure to 100 lux did not suppress nocturnal melatonin (Brainard et al. 1994a).

the same (Gaddy et al. 1993; Brainard et al. 1994a). On face value, it might be hard to imagine why all these similarities in experimental approach would not yield similar results. Results from various animal species are very clear about the influence of light intensity on the melatonin suppression response: As the light exposure increases, pineal melatonin synthesis is increasingly suppressed following a conventional fluence–response or dose–response function (Minneman et al. 1974; Brainard et al. 1983; Podolin et al. 1987; Nelson and Takahashi 1991). The results in Figure 1, however, are *not* reminiscent of a dose–response relationship between intensity and melatonin suppression in humans.

When confronted by such apparent contradictory data, the skeptical investigator may be tempted to question the overall capacity of light to regulate melatonin in humans. In fact, the literature on the effects of EMF on melatonin suppression may appear to be parallel to the data illustrated in Figure 1. Repeated EMF studies on melatonin within the same laboratory and between different laboratories some-times demonstrate melatonin suppression and sometimes do not (Brainard 1992). At least for melatonin regulation by electromagnetic energy in the visible spectrum, and portions of the ultraviolet spec-trum, the results are not as paradoxical as they might seem in Figure 1. A simple resolution to those enigmatic data can be achieved by under-standing the physiology involved in signal transduction to the pineal gland. Before discussing those ocular and neural mechanisms, it is use-ful to briefly review what is known about the melatonin suppression response in humans and animals.

THE LIGHT-INDUCED MELATONIN SUPPRESSION RESPONSE IN HUMANS

Klein and Weller (1972) were the first to demonstrate acute light-induced suppression of nocturnal melatonin synthesis in rats. Since that time, numerous animal studies have used the melatonin suppres-sion response to help determine the neural and biochemical mecha-nisms of melatonin regulation (Rollag et al. 1980; Klein et al. 1983). In addition, this response has been used as a model for testing the capac-ity of different light parameters for their relative influence on neu-roendocrine and/or circadian physiology (Vaněček and Illnerová 1982; Brainard et al. 1983, 1984, 1986a, 1994b; Bronstein et al. 1987). Complete dose–response curves show that exposure to 1.2 lux and 0.06 μW/cm^2 (0.2 lux) of white light during the night is sufficient to suppress mela-tonin in rats and hamsters, respectively (Minneman et al. 1974; Brainard et al. 1983). Further studies in hamsters demonstrate that even lower illuminances at 0.022 μW/cm^2 (0.05 lux) of monochromatic (500 nm) green light can suppress pineal melatonin (Podolin et al. 1987; Nelson and Takahashi 1991). Other studies testing relatively few illuminances of white light have shown a wide range of sensitivity for melatonin suppression among different species (Reiter 1993).

A set of early human studies failed to demonstrate the acute sup-pressive influence of light on melatonin in humans that had been demonstrated in other mammalian species (Vaughan et al. 1976, 1979; Jimerson et al. 1977; Wetterberg 1978; Lynch et al. 1978; Akerstadt et al. 1979). In those studies, illuminances ranging from 100–800 lux of white light failed to induce any significant melatonin suppression. A major breakthrough was made in 1980 when Lewy and colleagues demonstrated that exposure of the eyes of normal volunteers to 2500 lux of white light during the night induced an 80% decrease in circulating melatonin within 1 hour. In contrast, no significant melatonin suppression was observed in subjects exposed to 500 lux of white light (Lewy et al. 1980). Quite simply, this seminal discovery demonstrated that it takes much more light to suppress melatonin in humans than is required for regulating the circadian and neuroendocrine systems in some animal species. The earlier attempts to suppress melatonin in humans failed when investigators used typical indoor light levels reported to be between 100–800 lux, illuminances which are ample for human vision and more than sufficient for suppressing melatonin in many animal species. The discovery that much brighter light is needed to suppress melatonin in humans led to numerous studies confirming that bright light (2500 lux) entering the eyes of humans is a potent stimulus for controlling circadian rhythms (Czeisler et al. 1986, 1990; Lewy et al. 1987; Minors et al. 1991; Eastman 1992). It is not *entirely* accurate, however, that only "bright" light can suppress melatonin or regulate circadian rhythms in humans.

Following the landmark study of Lewy and colleagues (1980), a study was done to determine more precisely the dosages of light needed to suppress melatonin in normal volunteers (Brainard et al. 1988). In that study, healthy male volunteers were exposed to carefully controlled intensities of monochromatic green light at 509 nm (10 nm half-peak bandwidth) for 1 hour during the night. These volunteers were continuously exposed to the experimental light between 0200 and 0300 hours with their pupils fully dilated and their heads held steady relative to the light source by an ophthalmic head holder. To produce a uniform illumination of the whole retina, the volunteers had translucent white integrating hemispheres covering both eyes throughout the experimental light exposure. As shown in Figure 2, the results of this experiment demonstrated that light affects human melatonin in a dose–response fashion; i.e., the brighter the photic stimulus the greater the suppression of melatonin (Brainard et al. 1988). Other human studies have confirmed the dose–response relationship between light and melatonin suppression (McIntyre et al. 1989a, b).

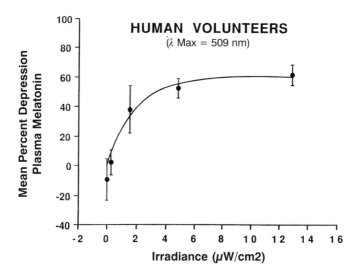

FIG. 2. The dose–response relationship between green monochromatic light (509 nm) exposure of normal volunteers' eyes and suppression of the hormone melatonin. Data points indicate mean ± SEM. (Reprinted from Brainard et al. 1988 with permission from Elsevier Science, the Netherlands.)

It is important to note that all of the stimuli used in this study activated the visual system; i.e., both the volunteers and the experimenters visually discerned the different light intensities and accurately reported them to appear green. The lower light intensities, however, did not change melatonin levels, whereas the higher intensities induced a 60–80% decrease in melatonin. Thus, light that is adequate to activate vision does not necessarily cause neuroendocrine or circadian change. It seems generally true in humans that considerably more light is needed for biological effects than for vision (Vaughan et al. 1976, 1979; Jimerson et al. 1977; Wetterberg 1978; Lynch et al. 1978; Akerstadt et al. 1979; Lewy et al. 1980; Czeisler et al. 1986, 1990; Lewy et al. 1987; Brainard et al. 1988; Minors et al. 1991; Eastman 1992).

The human melatonin dose–response curve shown in Figure 2 demonstrates a concept that may not be readily apparent: *Very "bright" light is not necessarily needed for melatonin suppression.* Table 1 illustrates both the photometric and radiometric measurements for light used in that experiment. Those data reveal that the threshold illuminance for producing a statistically significant melatonin suppression was between 5 and 17 lux in normal volunteers—an illuminance equal to civil twilight and well below typical indoor light. Thus, when the exposure of the human eye is carefully controlled, 25–100 times *less* light can suppress melatonin than originally believed (Lewy et al. 1980; Brainard et al. 1988).

The data illustrated in Figure 2 show mean melatonin suppression values from a group of six healthy volunteers. When data from the individual volunteers are examined, it becomes clear that some subjects may be considerably more sensitive to light in terms of melatonin suppression than others. The results shown in Figure 3 show the individual data from two of the volunteers in that study. Data from volunteer #5 shows that this individual exhibited a 60–61% decrease in plasma melatonin after exposure to an illuminance of 5.5 lux. In contrast,

TABLE 1
Dose–Response Curve for Melatonin Suppression by Monochromatic Light at 509 nm[a]

Quanta (photons/ second/cm^2)	Irradiance (μW/cm^2)	Illuminance (lux)		% Melatonin suppression
		photopic	scotopic	
9.2×10^{13}	0.01	0.03	0.17	−9.67
2.8×10^{15}	0.30	1.03	5.25	1.83
1.5×10^{16}	1.60	5.50	27.98	37.33
4.6×10^{16}	5.00	17.18	85.90	51.67
1.2×10^{17}	13.00	44.66	227.37	60.67

[a] Brainard et al. 1988

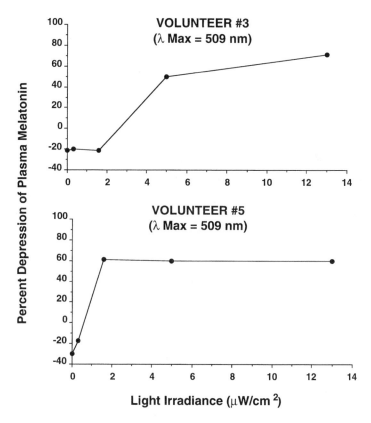

FIG 3. Data concerning the effects of different irradiances of monochromatic light (509 nm) on plasma melatonin in two different volunteers. Volunteer #3 had a threshold for light-induced melatonin 3–17 times higher than volunteer #5. (Reprinted from Brainard et al. 1988 with permission from Elsevier Science, the Netherlands.)

volunteer #3 exhibited no melatonin suppression after exposure to 5 lux. Hence, volunteer #3 showed a 3–17 times higher threshold for melatonin suppression than subject #5. When considering the biological effects of light in humans, it is important to recall that there may be very different light sensitivities between individuals. Furthermore, low illuminances do not necessarily need to comprise a monochromatic green wavelength to have a strong influence on melatonin regulation. Other experiments have shown that: (1) illuminances from 100–630 lux of white light can suppress plasma melatonin levels in humans when exposure conditions are more carefully controlled (Bojkowski et al. 1987; McIntyre et al. 1989a, b; Gaddy et al. 1992, 1993; Brainard et al. 1994c, d), (2) lower illuminances can influence the duration of the melatonin and sleep rhythms (Wehr 1991; Wehr et al. 1993), and (3) lower illuminances of light can phase-shift the human circadian pacemaker (Boivin et al. 1996).

The demonstration that relatively dim illuminances can suppress melatonin in normal humans created the same paradox illustrated in Figure 1. Why did early attempts to suppress melatonin in humans fail when illuminances from 100–800 lux were tested, while later studies elicited full melatonin suppression with illuminances between 5 and 100 lux? This paradox created an open door for clarifying the ocular physiology involved in transducing light stimuli to the circadian system and pineal gland.

THE ROLE OF OCULAR PHYSIOLOGY IN MELATONIN REGULATION

The eyes are the exclusive mediators of vision in all mammalian species. In addition, there is considerable evidence from human and animal studies that the biological, behavioral, and therapeutic effects of light are mediated via a photoreceptive mechanism in the eye as opposed to photoreceptive mechanisms in the skin or some other part of the body. Experimental data support this assumption, specifically, in terms of light stimulation of the circadian and neuroendocrine systems (Aschoff 1981; Binkley 1990; Klein et al. 1991; Wetterberg 1993), and in terms of light therapy for winter depression (Wehr et al. 1987).

Several research groups are working to clarify the details of how light is processed by the human eye to produce nonvisual biological and therapeutic effects. Figure 4 portrays some of the physical and anatomical elements involved in photic regulation of the melatonin generating system. This simplified illustration represents the human eye as the common site for transducing light stimuli to both the visual and circadian systems. An extremely complex rendering would be required to show all the neural elements involved in visual and circadian processing. Extensive neuroanatomical detail related to the

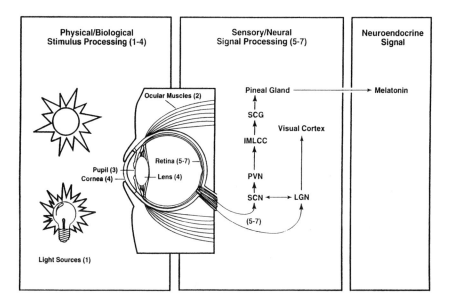

FIG. 4: This diagram portrays the human eye as the common site for trans-ducing light stimuli to both the visual cortex and the pineal gland. Understanding this ocular and neural physiology can resolve the paradox of why relatively dim light can suppress melatonin in one circumstance but not in another. The numbers in the illustration provide a cross reference to Table 2 for access to literature pertinent to the elements in this diagram. The abbreviations are: SCN = suprachiasmatic nuclei; LGN = lateral geniculate nuclei; PVN = paraventricular nuclei; IMLCC = intermediolateral cell column; SCG = superior cervical ganglion. (Reprinted from Brainard et al. 1996 with permission from Walter de Gruyter & Co.)

retinohypothalamic tract, suprachiasmatic nuclei, and the general circadian system can be found in the text edited by Klein and colleagues (1991).

The model system shown in Figure 4 comprises two general categories of elements: (1) components for physical/biological stimulus processing, and (2) structures involved in sensory/neural signal processing. To resolve the paradox of why dim light can suppress melatonin in one experiment but not in another, it is important to consider the physics of the light stimulus, the geometric relationship of the eyes to the light stimulus, gaze direction, status of the ocular media, pupil-lary dilation, retinal field exposure, photoreceptor sensitivity, the capacity of the system to integrate photic stimuli over time and space, and the adaptational state of the system. Each of these elements con-tributes to determining the effectiveness of a photic stimulus in mela-tonin regulation.

It is beyond the scope of this chapter to provide a complete descrip-tion of how the eye processes light for biological, behavioral, and ther-apeutic effects, but three reviews provide more detailed reports on this subject (Brainard et al. 1993, 1994c; Brainard in press), and Table 2 pro-vides access to some of the pertinent original literature. This table lists specific reports germane to the biological or therapeutic effects of light, as well as selected references on light and the ocular physiology of vision. The graphs collected in Figure 5 provide a sampling of the data that address the ocular and neural elements responsible for signal transduction in the melatonin generating system.

It is significant to note that the portions of the eye which process light to produce visual stimulation may or may not overlap with those parts of the eye that mediate the biological and behavioral effects of light. Similarly, there may or may not be different physiological processes for modulating the biological and behavioral responses to light. For example, the ocular media of the eye may modify the char-acteristics of light emitted from a lamp before it reaches the photore-ceptors. The cornea, aqueous humor, and vitreous humor of the healthy human eye are clear tissues which transmit nearly 100% of vis-ible and ultraviolet wavelengths down to 300 nm to the retina, with lit-tle age-related change in the transmission characteristics (Boettner and Wolter 1962; Lerman 1987). The crystalline lens, however, yellows with age and acts as a filter that significantly reduces the total transmission of radiant energy to the retina—particularly in the shorter wavelength portion of the spectrum (Lerman 1987).

The data shown in Figure 5A illustrate lenticular transmission of three different age groups of humans (Barker and Brainard 1991; Brainard et al. 1994c). These data demonstrate that the lens helps determine both the quantity and quality of photic stimuli that can reach photoreceptors for the circadian and neuroendocrine systems.

TABLE 2
Literature Pertinent to Ocular Physiology that Mediates the
Biological and Therapeutic Effects of Light in Humans

Photobiological variable	Anatomical site	Fig. 4 key	References[a]
Light source geometry	External environment	1	IESNA 1993 Dawson and Campbell 1990 Gaddy 1990
Gaze direction and movement	Ocular muscles	2	Sliney and Wolbarsht 1980 Brainard et al. 1988 Dawson and Campbell 1990 Gaddy 1990
Pupil diameter	Iris	3	Lowenstein and Loewenfeld 1962 Brainard et al. 1988 Gaddy et al. 1993
Ocular media transmission	Cornea, lens, aqueous, vitreous	4	Boettner and Wolter 1962 Barker and Brainard 1991 Brainard et al. 1993 Brainard et al. 1994c
Spatial integration of light	Retina–neural structures	5–7	Riggs 1965 Adler et al. 1992 Gaddy et al. 1992 Gaddy et al. 1994 Brainard et al. 1996
Temporal integration of light	Retina–neural structures	5–7	Riggs 1965 Brainard et al. 1994d
Wavelength sensitivity to light/ photoreceptors	Retina–neural structures	5–7	Gouras 1991 Brainard et al. 1988 Brainard et al. 1990 Oren et al. 1991 Stewart et al. 1991 Czeisler et al. 1995 Ruberg et al. 1996

[a] The first reference in each row is a classic citation from the literature on light or the ocular physiology of vision.

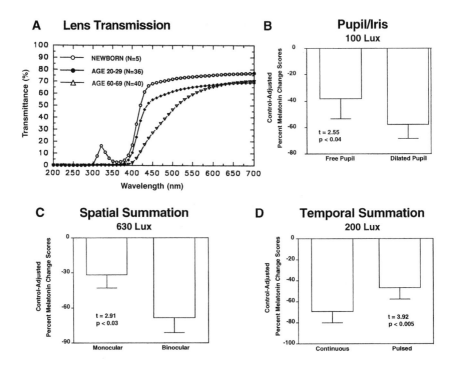

FIG. 5. These figures show data pertinent to ocular and neural physiology mediating the effects of light on melatonin in humans. Panel 5A shows the mean percent transmittance data from three age groups: 0–2 years, 20–29 years, and 60–69 years old (Barker and Brainard 1991; Brainard et al. 1994c). These data demonstrate significant decreases in ultraviolet, violet, indigo, blue, and green wavelengths reaching the retina over the human life span. Panels 5B–D illustrate control-adjusted, percent melatonin changes scores after exposure to a 90-minute, full-visual-field, white-light stimulus from a ganzfeld dome. Data in panel 5B confirm that melatonin suppression is significantly greater when volunteers' pupils are pharmacologically dilated versus when they are freely reactive to light (Gaddy et al. 1993). Data in 5C illustrate that input from two whole retinas produce a significantly stronger melatonin suppression than input from a single retina. Thus, there appears to be a summation of light stimuli across volunteers' retinas for melatonin regulation (Gaddy et al. 1994; Brainard in press). Data in 5D show that over a 90-minute exposure period, a series of 10-minute light pulses is not as effective as a continuous exposure for suppressing melatonin (Brainard et al. 1994d). More work is needed to clarify how the retinal/neural system for regulating the pineal gland integrates photic stimuli over time. (Fig. 5A is reprinted from Brainard et al. 1994c with permission from John Libbey & Co. Ltd. Fig. 5C is reprinted from Brainard in press with permission from the American Psychiatric Press.)

Thus, measures of corneal illumination are not necessarily equivalent to retinal illumination.

Like the lens, the iris of the eye is capable of modifying a photic stimulus before it reaches the retina. The iris can modify the illuminance or intensity of light that reaches the retina by adjusting pupillary diameter from 2–9 mm relative to the brightness of the light. Pupil constriction decreases retinal illumination while dilation increases retinal light exposure. Although it is well known that the iris can enhance vision, provide visual comfort, and protect the retina (Lowenstein and Loewenfeld 1962; Sliney and Wolbarsht 1980), little research has assessed the role of the iris and pupil in modulating the biological effects of light.

To determine if pupillary dilation affects melatonin regulation, subjects were studied on 3 separate nights with at least 1 week between each night of study (Gaddy et al. 1993). On the test nights, healthy volunteers were exposed to (1) darkness only; (2) a 100-lux, spatially uniform white light stimulus that filled the visual field while their pupils were pharmacologically dilated; or 3) the same 100-lux stimulus while their pupils were free to constrict. The light exposures were done with volunteers' heads held steady by an ophthalmic head holder in a ganzfeld dome for the entire exposure period. During the light exposures, the pharmacologically dilated pupils (mean diameter = 7.3 mm) were significantly larger ($p < 0.001$) than when the pupils were free to constrict (mean diameter = 3.3 mm). Plasma melatonin levels were significantly suppressed after light exposure in both the dilated and free pupil conditions compared to the dark exposure control condition ($p < 0.001$). As shown in Figure 5B, there was a significantly greater drop in melatonin when the pupils were dilated versus free to constrict ($p < 0.04$). These data confirm that the iris can modify the biological effectiveness of a photic stimulus for melatonin regulation (Gaddy et al. 1993).

Beyond the physical/biological stimulus processing of light stimuli by the ocular media and the iris, there is sensory and neural signal processing for the biological effects of light. For example, in the psychophysics of the visual system, the retina exhibits spatial summation of photic stimuli. Specifically, the area of retinal stimulation determines the minimum intensity needed for light perception (Riggs

1965). Recent data suggested that stimulation of a larger portion of the bilateral visual field resulted in greater melatonin suppression in healthy human subjects (Gaddy et al. 1992). Given the possibility that photic stimuli were spatially summated within the retinas, the following experiment tested the prospect of spatial summation between the two retinas (Gaddy et al. 1994; Brainard in press). Employing methods similar to those used in the pupillary studies, light-induced melatonin suppression was determined in normal volunteers on 3 different nights separated by 1-week intervals. On different nights, subjects were exposed to: (1) darkness only, (2) a monocular corneal illuminance of 630 lux of white light, or (3) a binocular exposure to 630 lux of white light. Melatonin was significantly suppressed by both monocular and binocular light exposure ($p < 0.001$). The data shown in Figure 5C indicate that plasma melatonin levels demonstrated a significantly greater suppression in the binocular condition than in the monocular condition ($p < 0.03$). Thus, there appears to be an additive effect of the two retinal inputs to the suprachiasmatic nuclei for melatonin control. These results suggest that there is cross-retina as well as within-retina summation for neuroendocrine regulation.

While these data indicate that, for control of human melatonin, light is summated over the area of retina that it reaches, it is unclear if photic stimuli are also summated over time. In animal studies, light pulses or "skeleton" photoperiods can entrain circadian behavioral rhythms and modulate seasonal reproduction similar to full cycles of light and dark (Pittendrigh and Daan 1976; Evered and Clark 1985). In light therapy for winter depression, a standard patient instruction is to "engage in such activities as reading, writing or eating" while concentrating the eyes "on the surfaces illuminated by the lights and not the lights themselves" (Society for Light Treatment and Biological Rhythms 1994). Although this procedure can be clinically effective, such an exposure method can introduce a wide variability in the actual dose of photons that reach patients' retinas (Gaddy 1990; Dawson and Campbell 1990; Brainard in press). Do the retinas and associated neural structures integrate variable photic stimuli over the treatment period?

The following study tested if constant-light stimuli are equivalent to intermittent stimuli for suppressing melatonin. Again, using methods similar to those used in the pupillary study, 12 healthy subjects were exposed on separate nights to (1) darkness only; (2) continuous, full-field, 200-lux white light; or (3) pulsed, full-field, 200-lux white light with lights on and off in 10-minute intervals (Brainard et al. 1994d). Both pulsed and continuous light exposures at 200 lux significantly suppressed plasma melatonin (p < 0.001). As shown in Figure 5D, continuous light exposure caused a significantly greater suppression of melatonin compared to the pulsed exposure (p < 0.005). These data show that over a 90-minute exposure period, a series of 10-minute light pulses is not as effective for suppressing melatonin as a continuous exposure. Further experiments are needed to characterize how the melatonin system integrates photic stimuli over time, and if similar responses are shared for other circadian or therapeutic effects of light.

RESOLVING THE PARADOXICAL LIGHT INTENSITY EFFECTS ON MELATONIN SUPPRESSION

It is now appropriate to return to the paradox discussed at the beginning of this chapter. As shown in the data presented in Figure 1, exposure to 100 lux of white light had completely different effects in two studies with many similarities. The data in this figure mirror the broader published literature. Some studies have shown no significant melatonin suppression after exposure of humans to 100–800 lux of white light (Vaughan et al. 1976; Jimerson et al. 1977; Wetterberg 1978; Lynch et al. 1978; Akerstadt et al. 1979; Vaughan et al. 1979; Lewy et al. 1980) while other studies have demonstrated significant melatonin suppression with illuminances considerably below 800 lux of white light (Bojkowski et al. 1987; McIntyre et al. 1989a, b; Gaddy et al. 1992, 1993, 1994; Brainard et al. 1993, 1994c, d; Brainard in press; Ruberg et al. 1996). The resolution to this variance lies in the specific physics of the light stimulus, the relationship of the light stimulus to the human eye, and the operation of the underlying ocular physiology.

For all their similarities, the two studies illustrated in Figure 1 had different empirical purposes which required key differences in light measurement and exposure. These key differences ultimately led to great differences in results. The first study was aimed at understanding the role of pupillary dilation in the biological effects of light while the second study sought to quantify the biological impact of built-in architectural light. To begin with, light measurement techniques differed significantly between the two studies. In the first experiment, illuminance was measured at the cornea of the observer while in the second study illuminance was measured at desktop. Desktop measurement is a standard technique for specifying architectural illuminance (IESNA 1993), but it can greatly underestimate or overestimate the amount of light actually reaching the volunteers' retina—the biologically effective illuminance. As one reviews the literature on the biological effects of light, it is striking how often investigators do not specify the details of the light measurement technique. Even among those investigators who are clear about their measurement approach, the methods vary widely. Thus, the discerning reader should look beyond simple reports of a given lux level having a specific biological effect and ask how was that lux level measured.

Another key difference between the two studies illustrated in Figure 1 lies in the behavior of the two groups of experimental subjects. In the first study, volunteers' heads were held steady with a constant orientation to a uniform, full-visual-field light stimulus for the entire exposure period. In the second study, volunteers were free to move their head and eyes throughout the exposure period. Normally, the behavior of the human eye is dynamic—our head and eyes are in constant motion relative to light stimuli. Studies have shown that when volunteers are free to alter their gaze and/or distance from a light source, they can lose 80–99% of their putative corneal irradiance (Dawson and Campbell 1990). In addition, the loss of corneal illuminance is compounded by the eye's optics, which focus an image of the light source on the retina rather than diffusing the light across it (Gaddy 1990). Hence, in a "typical" room with a desktop illuminance of 100 lux, the occupants may be able to see 100 lux or more when they look up directly toward the light fixtures, but if they look at the floor or walls, the light reaching their eyes may drop to 10 lux or less. Light entering the eyes can be decreased even more if the volunteers close their eyes, squint, or gaze into shadowy areas. Gaze aversion not only reduces general corneal illuminance, it also reduces the total area of the retinal image produced by a discrete light source. As shown in Figures 5C and 5D, the more total retinal area that is exposed and the more constant the light exposure, the greater the suppression of melatonin (Brainard et al. 1994d; Brainard in press).

A final important difference between the two studies illustrated in Figure 1 lies in the status of subjects' pupils. In the first study, the volunteers had their pupils fully dilated during the light exposure; in the second study, the volunteers' pupils were freely reactive to light. As shown in Figure 5B, a fully dilated pupil permits a greater melatonin suppression with 100 lux compared to when the pupil is free to constrict. Thus, the apparent paradox presented in Figure 1—why 100 lux can suppress melatonin in some circumstances but not in others—can be resolved by careful understanding of the specific physics of the light stimulus, its relationship to the human eye, and the operation of the underlying ocular physiology.

THE ROLE OF LIGHT WAVELENGTH IN MELATONIN REGULATION

Currently, it is not known what photoreceptors transduce light stimuli for circadian and neuroendocrine regulation. The retinal photoreceptor cells that mediate vision in humans include rod cells and three different cone cells. The relative spectral sensitivity of the visual photoreceptors has been well established (Wald 1955; Gouras 1991). It is useful to note that while the rodent retina contains both cone and rod photoreceptors (Cicerone 1976; Carter-Dawson et al. 1979; Jacobs et al. 1991; Szel et al. 1992), there is considerable variability in the retinal structure and physiology across mammalian species (Rodieck 1973). Studies on rodents and humans suggest that wavelengths in the blue and green portion of the spectrum have the strongest capacity for regulating pineal melatonin secretion (Cardinali et al. 1972a, b; Brainard et al. 1984, 1988; Thiele and Meissl 1987; Bronstein et al. 1987; Podolin et al. 1987) as well as the general circadian system (Takahashi et al. 1984). Similarly, results from a small set of studies using different wavelengths to treat winter depression suggest that blue and green wavelengths may provide the strongest therapeutic light stimulus (Brainard et al. 1990; Oren et al. 1991; Stewart et al. 1991). Although the peak sensitivity may be in the blue–green spectral range for melatonin regulation, this does not preclude other wavelengths from influencing pineal and circadian responses. Given sufficient intensity, short wavelengths in the "nonvisible" ultraviolet region of the spectrum (Brainard et al. 1986a, b, 1994b; Podolin et al. 1987) and longer wavelengths in the red end of the spectrum (McCormack and Sontag 1980; Vaněček and Illnerová 1982; Nguyen et al. 1990) are quite capable of modulating melatonin and rhythms in some rodents species. A complete action spectrum, however, has not been defined for melatonin regulation in animals or humans.

Recent findings suggest that neither the rods nor cones used for vision participate in regulating the circadian and neuroendocrine systems. A study demonstrated that exposure to light at night still induced acute melatonin suppression and the ambient light:dark cycle still entrained the melatonin rhythms in rats with total or near-total destruction of retinal photoreceptors (Webb et al. 1985). Other studies on retinally degenerate mice (rd/rd) showed that these animals retained normal circadian responses to light pulses (515 nm) despite a near-total loss of the classic visual photoreceptors (Foster et al. 1991; Provencio et al. 1994; Provencio and Foster 1995). Finally, light-induced melatonin suppression has been demonstrated in some humans with complete visual blindness (Czeisler et al. 1995). In that study, blind subjects with loss of pupillary reflex, no conscious perception of the light stimuli, and no outer retinal functioning (as determined by electroretinographic testing) exhibited neuroendocrine sensitivity to light and circadian entrainment (Czeisler et al. 1995).

One approach for identifying the photoreceptors involved in melatonin regulation is to study whether a genetic deficiency in retinal photoreceptors affects the influence of light on melatonin regulation. In one such study, 14 volunteers with red–green color vision deficiencies were compared to 7 volunteers with normal color vision for their response to light suppression of melatonin. Melatonin suppression was observed in the control subjects, the whole group of color vision-deficient subjects, a subgroup of protanopic observers (individuals functionally lacking the "red" cone pigment), and a subgroup of deuteranopic observers (individuals functionally lacking the "green" cone pigment). There were no significant differences in the magnitude of acute light-induced melatonin suppression between the normal control group and the groups of color vision-deficient volunteers (Ruberg et al. 1996). In a second study, hourly profiles of the melatonin rhythm were compared in six red/green color vision-deficient male subjects and six normal control subjects. Light exposure elicited no immediate differences between these two groups in terms of nocturnal melatonin onset, offset, duration, or acrophase (Ruberg et al. 1996). These findings suggest that a normal three-cone visual system is not necessary for light-mediated regulation of the human pineal gland and melatonin.

Currently, it is premature to rule out the classic visual photoreceptors from mediating the effects of light on melatonin regulation in humans. What, however, are the implications that a normal trichromatic visual system is not necessary for melatonin regulation, and perhaps for other circadian and therapeutic effects of light? Predominantly, scientists and clinicians working on the biological and therapeutic effects of light have used photometric measurement techniques and terminology (lux, candelas, lumens) for specifying light stimuli and characterizing light-producing equipment. Photometric measures and descriptors are based on the "standard observer"—a standard, normal three-cone visual system adapted to daytime light levels (CIE 1987). If the normal, three-cone visual system does not mediate the effects of light on the neuroendocrine circadian systems, as has been suggested by the studies discussed previously (Czeisler et al. 1995; Ruberg et al. 1996), then the use of "lux" or other photopic measures becomes questionable. At this time, the photopic system remains serviceable for describing light stimuli for melatonin regulation, but the community of professionals involved in this field may need to eventually change in their use of this nomenclature and measurement technique.

CONCLUSION

Along with supporting vision, light detected by the eyes is a potent stimulus for controlling the circadian and neuroendocrine systems in mammals. This chapter focused on the regulation of human melatonin by light because it has been hypothesized that melatonin suppression due to exposure to light at night and/or EMF may lead to an increased risk of cancer in industrialized societies. There can be no doubt that exposing a human's eyes to light at night will induce a rapid suppression of melatonin synthesis and secretion. In general, considerably more light is needed for melatonin suppression than for vision. Some studies, however, showed that light ranging from 100–800 lux did not suppress melatonin, while other studies showed that low illuminances of 5–100 lux did suppress melatonin in healthy volunteers. That apparent paradox can be resolved by understanding the specific physics of the light stimulus, the relationship of the light stimulus to the human eye, and the operation of the underlying ocular physiology.

It is important to recognize that portions of the human eye which process light to produce visual stimulation may or may not overlap with those parts of the eye that mediate the biological, behavioral, and therapeutic effects of light. Simply put, humans appear to "see" light in more than one way—for visual perception of the world as well as for detecting illumination that influences nonvisual biology. It is a relatively recent discovery that our species "sees" light for circadian regulation, and much work remains to be completed to define the physiology that supports this sensory system. Do humans possess other sensory capacities yet to be revealed? More specifically, are humans equipped to "see" or detect EMF outside the visible or near-visible ranges? These and many other questions await further experimental exploration.

ACKNOWLEDGMENTS

The author would like to acknowledge the steadfast assistance of John P. Hanifin for his careful preparation of the figures, tables, and document layout, as well as for his attentive editing of the text. This research was supported, in part, by U.S. FDA Grant #785346, NIMH Grant #MH-44890, NASA Grant #NAGW1196, the National Electrical Manufacturer's Association (#LRI 89:DR:1), the Lighting Research Institute (#LRI 88:SP:LREF:6), USUHS Grant # R07049, Jefferson's Dean's Overage Research Program, and the Philadelphia Chapter of the Illuminating Engineering Society.

REFERENCES

Adler, J.S., D.F. Kripke, R.T. Loving, S.L. Berga. 1992. Peripheral vision suppression of melatonin. *J. Pineal Res.* 12:49–52.

Akerstadt, T., J.E. Froberg, Y. Friberg, L. Wetterberg. 1979. Melatonin excretion, body temperature and subjective arousal during 64 hours of sleep deprivation. *Psychoneuroendocrinology* 4:219–225.

Aschoff, J., ed. 1981. *Handbook of Behavioral Neurobiology, Biological Rhythms.* New York: Plenum Press.

Barker, F.M., G.C. Brainard. 1991. *The Direct Spectral Transmittance of the Excised Human Lens as a Function for Age.* U.S. Food and Drug Administration: Order # FDA 785345 0090 RA.

Binkley, S. 1988. *The Pineal: Endocrine and Nonendocrine Function.* Englewood Cliffs, New Jersey: Prentice Hall.

Binkley, S. 1990. *The Clockwork Sparrow.* Englewood, New Jersey: Prentice Hall.

Boettner, E.A., J.R. Wolter. 1962. Transmission of the ocular media. *Invest. Ophthalmol. Vis. Sci.* 1:776–783.

Boivin, D.B., J.F. Duffy, R.E. Kronauer, C.A. Czeisler. 1996. Dose–response relationships for resetting of human circadian clock by light. *Nature* 379:540–542.

Bojkowski, C.J., M.E. Aldhous, J. English, C. Franey, A.L. Poulton, D.J. Skene, J. Arendt. 1987. Suppression of nocturnal plasma melatonin and 6-sulphatoxymelatonin by bright and dim light in man. *Horm. Metab. Res.* 19:437–440.

Brainard, G.C. 1992. Project Review of Electric and Magnetic Fields and Melatonin. Palo Alto, California: Electric Power Research Institute.

Brainard, G.C. The healing light: Interface of physics and biology. In: *Beyond Seasonal Affective Disorder: Light Treatment for SAD and Non-SAD Disorders*, R.W. Lam, ed. Washington, D.C.: American Psychiatric Press, Inc. (in press).

Brainard, G.C., B.A. Richardson, T.S. King, S.A. Matthews, R.J. Reiter. 1983. The suppression of pineal melatonin content and N-acetyl-transferase activity by different light irradiances in the Syrian hamster: A dose–response relationship. *Endocrinology* 113:293–296.

Brainard, G.C., B.A. Richardson, T.S. King, R.J. Reiter. 1984. The influence of different light spectra on the suppression of pineal melatonin content in the Syrian hamster. *Brain Res.* 294:333–339.

Brainard, G.C., P.L. Podolin, S.W. Leivy, M.D. Rollag, C. Cole, F.M. Barker. 1986a. Near ultraviolet radiation (UV-A) suppresses pineal melatonin content. *Endocrinology* 119:2201–2205.

Brainard, G.C., M.K. Vaughan, R.J. Reiter. 1986b. Effect of light irradiance and wavelength on the Syrian hamster reproductive system. *Endocrinology* 119:648–654.

Brainard, G.C., A.J. Lewy, M. Menaker, R.H. Fredrickson, L.S. Miller, R.G. Weleber, V. Cassone, D. Hudson. 1988. Dose–response relationship between light irradiance and the suppression of plasma melatonin in human volunteers. *Brain Res.* 454:212–218.

Brainard, G.C., N.E. Rosenthal, D. Sherry, R.G. Skwerer, M. Waxler, D. Kelly. 1990. Effects of different wavelengths in seasonal affective disorder. *J. Affective Disord.* 20:209–216.

Brainard, G.C., J.R. Gaddy, F.M. Barker, J.P. Hanifin, M.D. Rollag. 1993. Mechanisms in the eye that mediate the biological and therapeutic effects of light in humans. In: *Light and Biological Rhythms in Man*, L. Wetterberg, ed., pp. 29–53. Stockholm: Pergamon Press.

Brainard, G.C., R.R. Long, J.P. Hanifin, F.L. Ruberg, J.R. Gaddy, C.A. Bernecker, F.J. Fernsler, M.D. Rollag. 1994a. Architectural lighting: Balancing biological effects with utility costs. In: *The Biologic Effects of Light*, M.F. Holick, E.G. Jung, eds., pp. 169–185. New York: Walter de Gruyter & Co.

Brainard, G.C., F.M. Barker, R.J. Hoffman, M.H. Stetson, J.P. Hanifin, P.L. Podolin, M.D. Rollag. 1994b. Ultraviolet regulation of neuroendocrine and circadian physiology in rodents. *Vision Res.* 34:1521–1533.

Brainard, G.C., J.R. Gaddy, F.L. Ruberg, F.M. Barker, J.P. Hanifin, M.D. Rollag. 1994c. Ocular mechanisms that regulate the human pineal gland. In: *Advances in Pineal Research: 8*, M. Møller, P. Pévet, eds., pp. 415–432. London: John Libbey and Co. Ltd.

Brainard, G., J. Hanifin, S. Leibowitz, S. Tirney, J. Georgiou, M. Rollag. 1994d. Constant versus intermittent ocular exposure during light treatment: Is there temporal summation of photic stimuli? *Soc. Light Treatment Biol. Rhythms Abst.* 6:14.

Brainard, G.C., J.P. Hanifin, P.R. Hannon, W. Gibson, J. French, M.D. Rollag. 1996. The biological and behavioral effects of light in humans: From basic physiology to application. In: *The Biologic Effects of Light 1995*, M.F. Holick, E.G. Jung, eds., pp. 380–397. New York: Walter de Gruyter & Co.

Bronstein, D.M., G.H. Jacobs, K.A. Haak, J. Neitz, L.D. Lytle. 1987. Action spectrum of the retinal mechanism mediating nocturnal light-induced suppression of rat pineal gland N-acetyltransferase. *Brain Res.* 406:352–356.

Cardinali, D.P., F. Larin, R.J. Wurtman. 1972a. Control of the rat pineal gland by light spectra. *Proc. Natl. Acad. Sci. U.S.A.* 69:2003–2005.

Cardinali, D.P., F. Larin, R.J. Wurtman. 1972b. Action spectra for effects of light on hydroxyindole-O-methyltransferase in rat pineal, retina and harderian gland. *Endocrinology* 91:877–886.

Carter-Dawson, L.D., M.M. LaVail. 1979. Rods and cones in the mouse retina. I. Structural analysis using light and electron microscopy. *J. Comp. Neurol.* 188:245–262.

Cicerone, C.M. 1976. Cones survive rods in the light-damaged eye of the albino rat. *Science* 194:1183–1185.

Commission Internationale de l'Eclairage (CIE). 1987. International Lighting Vocabulary, CIE Publication No. 17.4. Vienna.

Czeisler, C.A., J.S. Allan, S.H. Strogatz, J.M. Ronda, R. Sanchez, C.D. Rios, W.O. Freitag, G.S. Richardson, R.E. Kronauer. 1986. Bright light resets the human circadian pacemaker independent of the timing of the sleep–wake cycle. *Science* 233:667–671.

Czeisler, C.A., M.P. Johnson, J.F. Duffy, E.N. Brown, J.M. Ronda, R.E. Kronauer. 1990. Exposure to bright light and darkness to treat physiologic maladaptation to night work. *N. Engl. J. Med.* 322:1253–1259.

Czeisler, C.A., T.J. Shanahan, E.B. Klerman, H. Martens, D.J. Brotman, J.S. Emens, T. Klein, J.F. Rizzo III. 1995. Suppression of melatonin secretion in some blind patients by exposure to bright light. *N. Engl. J. Med.* 332:6–11.

Dawson, D., S.S. Campbell. 1990. Bright light treatment: Are we keeping our subjects in the dark? *Sleep* 13:267–271.

Eastman, C.I. 1992. High-intensity light for circadian adaptation to a 12-h shift of the sleep schedule. *Am. J. Physiol.* 263:R428–R436.

Evered, D., S. Clark, ed. 1985. *Photoperiodism, Melatonin and the Pineal.* London: Pitman Publishing Ltd.

Foster, R.G., I. Provencio, D. Hudson, S. Fiske, W. DeGrip, M. Menaker. 1991. Circadian photoreception in the retinally degenerate mouse (rd/rd). *J. Comp. Physiol. [A]* 169:39–50.

Gaddy, J.R. 1990. Sources of variability in phototherapy. *Sleep Res.* 19:394.

Gaddy, J.R., M. Edelson, K. Stewart, G.C. Brainard, M.D. Rollag. 1992. Possible retinal spatial summation in melatonin suppresion. In: *Biologic Effects of Light*, M.F. Holick, A.M. Kligman, eds., pp. 196–204. New York: Walter de Gruyter & Co.

Gaddy, J.R., M.D. Rollag, G.C. Brainard. 1993. Pupil size regulation of threshold of light-induced melatonin suppression. *J. Clin. Endocrinol. & Metab.* 77:1398–1401.

Gaddy, J.R., F.L. Ruberg, G.C. Brainard, M.D. Rollag. 1994. Pupillary modulation of light-induced melatonin suppression. In: *The Biologic Effects of Light*, M.F. Holick, E.G. Jung, eds., pp. 159–168. Berlin: Walter de Gruyter & Co.

Gouras, P. 1991. Color Vision. In: *Principle of Neuroscience 3rd Edition*, C.E.R. Vandel, J.H. Schswarty, T.M. Jessel, eds., pp. 467–480. New York: Elsevier.

Illuminating Engineering Society of North America (IESNA). 1993. *Lighting Handbook: Reference & Application.* New York: Illuminating Engineering Society of North America.

Jacobs, G. H., J. Neitz, J.F. Deegan. 1991. Retinal receptors in rodents maximally sensitive to ultraviolet light. *Nature* 353:655–656.

Jimerson, D.C., H.J. Lynch, R.M. Post, R.J. Wurtman, W.E. Bunney Jr. 1977. Urinary melatonin rhythms during sleep deprivation in depressed patients and normals. *Life Sci.* 20:1501–1508.

Kitay, J. I., M.D. Altschule. 1954. *The Pineal Gland.* Cambridge, Massachusetts: Harvard University Press.

Klein, D. C., J.L. Weller. 1972. Rapid light-induced decrease in pineal serotonin N-acetyltransferase activity. *Science* 177:532–533.

Klein, D.C., R. Smoot, J.L. Weller, S. Higa, S.P. Markey, G.J. Creed, D.M. Jacobowitz. 1983. Lesions of the paraventricular nucleus area of the hypothalamus disrupt the suprachiasmatic spinal cord circuit in the melatonin rhythm generating system. *Brain Res. Bull.* 10:647–652.

Klein, D.C., R.Y. Moore, S.J. Reppert, eds. 1991. *Suprachiasmatic Nucleus: The Mind's Clock.* Oxford: Oxford University Press.

Lam, R.W., ed. *Beyond Seasonal Affective Disorder: Light Treatment for SAD and Non-SAD Disorders.* Washington, D.C.: American Psychiatric Press, Inc. (in press).

Lerman, S. 1987. Chemical and physical properties of the normal and aging lens: Spectroscopic (UV, fluorescence, phosphorescence, and NMR) analyses. *Am. J. of Optom. Physiol. Opt.* 64:11–22.

Lewy, A.J., T.A. Wehr, F.K. Goodwin, D.A. Newsome, S.P. Markey. 1980. Light suppresses melatonin secretion in humans. *Science* 210:1267–1269.

Lewy, A.J., R.L. Sack, S. Miller, T.M. Hoban. 1987. Antidepressant and circadian phase-shifting effects of light. *Science* 235:352–354.

Lowenstein, O., I.E. Loewenfeld. 1962. The pupil. In: *The Eye*, H. Davson, ed., pp. 231–267. New York: Academic Press.

Lynch, H.J., D.C. Jimerson, Y. Ozaki, R.M. Post, W.E. Bunney, R.J. Wurtman. 1978. Entrainment of rhythmic melatonin secretion in man to a 12-hour phase shift in the light/dark cycle. *Life Sci.* 23:1557–1563.

McCormack, C.E., C.R. Sontag. 1980. Entrainment by red light of running activity and ovulation rhythms of rats. *Am. J. Physiol.* 239:R450–R453.

McIntyre, I.M., T.R. Norman, G.D. Burrows, S.M. Armstrong. 1989a. Human melatonin suppression by light is intensity dependent. *J. Pineal Res.* 6:149–159.

McIntyre, I.M., T.R. Norman, G.D. Burrows, S.M. Armstrong. 1989b. Quantal melatonin suppression by exposure to low intensity light in man. *Life Sci.* 45:327–332.

Minneman, K.P., H. Lynch, R.J. Wurtman. 1974. Relationship between environmental light intensity and retina-mediated suppression of rat pineal serotonin-N-acetyltransferase. *Life Sci.* 15:1791–1796.

Minors, D.S., J.M. Waterhouse, A. Wirz-Justice. 1991. A human phase-response curve to light. *Neurosci. Lett.* 133:36–40.

Nelson, D.E., J.S. Takahashi. 1991. Comparison of visual sensitivity for suppression of pineal melatonin and circadian phase-shifting in the golden hamster. *Brain Res.* 554:272–277.

Nguyen, D.C., J.P. Hanifin, M.D. Rollag, M.H. Stetson, G.C. Brainard. 1990. The influence of different photon densities of 620 nm light on pineal melatonin in Syrian hamsters. *The Anatomical Record* 226:72A.

Oren, D.A., G.C. Brainard, J.R. Joseph-Vanderpool, S.H. Johnston, E. Sorek, N.E. Rosenthal. 1991. Treatment of seasonal affective disorder with green light versus red light. *Am. J. Psychiatry* 148:509–511.

Pittendrigh, C.S., S. Daan. 1976. A functional analysis of circadian pacemakers in nocturnal rodents. IV. Entrainment: Pacemaker as clock. *J. Comp. Physiol.* 106:291–331.

Podolin, P.C., M.D. Rollag, G.C. Brainard. 1987. The suppression of nocturnal pineal melatonin in the Syrian hamster: Dose–response curves at 500 nm and 360 nm. *Endocrinology* 121:266–270.

Provencio, I., R.G. Foster. 1995. Circadian rhythms in mice can be regulated by photoreceptors with cone-like characteristics. *Brain Res.* 694:183–190.

Provencio, I., S. Wong, A.B. Lederman, S.M. Argamaso, R.G. Foster. 1994. Visual and circadian responses to light in aged retinally degenerate mice. *Vision Res.* 34:1799–1806.

Reiter, R.J. 1993. The mammalian pineal gland as an end organ of the visual system. In: *Light and Biological Rythms in Man*, L. Wetterberg, ed., pp. 145–160. Stockholm: Pergamon Press.

Riggs, L.A. 1965. Light as a stimulus for vision. In:*Vision and Visual Perception*, C. Graham, ed., pp. 1–38. New York: John Wiley & Sons.

Rodieck, R.W. 1973. *The Verterbrate Retina.* San Franscisco: W.H. Freeman and Co.

Rollag, M.D., G.D. Nieswender. 1976. Radioimmunoassay of serum concentrations of melatonin in sheep exposed to different lighting regimens. *Endocrinology* 98:482–489.

Rollag, M.D., E.S. Panke, W. Trakulrungski, C. Trakulrungski, R.J. Reiter. 1980. Qualification of daily melatonin synthesis in the hamster pineal gland. *Endocrinology* 106:231–236.

Rosenthal, N.E., M.C. Blehar, eds. 1989. *Seasonal Affective Disorders and Phototherapy.* New York: The Guilford Press.

Ruberg, F.L., D.J. Skene, J.P. Hanifin, M.D. Rollag, J. English, J. Arendt, G.C. Brainard. 1996. Melatonin regulation in humans with color vision deficiencies. *J. Clin. Endocrinol. & Metab.* 81:2980–2985.

Sliney, D., M. Wolbarsht. 1980. *Safety with Lasers and Other Optical Sources.* New York: Plenum Press.

Society for Light Treatment and Biological Rhythms. 1994. *Questions and Answers About Light Therapy.*

Stevens, R.G., S. Davis, D.B. Thomas, L.E. Anderson, B.W. Wilson. 1992. Electric power, pineal function, and the risk of breast cancer. *FASEB J* 6:853–860.

Stewart, K.T., J.R. Gaddy, B. Byrne, S. Miller, G.C. Brainard. 1991. Effects of green or white light for treatment of seasonal depression. *Psychiatry Res.* 38:261–270.

Szel, A., P. Rohlich, A.R. Caffe, B. Juliusson, G. Aguirre, T. Van Veen. 1992. Unique topographic separation of two spectral classes of cones in the mouse retina. *J. Comp. Neurol.* 325:327–342.

Takahashi, J.S., P.J. DeCoursey, L. Bauman, M. Menaker. 1984. Spectral sensitivity of a novel photoreceptive system mediating entrainment of mammalian circadian rhythms. *Nature* 308:186–188.

Thiele, G., H. Meissl. 1987. Action spectra of the lateral eyes recorded from mammalian pineal glands. *Brain Res.* 424:10–16.

Vaněček, J., H. Illnerová. 1982. Night pineal N-acetyltransferase activity in rats exposed to white or red light pulses of various intensities and duration. *Experientia* 38:1318–1320.

Vaughan, G.M., R.W. Pelham, S.F. Pang, L.L. Loughlin, K.M. Wilson, K.L. Sandock, M.K. Vaughan, S.H. Koslow, R.J. Reiter. 1976. Nocturnal elevation of plasma melatonin and urinary 5-hydroxyindoleacetic acid in young men: Attempts at modification by brief changes in environmental lighting and sleep by autonomic drugs. *J. Clin. Endocrinol. & Metab.* 42:752–764.

Vaughan, G. M., R. Bell, A. de la Pena. 1979. Nocturnal plasma melatonin in humans: Episodic pattern and influence of light. *Neurosci. Lett.* 14:81–84.

Wald, G. 1955. The photoreceptor process in vision. *Am. J. Ophthalmol.* 40:18–41.

Webb, S.M., T.H. Champney, A.K. Lewinski, R.J. Reiter. 1985. Photoreceptor damage and eye pigmentation: Influence on the sensitivity of rat pineal N-acetyltransferase activity and melatonin levels to light at night. *Neuroendocrinology* 40:205–209.

Wehr, T.A. 1991. The durations of human melatonin secretion and sleep respond to changes in daylength (photoperiod). *J. Clin. Endocrinol. & Metab.* 73:1276–1280.

Wehr, T.A., R.G. Skwerer, F.M. Jacobsen, D.A. Sack, N.E. Rosenthal. 1987. Eye versus skin phototherapy of seasonal affective disorder. *Am. J. Psychiatry* 144:753–757.

Wehr, T.A., D.E. Moul, G. Barbato, H.A. Giesen, J.A. Seidel, C. Barker, C. Bender. 1993. Conservation of photoperiod-responsive mechanisms in humans. *Am. J. Physiol.* 265:R846–R857.

Wetterberg, L. 1978. Melatonin in humans: Physiological and clinical studies. *J. Neural Transm.* (Suppl) 13:289–310.

Wetterberg, L., ed. 1993. *Light and Biological Rhythms in Man.* New York: Pergamon Press.

Wurtman, R.J., M.J. Baum, J. Potts. eds. 1985. *The Medical and Biological Effects of Light.* New York: The New York Academy of Sciences.

11 Response of Mammalian Pineal Gene Expression to Light and Magnetic Field Exposure

WENDY HAGGREN
Pettis Veterans Affairs Medical Center,
Loma Linda, California

CONTENTS

INTRODUCTION
REGULATION OF PINEAL MELATONIN SYNTHESIS
EFFECTS OF LIGHT EXPOSURE ON PINEAL GENE EXPRESSION
EFFECTS OF MAGNETIC FIELD EXPOSURE ON
    PINEAL GENE EXPRESSION
FINAL COMMENT
ACKNOWLEDGMENTS
REFERENCES

The nightly production of melatonin in the mammalian pineal gland is a rhythmic phenomenon occurring in response to signals from an endogenous oscillator, the circadian clock, which resides in the suprachiasmatic nucleus (Takahashi and Zatz 1982). While many aspects of the process by which the onset of darkness stimulates melatonin production are reasonably well understood, the molecular mechanisms underlying the regulation of pineal melatonin synthesis are only now being characterized. Throughout the hours of darkness, light will always have a suppressive effect on pineal melatonin synthesis. However, different mechanisms appear to regulate pineal gene expression in the first half of the night as compared to those that function in the later hours.

Study of effects of environmental agents on pineal gene expression will lead to determining the molecular mechanisms producing this response; namely, the specific signal-transduction pathways involved in regulation. Essential for completing these studies, however, is the cloning of genes for critical enzymes. Fortunately, this process has now been accomplished. In addition to two recent papers that discuss cloning the gene for the rate-limiting enzyme in pineal melatonin synthesis (Borjigin et al. 1995; Coon et al. 1995), two timely reviews provide excellent summaries of the cloning and characterization of many of the genes for enzymes and proteins involved in pineal melatonin synthesis (Craft 1993; Stehle 1995). Moreover, these reviews emphasize the role that molecular biology has played in advancing our knowledge in this important area of biology, advances which may lead to an understanding of the bases of human pathologies. For instance, determination of mechanisms by which changes in the expression of specific genes in the suprachiasmatic nucleus and pineal can influence melatonin production may provide an explanation of the variability of human response to different intensities of light. This knowledge could broaden our ability to treat such diseases as seasonal affective disorder (Partonen 1994).

Physical agents other than visible light have been shown to affect pineal melatonin production (reviewed in Reiter 1992). Understanding the role of light in entraining the mammalian circadian rhythm will provide explanations of mechanisms involved in the actions of other physical agents affecting melatonin production and circadian timing. Exposure to a magnetic field in late afternoon or early evening has been shown to suppress pineal melatonin synthesis (Matt et al. 1994; Kato et al. 1994; Selmaoui and Touitou 1995). In our laboratory, using a whole animal model, we are pursuing studies to test the hypothesis that light and magnetic fields are related but distinct physical environmental agents that will affect, in a similar manner, the expression of genes comprising the circadian clock. These findings are discussed in more detail following a brief review of pertinent literature, which will update our picture of the regulation of pineal melatonin synthesis.

REGULATION OF PINEAL MELATONIN SYNTHESIS

The mammalian pineal gland and retina are derived from similar tissues, are evolutionarily related, and share similar biochemical processes (Lolley et al. 1992; Craft 1993; Korf 1994). Both the retina and the pineal gland synthesize melatonin. In a recent study, Tosini and Menaker (1996) demonstrated that cultured retina from the golden hamster produced melatonin in a 24-hour circadian rhythm. These investigators showed that by introducing light into the incubator containing perfused retinas, the circadian oscillator(s) directing retinal melatonin synthesis could be entrained by light in vitro. However, there are significant differences between the pineal and the retina. For instance, the mammalian pineal gland is not photoreceptive, and melatonin synthesis appears to be regulated differently in the retina and the pineal (Steinlechner et al. 1995; Tosini and Menaker 1996). Nevertheless, the evolutionary relationship between the retina and the pineal gland is intriguing, because the retina is required to receive the light that transmits the signal for entrainment of the mammalian circadian rhythm. This signal passes through the suprachiasmatic nucleus in the anterior hypothalamus and is transmitted to the pineal gland. Thus, a neuronal pathway is established in which the control of circadian rhythms is embodied in three tissues: the retina, the hypothalamus, and the pineal gland (Craft 1993).

At the onset of darkness, the circadian clock in the suprachiasmatic nucleus transmits a neuronal signal through the superior cervical ganglion to sympathetic innervation of the pineal gland, thus releasing norepinephrine. This neurohormone interacts with ß- and α-adrenergic receptors, initiating a series of events which includes a rise in intracellular cyclic AMP (cAMP) and activation of an enzyme cascade that transforms tryptophan to serotonin and, finally, to melatonin. One of the first pieces of evidence that this process is controlled at the level of gene transcription came from studies showing that RNA transcription preceded, and quite possibly was required for, nightly pineal melatonin synthesis (Morrissey and Lovenberg 1978a, b). While the activity of several pineal enzymes has been shown to increase in the dark, only recently, with the cloning of the genes for these enzymes, have cyclic changes in mRNA levels been shown, suggesting control of melatonin synthesis at the level of gene transcription. Figure 1 presents a summary of these events.

As stated previously, melatonin is synthesized in the pineal gland from tryptophan, an essential amino acid. Pineal tryptophan hydroxylase, the first of two enzymes that convert tryptophan into serotonin, exhibits increased activity during the hours of darkness (Reiter 1991; Craft 1993). The gene for this enzyme has been cloned from rat and rabbit pineal cDNA libraries. Subsequent analysis demonstrated that tryptophan hydroxylase mRNA levels are highest at night (Craft 1993).

Serotonin is modified by pineal serotonin N-acetyltransferase (S-NAT) in what is considered to be the rate-limiting step in melatonin synthesis. This arylalkylamine NAT is expressed primarily in the

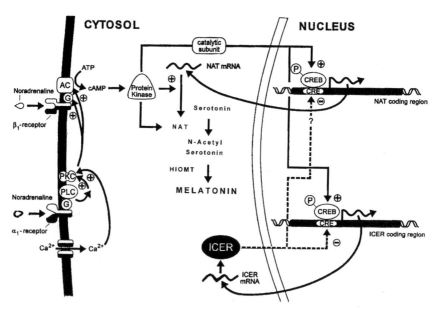

FIG. 1. Regulation of pineal melatonin synthesis by cAMP signaling pathways. Abbreviations not included in text: AC, adenylate cyclase; G, G protein; PLC, phospholipase C; PKC, protein kinase C. (Modified from Takahashi 1994 and reprinted with permission of Current Biology Ltd.)

pineal gland, and is evolutionarily and functionally divergent from the two forms of arylamine NAT cloned from liver (Craft 1993). Since 1970 (Klein and Weller 1970), substantial nocturnal increases in rat pineal S-NAT activity have been measured, yet the gene was cloned only recently from rat and sheep (Borjigin et al. 1995; Coon et al. 1995). S-NAT gene expression exhibits a circadian pattern, with transcript levels at night 2-fold higher than daytime levels in sheep (Coon et al. 1995), and about 150-fold higher in the rat (Borjigin et al. 1995; Coon et al. 1995). Although species-specific differences in pineal melatonin production and S-NAT enzyme activity have been known for some time (reviewed in Reiter 1991), data from gene expression studies will provide a molecular explanation for these differences based on transcriptional regulation and protein modification. The molecular cloning of the gene for S-NAT (Borjigin et al. 1995; Coon et al. 1995) will have an exciting influence on pineal research. Because S-NAT is considered the rate-limiting enzyme in melatonin synthesis, changes in pineal S-NAT gene expression now can be used as a model to assess directly the influence of extracellular signals on the regulation of transcription factors and subsequent gene expression.

The final step in melatonin synthesis is the methylation of modified serotonin by hydroxyindole-*O*-methyltransferase (HIOMT). In contrast to pineal S-NAT activity, the activity of HIOMT varies little from day to night. The gene encoding this enzyme has been cloned from chicken, bovine, and human pineal gland (Voisin et al. 1992; Craft 1993; Donohue et al. 1993).

As mentioned previously, depending on the species, melatonin synthesis appears to be regulated, wholly or in part, at the level of gene transcription. Consequently, it is essential to determine the role of transcriptional regulatory proteins in this process. For instance, the cAMP regulatory element binding protein (CREB) is expressed constitutively, and its transcriptional regulatory property occurs through differential phosphorylation by protein kinase A. CREB, which regulates genes whose promoters contain a cAMP response element (CRE), is probably the most critical and predominant transcriptional regulator in the pineal gland at the time of melatonin synthesis (Roseboom and Klein 1995; Tamotsu et al. 1995). Not surprisingly, sequence analysis of cloned genes for the physiologically relevant pineal enzymes and for a variety of membrane-bound receptors revealed that the CRE is found in the promoter region of many pineal genes (Stehle 1995). Closely related to CREB, the cAMP response element modulator (CREM) functions as both transcriptional activator and transcriptional repressor. Although CREM transcripts originating from the most upstream promoter have not been found in the pineal gland, a second promoter (located between coding sequences) inducibly expresses the sequences of CREM consisting only of DNA-binding domains. Known as the inducible cAMP early regulator (ICER; Stehle et al. 1993), this small protein consists only of a DNA-binding domain, and acts as a strong repressor of cAMP-induced gene expression. In rat pineal, transcription of the ICER gene is induced by rising cAMP levels such that nightly transcript levels of ICER increase as melatonin production peaks. As shown in cell culture and pineal organ culture, ICER protein represses transcription of CRE-regulated gene transcription (Molina et al. 1993; Stehle et al. 1993). The temporal pattern of ICER expression in the rat pineal gland, maximal at 1–2 hours after peak melatonin production and beginning to fall just before the onset of light, suggests a role for ICER in an autoregulatory feedback loop that creates an intrapineal timing mechanism whereby melatonin synthesis is down-regulated in anticipation of the onset of light (Stehle 1995). Studies of cAMP-induced gene expression and consequent repression of transcription have provided a molecular basis to explain the observation that while darkness is required for initiation of melatonin production, onset of light is not required to end pineal melatonin synthesis (Reiter 1991). The proposed involvement of CREB and ICER in the regulation of pineal melatonin synthesis is illustrated in Figure 1.

When cells are stimulated by various agents, either chemical (e.g., growth factors) or physical (e.g., magnetic fields), alterations in signal-transduction mechanisms result in the expression of a relatively small group of genes called immediate early or primary response genes (reviewed in Morgan and Curran 1991). The best-studied of these genes include *fos* and *jun*. These genes are characterized by the rapid and transient induction of their respective mRNAs and proteins, a process that is not dependent on prior protein synthesis. The immediate early genes encode proteins that serve as transcriptional regulators. (Induction or repression of gene transcription is possible, depending on the specific regulator involved.) Indeed, Curran and Morgan (1987) and Curran et al. (1989) formulated the concept of stimulus-transcription coupling (the transduction of extracellular signals to long-term changes in gene expression and cell adaptation) based on observations of the rapid and inducible expression of transcriptional regulators in response to ligand–receptor interactions. Activator protein-1 (AP-1) (Morgan and Curran 1991) is a transcriptional regulatory complex that exists as either a heterodimer (one member of the FOS family of proteins and one member of the JUN family of proteins) or a homodimer (JUN proteins only), and that recognizes a specific base sequence (i.e., an AP-1 site or response element) in the promoter region of AP-1-regulated genes (Angel and Karin 1991). Importantly, the FOS and JUN family members that constitute AP-1 demonstrate different expression dynamics, thus allowing the composition of AP-1 to change with the state of the cell. As a consequence, the function of AP-1 may change, because FOS-related antigen-2 (FRA-2) and JUNB serve as transcriptional repressors rather than transcriptional activators (Baler and Klein 1995). In the pineal, AP-1 binding activity occurs throughout the nighttime hours of darkness, rising and falling in much the same time frame as melatonin production (Carter 1994). As has been found in other regions of brain (Hope et al. 1992; Takeuchi et al. 1993), a picture begins to emerge of turnover in proteins functioning in tandem at the AP-1 binding site, which is thought to confer specificity of function (i.e., different protein combinations bind to same region of promoter DNA, although these combinations may have different actions).

To date, c-*fos* gene expression in response to light entrainment of the mammalian circadian rhythm has been studied primarily in the suprachiasmatic nucleus, the proposed site of the mammalian circadian clock. Expression of the c-*fos* gene exhibits a circadian rhythm in the light-receptive region of the rat suprachiasmatic nucleus when animals are entrained to a 12:12 light:dark cycle, with c-*fos* expression apparently regulated by ambient light (Schwartz et al. 1994). Using in situ hybridization techniques, Schwartz et al. (1994) showed that following a low level of expression during darkness, c-*fos* transcript level peaked about 2 hours after onset of light, then dropped to an intermediate level for the remainder of the daytime. Numerous reports describe the strong induction of c-*fos* expression in the rodent suprachiasmatic nucleus caused by a pulse of light in the early-evening hours (reviewed in Schwartz et al. 1994). Photic stimulation of c-*fos* in the suprachiasmatic nucleus is restricted to those times of day (e.g., early evening) when light is capable of shifting the timing of the circadian rhythm, a phenomenon termed "gating" (Schwartz et al. 1994). While gating of the response to light has a clear physiological basis, the mechanism is unknown.

The role of FOS protein in the pineal has not been established. Recent reports show that induction of pineal c-*fos* gene expression occurs through the α-adrenergic receptor by mechanisms involving intracellular calcium (Ca^{2+}) (Carter 1992; Yu et al. 1993; Baler and Klein 1995; Roseboom and Klein 1995). Induction of the expression of two other pineal immediate early genes, *jun*B and *fra*-2, occurs primarily through the ß-adrenergic receptor (Carter 1992; Baler and Klein 1995). Activation of the pineal ß-adrenergic receptor produces the increases in cAMP that have been shown to drive melatonin synthesis (Reiter 1991; Roseboom and Klein 1995). Consequently, c-*fos* expression is thought to have a role in potentiating melatonin synthesis. Baler and Klein (1995) showed recently that in the Sprague-Dawley rat, pineal FOS protein was expressed at a relatively constant level throughout daytime and nighttime under both light–dark and constant-darkness conditions. However, in the same study, there was a strong temporal correlation of *fra*-2 gene expression with both FRA-2 protein expression and NAT enzyme activity, under both light–dark and constant-darkness conditions. Thus, *fra*-2, which is thought to have a role as a repressor of gene transcription, is expressed in a circadian pattern and is closely associated with nightly pineal melatonin synthesis.

Key times of night in the regulation of mammalian pineal melatonin production appear to be (1) a light-sensitive period during the first half of darkness, when light can shift the phase of the circadian rhythm, which is also characterized by a reversible decrease in pineal melatonin synthesis in response to light; and (2) a period during the last half of the dark hours, when a molecular intrapineal timing mechanism terminates melatonin synthesis whether or not a light cue for dawn is experienced. During the last half of dark hours, a light pulse as short as 1 minute will terminate pineal melatonin production, which does not resume when animals are returned to darkness (Illnerová and Vaněček 1979; Hoffmann et al. 1980).

EFFECTS OF LIGHT EXPOSURE ON PINEAL GENE EXPRESSION

This volume discusses, in part, a possible association between long-term residential and/or occupational exposure to low-level magnetic fields and an increased incidence of cancer in both children and adults. Unfortunately, a complete and plausible mechanism to explain how magnetic field exposure could be linked to the process of carcinogenesis has not yet been demonstrated. However, Stevens et al. (1992) proposed that magnetic field exposure may lower nighttime levels of melatonin, a powerful antioxidant and endogenous anti-cancer agent, thus predisposing individuals to the action of carcinogens or tumor promoting agents. Indeed, several research groups have reported that in vivo exposure of animal models to either static or alternating magnetic fields decreased both the nighttime production of melatonin and the activity of S-NAT (Matt et al. 1994; Kato et al. 1994; Selmaoui and Touitou 1995). The reported action of magnetic field exposure in animals bears similarity to the suppressive effects of another physical agent, light, on nightly melatonin synthesis. To understand how magnetic field exposure may alter melatonin production, it is important to understand how light affects this process.

A great deal of research on the molecular basis of pineal melatonin production has been done in the rat, an excellent model for studying melatonin production because nighttime levels of S-NAT activity and pineal melatonin production are more than 100-fold higher than daytime levels. However, in our laboratory, we find the seasonally breeding Djungarian hamster (*Phodopus sungorus*) a particularly good biological model for magnetic field exposure effects on circadian processes. In addition to a robust, well-characterized nighttime melatonin rhythm (Lerchl and Schlatt 1992; Lerchl and Nieschlag 1992), changes in day length cause Djungarian hamsters to exhibit a variety of physiological responses, such as changes in body weight, testicular size and weight, and coat color (Niklowitz et al. 1994).

Of particular interest in this laboratory is the molecular basis of circadian rhythm entrainment, essentially a perturbation of the timing of the endogenous clock. Because daily adjustments are necessary to maintain a 24-hour rhythm in mammals, the ability of photoperiod to entrain the clock allows animals in high-latitude, temperate climates to prepare for changing seasons (reviewed in Nelson et al. 1990). Thus, entrainment has significant evolutionary and survival value to a species. Much has been learned about the molecules constituting the endogenous clock, and the mechanisms by which light entrains these clocks, through research on the filamentous fungus *Neurospora* (Crosthwaite et al. 1995) and the fruit fly *Drosophila* (Hunter-Ensor et al. 1996; Zeng et al. 1996). Recent work has shown that the molecular mechanisms regulating entrainment are different in these two organisms, one relying primarily on transcription (*Neurospora*) and one on transcription and protein interactions (*Drosophila*). Along similar lines of evidence, Coon et al. (1995) proposed that differences in the regulation of S-NAT activity between the rat and the sheep stem from differences in contribution of transcriptional and post-transcriptional mechanisms.

During an uninterrupted light–dark cycle, c-*fos* mRNA appears to have a circadian expression pattern in Djungarian hamster pineal (Fig. 2). Furthermore, we find that pineal c-*fos* expression is sensitive to interruptions of darkness by light, an event which is known to cause a decrease in both pineal S-NAT activity and pineal melatonin production (Illnerová and Vaněček 1979 and references therein). We have studied pineal c-*fos* expression in long day-entrained hamsters that have 16 hours of light beginning at 0100 hours, and lights off at 1700 hours for 8 hours of darkness. Pineal c-*fos* expression (undetectable at 30 minutes following onset of darkness; data not shown) is strong at 1 hour after lights out. Levels of c-*fos* drop by 50% at 2 hours after lights out and drop by another 30% at 3 hours after lights out. One group of hamsters was exposed to a 20-minute pulse of light (300 lux) beginning 2.75 hours after the onset of darkness. Thirty minutes from the start of the light pulse, pineal c-*fos* levels were decreased to 10% or less of the levels found in hamsters that had been in uninterrupted darkness. This effect of light decreasing pineal c-*fos* expression also has been seen when the light pulse is administered at 1 hour after onset of darkness. We concluded that pineal c-*fos* is not expressed in the Djungarian hamster pineal gland in the presence of light.

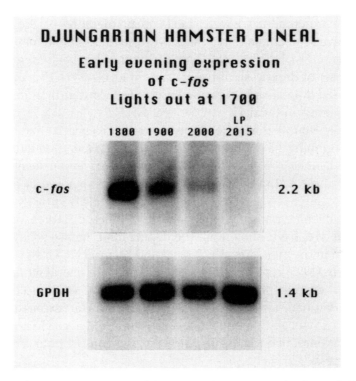

FIG. 2. Early-evening expression of Djungarian hamster pineal c-fos and effect of a light pulse. Molecular methods: Gene expression was determined using Northern blot analysis. Pineal glands were frozen in liquid nitrogen and stored at –80°C. Frozen pineals were homogenized in Ultraspec™ (Biotecx, Houston, Texas). Total pineal RNA, extracted according to manufacturer's instructions, was electrophoresed in a denaturing formaldehyde-agarose gel, then transferred to nylon membrane. The template for the probe for the c-fos gene was generated from Djungarian hamster pineal RNA using polymerase chain reaction (PCR) technology to produce a 400-base gene fragment. For hybridization to immobilized hamster RNA, the template was used to make a ^{32}P-labeled strand of RNA. Following quantification of c-fos hybridization to the blot, the c-fos probe was removed and the blot hybridized a second time to probe for the constitutively expressed gene, glyceraldehyde 3-phosphate dehydrogenase (GPDH). Our 1,000-base probe for GPDH was generated from rat tissue using PCR. This double-stranded DNA probe was labeled with ^{32}P for hybridization. Following hybridization, the blot was scanned in the AMBIS-4000 Radioanalytic Imager (Scanalytics, Billerica, Massachusetts), which computes the amount of radioactivity (counts per minute, cpm) in each band due to hybridization of the gene probe to complementary immobilized RNA. Levels of c-fos gene expression in each lane are determined as the ratio c-fos cpm over GPDH cpm.

In one experiment, we were able to obtain measures of serum melatonin levels in animals in which we also determined pineal c-*fos* expression. At 1 hour after a 20-minute light pulse (beginning 3 hours after onset of darkness), serum melatonin levels were 27% of that in unexposed animals and pineal c-*fos* was 14% of that in animals that had remained in the dark.

We also found that when animals were given a 20-minute light pulse beginning 3.5 hours after onset of darkness and then returned to darkness, pineal c-*fos* expression returned 2 hours later to levels equivalent to those found in hamsters that were not exposed to the light pulse.

Early-evening transcriptional patterns of pineal c-*fos* that are similar to what we have shown in the Djungarian hamster have been reported in the rat (Carter 1992; Baler and Klein 1995). However, Baler and Klein (1995) reported only a twofold increase over daytime levels in pineal c-*fos* at 2 hours after onset of darkness. Our results in the Djungarian hamster showed greater changes in c-*fos* expression during the early-evening hours, increasing from undetectable at 30 minutes after onset of darkness to a strong expression at 1 hour after onset of darkness.

A further consideration in determining the possible role of c-*fos* in pineal melatonin synthesis is whether or not pineal c-*fos* gene expression has a circadian rhythm; that is, "What is the pattern of pineal c-*fos* expression when hamsters are kept in complete darkness?" For example, Baler and Klein (1995) showed that during the night, expression levels of *fra*-2 increased and decreased at the same time as the activity of NAT increased and decreased, even when rats were housed in complete darkness. Thus, pineal *fra*-2 expression does not require light cues, but maintains an expression pattern based on the entrained photoperiod. This finding indicates that FRA-2 protein and *fra*-2 mRNA are regulated in a true circadian manner. In contrast, Baler and Klein (1995) showed that FOS protein had a constant expression over a 24-hour period when the rats were in constant darkness. Our results with the Djungarian hamster were quite different. We found that on day 6 of constant darkness, Djungarian hamster pineal c-*fos* clearly maintained an expression pattern exactly the same as found in hamsters on a light–dark regimen (unpublished data). We concluded that in the

Djungarian hamster, pineal c-*fos* is not expressed during those hours of the day that the hamsters would be exposed to light.

Our data may be indicative of a species-specific difference between the genetically homogeneous albino lab rat used in other studies and our outbred Djungarian hamsters. Pineal c-*fos* expression may be regulated differently in this nonseasonally breeding rat, while the potentiating effect of pineal FOS protein may be more critical in a photoperiodic breeder such as the Djungarian hamster. The sensitivity to light of Djungarian hamster pineal c-*fos* expression may indicate a role in entrainment, much the same as was recently proposed for the suprachiasmatic nucleus clock: c-*fos* expression is not required for normal function of the circadian rhythm, but is activated during perturbation (that is, light-induced entrainment) of the mammalian biological clock (Honrado et al. 1996).

EFFECTS OF MAGNETIC FIELD EXPOSURE ON PINEAL GENE EXPRESSION

Just as light-pulse effects on suprachiasmatic nucleus c-*fos* expression are restricted to times when light will shift the phase of the circadian rhythm, we also expect that magnetic field exposure will have effects on circadian processes only if such exposure is administered at specific times of day.

Our work on the effects of magnetic field exposure on gene expression in the mammalian pineal gland has been guided by two lines of research. First was evidence showing that magnetic field exposure may act similarly to light. Indeed, reports to date have indicated that magnetic field exposure, like light, produced a decrease in melatonin synthesis in rodents (Matt et al. 1994; Kato et al. 1994; Selmaoui and Touitou 1995). Second, in vitro studies have shown evidence of magnetic field-induced changes in gene expression that are relevant to our studies. For instance, c-*fos* expression was shown to be increased 2.5-fold in CEM-CM3 T-lymphoblastoid cells exposed for 30 minutes to a 1-G, 60-Hz, sinusoidally varying magnetic field (Phillips et al. 1992). Other studies have shown that ICER expression was increased two- to fourfold in magnetic field-exposed cultures of rat PC12 cells (Haggren et al. 1995).

In our studies, we use the long day-entrained Djungarian hamster (light:dark 16:8) to investigate the effects of magnetic field exposure on pineal gene expression. Our exposure room contains two identical magnetic field exposure coils. We expose the hamsters in their plastic cages (with stainless steel wire lids) to a 1-G, 60-Hz, sinusoidal magnetic field using a modified Merritt coil. The exposure equipment is positioned such that during a 1-G exposure, the unenergized coil receives stray magnetic fields amounting to 6–8 mG. Because we have focused on early-evening pineal gene expression, which we have studied extensively with light, we routinely include a group of hamsters that receive light exposure. In our experiments, pineal gene expression in magnetic field-exposed hamsters can be compared to pineal gene expression in animals that have been either sham- or light-exposed. When magnetic field exposures are performed after onset of darkness, the caged hamsters are transported in a light-proof cart to the light-locked exposure facility. All magnetic field exposures occurring after darkness are conducted in dim red light, which we have measured to produce less than 3 lux at a distance of 0.5 m.

We have conducted magnetic field exposures at two times of day: for 15 minutes beginning 2 hours before onset of darkness (late afternoon) and for 15 minutes beginning 3 hours after onset of darkness (early evening). For the late-afternoon exposures, we examined pineal c-*fos* expression at 3 hours after lights out (5 hours after magnetic field/sham exposure) and at 5 hours after lights out (7 hours after magnetic field/sham exposure). For the early-evening exposures, we examined pineal c-*fos* expression at 30 minutes and at 1 hour after magnetic field/sham exposure. In none of our experiments was there a difference between magnetic field- and sham-exposed pineal c-*fos* expression. Having repeated these magnetic field and sham exposures several times, we concluded that this field exposure has no effect on early-evening pineal c-*fos* expression in the long day-entrained Djungarian hamster.

We also asked whether pineal expression of a repressor protein, such as ICER, might be increased by magnetic field exposure, producing a delay in the initiation of nightly melatonin synthesis. Thus, we investigated the possibility that an in vivo system would produce results similar to our in vitro observations (Haggren et al. 1995). Our results with the long day-entrained Djungarian hamsters, however, showed no effect, as compared to sham-exposed hamsters, of our magnetic field exposure treatment on pineal ICER expression.

A recent abstract by Matt et al. (1994) reported that magnetic field exposure delayed the onset of melatonin production in short day-entrained, but not in long day-entrained, Djungarian hamsters. We currently are investigating molecular effects in a short day-entrained Djungarian hamster, which receives 8 hours of light and 16 hours of darkness.

FINAL COMMENT

Because of the apparent effect of magnetic field exposure on melatonin production, it is essential to define the mechanism by which alterations in the production of this physiologically important molecule occur. A key question in trying to characterize the mechanism is, "What tissue is the target for magnetic fields?" Several studies have pointed to the retina as essential for the response of the mammalian circadian system to magnetic field exposure (Olcese et al. 1985; Reuss and Olcese 1986; Schneider and Semm 1992). Alternatively, it may be that magnetic field exposure targets the suprachiasmatic nucleus, producing signals similar to those produced in the retina by light, and that these signals are then sent along appropriate pathways to the pineal. Still another possibility is that the pineal itself may be the primary target for magnetic field exposure.

Another key question is, "What is the molecular target for magnetic field exposure?" It is reasonable that this exposure, like light, will result in changes in the expression of genes that encode transcriptional regulators and key enzymes. Consequently, identifying such sensitive genes is an immediate priority. Recent advances in circadian molecular biology, described in the foregoing discussion, make this task an exciting and achievable challenge. Additionally, new techniques in molecular biology should make significant contributions to this area. For instance, the technique of differential display potentially allows the identification of genes that are expressed under one condition (for instance, magnetic field exposure) and not under another (for instance, no field exposure). Indeed, this technique has been used in studies of light- and dark-cycle-specific pineal gene expression (Gauer et al. 1995). Furthermore, differential display may have great value in determining which tissue is the target for magnetic field exposure.

ACKNOWLEDGMENTS

I would like to extend my heartfelt thanks to Tsehay E. Mekonnen and Tamako Ishida-Jones, who have conducted the laboratory work. I thank Dr. W. Ross Adey, who has been unfailing in his support, both personally and scientifically. Dr. Kathleen S. Matt, Arizona State University, provided the Djungarian hamsters used to start the breeding colony that is housed at the Animal Research Facility in the Jerry L. Pettis Veterans Affairs Medical Center, Loma Linda, California. I thank Dr. Jerry L. Phillips for his critical reading of the manuscript. This work has been supported by the U.S. Department of Energy, Office of Energy Management under contracts DE-AI01-90CE35035 and DE-AI01-95EE34020 to Dr. W. Ross Adey; by funds from the Department of Veterans Affairs; and by Loma Linda University Research Support Funds.

REFERENCES

Angel, P., M. Karin. 1991. The role of JUN, FOS and the AP-1 complex in cell-proliferation and transformation. *Biochim. Biophys. Acta* 1072:129–157.

Baler, R., D.C. Klein. 1995. Circadian expression of transcription factor FRA-2 in the rat pineal gland. *J. Biol. Chem.* 270:27319–27325.

Borjigin, J., M.M. Wang, S.H. Snyder. 1995. Diurnal variation in mRNA encoding serotonin. N-acetyltransferase in pineal gland. *Nature* 378:783–785.

Carter, D.A. 1992. Neurotransmitter-stimulated immediate-early gene responses are organized through differential post-synaptic receptor mechanisms. *Mol. Brain Res.* 16:111–118.

Carter, D.A. 1994. A daily rhythm of activator protein-1 activity in the rat pineal is dependent upon trans-synaptic induction of JUNB. *Neuroscience* 62:1267–1278.

Coon, S.L., P.H. Roseboom, R. Baler, J.L. Weller, M.A.A. Namboodiri, E.V. Koonin, D.C. Klein. 1995. Pineal serotonin N-acetyltransferase: Expression cloning and molecular analysis. *Science* 270:1681–1683.

Craft, C.M. 1993. Molecular biology of the pineal gland: Melatonin synthesizing enzymes. In: *Melatonin*, H.-S. Yu, R.J. Reiter, eds., pp. 17–38. London: CRC Press.

Crosthwaite, S.K., J.L. Loros, J.C. Dunlap. 1995. Light-induced resetting of a circadian clock is mediated by a rapid increase in *frequency* transcript. *Cell* 81:1003–1012.

Curran, T., J.I. Morgan. 1987. Memories of *fos*. *Bioessays* 7:255–258.

Curran T., D. Cohen, J. Hempstead, J.I. Morgan. 1989. Stimulus-transcription coupling in neuronal cells. In: *Allosteric Modulation of Amino Acid Receptors: Therapeutic Implications*, E. Barnard, E. Costa, eds., pp. 335–345. New York: Raven Press, Ltd.

Donohue, S.J., P.H. Rosebloom, H. Illnerová, J.L. Weller, D.C. Klien. 1993. Human hydroxyindole O-methyltransferase: Presence of LINE-1 fragment in a cDNA clone and pineal mRNA. *DNA Cell Biol.* 12:715–727.

Gauer, F., W. Kedzierski, C.M. Craft. 1995. Identification of circadian gene expression in the rat pineal gland and retina by mRNA differential display. *Neurosci. Lett.* 187:69–73.

Haggren, W., J.L. Phillips, T.E. Mekonnen, M. Campbell-Beachler, T. Ishida-Jones, O.I. Ivaschuk, W.R. Adey. 1995. Effects of 60 Hz magnetic field exposure in vitro and in vivo on the expression of the transcriptional repressor, ICER. In: Abstracts of the 17th Annual Bioelectromagnetics Society Meeting, Boston, Massachusetts, p. 3.

Hoffmann, K., H. Illnerová, J. Vaněček. 1980. Pineal N-acetyltransferase activity in the Djungarian hamster. *Naturwissenschaften* 67:408–409.

Honrado, G.I., R.S. Johnson, D.A. Golombek, B.M. Spiegelman, V.E. Papaioannou, M.R. Ralph. 1996. The circadian system of c-*fos* deficient mice. *J. Comp. Physiol. A Sens. Neural Behav. Physiol.* 178:563–570.

Hope, B., B. Kosofsky, S.E. Hyman, E.J. Nestler. 1992. Regulation of immediate early gene expression and AP-1 binding in the rat nucleus accumbens by chronic cocaine. *Proc. Natl. Acad. Sci. USA* 89:5764–5768.

Hunter-Ensor, M., A. Ousley, A. Sehgal. 1996. Regulation of the *Drosophila* protein *timeless* suggests a mechanism for resetting the circadian clock by light. *Cell* 84:677–685.

Illnerová, H., J. Vaněček. 1979. Response of rat pineal serotonin N-acetyltransferase to one minute light pulse at different night times. *Brain Res.* 167:431–434.

Kato, M., K. Honma, T. Shigemitsu, Y. Shiga. 1994. Circularly polarized 50-Hz magnetic field exposure reduces pineal gland and blood melatonin concentrations of Long-Evans rats. *Neurosci. Lett.* 166:59–62.

Klein, D.C., J.E. Weller. 1970. Indole metabolism in the pineal gland. A circadian rhythm in N-acetyltransferase activity. *Science* 169:1093–1095.

Korf, H.-W. 1994. The pineal organ as a component of the biological clock: Phylogenetic and ontogenetic consideration. In: *The Aging Clock*, W. Pierpaoli, W. Regelson, and N. Fabris, eds., pp. 13–42. Annals of the New York Academy of Sciences.

Lerchl, A., E. Nieschlag. 1992. Interruption of nocturnal pineal melatonin synthesis in spontaneous recrudescent Djungarian hamsters (*Phodopus sungorus*). *J. Pineal Res.* 13:36–41.

Lerchl, A., A. Schlatt. 1992. Serotonin content and melatonin production in the pineal gland of the male Djungarian hamster (*Phodopus sungorus*). *J. Pineal Res.* 12:128–134.

Lolley, R.N., C.M. Craft, R.H. Lee. 1992. Photoreceptors of the retinal and pinealocytes share common components of signal transduction. *Neurochem. Res.* 17:81–89.

Matt, K.S., B.W. Wilson, J.E. Morris, L.B. Sasser, D.L. Miller, L.E. Anderson. 1994. The effect of EMF exposure on neuroendocrine mechanisms of environmental integration. In: Abstracts of the 16th Annual Bioelectromagnetics Society Meeting, Copenhagen, Denmark, June 12–17, p. 49. Frederick, Maryland: The Bioelectromagnetics Society.

Molina, C.A., N.S. Foulkes, E. Lalli, P. Sassone-Corsi. 1993. Inducibility and negative autoregulation of CREM: An alternative promoter directs the expression of ICER, an early response repressor. *Cell* 75:875–886.

Morgan, J.I., T. Curran. 1991. Stimulus-transcription coupling in the nervous system: Involvement of the inducible proto-oncogenes *fos* and *jun*. *Annu. Rev. Neurosci.* 14:421–451.

Morrissey, J.J., W. Lovenberg. 1978a. Synthesis of RNA in the pineal gland during N-acetyltransferase induction. *Biochem. Pharmacol.* 27:551–555.

Morrissey, J.J., W. Lovenberg. 1978b. Synthesis of RNA in the pineal gland during N-acetyltransferase induction: The effects of actino-mycin D, a-amanitin and cordycepin. *Biochem. Pharmacol.* 27:557–562.

Nelson, R.J., L.L. Badura, B.D. Goldman. 1990. Mechanisms of seasonal cycles of behavior. *Annu. Rev. Psychol.* 41:81–108.

Niklowitz, P., A. Lerchl, E. Nieschlag. 1994. Photoperiodic responses in Djungarian hamsters (*Phodopus sungorus*): Importance of light his-tory for pineal and serum melatonin profiles. *Biol. Reprod.* 51:714–724.

Olcese, J., S. Reuss, L. Vollrath. 1985. Evidence for the involvement of the visual system in mediating magnetic field effects on pineal melatonin synthesis in the rat. *Brain Res.* 333:382–384.

Partonen, T. 1994. The molecular basis for winter depression. *Ann. Med.* 26:239–243.

Phillips, J.L., W. Haggren, W.J. Thomas, T. Ishida-Jones, W.R. Adey. 1992. Magnetic field-induced changes in specific gene transcription. *Biochim. Biophys. Acta* 1132:140–144.

Reiter, R.J. 1991. Pineal melatonin: Cell biology of its synthesis and of its physiological interactions. *Endocrine Rev.* 12:151–180.

Reiter, R.J. 1992. Alterations of the circadian melatonin rhythm by the electromagnetic spectrum: A study in environmental toxicology. *Regul. Toxicol. Pharmacol.* 15:226–244.

Reuss, S., J. Olcese. 1986. Magnetic field effects on the rat pineal gland: Role of retinal activation by light. *Neurosci. Lett.* 64:97–101.

Roseboom, B.H., D. Klein. 1995. Norepinephrine stimulation on pineal cyclic AMP response element-binding protein phosphorylation: Primary role of a ß-adrenergic receptor/cyclic AMP mechanism. *Mol. Pharmacol.* 47:439–449.

Schneider, T., P. Semm. 1992. The biological and possible clinical significance of magnetic influences on the pineal melatonin synthesis.
Exp. Clin. Endocrinol. 11:251–258.

Schwartz, W.J., J. Takeuchi, W. Shannon, E.M. Davis, N. Aronin. 1994.
Temporal regulation of light-induced FOS and FOS-like protein
expression in the ventrolateral subdivision of the rat suprachiasmatic nucleus. *Neuroscience* 58:573–583.

Selmaoui, B., Y. Touitou. 1995. Sinusoidal 50-Hz magnetic fields
depress rat pineal NAT activity and serum melatonin. Role of duration and intensity of exposure. *Life Sci.* 57:1351–1358.

Stehle, J.H. 1995. Pineal gene expression: Dawn in a dark matter. *J.
Pineal Res.* 18:179–190.

Stehle, J.H., N.S. Foulkes, C.A. Molina, V. Simonneaux, P. Pévet, P.
Sassone-Corsi. 1993. Adrenergic signals direct rhythmic expression
of transcriptional repressor CREM in the pineal gland. *Nature*
365:314–320.

Steinlechner, S., I. Baumgartner, G. Klante, R.J. Reiter. 1995. Melatonin
synthesis in the retinal and pineal gland of Djungarian hamsters at
different times of the year. *Neurochem. Int.* 27:245–251.

Stevens, R.G., S. Davis, D.B. Thomas, L.E. Anderson, B.W. Wilson. 1992.
Electric power, pineal function, and the risk of breast cancer. *FASEB
J.* 6:853–660.

Takahashi, J.S. 1994. ICER is nicer at night (sir!). *Curr. Biol.* 4:165–168.

Takahashi, J.S., M. Zatz. 1982. Regulation of circadian rhythmicity.
Science 217:1104–1111.

Takeuchi, J., W. Shannon, N. Aronin, W.J. Schwartz. 1993. Com-
positional changes of AP-1 DNA-binding proteins are regulated by
light in a mammalian circadian clock. *Neuron* 11:825–836.

Tamotsu, S., C. Schomerus, J.H. Stehle, P.H. Roseboom, H.-W. Korf.
1995. Norepinephrine-induced phosphorylation of the transcription factor CREB in isolated rat pinealocytes: An immunocytochemical study. *Cell Tissue Res.* 282:219–226.

Tosini, G., M. Menaker. 1996. Circadian rhythms in cultured mammalian retina. *Science* 272:419–421.

Voisin, P., J. Guerlotté, M. Bernard, J.-P. Collin, M. Cogné, M. 1992.
Molecular cloning and nucleotide sequence of a cDNA encoding

hydroxyindole-*O*-methlytransferase from chicken pineal gland. *Biochem. J.* 282:571-576.

Yu, L., N.C. Schaad, D.C. Klein. 1993. Calcium potentiates cyclic AMP stimulation of pineal arylalkylamine N-acetyltransferase. *J. Neurochem.* 60:1436–1443.

Zeng, H., Z. Qian, M.P. Myers, M. Rosbash. 1996. A light-entrainment mechanism for the *Drosophila* circadian clock. *Nature* 380:129–135.

12 Daytime Melatonin in Postmenopausal Japanese-American Women

MICHINORI KABUTO
  Environmental Risk Research Division, National Institute
  for Environmental Studies, Tsukuba City, Japan

CONTENTS

BACKGROUND
CORRELATIONS AMONG THE PARAMETERS
  OF MELATONIN STATUS
DAYTIME ESTRADIOL LEVELS IN POSTMENOPAUSAL WOMEN
DAYTIME SERUM MELATONIN
IMPLICATIONS FOR FUTURE RESEARCH
REFERENCES

BACKGROUND

Melatonin, an indoleamine produced primarily by the pineal gland, has been suggested to have antitumor activities. In addition, evidence has accumulated that melatonin, at least when administered exogenously, may suppress estrogen synthesis possibly through reducing luteinizing hormone/follicle stimulating hormone (LH/FSH) secretion (Voordouw et al. 1992), may interfere with the binding of estrogen to its receptors expressed in breast cancer cells in vitro (Hill et al. 1992; Wilson et al. 1992; Liburdy et al. 1993), may ameliorate immune function (Finocchiaro et al. 1988), and may act as a scavenger of free radicals (Reiter et al. 1994). These pharmacological and clinical findings (Lissoni et al. 1991, 1992) led to a hypothesis that elevated endogenous melatonin can exert oncostatic action via immunomodulation and/or alterations of reproductive hormones or free radicals. In this context, research on how exposure to extremely low frequency (ELF) electric and magnetic fields (EMF) affects melatonin secretion becomes critically important. It has been shown for animals (Kato et al. 1993, 1994a, b; Lerchl et al. 1991; Reiter 1993; Löscher et al. 1994) and suggested for humans (Wilson and Anderson 1990; Graham et al. 1994) that exposure to ELF EMF can suppress the nocturnal increase of melatonin production. This suppression, therefore, has been assumed as the underlying mechanism for the suggested association between increased breast cancer risk and exposure to ELF EMF (Stevens 1993; Loomis et al. 1994).

Recent epidemiologic studies have reported that estrogen status in postmenopausal women is significantly associated with subsequent breast cancer risk (Kabuto et al. 1994; Toniolo et al. 1995). These studies suggest that estrogen during the postmenopausal period may be a factor that promotes (or accelerates) breast cancer development. Such association has been unclear for premenopausal women; melatonin may influence estrogen in premenopausal women.

The study reported in this chapter examined the question of whether melatonin is involved in regulating estrogen status in post-menopausal women, whose estrogen status is no longer regulated by the pituitary-gonadal axis or LH/FSH but depends on the androgens produced by the adrenal. Melatonin levels in sera were determined in postmenopausal women selected randomly from Japanese Americans and Caucasians in Los Angeles, and from Japanese in Japan.

CORRELATIONS AMONG THE PARAMETERS OF MELATONIN STATUS

Melatonin is produced with a large day–night rhythm as well as a seasonal rhythm. Therefore, melatonin status could be expressed in many different ways; e.g., peak level during the night, average daytime or nighttime level, cumulative level for a day, or average annual level. Melatonin also can fluctuate based on the menstrual cycle, although this is not a factor in postmenopausal women. Because of this complexity of melatonin synthesis, it is not clear that a single daytime serum level of melatonin is useful for studies of the relationship of melatonin on risk of diseases such as breast cancer. We have conducted a preliminary examination on the possible correlations among the parameters of melatonin status using urinary melatonin levels.

Urinary excretion rates of melatonin (UERM) were determined for urine specimens collected from seven healthy Japanese students. Melatonin in urine was determined by radioimmunoassay (RIA) using the commercial, ultrasensitive RIA kits for melatonin (Bühlmann Laboratories AG, Switzerland). The students remained in an experimental room from 1800–2400 hours, free from hard physical activities, then slept in almost completely dark conditions from 2400–0800 hours in a sound-insulated room located within the experimental room. The temperature in both rooms was kept constant at 23°C. Light intensity within the experimental room was consistently around 500 lux after sunset; the intensity varied at higher levels due to sunlight during the day. The specimens were collected during five time periods from 1800–2400, 2400–0400, 0400–0800, 0800–1200, and 1200–1800 hours. The sample collected at 0400 hours involved a brief waking; for the daytime samples, the students returned to the laboratory. In another study with the same subjects (data not shown), similar levels and rhythm of UERM were observed when they were kept sleep-deprived in the 500-lux experimental room for the entire 24-hour period; the amplitude was lower (1.4 ng/hr versus 1.76) and the acrophase later (0408 hours versus 0305 hours) though neither difference was statistically significant. These findings show that, at least among this group of young Japanese volunteers, 500-lux light did not have a dramatic effect on melatonin production.

As shown in Table 1 and illustrated in Figure 1, mean UERM values obtained for each of the time periods showed a marked and significant peak in samples collected from 2400–0400, as expected. This finding validated the assay methods adopted as well as the time schedule for urine collection. The UERM for 8 hours of nighttime (2400–0800 hours) when subjects were sleeping varied from 1.86–6.39 ng/hour; UERM for 16 hours of daytime (0800–2400 hours), when subjects were awake, varied from 0.45–1.21 ng/hour.

TABLE 1
Means (± SD) UERM According to Time Periods of Urine Collection

Time period	Mean (± SD) UERM, ng/hour
1800–2400 hours (daytime)	0.90 (0.69)
2400–0400 hours (nighttime)	3.88 (2.35)
0400–0800 hours (nighttime)	2.65 (1.28)
0800–1200 hours (daytime)	0.81 (0.40)
1200–1800 hours (daytime)	0.36 (0.15)

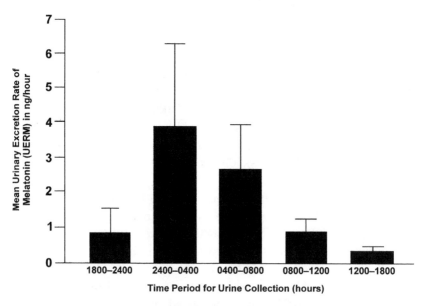

FIG. 1. Means (± SD) of UERM by time periods of urine collection.

An analysis of the day–night rhythm for these UERM values using the Cosinor method showed that the acrophase was, on average, 0305 hours. This finding may suggest that the timing of urine collection during sleep should be shifted from 0400 hours to, for example, 0300 hours so that UERM would reflect more accurately the peak melatonin production expected around 0200 hours. The correlation coefficients (excluding the UERM for 0800–1200 hours) summarized in Table 2 show, however, that other daytime UERM were highly correlated with the peak UERM for 2400–0400 hours, or with either of the cumulative doses for nighttime or a whole day (Table 3). The correlation data also suggest that cumulative dose for daytime, when UERM are much lower than those during nighttime, may substantially contribute to the cumulative dose for a whole day, as indicated by the mean values; the cumulative dose for daytime was 38% (15.94 ng) of that for a whole day (42.08 ng).

The morning UERM for 0800–1200 hours was not related to night-time melatonin. This UERM may have been affected by exposures to sunlight after the subjects awakened at 0800 hours, because subjects were exposed to sunlight randomly after waking up and the intensity of sunlight varied daily according to the weather.

In summary, the data from this preliminary study of UERM suggest that a measure of serum melatonin from an afternoon collection, 1200–1800 hours, might reflect melatonin status as a whole in terms of the peak level at the acrophase of its day–night rhythm, and cumulative dose for nighttime or a whole day. It should be noted that human plasma melatonin correlates with urinary 6-hydroxymelatonin excretion (Markey et al. 1985), which is also expected to correlate with urinary melatonin excretion.

DAYTIME ESTRADIOL LEVELS IN POSTMENOPAUSAL WOMEN

Midafternoon blood samples were taken from postmenopausal women (Kabuto et al. 1994) randomly selected from Japanese-Americans in Los Angeles (LA-J; parents are mostly Japanese), Caucasians in Los Angeles (LA-W), and Japanese in a rural area of Japan (J-J). Numbers of LA-J, LA-W, and J-J were 32, 31, and 65, respectively. Brief profiles of these subjects are summarized in Table 4. Additional measurements were

TABLE 2
Pearson's Correlation Coefficients Among the Parameters of Melatonin Status

	UERM from 2400 to 0400 hours	Cumulative dose for nighttime	Cumulative dose for a whole day
UERM from 0800 to 1200 hours	−0.260[a]	0.253[a]	0.405[a]
UERM from 1200 to 1800 hours	0.888 ($p < 0.01$)	0.978 ($p < 0.001$)	0.769 ($p < 0.05$)
UERM from 1800 to 2400	0.928 ($p < 0.01$)	0.893 ($p < 0.01$)	0.741 ($p = 0.057$)
Cumulative dose for daytime	0.123[a]	0.124[a]	0.721 ($p = 0.068$)
Cumulative dose for nighttime	0.954 ($p < 0.001$)	—	0.777 ($p < 0.05$)

[a] Not significant.

TABLE 3
Cumulative Dose of Melatonin

Time period	Mean ($\pm$ SD) cumulative dose melatonin, ng
Daytime	15.9 (13.0)
Nighttime	26.1 (14.3)
Whole day	42.1 (20.5)

performed for sera collected two times in the follicular and luteal phases (on the 11th and 22nd day after the last menstruation, respectively) from 14 premenopausal Japanese women.

Kabuto et al. (1994) reported a strong association between the serum status of estradiol (E_2) [serum levels of total E_2, E_2 unbound, and E_2 bound to sex-hormone-binding globulin (SHBG)] and breast cancer incidence rate among the three groups. Figure 2 (data adjusted for age and smoking) shows a strong correlation of each of the three groups with breast cancer risk as estimated from tumor registries in Los Angeles and Japan. E_2 unbound to SHBG, which consists of the free fraction and fraction bound to albumin, is thought to be biologically active and related directly to the risk of breast cancer. E_2 bound to SHBG seems to be much less active, as has been observed in nested case–control studies of Japanese (Kabuto et al. unpublished data) and of Caucasians (Toniolo et al. 1995). The strong correlation between E_2 bound to SHBG and breast cancer incidence rate in Figure 2, therefore, seems to be a reflection of the extremely high levels of total E_2 in LA-J and LA-W. In the same study (Kabuto et al. 1994), however, no correlation with breast cancer incidence rate was found for dehydroepiandrosterone-sulfate (DHEA), prolactin, and progesterone (data not shown).

The serum levels in LA-W and LA-J groups of total E_2, SHBG-unbound E_2, and SHBG-bound E_2 were significantly elevated in

TABLE 4
Major Profiles of the Study Subjects

Category	LA-W	LA-J	J-J
Number of participants	31	32	65
Age (years)	65.3 (3.7)	61.9 (4.6)[a, b]	61.2 (6.0)[c]
Weight (kg)	69.0 (11.0)	54.4 (7.6)[b,c]	51.4 (7.1)[c]
Height (cm)	163.1 (6.7)	155.3 (5.6)[b,c]	151.6 (5.4)[c]
Body mass index	25.9 (3.4)	22.6 (3.6)	22.3 (2.7)
% current + ex-smokers	41.9%	40.6%	10.2%
% estrogen replacement therapy	30.2%	33.3%	1.5%
% age at menarche < 12 years	34.8%	50.0%	2.9%
% age at menopause > 55 years	16.7%	9.47%	2.9%

LA-W = Caucasians in Los Angeles.
LA-J = Japanese in Los Angeles.
J-J = Japanese in Japan.
The values other than % values indicate mean ($\pm$ SD).
[a] The mean difference is significant compared to LA-W with $p < 0.01$.
[b] The mean difference is significant compared to J-J with $p < 0.001$.
[c] The mean difference is significant compared to LA-W with $p < 0.001$.

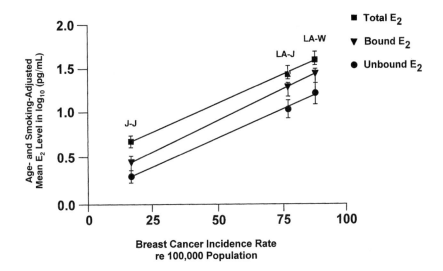

FIG. 2. Correlations between breast cancer incidence rate and estradiol status among three groups of postmenopausal women. Mean (± SD) levels of total E_2, SHBG-bound E_2, and SHBG-unbound E_2, adjusted for age and smoking status, are indicated by the closed square, triangle, and circle, respectively. The lines in the figure are the regression lines for each of the three parameters. See text for details.

women who were at the time on estrogen replacement therapy or smoking, and in women who reached menarche at an early age compared to women in the J-J group. No such differences were found for body mass index, number of children, or parous/nulliparous. Although the data illustrated in Figure 2 were adjusted only for age and smoking, the correlations were consistent regardless of further adjustment for estrogen replacement therapy and age at menarche. An unexpected finding was that, especially for LA-J women, postmenopausal serum E_2 status was still strongly associated with age at menarche over a period of more than 40 years. This suggests that some environmental factors, such as diet, may have caused earlier menarche as well as the long-lasting enhancement of E_2 level.

DAYTIME SERUM MELATONIN

Serum melatonin levels were directly measured with ELISA assay kits (Bühlmann Laboratories AG). Mean serum levels of melatonin were significantly higher in LA-W and LA-J women than in J-J women (Table 5). The values were higher compared to the reported values of daytime melatonin (~10 pg/mL) for Caucasians. We attribute the difference to the ELISA assay methods used. That daytime serum melatonin levels may be higher in early morning or late afternoon than in midafternoon (reference data by Bühlman Laboratories AG) does not explain the variation of melatonin levels, because blood was collected mostly during midafternoon. The melatonin levels in LA-W and LA-J women were in the same range as those in premenopausal Japanese women.

Melatonin levels were not correlated with levels of total E_2, SHBG-unbound E_2, or SHBG-bound E_2—on an individual basis—among the postmenopausal women in our study. No correlation between melatonin and total E_2 levels was observed for the premenopausal Japanese

TABLE 5
Mean Levels of Melatonin in the Three Groups of
Postmenopausal Women and a Group of
Premenopausal Japanese Women

Subjects	Mean (± SD) melatonin level
Postmenopausal women	
Caucasians (LA-W)	43.3 (16.9)
Japanese-Americans (LA-J)	25.8 (16.1)
Japanese in Japan (J-J)	12.8 (6.9)
Premenopausal Japanese women	
Follicular phase	45.6 (24.7)
Luteal phase	36.8 (20.9)

women, either, although mean total E_2 level was slightly lower in the follicular phase than in the luteal phase (78.9 versus 87.0 pg/mL), thus showing a weak negative correlation with the mean levels of melatonin. Because melatonin seems to affect the pituitary-gonadal axis primarily through a suppression of LH/FSH surge in premenopausal women (Voordouw et al. 1992), these results might indicate an importance of melatonin status during the period closer to LH/FSH surge.

As stated previously, E_2 levels were observed to be significantly elevated in women on estrogen replacement therapy and in women who smoked (more than 11 cigarettes/day) compared to women who were not on estrogen replacement and who did not smoke. In contrast, melatonin levels in subjects on estrogen replacement or who smoked (both of which were more common among LA-W and LA-J than among J-J) were not different.

IMPLICATIONS FOR FUTURE RESEARCH

Melatonin has been suggested experimentally and clinically to reduce risk, or inhibit development, of breast cancer via several possible pathways, including effects on estrogen metabolism, effects on the immune system, and effects as a free radical scavenger. We have presented evidence that in postmenopausal women, daytime melatonin level is not correlated with estradiol level, and that daytime melatonin levels are higher in women drawn from populations with a higher risk of breast cancer, contrary to expectation if melatonin inhibits the disease. These data must be interpreted cautiously, however, because this was a study of healthy women without breast cancer, and because conclusions regarding the relationship of melatonin level to breast cancer require studies of women with breast cancer and appropriate controls within well-defined populations. Absolute melatonin levels may differ for many reasons across national and ethnic boundaries, but variations within populations may still be important.

Our results have supported the view that daytime urinary melatonin level can be used to estimate total melatonin production. This would make possible the study of the relationship of melatonin to risk of breast cancer, particularly in cohort studies. A morning void urine sample could be collected and saved from a large number of healthy women. These women could be studied over time, and definitive studies conducted.

We are not able to say whether daytime serum melatonin level is related to nocturnal production. However, we have shown that the daytime level is higher in Caucasian women in the United States than in Americans of Japanese descent, and that levels in both of these groups are higher than in Japanese women.

Possible underlying causes of the elevation of daytime melatonin levels among LA-J (who are Japanese genetically) and LA-W compared to those in J-J should be considered. There seems to be at least three possibilities that need further clarification:

- A possible difference in dietary tryptophan intake, which recently has been shown to affect directly the amount of melatonin synthesis (Sielaff et al. 1991; Bubenik et al. 1992; Huether 1993; Yaga et al. 1993; Zimmermann et al. 1993). No data are available whether there is any substantial difference in the tryptophan intake between citizens of the United States and Japan.

- A possible difference in aging of the physiological functions in both pineal and gonadal glands, not only by the higher levels of both melatonin and E2, but by the later age at menopause of LA-J and LA-W compared to that of J-J (Table 4).

- A possible homeostatic response of melatonin to the possible increase of free radicals through the suggested interaction (Reiter et al. 1994), if the higher risk for breast cancer in LA-J and LA-W compared to that in J-J could be attributed to amount of free radicals.

In patients with cancer at various sites, it has been shown that daytime melatonin levels exhibit a nonspecific elevation (Falkson et al. 1990). This may be through a link between the cancer and the pineal via tumor-induced interferon, which is expected to stimulate melatonin synthesis in the pineal both indirectly via sympathetic nerves and directly on the pinealocytes (Withyachumnarnkul et al. 1991). However, in a recent study using a newly developed, chemiluminescence-ELISA method (Satoh et al. 1995), no difference in mean levels of interferon and other cytokines were observed between two groups of normal male subjects selected from Japanese in Japan and

Caucasians in the United States. Thus, interferon seems not to be involved in the melatonin increase among LA-J, suggesting also that it does not have a physiological role in regulating pineal melatonin synthesis under normal situations.

There remains the question of what parameter of melatonin status is the best to use in studies of breast cancer, especially in connection with the suggested effects of ELF EMF exposure. In those animal experiments showing a breast cancer inhibition by melatonin (see Blask, this volume), melatonin is expected to exert its effects temporarily as the serum melatonin level is enhanced by the manual administration. This suggests that the resultant peak level and/or timing of the peak may be important, which may have critical importance if ELF EMF exposures reduce the nocturnal peak level of melatonin. Therefore, large cohort studies will be essential to clarify the relationships among EMF exposure, various aspects of melatonin status, and subsequent breast cancer risk.

REFERENCES

Bubenik, G.A., R.O. Ball, S-F. Pang. 1992. The effect of food deprivation on brain and gastro-intestinal tissue levels of tryptophan, serotonin, 5-hydroxyindoleacetic acid, and melatonin. *J. Pineal Res.* 12(1):7–16.

Falkson, G.F., H.C. Falkson, M.E. Steyn, B.L. Rapoport, B.J. Meyer. 1990. Plasma melatonin in patients with breast cancer. *Oncology* 47:401–405.

Finocchiaro, L.M., E.S. Arzt, S. Fernandez-Castelo, M. Criscuolo, S. Finkielman, V.E. Nahmod. 1988. Serotonin and melatonin synthesis in peripheral blood mononuclear cells: Stimulation by interferon-γ as part of an immunomodulatory pathway. *J. Interferon Res.* 8:705–716.

Graham, C., M.R. Cook, H.D. Cohen, D.W. Riffle. 1994. Nocturnal melatonin levels in men exposed to magnetic fields: A replication study. In: Abstracts of the Annual Review of Research on Biological Effects of Electric and Magnetic Fields from the Generation, Delivery, and Use of Electricity, Albuquerque, New Mexico, November 610, A-51, pp. 51–52. Frederick, Maryland: W/L Associates, Ltd.

Hill, S.M., L.L. Spriggs, M.A. Simon, H. Muraoka, D.E. Blask. 1992. The growth inhibitory action of melatonin on human breast cancer cells is linked to the estrogen response system. *Cancer Lett.* 64:249–256.

Huether, G. 1993. The contribution of extrapineal sites of melatonin synthesis to circulating melatonin levels in higher vertebrates. *Experientia* 49:665–670.

Kabuto, M., H. Shimizu, H. Imai, L. Bernstein, R. Roth, B.E. Henderson. 1994. Postmenopausal serum estradiol among Japanese- and White-American women in Los Angeles and Japanese women in Japan. *Int. J. Oncol.* 5(Suppl):399.

Kato, M., K. Honma, T. Shigemitsu, Y. Shiga. 1993. Effects of exposure to a circularly polarized 50-Hz magnetic field on plasma and pineal melatonin levels in rats. *Bioelectromagnetics* 14:97–106.

Kato, M., K. Honma, T. Shigemitsu, Y. Shiga. 1994a. Circularly polarized 50-Hz magnetic field exposure reduces pineal gland and blood melatonin concentrations of Long-Evans rats. *Neurosci. Lett.* 166:59–62.

Kato, M., K. Honma, T. Shigemitsu, Y. Shiga. 1994b. Horizontal or vertical 50-Hz, 1-μT magnetic fields have no effect on pineal gland or plasma melatonin concentration of albino rats. *Neurosci. Lett.* 168:205–208.

Lerchl, A., R.J. Reiter, K.A. Howes, K.O. Nonaka, K.-A. Stokkan. 1991. Evidence that extremely low frequency Ca^{2+}-cyclotron resonance depresses pineal melatonin synthesis in vitro. *Neurosci. Lett.* 124:213–215.

Liburdy, R.P., T.R. Sloma, R. Sokolic, P. Yaswen. 1993. ELF magnetic fields, breast cancer, and melatonin: 60-Hz fields block melatonin's oncostatic action on ER^+ breast cancer cell proliferation. *J. Pineal Res.* 14(2):89–97.

Lissoni, P., S. Barni, G. Cattaneo, G. Tancini, G. Esposti, D. Esposti, F. Fraschini. 1991. Clinical results with the pineal hormone melatonin in advanced cancer resistant to standard antitumor therapies. *Oncology* 48:448–450.

Lissoni, P., S. Barni, A. Ardizzoia, F. Paolorossi, S. Crispino, G. Tancini, E. Tisi, C. Archili, D. De Toma, G. Pipino, A. Conti, G.J.M. Maestroni. 1992. Randomized study with the pineal hormone melatonin versus supportive care alone in advanced nonsmall cell lung cancer resistant to a first-line chemotherapy containing cisplatin. *Oncology* 49:336–339.

Loomis, D.P., D.A. Savitz, C.V. Ananth. 1994. Breast cancer mortality among female electrical workers in the United States. *J. Natl. Cancer Inst.* 86:921–925.

Löscher, W., U. Wahnschaffe, M. Mevissen, A. Lerchl, A. Stamm. 1994. Effects of weak alternating magnetic fields on nocturnal melatonin production and mammary carcinogenesis in rats. *Oncology* 51:288–295.

Markey, S.P., S. Higa, M. Shih, D.N. Danforth, L. Tamarkin. 1985. The correlation between human plasma melatonin levels and urinary 6-hydroxymelatonin excretion. *Clin. Chim. Acta.* 150:221–225.

Reiter, R.J. 1993. Electric and magnetic fields and melatonin production. *Biomed. & Pharmacother.* 47:439–444.

Reiter, R.J., D.-X. Tan, B. Poeggeler, A. Menendez-Pelaez, L.D. Chen, S. Saarela. 1994. Melatonin as a free radical scavenger: Implications for aging and age-related diseases. *Ann N.Y. Acad Sci.* 719:1–12.

Satoh, T., D.J. Tollerud, L. Guevarra, Y. Rakue, T. Nakadate, J. Kagawa. 1995. Chemiluminescence assays for cytokines in serum: Influence of age, smoking, and race in healthy subjects. *Allergy* (Japanese) 44(7):661–669.

Sielaff, T., L. Demisch, P. Gebhart, A. Blumhofer, A. Khazai, B. Lemmer. 1991. Chronobiological effects of L-tryptophan in humans: Influence on melatonin secretion. *Adv. Exp. Med. Biol.* 294:489–491.

Stevens, R.G. 1993. Breast cancer and electric power. *Biomed. & Pharmacother.* 47:435–438.

Toniolo, P.G., L. Mortimer, A. Zeleniuch-Jacquotte, S. Banerjee, K.L. Koenig, R.E. Shore, P. Strax, B.S. Pasternack. 1995. A prospective study of endogenous estrogens and breast cancer in post-menopausal women. *J. Natl. Cancer Inst.* 87:190.

Voordouw, B.C., R. Euser, R.E. Verdonk, B.T. Alberda, F.H. de Jong, A.C. Drogendijk, B.C. Fauser, M. Cohen. 1992. Melatonin and melatonin-progestin combinations alter pituitary-ovarian function in women and can inhibit ovulation. *J. Clin. Endocrinol. & Metab.* 74:108–117.

Wilson, B.W., L.E. Anderson. 1990. ELF electromagnetic-field effects on the pineal gland. In: *Extremely Low Frequency Electromagnetic Fields:*

The Question of Cancer, B.W. Wilson, R.G. Stevens, L.E. Anderson, eds., pp. 159–186. Columbus, Ohio: Battelle Press.

Wilson, S.T., D.E. Blask, A.M. Wilson. 1992. Melatonin augments the sensitivity of MCF-7 human breast cancer cells to tamoxifen in vitro. *J. Clin. Endocrinol. & Metab.* 75:669–671.

Withyachumnarnkul, B., R.J. Reiter, A. Lerchl, K.O. Nonaka, K.-A. Stokkan. 1991. Evidence that interferon-gamma alters pineal metabolism both indirectly via sympathetic nerves and directly on the pinealocytes. *Int. J. Biochem.* 23(12):1397–1401.

Yaga, K., R.J. Reiter, B.A. Richardson. 1993. Tryptophan loading increases daytime serum melatonin levels in intact and pinealectomized rats. *Life Sci.* 52:1231–1238.

Zimmermann, R.C., C.J. McDugle, M. Schumacher, J. Olcese, J. W. Mason, G.R. Heninger, L.H. Price. 1993. Effects of acute tryptophan depletion on nocturnal melatonin secretion in humans. *J. Clin. Endocrinol. & Metab.* 76:1160–1164.

PART III
Circumstantial Case

SECTION 3
EMF Effects on Melatonin

13 Effects of 50-Hz Magnetic Fields on Pineal Function in the Rat

Masamichi Kato
Department of Physiology, Hokkaido University
School of Medicine, Sapporo, Japan
Tsukasa Shigemitsu
Abiko Research Laboratory, Central Research
Institute of Electric Power Industry, Abiko,
Chiba, Japan

Contents

Introduction
Neuroendocrine Transducer
Effects of Manipulation of Geomagnetic Field on Melatonin
Effects of 60-Hz Electric Fields on Melatonin
Effects of Power-Frequency Magnetic Fields on Melatonin
Effects in Nonrodent Species
Mechanism of Magnetic Field Effects on Melatonin
Current Experiments with 50-Hz Magnetic Fields
Exposure Facility Design and Operating Characteristics
Design
Magnetic Field Readings
Lighting
Other Experimental Environmental Conditions
Melatonin Assay
Sample Handling
Assay

(continued)

CONTENTS (continued)

EXPERIMENTAL DESIGN AND STATISTICS
  Summary of Completed Experiments
  Sampling Protocol
  Statistical Analysis
RESULTS OF EXPERIMENTS WITH WISTAR-KING RATS
  Control Conditions
  Control, and 7 and 350 μT
  Sequential Experiments Across Time
  Linearly Polarized Magnetic Field
PIGMENTED AND ALBINO RATS
DISSOCIATION OF DATA BETWEEN SERUM AND PINEAL GLAND
BIOPHYSICAL MECHANISMS
  Magnetic Field Orientation and Intensity
  Possible Biophysical Mechanisms of Interaction
  Intra- and Interspecies Differences
CONCLUSIONS
ACKNOWLEDGMENT

INTRODUCTION

Neuroendocrine Transducer

The pineal gland is regarded as a neuroendocrine transducer that converts a neural signal, initiated by light, into an endocrine output, melatonin (Wurtman and Axelrod 1965). In mammals, information about the light–dark environment is detected at the retina and transferred, via optic nerve, to the suprachiasmatic nuclei. These nuclei generate the melatonin rhythm, along with many other circadian rhythms (Moore and Eichler 1972; Moore 1973). The timing signal is conveyed from the nuclei to the pineal gland via thoracic spinal cord, superior cervical ganglia, and post-sympathetic fibers. Main functions of the pineal hormone melatonin are to (1) inhibit the hypothalamic-pituitary-gonadal axis (Reiter 1980); (2) exert an oncostatic effect

(Nakatani et al. 1940; Liburdy 1992); and (3) stimulate immune function (Maestroni et al. 1986).

However, the possibility now exists that this system has a broad sensitivity to electromagnetic stimuli, including the electric and magnetic fields associated with the use of AC electric power (Wilson and Anderson 1990).

Effects of Manipulation of Geomagnetic Field on Melatonin

Semm et al. (1980) provided the first evidence that the pineal gland can respond to stimuli other than light. These investigators demonstrated a significant diminution of single-unit electrical activity of guinea pig pineal gland cells following acute, in vivo inversion of the vertical component of the Earth's geomagnetic field by means of a Helmholz coil. This finding suggested that pineal melatonin synthesis might be affected by magnetic fields. Welker et al. (1983) demonstrated that unrestrained rats, exposed to a 15-minute inversion of the horizontal component of the Earth's DC magnetic field during the nighttime hours in the presence of dim red light, had a significantly decreased pineal melatonin synthesis as compared to unexposed control animals. Olcese and Reuss (1986) reported that, in both hooded (pigmented) and albino rats, melatonin synthesis was markedly inhibited following a single, 30-minute exposure to a magnetic field stimulus consisting of a 50° rotation of the Earth's horizontal geomagnetic field.

Effects of 60-Hz Electric Fields on Melatonin

Wilson et al. (1981) reported that, after 21 days of exposure to 60-Hz electric fields between approximately 2 and 40 kV/m, the normal nocturnal peak in pineal melatonin rhythm in male rats was greatly reduced. In another experiment, Wilson et al. (1986) found that 3 days after cessation of exposure to 39 kV/m, 60-Hz electric fields for 4 weeks, nocturnal melatonin concentration had returned to normal. Reiter et al. (1988) demonstrated melatonin reductions in rats exposed to 10, 65, or 130 kV/m in utero through weanling. Collectively, these studies suggested an all-or-none effect rather than a graded dose–response effect.

Effects of Power-Frequency Magnetic Fields on Melatonin

Other investigators soon reported that 60-Hz magnetic fields also could inhibit melatonin. Yellon (1994) reported that 15-minute exposure to a 60-Hz, 0.1-mT magnetic field starting 2 hours before lights off resulted in suppression of nighttime melatonin of Djungarian hamsters in some but not all experiments. McCormick et al. (1994) saw no effect on melatonin of 10 weeks exposure to 60-Hz horizontal magnetic fields of $2\,\mu T$, $100\,\mu T$, or 1 mT in F344 rats and B6C3F1 mice. Lerchl et al. (1990) reported that pineal N-acetyltransferase (NAT) activity of rats was depressed by intermittent exposure to quasi-rectangular magnetic fields with 200 millisecond duration. This observation highlighted the possibility that specific aspects of magnetic field exposure might critically affect the melatonin response.

Effects in Nonrodent Species

The significance of these rodent effects for human health is not known. Wilson et al. (1990) reported that some human subjects using a particular type of electric blanket showed statistically significant changes in mean nighttime urinary excretion of the melatonin metabolite, 6-hydroxy melatonin sulfate (6-OHMS). Graham et al. (1993) reported that human subjects with low base-line melatonin concentration showed significantly suppressed nocturnal serum melatonin concentration after exposure to a $20\text{-}\mu T$, circularly polarized magnetic field for 1 night.

Rogers et al. (1993) investigated effects of exposure to a combined 60-Hz vertical electric field and 60-Hz horizontal magnetic field for 6 weeks on nonhuman primates (*Papio cynocephalus*). Using indwelling venous catheters and an automatic blood sampling system, they collected blood samples from the baboons at 2-hour intervals for 24-hour periods before, during, and following the regularly scheduled, 6-week exposure to the electric and magnetic fields (EMF). No sign of a reduction in serum melatonin concentration was detected in a series of three experiments using a consistent protocol (Rogers et al. 1995b). However, in another small experiment (Rogers et al. 1995a), in which electromagnetic fields were turned on and off irregularly and in a manner that allowed presence of transients, dramatic reductions in melatonin were observed. Lee et al. (1993) did not see any effect on melatonin in female lambs exposed to environmental EMF beneath a commercial, 60-Hz, 500-kV transmission line. In this case, the magnetic field presumably was a near-horizontal, flat, elliptical field.

Mechanism of Magnetic Field Effects on Melatonin

There are two main hypotheses concerning the mechanisms of "magnetosensitivity," the "brain hypothesis" or the "retina hypothesis." The former hypothesis assumes a direct effect of magnetic field on central nervous structures such as the pineal gland and/or suprachiasmatic nuclei. Presumably the effect is a result of induced electric (eddy) currents (Lerchl et al. 1991). We will discuss this point later.

It has long been known that extremely low frequency (ELF) and transient magnetic fields of moderate flux densities generate visual phenomena known as magnetophosphenes (d'Arsonval 1896). Lövsund et al. (1979, 1980) reported that magnetophosphenes are generated in the retina, and that the threshold values varied with the frequency of the magnetic field and the luminance level of the background light, the maximum sensitivity being at 20 Hz and about 8 mT. Lövsund et al. (1981) further studied retinal ganglion cells that responded to both light and magnetic field; the authors assumed the eddy current gave rise to the effects produced by the magnetic field. These results suggest that the retinal photoreceptors and/or synaptic connections within the retina are likely sources of magnetic field stimulation. Once elicited, the neuronal signals propagate in the same channels that normally convey action potentials initiated by light.

Olcese and coworkers (Olcese 1990; Olcese and Reuss 1986; Schneider and Semm 1992; Stehle et al. 1988) have emphasized the role of the retina in responding to magnetic fields. Olcese et al. (1985) reported that acutely blinded rats showed no inhibition of pineal melatonin synthesis produced by magnetic stimulation as compared with intact subjects, and Reuss and Olcese (1986) reported that pineal responsiveness to a magnetic field stimulus was absent in intact rats housed in total darkness. From these results, the authors hypothesized that retinal photoreceptors might be capable of responding to a magnetic field. On this point, Syrian Golden hamsters exposed to a circularly polarized magnetic field of 350 μT for 7 weeks in total darkness did not show any melatonin reduction (Karube, personal communication). This result supports Reuss and Olcese's hypothesis.

Recognizing that ocular pigmentation diminishes the proportion of incident light reaching retinal photoreceptive cells, Olcese and Reuss (1986) compared inhibition of pineal melatonin synthesis of albino Sprague-Dawley and pigmented Long-Evans rats following a single, 30-minute, 50° rotation of the horizontal component of the Earth's geomagnetic field. Finding similar sensitivity to magnetic field-induced disruption of melatonin synthesis in the two strains, the authors concluded that the fact that rats, regardless of their pigmentation, are still capable of responding to an artificial magnetic field "suggests that pigmentation—or lack thereof—may not be a significant factor in the mediation of magnetic field information to other components of the magnetosensitivity system, e.g. the pineal organs." However, in a later experiment, Olcese demonstrated that magnetic field stimulation did not depress melatonin in ACI rats, a fully pigmented strain. The author reported that "it would seem that pigmentation is in fact an important factor in determining pineal sensitivity to magnetic field" (Olcese 1990).

Lynch et al. (1984) compared thresholds of light intensity required to suppress pineal and serum melatonin concentration for Sprague-Dawley and Long-Evans strains, anticipating that the "albino's inability to attenuate light impinging on its retinae would increase its sensitivity to the photic suppression of pineal melatonin content and of circulating melatonin levels." Contrary to their expectation, they found that the pigmented Long-Evans rat is more sensitive to light; threshold intensities were lower (0.022 μw/cm^2) in the Long-Evans than in the Sprague-Dawley (0.110 μw/cm^2).

Raybourn (1983) reported that DC magnetic fields at 5–10 mT suppress the b-wave of an electroretinogram, providing further evidence that either photoreceptors or synaptic processes in the retina are involved in magnetoreception. Baylor et al. (1979a, b) used a suction electrode to record the membrane current of single photoreceptor (rod) outer segments and showed that the receptor was sensitive enough to respond to single photon stimulation at wavelengths of 400–600 nm. One remaining question is: Do photons with energy at ELF wavelengths have enough strength to stimulate either retinal photoreceptors or a magnetoreceptor, be it the photoreceptor itself or a different kind of still-unknown cell?

Based on behavioral experiments conducted with newts, Phillips and Borland (1992) suggested that magnetic compass orientation is affected by the wavelength of light, again indicating that photoreceptors are responsible for detecting magnetic field information.

Current Experiments with 50-Hz Magnetic Fields

Kato et al. (1993, 1994a–d) have completed the most extensive series of experiments reported to date describing the effects of 6 weeks of exposure to 50-Hz magnetic fields on melatonin in rodents. In this paper, we summarize these experiments as a set and attempt to identify possible biological and biophysical mechanisms by which magnetic fields produce effects on melatonin.

EXPOSURE FACILITY DESIGN AND OPERATING CHARACTERISTICS

Design

Our cubic exposure system, which is based on a modification of the Helmholz coil, consists of five equally spaced, square coils (Shigemitsu et al. 1993). This exposure facility can generate either horizontal or vertical magnetic fields up to 0.3 mT. Circularly polarized or elliptically polarized fields also can be generated by changing the current and phase differences between the two sets of coils. Two identical systems allow simultaneous magnetic field and sham exposure within the same animal room (Fig. 1). For these experiments, the x, y, z directions were set in relation to the walls, which are oriented south-north and east-west. This arrangement provides the horizontal magnetic fields in the x direction and the vertical fields in the z direction. Each exposure device includes three 1-m^2 wooden shelves, each of which can hold eight plastic cages. These cage shelves are isolated from the coils,

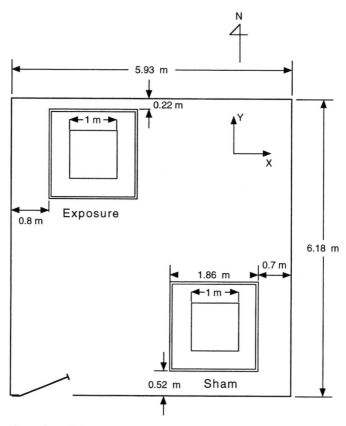

FIG. 1. Floor plan of the experimental room containing the two exposure systems. Both devices were constructed in the same manner, but the sham-exposure device was not connected to the magnetic field source. The field-generation equipment was housed in the room outside the doorway. The coil set in the upper left, or northwest corner, was used as the field-exposure device in most of the experiments; the coil set in the lower right, or southeast corner, was used as the concurrent sham-exposure device. (Reprinted from Shigemitsu et al. 1993 by permission of John Wiley & Sons, Inc.)

which are supported by separate wooden frames; this isolation eliminates mechanical vibration of the cages. With two devices holding 24 cages, the maximum number of subjects the exposure facility accommodates is 48 (two rats per cage). The sham-exposure facility also holds 48 rats.

Magnetic Field Readings

Because our exposure and sham-exposure facilities are in the same room, the magnetic fields of the exposure system spill over into the sham-exposure facility. During these experiments, measurements were made occasionally to assess the stray field by using an MFM-14A meter (Shoden, Tokyo) at eight points corresponding to cage placements on each shelf of the sham system. The intensity of the stray fields was less than 2% of the strength in the exposure system (Fig. 2). Because of the spill-over, the waveform of the stray field was somewhat depressed to an ellipsoidal form. When the field was circularly polarized, this depression ratio was 0.6 [B_V = 0.6 B_H where B_V and B_H are the root mean square (RMS) values of the vertical and horizontal components of the magnetic field, respectively]. In an elliptically polarized field with an axis ratio of 4:1 (B_H = 4 B_V), the depression ratio was 0.15. There was no depression in linearly polarized fields.

The background level of the 50-Hz magnetic field in the experimental room was measured by using the MFM-14A meter. The average levels were 0.014 - 0.024 μT, varying among different sets of measurements.

The value of the horizontal component of the magnetic field was in the range of 25–27 μT, and its orientation was parallel to direction y. The vertical component was in the range of 38–42 μT. There was no difference in static fields between the exposure and the sham-exposure facilities (Fig. 3).

According to the recommendation of the Institute of Electrical and Electronics Engineers (1994), the magnetic field can be expressed by the resultant strength, B_R. B_R can be obtained by the expression

$$B_R = \sqrt{(B_H^2 + B_V^2)}$$

where B_H and B_V are the RMS values of the horizontal and vertical components of the magnetic field, respectively. If the magnetic field is circularly polarized (B_H = B_V), the resultant B_R is 1.4 × B_H (or 1.4 × B_V). In elliptically polarized fields with an axis ratio of 1:4, B_R = | (1/16 B_H^2 + B_H^2) = 1.03 × B_H. If the magnetic field is linearly polarized, B_R= B_H (or = B_V). In this text, in experiments with both

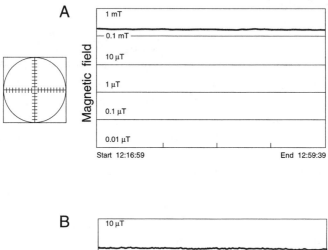

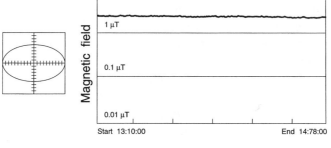

FIG. 2. Sample of recorded magnetic field strengths and Lissajous figures for the field-exposure (panel A) and sham-exposure (panel B) areas. In this case, the exposure coils were set to produce 0.28 mT circularly polarized field. The value in the center of the sham-exposure device was 4.3 μT. The Lissajous figure in the sham-exposure system is somewhat distorted to ellipsoidal polarization (in this case, the ratio of major:minor axes is 5:3) compared with the circularly polarized field in the exposure system. (Reprinted from Shigemitsu et al. 1993 by permission of John Wiley & Sons, Inc.)

circularly and elliptically polarized magnetic fields, the magnetic field vector loci are shown in each corresponding figure (Figs. 7, 8, 15). The total harmonic distortion of the generated 50-Hz magnetic field was about 0.03%.

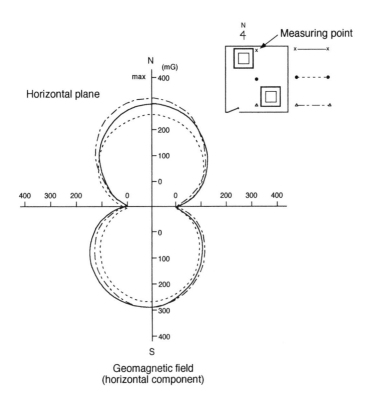

FIG. 3. Horizontal component of geomagnetic field in the laboratory.

Lighting

A 12:12 light:dark cycle was used; lights were turned on at 0600 hours and turned off at 1800 hours. Eight tubes of 40-watt, straight, fluorescent lights were installed on the ceiling 3.5 m above the floor, and four tubes of 40-watt fluorescent lights were set up beside each system 1 m apart and 1 m above the floor. Light-scattering panels were set up on top of the exposure systems. Under these conditions and with eight cages placed in each shelf, the overall light intensity was between 20.4 and 84.4 lux, depending on cage location. The cage position of all subjects was systematically rotated on Monday and Thursday.

Other Experimental Environmental Conditions

Temperature was maintained at 21.0 ± 2.0°C. Relative humidity varied from 40–60% depending on changes in the air conditioning cycle and the seasons. Although the air conditioner was the main contributor to audible noise, the average sound pressure was about 70 dB, which was the general room background noise. There was no difference in the sound level whether or not the exposure system was energized.

MELATONIN ASSAY

Sample Handling

Rats were sacrificed by decapitation and trunk blood was collected in heparinized glass tubes. When samples were collected at night, only dim red light was used. Plasma was separated by centrifugation at 4°C and stored at –80°C until determination of melatonin. The pineal glands were removed immediately after decapitation and transferred into an ice-cold microhomogenizer containing 0.1 M Tris-HCl buffer (pH = 7.4). After homogenization, the pineal samples were centrifuged (in 4°C, 10,000 g × 30 minutes); the supernatant was stored at –80°C until assay.

Assay

Melatonin was extracted by reverse-phase chromatography (Sep-Pak C_{18}) before the assay (Kawashima et al. 1984). Then 1 mL (0.5 mL for night samples) of plasma, or 50 μL (10 μL for night samples) of the pineal supernatant were applied to the column, and melatonin was eluted with methanol. The eluant was dried by vacuum centrifugation and reconstituted with 0.1 M Tris buffer (pH = 7.4). A specific antibody for melatonin was kindly supplied by Prof. K Kawashima. After 24-hour incubation with antibody and ^{4}H-melatonin at 4°C, the bound fraction of melatonin was separated by an ammonium sulfate method. Radioactivity was counted by liquid scintillation; the sensitivity of this assay was 1.6 pg/tube. The recovery rate was about 97%. The intra- and interassay coefficients of variance were 4.0 and 4.7, respectively.

EXPERIMENTAL DESIGN AND STATISTICS

Summary of Completed Experiments

We have completed 18 experiments in which melatonin was assayed (Fig. 4); 15 experiments involved simultaneous magnetic field and sham exposure. Albino Wistar-King rats were used for 16 experiments and pigmented Long-Evans rats for the remaining two experiments (#10 and #11). Among the 15 exposure experiments, we performed 5 using a circularly polarized field and with the experimental group at 1.4 μT (B_R). The rotating plane was perpendicular to the horizontal component of the geomagnetic field. In each of these experiments, the sham-exposed control group was exposed to 0.02 μT. The intent here was to establish across time the continuing efficacy of the critical "positive control" experiment. In addition, three complete "negative control" experiments (#2, #9, and #10) were conducted in which the exposure coils were not activated. These were spread out during the research program, providing "historical control" data for comparison with data of other experiments.

To investigate the effects of magnetic field intensity, other exposure experiments were conducted in which the experimental group was exposed to circularly polarized fields of 7, 70, or 350 μT. In these experiments, the sham-exposed controls received exposures of 0.1, 1.4 or 7 μT, respectively. To assess the effect of orientation of the circularly polarized field, one experiment (#18) was completed in which the rotating plane was parallel to the horizontal component of the geomagnetic field. The experimental group received 1.4 μT, and the sham-exposed control group received 0.02 μT. Also, to test the effects of polarization of the magnetic fields, a vertical field of 1 μT (#14), and horizontal fields of 5 μT (#12) and 1 μT (#8) were used in single experiments. The sham-exposed control groups received 0.1 or 0.02 μT, respectively.

Sampling Protocol

In the initial two experiments, samples were collected every 4 hours, meaning the sample sizes per group—typically six or seven—were smaller than the later ones. In the later 16 experiments, the sample size

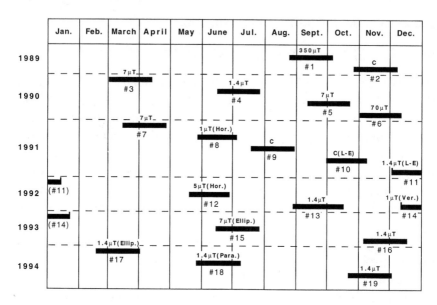

FIG. 4. Summary of the chronological sequence for the 19 experiments. Melatonin was assayed in 18 experiments; experiment #5 was exclusively for histological investigation (Matsushima et al. 1993) and no melatonin assay was carried out. All experiments lasted 6 weeks, and used a common exposure and analysis protocol. The only differences were in strain of rat and magnetic field condition, as summarized. Wistar-King rats were used in all experiments except #10 and #11. The indicated experiment numbers are used as a key to citations of experiments in the text. Abbreviations used are: Hor. = horizontal, L-E = Long-Evans, Ellip. = elliptical, Ver. = vertical, and C = control. The rotating plane of the magnetic field was perpendicular to the horizontal component of the local geomagnetic field, except for #18 where it is indicated (Para.), which means the rotating plane was parallel to the horizontal component of the geomagnetic field.

was about 24 per group per timepoint. In all experiments after #1 and #2, only daytime (at 1200 hours) and nighttime (at 2400 hours) samples were obtained.

Statistical Analysis

Using the Smirnoff test, data sets were examined for extreme values, and the few "outliers" detected were deleted. The Student t-test was used to compare pairs of means; within- or between-subject tests were used as appropriate. At $p < 0.05$, a difference was regarded as statistically significant.

RESULTS OF EXPERIMENTS WITH WISTAR-KING RATS

Control Conditions

Plasma melatonin concentration of the control group, which received no 50-Hz magnetic field because the facility was not energized, showed circadian rhythm, an effect already reported by many authors (Fig. 5). Melatonin content of the pineal gland also showed a similar circadian rhythm (Fig. 6).

In another control experiment (see Fig. 9, p. 355), the subjects also showed circadian melatonin rhythms; plasma concentration was about 40 pg/mL at 1200 hours and about 110 pg/mL at 2400 hours. Melatonin content of the pineal gland was about 200 pg/gland in the day and about 1250 pg/gland at night (see Fig. 10, p. 356).

Control, and 7 and 350 μT

Whether examining plasma or pineal gland melatonin, the concentrations were significantly less, at nearly all timepoints, in field-exposed subjects. Significant differences were recognized between the control and 350-μT groups at 800, 1200, 1600, and 2400 hours, and also between the control and 7-μT stray field groups at 800, 1200, 2000, and 2400 hours. No statistical difference was found between 350- and 7-μT sham-exposed rats at any timepoint. Similar results were obtained from pineal gland melatonin concentration (Fig. 6). Significant differences between control and 350 μT-exposed rats, and between control and the sham-exposed groups are noted in the figure.

Sequential Experiments Across Time

Figures 7 and 8 show the combined control (no exposure) data (#9) and the results of three different exposure experiments (#4, #6, and #7). In general, any magnetic field intensity exceeding 1.4 μT produced a suppression of melatonin in both plasma (Fig. 7) and pineal gland (Fig. 8). Furthermore, the degree of melatonin suppression was

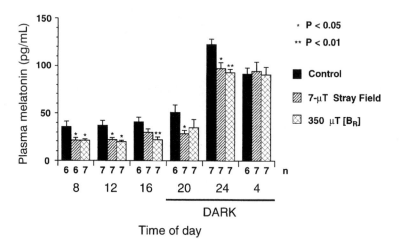

FIG. 5. Plasma melatonin concentrations through the light:dark cycle; the period of darkness, 1800–0600 hours, is indicated. Standard errors (SEs) are shown; number of sample (n) is indicated. Stars indicate timepoints at which differences from the control mean are statistically significant. The 7- and 350-μT data came from experiment #1, and the control data came from experiment #2. (Reprinted from Kato et al. 1993 by permission of John Wiley & Sons, Inc.)

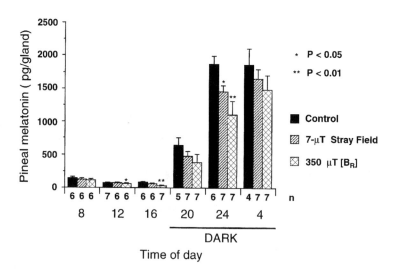

FIG. 6. Melatonin contents for pineal gland through the light:dark cycle. All other aspects of Figure 6 are as in Figure 5. The data came from the same subjects providing data for Figure 5. (Reprinted from Kato et al. 1993 by permission of John Wiley & Sons, Inc.)

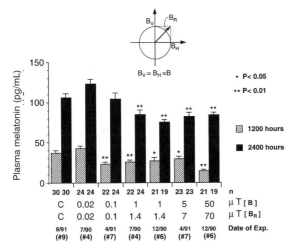

FIG. 7. Melatonin contents at 1200 (lights on) and 2400 (lights off) hours at different strengths of magnetic fields. Means and SEs are provided; stars indicate statistically significant differences between the values at control (C) and other strengths. Significant decrease of melatonin concentration is recognized at fields stronger than 1.4 μT. (Reprinted from Kato et al. 1993 by permission of John Wiley & Sons, Inc.)

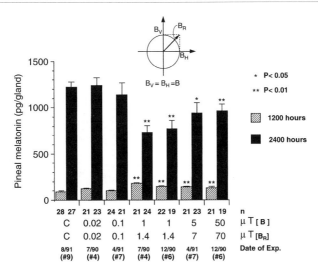

FIG. 8. Melatonin concentrations in the pineal gland at 1200 and 2400 hours at different flux densities of circularly polarized magnetic fields across time. Experimental conditions were the same as in Figure 7. The data came from the same subjects providing data for Figure 7. (Reprinted from Kato et al. 1993 by permission of John Wiley & Sons, Inc.)

the same for magnetic field intensities between 1.4 and 70 μT. These results suggest a sharp, all-or-none (i.e., step–function) relationship, rather than a more gradual dose–response relationship, between magnetic field intensity and melatonin suppression. The possibility of "window" effects might be offered by some observers. We have not conducted experiments specifically designed to search for such effects.

Plasma

No statistically significant differences were observed among the nighttime plasma values for control, 0.02- and 0.1-μT groups (Fig. 7). Compared with the control, there was a significant decrease in melatonin concentration at 1200 hours for a magnetic field greater than 0.1 μT, and at 2400 hours for a magnetic field greater than 1.4 μT. For a magnetic field stronger than 1.4 μT, there were no significant differences among the values at 2400 hours. At 1200 hours, a significant decrease was observed for a magnetic field stronger than 0.1 μT.

Pineal gland

The results for the pineal gland (Fig. 8) were highly similar to those described for plasma. Pineal gland melatonin assays showed statistically significant reductions at 2400 hours with a magnetic field stronger than 1.4 μT.

Repeatability of results

Some authors, such as Yellon (1994) and Reiter et al. (1994) have noted that positive results in their initial melatonin suppression experiments have not been substantiated as more experiments were completed. As possible explanations, variables such as (1) age or species of subjects; (2) assay methodology; (3) exposure parameters, such as duration, field intensity, presence of transients, and vector alignment; and (4) photoperiod or season, have been offered (Rogers et al. 1993).

Because of such concerns about repeatability, we have conducted replicate experiments. We conducted our "positive control," 1.4-μT experiment five times; we saw the effect in four out of the five experiments, including one done with Long-Evans rats (see p. 361). Comparison of long-term trends was made somewhat difficult because we began to use a new specific antibody for melatonin in experiment #14.

At 1.4 μT, plasma melatonin values (Fig. 9) were reduced significantly at both 1200 and 2400 hours in experiments #4, #13, and #19. However, the effect was not seen in experiment #16. At this flux density, the pineal gland melatonin values also showed statistically significant reduction in two of three experiments (Fig. 10). The effect occurred in experiments #4, #11, and #16, but not #19. Interestingly, these results showed a "dissociation" of plasma and pineal gland results in two of the five experiments (see p. 363). Experiment #16 did not show the suppression in plasma melatonin, but did show suppression in pineal gland melatonin. Conversely, experiment #19 did not show the effect in the gland but did in the plasma.

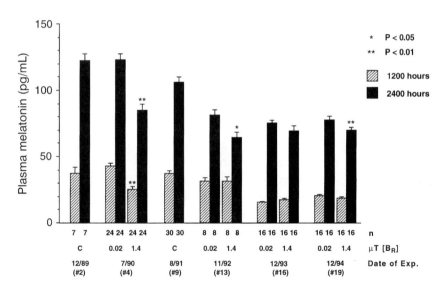

FIG. 9. Results from four experiments with field-exposed (1.4 μT) groups and sham-exposed (0.02 μT) groups, and from two control experiments without energized exposure coils. Mean plasma melatonin concentrations at 1200 and 2400 hours are provided, along with SEs. Statistically significant differences can be observed between the mean values of control (#2, #9) and other experiments at the two timepoints. In each case, number of samples, magnetic field strength, and experiment number are provided.

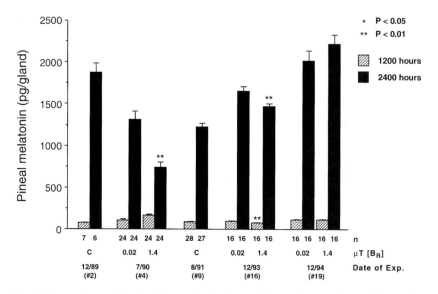

FIG. 10. Melatonin levels of pineal gland at 1200 and 2400 hours from either control (C) or 1.4-μT exposure experiments. Data were obtained from the same rats from those in Figure 9.

We believe these results show very good reproducibility of the effect. Ignoring the dissociation effect, all five experiments showed statistically significant suppression of either pineal gland or plasma melatonin concentrations as a result of 6 weeks of exposure to a 1.4-μT, circularly polarized magnetic field. In summary, the effect is reproducible, but there is variation that remains to be explained.

Recovery

Melatonin concentrations in pineal gland and plasma were suppressed following 6 weeks of exposure to a circularly polarized, 50-Hz, 1.4-μT magnetic field. To examine the time-course of recovery, melatonin concentrations of separate groups were assayed at the end of 6 weeks of exposure, at 1 week after cessation of exposure, and at 4 weeks after cessation of exposure. Nocturnal melatonin concentration was decreased significantly at the end of the exposure period but was normal at both 1 and 4 weeks after cessation of exposure (Fig. 11). As suggested by Wilson et al. (1986), our results indicate that the magnetic field-induced melatonin suppression effect is both short-lived and fully reversible.

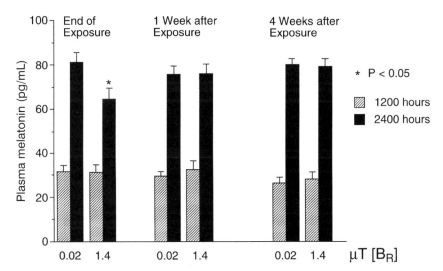

FIG. 11. Plasma melatonin concentrations at the end of 6 weeks of exposure and at either 1 or 4 weeks following termination of exposure. Mean values, with SEs, for 1200 and 2400 hours are provided. Exposure to 1.4 μT reduced nighttime melatonin significantly, but the difference had disappeared with cessation of exposure. (Reprinted from Kato et al. 1994d by permission of John Wiley & Sons, Inc.)

Linearly Polarized Magnetic Field

Contrasting our positive outcomes obtained with rats exposed to circularly polarized magnetic fields with the negative outcome observed in primates exposed to a horizontal magnetic field (Rogers et al. 1995b), we wondered if species differences or some specific aspect of exposure parameters, such as field orientation, might be important. Therefore, we conducted an experiment within our laboratory, using the same species and a consistent protocol, to determine if horizontal or vertical magnetic field exposure produced effects different from those produced by circularly polarized magnetic field exposure.

Horizontal field

Comparison of the plasma melatonin concentrations of the 1-μT exposed group and sham-exposed group (#8), and historical control group (#9) indicated there were no statistically significant differences among the three groups (Fig. 12). After exposure to 5 μT in experiment #12, plasma melatonin showed a significant reduction but pineal melatonin did not (Fig. 12). In our laboratory, a horizontal magnetic field is not nearly as potent a stimulus at inducing melatonin suppression in rats as is a circularly polarized magnetic field.

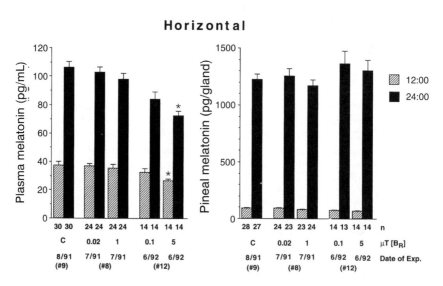

Horizontal

FIG. 12. Plasma (left) and pineal gland (right) melatonin concentrations in one control and two exposure experiments conducted with horizontal magnetic fields. Only at 5 μT did the values of the exposed groups differ significantly from those of the control group from plasma, but not from pineal gland. In each case, the sample size, the magnetic field intensity, and the experimental numbers are provided.

Vertical field

Exposure to 1 μT or 0.02 μT did not produce significant differences in either plasma or pineal melatonin concentration (Fig. 13). On this point, Löscher et al. (1994) reported that serum melatonin was suppressed after 8–9 weeks of 50-Hz vertical magnetic field exposure at strengths of 0.3–1 μT to Sprague-Dawley rats that were pretreated with 7,12 dimethylbenz(a)anthracene (DMBA).

Elliptically polarized magnetic field

To test if differences of exposure parameters were important, the effect of a 50-Hz, ellipsoidal magnetic field exposure for 6 weeks on plasma and pineal gland melatonin concentration was investigated as a continuation of the abovementioned horizontally or vertically polarized magnetic field exposures. The ellipsoidal magnetic field was simulated to be equivalent to ground-level exposure in the vicinity of a double-circuit transmission line of low reactance phase arrangement (Fig. 14).

In our exposure experiments, the magnetic field was ellipsoidal, the ratio of the major:minor axis was 4:1, and the field intensities were 1.4

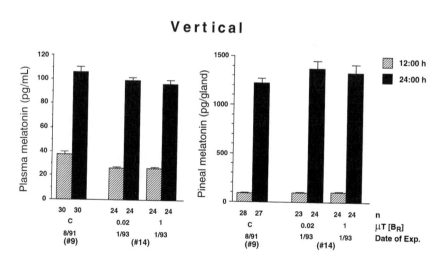

FIG. 13. Concentration of melatonin in plasma (left) and in the pineal gland (right) at 1200 and 2400 hours at the end of 6 weeks of exposure to a 1-μT vertical magnetic field. (Reprinted from Kato et al. 1994c with permission from Elsevier Science Ireland Ltd.)

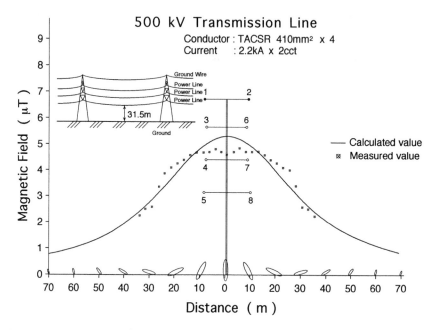

FIG. 14. An example of magnetic fields profile under double circuit transmission lines. Magnetic fields 1 m above the ground were calculated by Biot-Savart's law as well as measured by Gaussmeters. Voltage and current values, as well as number of conductors, are indicated. (Provided by M. Yasui, Tokyo Electric Power Company.)

(B_R) and 7.0 μT (B_R); a concurrent sham-exposure group was exposed to a stray field of 0.02 (#17) and 0.1 μT (#15), respectively. There were no statistically significant differences in plasma melatonin concentration between the values at 1200 hours, nor between the values at 2400 hours, at the two strengths tested (Fig. 15). These results indicate that exposure for 6 weeks to ellipsoidal magnetic fields at 1.4 and 7.0 μT has no effect on pineal gland function.

Conclusion

We conclude from these experiments that, in contrast to the highly effective, circularly polarized magnetic field, exposure to vertical, horizontal, and 4:1 elliptical magnetic field does not result in suppression of melatonin.

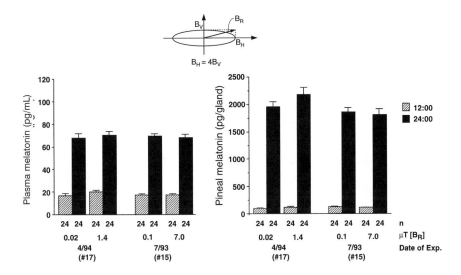

FIG. 15. An elliptically polarized magnetic field, with an axis ratio of 4:1, does not produce melatonin suppression. Plasma (left) and pineal gland (right) melatonin content are shown. Means, with SEs, are provided for both 1200 and 2400 hours. All means are based on a sample size of 24. There were no statistically significant differences. These data are from experiment #17, in which the experimental group received 1.4 μT (B_R) and sham-control group received 0.02 μT (B_R), and from experiment #15, in which the experimental group received 7 μT (B_R) and the sham-control group received 0.1 μT (B_R).

PIGMENTED AND ALBINO RATS

We exposed pigmented Long-Evans rats to a circularly polarized, 50-Hz magnetic field for 6 weeks to contrast effects with those observed previously in albino Wistar-King rats. In experiment #11, the magnetic field-exposed group was exposed to 1.4 μT (B_R) and the control group received 0.02 μT (B_R). Compared with the historical control group (#10), both magnetic field-exposed groups showed statistically significant reductions in plasma and pineal melatonin concentration at both 1200 and 2400 hours (Fig. 16). Furthermore, at 2400 hours, the melatonin values of 1.4-μT subjects were less than those of the 0.02-μT group.

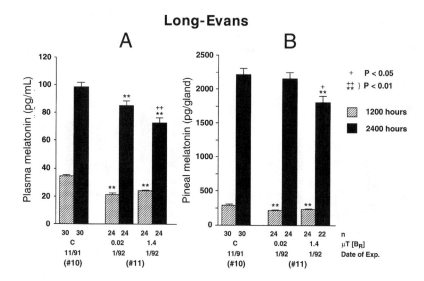

FIG. 16. Effects of 1.4-μT, circularly polarized magnetic field exposure in pigmented, Long-Evans rats. Mean plasma (left) and pineal gland (right) melatonin concentrations are provided, with SEs, at both 1200 and 2400 hours. Statistically significant differences from control values are indicated. These data came from experiments #10 and #11. In each case, the sample size, magnetic field intensity, and experiment number are provided. (Reprinted from Kato et al. 1994a with permission from Elsevier Science Ireland Ltd.)

These results clearly indicate that 50-Hz, circularly polarized magnetic field exposure reduces melatonin in pigmented rats, just as in albino rats. Furthermore, the fact that the pigmented rats showed differential effects in response to 0.02 and 1.4 μT, something the albino rats did not do, suggests that the "threshold" magnetic field strength required for magnetic field-induced melatonin reduction is lower in pigmented than in albino rats.

Taking into account both our results with magnetic fields and the results of Lynch et al. (1984) with light stimulation, it would be reasonable to assume that some common, or similar, mechanism exists between photo- and magnetosensitivity. However, it also is possible that pigmented and nonpigmented rat strains differ in other important respects besides pigmentation that complicate elucidation of photoreceptor and magnetoreceptor inter-relationships.

DISSOCIATION OF DATA BETWEEN SERUM AND PINEAL GLAND

In 5 of the 18 exposure experiments there was dissociation between the data of serum and of pineal gland. Serum melatonin was suppressed in four experiments while there was no significant reduction in pineal gland melatonin. In the remaining one experiment, pineal melatonin was significantly suppressed without a similar reduction in the serum concentration, although the value was smaller as compared to the sham-control value. These five experimental results may represent a certain aspect of biological effects of magnetic fields, because this number is too significant to be ignored.

In the pineal gland, most synthesized serotonin is stored in the granular vesicles, and it was pointed out that melatonin may likewise exist in the granular vesicles (Pévet 1983), though the melatonin may be contained in lipid droplets (De Martino 1963). Melatonin is secreted into the bloodstream through the pinealocyte membrane by exocytosis. However, because no reliable antibody for immunohistochemical staining of melatonin has been developed yet, the process of how melatonin is transported from the granular vesicles into blood is still unclear (Matsushima, personal communication). Once melatonin reaches target cells, it combines with G protein-coupled, membrane-bound receptors, and subsequently the second-messenger system mediates the effects of melatonin (Morgan et al. 1994).

If magnetic field exposure delays the process of movement of melatonin from the granular vesicles to release from the pinealocyte, there can be no measurable changes in melatonin content in the pineal gland even if the synthesis itself were reduced. On the other hand, plasma melatonin is taken up by the melatonin receptors, thus reducing the concentration of melatonin in blood.

In our studies, exposure to stronger magnetic fields, such as 7 μT (#3, #7), 70 μT (#6), or 350 μT (#1), resulted in reduction of both plasma and pineal gland melatonin compared to controls (such as #2, #9). In these cases, it is possible that the stronger fields affected melatonin synthesis more effectively than the delaying process; thus both pineal gland and plasma melatonin were reduced. The strength of 1.4 μT of circularly polarized field may be near threshold value.

Grota et al. (1994) observed a similar phenomenon following electric field exposure for 30 days. They suggested stimulated melatonin degradation, sampling time, and other factors as possible reasons for such phenomenon.

BIOPHYSICAL MECHANISMS

Magnetic Field Orientation and Intensity

Our experiments establish that 6 weeks of exposure to a circularly polarized magnetic field, at intensities exceeding 1.4 μT (B_R), suppresses plasma and pineal melatonin concentration. Horizontal and vertical fields, at intensities up to 1 μT, do not suppress melatonin. However, it appears that field intensity and orientation might interact; with a magnetic field intensity of 5 μT, horizontal field exposure suppressed plasma melatonin but not pineal melatonin.

Degree of circular polarization also appears to be an important variable. Elliptically polarized fields of 1.4 μT, with a major:minor axis ratio of 5:3 or 5:4 (see Fig. 2 and Figs. 7–10), also effectively reduced melatonin. However, an elliptically polarized field of 1.4 μT with a ratio of 4:1 was ineffective. Once again, field intensity might interact with degree of ellipticity; at 5 μT, a 4:1 field, which is largely horizontal, did suppress melatonin.

Our experiments show that field orientation and shape, possibly interacting with field intensity, determine whether or not melatonin suppression will result. Electric currents are induced in the body by alternating magnetic fields. The induced currents circulate in a closed loop, located in the plane perpendicular to the direction of the magnetic field. We calculated induced current density and absorbed power density (W/cm^2) of circularly polarized, elliptically polarized, and linearly polarized magnetic fields (Table 1). The computations assumed the body is a spherical object with uniform conductivity. When the magnetic field is circularly polarized, the induced current density (J_c) remains constant throughout the 50-Hz cycle. However, when linearly polarized or elliptically polarized magnetic fields are applied, the

TABLE 1

Equations Used to Describe Alternating Magnetic Fields
of Various Polarities and Formulae Used to Estimate
Induced Current and Power Densities

	Linear (Horizontal) $B_H=B_0, B_V=0, \beta=0$	Circular $B_H=B_V=B_0, \beta=-\pi/2$	Elliptical $B_H=4B_V=B_0, \beta=-\pi/2$
Magnetic field			
Vector **B**	$B=\sqrt{2}B_0\sin(\omega t)e_H$	$B=\sqrt{2}B_0\{\sin(\omega t)e_H+\sin(\omega t-\pi/2)e_V\}$	$B=\sqrt{2}B_0\{\sin(\omega t)e_H+\frac{1}{4}\sin(\omega t-\pi/2)e_V\}$
rms B_{rms}	$B_L=B_0$	$B_C=\sqrt{2}B_0\fallingdotseq1.41B_L$	$B_E=\frac{\sqrt{17}}{4}B_0\fallingdotseq1.03B_L$
Induced current			
Vector **J**	$J=\frac{\rho\omega\sigma}{\sqrt{2}}B_0\cos(\omega t)e_V$	$J=-\frac{\rho\omega\sigma}{\sqrt{2}}B_0\{\sin(\omega t)e_H-\cos(\omega t)e_V\}$	$J=-\frac{\rho\omega\sigma}{\sqrt{2}}B_0\{\frac{1}{4}\sin(\omega t)e_H-\cos(\omega t)e_V\}$
Strength |J|	$\|J\|=\frac{\rho\omega\sigma}{\sqrt{2}}B_0\|\cos(\omega t)\|$	$\|J\|=\frac{\rho\omega\sigma}{\sqrt{2}}B_0$	$\|J\|=\frac{\rho\omega\sigma}{\sqrt{2}}B_0\sqrt{\frac{1}{16}\sin^2(\omega t)+\cos^2(\omega t)}$
rms J_{rms}	$J_L=\frac{\rho\omega\sigma}{2}B_0$	$J_C=\frac{\rho\omega\sigma}{2}B_0\sqrt{2}\fallingdotseq1.41J_L$	$J_E=\frac{\rho\omega\sigma}{2}B_0\frac{\sqrt{17}}{4}\fallingdotseq1.03J_L$
Power density			
Strength P	$P=\frac{\rho^2\omega^2\sigma}{2}B_0^2\cos^2(\omega t)$	$P=\frac{\rho^2\omega^2\sigma}{2}B_0^2$	$P=\frac{\rho^2\omega^2\sigma}{2}B_0^2\{\frac{1}{16}\sin^2(\omega t)+\cos^2(\omega t)\}$
rms P_{rms}	$P_L=\frac{\rho^2\omega^2\sigma}{4}B_0^2$	$P_C=\frac{\rho^2\omega^2\sigma}{4}B_0^2\times2=2P_L$	$P_E=\frac{\rho^2\omega^2\sigma}{4}B_0^2\frac{17}{16}\fallingdotseq1.06P_L$

Magnetic field (mT), induced current (mA/m^2) and power density (W/m^3) at linearly polarized, circularly polarized, and elliptically-polarized ($B_h=4B_v=B_o$) fields were calculated. $\omega=2\pi f$; f = frequency, ρ = radius of spherical object; σ = conductivity of spherical object.

induced current densities, J_L or J_E, oscillate. Furthermore, in a linearly polarized field, the induced current crosses the zero current level, but in an elliptically polarized field, the induced current does not reach zero voltage. In both cases, the oscillating frequency of the induced current is twice that of the frequency of the applied magnetic field. The calculations show that the current density produced by a circularly polarized magnetic field is about 40% greater than that induced by either a linearly polarized or elliptically polarized magnetic field of the same intensity (Table 1 and Fig. 17). Also, the absorbed power density is about 2 times greater for the circularly polarized magnetic field than for the elliptically polarized or linearly polarized magnetic field. Both induced current density and absorbed power density are nearly equal for linearly polarized and elliptically polarized magnetic fields.

Induced Current Density

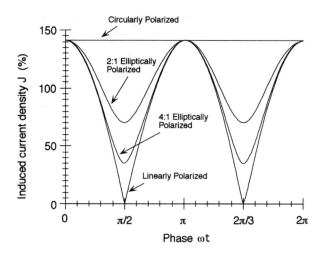

Power   Density

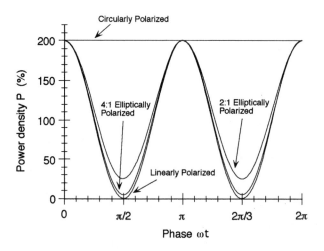

FIG. 17. Profiles of induced current density (top panel) and absorbed power density (bottom panel) of circularly polarized, elliptically polarized ($B_H = 4B_V = B_0$), and linearly polarized magnetic fields. The abscissa shows phase angle (ωt); the ordinate of the upper graph represents induced current (A/m^2) and the ordinate of the lower graph represents power density (W/m^3) at percent value (%).

These differences in induced current and absorbed power density might explain differences in results in our experimental data. In summary, we found that a circularly polarized magnetic field is a far more potent stimulus for reducing melatonin than is either a linearly or elliptically polarized magnetic field.

Possible Biophysical Mechanisms of Interaction

We propose two mechanisms by which such differences in induced current might produce different biological effects.

Membrane potentials

At the biophysical level, induced currents can affect the membrane potential of cells. If the cell is an electrically excitable tissue, such as a neuron, the partial hyper- or depolarization evoked by the magnetic field might alter the probability of cell firing, produced by depolarization below the threshold, occurring as a result of normal biological activity. If a neuron is depolarized by the induced current, it will be more sensitive to other depolarizing cellular inputs; at times when it is partially hyperpolarized by the induced current, it will become resistant to other normal physiological inputs. Thus it might be possible, for example, that the response of the pinealocytes to activity in the superior cervical ganglion might be altered by magnetic field-induced electric currents at the pineal gland. The same possibility exists, of course, at any point in the chain of electrically excitable structures from retina to pineal gland.

Let us assume that the pineal gland of a rat is a sphere with a diameter of 1 mm and homogeneous conductivity of 0.1 S/m. If a circularly polarized magnetic field of 1.4 μT is applied, we calculate that the induced current density in the pineal gland will be 11.1 nA/m^2 or 1.11 pA/cm^2; a circular field of 7 μT induces 5.55 pA/cm^2. When a linearly polarized magnetic field of 1 μT is applied, induced current density is calculated as 0.785 pA/cm^2. In reality, however, biological tissues inside the skull are not homogeneous in conductivity. The skull contains such tissues as bone, dura mater, pia mater, brain, blood vessels, and peripheral nerve fibers with different shapes and conductivities. Yamazaki et al. 1996 developed measuring and analyzing methods to estimate the distribution and strength of the induced current within these complex tissue structures. Using the plural medium model, they are planning to estimate the characteristics of induced current. When an action potential is produced in a neuron, a membrane current of the order of mA/cm^2 is recorded (Hodgkin and Huxley 1952). Therefore, the induced current density of the order of pA/cm^2, if it were obtained by the simple calculation mentioned previously, is considerably smaller. The problem remains of finding mechanisms by which these weak induced currents can act effectively as agents influencing resting potential, or ion-channels of the membrane. This is the most fundamental issue when we think about mechanisms of interaction of weak ELF EMF with cells.

Wiesenfeld and Moss (1995), Collins et al. (1995), and Moss and Pei (1995) recently discussed a phenomenon called stochastic resonance. Stochastic resonance has been proposed as a means for improving signal detection in certain nonlinear systems, including sensory neurons. It concerns the problem of detecting weak signals in a noisy environment. As described for crayfish mechanoreceptors, the system becomes a more sensitive detector as more noise is added, at least up to a point; it is optimally sensitive to externally applied signals at some nonzero level of the residual internal noise (Wiesenfeld and Moss 1995). Moss and Pei (1995) exemplified muscle spindle afferents and parallel-arrayed ion channels as likely systems for stochastic resonance. Kruglikov and Dertinger (1994) mentioned that "... signal quality plays an important role in the appearance of stochastic resonance. Long-term correlation of the input signal is one of the necessary conditions for the existence of signal amplification."

It is possible that stochastic resonance takes place either in pineal gland cells or retina, or in elements in nerve chains connecting these two sites. Of course, this must be proven experimentally in the future.

Anatomical considerations
At the anatomical level, another set of possible mechanisms becomes relevant. Electric currents induced by magnetic fields tend to be distributed in a loop around the outer edges of the body. Furthermore, anatomic boundaries, especially those between tissues with different conductivities, will alter current density. In the rat, the pineal gland is located just under the dura and skull; i.e., at the "periphery" where induced currents will be strongest. The boundary between relatively

low conductivity skull/dura and high conductivity brain might be a location of current flow greatly exceeding the 11 nA/m^2 computed above. Thus the currents which appear to be "too weak to be effective" might be stronger and more effective than suggested by simple calculations of homogenous, symmetric bodies. Reilly (1992) notes that currents oriented parallel to neurons are 5–10 times more effective at stimulating neurons than are currents oriented perpendicular to the neuron. Furthermore, depolarization is much more readily produced at "bends and ends" of neurons. Additionally, it has been suggested that the position of the superior cervical ganglia, in the neck next to the carotids, might make these ganglia vulnerable to stimulation by external electric field (Kaune 1985). The small cross section of the neck, and the presence of large arteries filled with rapidly flowing, highly conductive solutions, might produce local induced currents sufficient to be effective physiological stimuli.

The pineal gland of other mammals, such as cat, dog, horse, monkey and human, is located deep inside the brain. It might be that most of the induced currents flow around the periphery of the relatively homogeneous brain and thus do not stimulate the pineal gland as effectively in these species as it does in the rat. Thus, anatomic considerations might be very important. In summary, differences in distributions of induced currents among different mammalian species might be one factor explaining differing outcomes in in vivo experiments conducted with various species.

Intra- and Interspecies Differences

There are substantial differences among species in the sensitivity of the pineal gland response to light. Nozaki et al. (1990) reviewed relationships between melatonin suppression and light intensity and/or duration of exposure among different mammalian species. Rodents are more sensitive to light-induced melatonin suppression than are monkeys or humans. Differences also exist among individuals of a single species. In humans, physiologic changes associated with certain depressive illnesses are reported to alter the sensitivity of the pineal gland to light as perceived by the eye (McIntyre et al. 1990).

Just as there are species-specific variations in sensitivity to light, it is likely that there are variations in the sensitivity of various species to electric and/or magnetic fields. In the two electromagnetic field and melatonin experiments conducted to date with human subjects, both Wilson et al. (1990) and Graham et al. (1993) reported that subsets of their study samples showed melatonin reductions. These findings indicate that periodic exposure to pulsed electric and magnetic fields of sufficient intensity and duration can affect pineal gland functions in certain individuals.

If the biophysical and biological mechanisms of magnetic field exposure on the living body were clearly understood, it would be beneficial not only for basic science but also for epidemiologic study and applied sciences.

CONCLUSIONS

Using the same exposure facility and a consistent protocol, we completed 18 experiments examining the effects of 6 weeks of exposure to different parameters of 50-Hz magnetic fields on melatonin in the plasma and pineal gland of rats. Results are summarized as follows:

1. Circularly polarized magnetic fields stronger than $1.4\,\mu T$ (B_R) suppressed plasma and pineal melatonin.
2. This finding has been replicated consistently in 5 experiments completed over a period of 3 years.
3. Elliptically polarized magnetic fields of either 1.4 or $7\,\mu T$ (B_R) did not suppress melatonin.
4. Linearly polarized magnetic fields of either horizontal or vertical orientation did not suppress melatonin at $1\,\mu T$, although $5\,\mu T$ reduced plasma melatonin concentrations.
5. Relative densities of induced current and absorbed power exposure to magnetic fields were substantially greater with circularly polarized exposure.

ACKNOWLEDGMENT

Walter R. Rogers of San Antonio has continuously given us invaluable suggestions and advice during the current series of experiments, and in editing the manuscript. The authors express their cordial thanks to him.

REFERENCES

Baylor, D.A, T.D. Lamb, K.W. Yau. 1979a. Responses of retinal rods to single photons. *J. Physiol.* 288:613–634.

Baylor, D.A, T.D. Lamb, K.W. Yau. 1979b. The membrane current of single rod outer segments. *J. Physiol.* 288:589–611.

Collins, J.J., C.C. Chow, T.T. Imhoff. 1995. Stochastic resonance without tuning. *Nature* 376:236–238.

d'Arsonval, M.A. 1896. Dispositifs pour la mesure des courants alternatifs de toutes frequences. *Compt. Rend. Soc. Biol.* 3:450–451.

De Martino, C., F. De Luca, F.M. Paluello, G. Tonietti, L. Orci. 1963. The osmiophilic granules of the pineal body in rats. *Experientia* 19:639–641.

Graham, C., M.R. Cook, H.D. Cohen, D.W. Riffle, S.J. Hoffman, F.J. McClernon, D. Smith, M.M. Gerkovich. 1993. EMF suppression of nocturnal melatonin in human volunteers. In: Abstracts of the Annual Review of Research on Biological Effects of Electric and Magnetic Fields from the Generation, Delivery, and Use of Electricity, Savannah, Georgia, October 31–November 4, A-31, pp. 98–99. Frederick, Maryland: W/L Associates, Ltd.

Grota, L.J., R.J. Reiter, P. Keng, S. Michaelson. 1994. Electric field exposure alters serum melatonin but not pineal melatonin synthesis in male rats. *Bioelectromagnetics* 15:427–437.

Hodgkin, A.L., A.F. Huxley. 1952. A quantitative description of membrane current and its application to conduction and excitation in nerve. *J. Physiol.* 117:500–544

Institute of Electrical and Electronics Engineers. 1994. Specifications for magnetic flux density and electric field strength meters—10 Hz to 3 kHz. In: *IEEE Recommended Practice for Instrumentation*, pp. 1308–1994.

Kato, M., K. Honma, T. Shigemitsu, Y. Shiga. 1993. Effects of exposure to a circularly polarized 50-Hz magnetic field on plasma and pineal melatonin levels in rats. *Bioelectromagnetics* 14:97–106.

Kato, M., K. Honma, T. Shigemitsu, Y. Shiga. 1994a. Circularly polarized 50-Hz magnetic field exposure reduces pineal gland and blood melatonin concentrations of Long-Evans rats. *Neurosci. Lett.* 166:59–62.

Kato, M., K. Honma, T. Shigemitsu, M.Yasui, T. Kikuchi. 1994b. Ellipsoidal magnetic field exposure for 6 weeks has no effect on pineal or plasma melatonin concentration of the rat. In: Abstracts of the 16th Annual Bioelectromagnetics Society Meeting, Copenhagen, Denmark, June 12–17, pp. 98–99. Frederick, Maryland: The Bioelectromagnetics Society.

Kato, M., K. Honma, T. Shigemitsu, Y. Shiga. 1994c. Horizontal or vertical 50-Hz, 1-mT magnetic fields have no effect on pineal gland or plasma melatonin concentration on albino rats. *Neurosci. Lett.* 168:205–208.

Kato, M., K. Honma, T. Shigemitsu, Y. Shiga. 1994d. Recovery of nocturnal melatonin concentration takes place within one week following cessation of 50 Hz circularly polarized magnetic field exposure for six weeks. *Bioelectromagnetics* 15:489–492

Kaune, W.T. 1985. Coupling of living organisms to ELF electric and magnetic fields. In: *Biological and Human Health Effects of Extremely Low Frequency Electromagnetic Fields*, pp. 25-60, Arlington, Virginia: American Institute of Biological Sciences.

Kawashima, K., A. Nagakura, R.J. Wurzburger, S. Spector. 1984. Melatonin in serum and the pineal of spontaneously hypertensive rats. *Clin. Exp. Hypertens. Part A Theory Pract.* A6:1517–1528.

Kruglikov, I.L., H. Dertinger. 1994. Stochastic resonance as a possible mechanism of amplification of weak electric signals in living cells. *Bioelectromagnetics* 15:539–548.

Lee, J.M. Jr., F. Stormshak, J.M. Thompson, P. Thinesen, L.J. Painter, E.G. Olenchek, D.L. Hess, R. Forbes, D.L. Foster. 1993. Melatonin secretion and puberty in female lambs exposed to environmental electric and magnetic fields. *Biol. Reprod.* 49:857–864.

Lerchl, A., K.O. Nonaka, K-A. Stokkan, R.J. Reiter. 1990. Marked rapid alterations in nocturnal pineal serotonin metabolism in mice and rats exposed to weak intermittent magnetic fields. *Biochem. Biophys. Res. Commun.* 169:102–108.

Lerchl, A., K.O. Nonaka, R.J. Reiter. 1991. Pineal gland "magnetosensitivity" to static magnetic fields is a consequence of induced electric currents (eddy currents). *J. Pineal. Res.* 10:109–116.

Liburdy, R.P. 1992. Biological interactions of cellular systems with time-varying magnetic fields. *Ann. N. Y. Acad. Sci.* 649:74–95

Löscher, W., U. Wahnschaffe, M. Mevissen, A. Lerchl, A. Stamm. 1994. Effects of weak alternating magnetic fields on nocturnal melatonin production and mammary carcinogenesis in rats. *Oncology* 51:288–295.

Lövsund, P., P.A. Öberg, S.E.G. Nilsson. 1979. Influence on vision of extremely low frequency electromagnetic fields. *Acta Ophthalmol.* 57:812–821.

Lövsund, P., S.E.G. Nilsson, P.A. Öberg, T. Reuter. 1980. Magneto-phosphenes: A quantitative analysis of thresholds. *Med. & Biol. Eng. & Comput.* 18:326–334.

Lövsund, P., S.E.G. Nilsson, P.A. Öberg. 1981. Influence on frog retina of alternating magnetic fields with special reference to ganglion cell activity. *Med. & Biol. Eng. & Comput.* 19:679–685.

Lynch, H.L., W.H. Deng, R.J. Wurtman. 1984. Light intensities required to suppress nocturnal melatonin secretion in albino and pigmented rats. *Life Sci.* 35:841–847.

Maestroni, G.J.M., A. Conti, W. Pierpaoli. 1986. Role of the pineal gland in immunity. *J. Neuroimmunol.* 13:19–30.

Matsushima, S., Y. Sakai, Y. Hira, M. Kato, T. Shigemitsu, Y. Shiga. 1993. Effect of magnetic field on pineal gland volume and pinealocyte size in the rat. *J. Pineal Res.* 14:145–150.

McCormick, D.L., M.A. Cahill, J.B. Harder, B.M. Ryan, J.C. Findlay, L.E. Pomerantz, R.R. Szymanski, G.A. Boorman. 1994. Pineal function assessment in F344 rats and B6C3F1 mice exposed to 60 Hz magnetic fields. In: Abstracts of the 16th Annual Bioelectromagnetics Society Meeting, Copenhagen, Denmark, June 12–17, p. 50. Frederick, Maryland: The Bioelectromagnetics Society.

McIntyre, I.M., T.R. Norman, G.B. Burrows, S.M. Armstrong. 1990. Melatonin supersensitivity to dim light in seasonal affective disorder. *Lancet* 335:488.

Moore, R.Y. 1973. Visual pathways and the central neural control of diurnal rhythms. In: *The Neurosciences Third Study Program*, F.O. Schmitt, F.G. Worden, eds., pp. 537–542. Cambridge, Massachusetts and London, England: The MIT Press.

Moore, R.Y., V.B. Eichler. 1972. Loss of a circadian adrenal corticosterone rhythm following suprachiasmatic lesions in the rat. *Brain Res.* 42:201–206.

Morgan, P.J., P. Barrett, H.E. Howell, R. Helliwell. 1994. Melatonin receptors: Localization, molecular pharmacology, and physiological significance. *Neurochem. Int.* 24:101–146.

Moss, F., X. Pei. 1995. Neurons in parallel. *Nature* 376:211–212.

Nakatani, M., Y. Ohara, E. Katagiri, K. Nakano. 1940. Studien über die zirbellosen wiblichen weissen Ratten (Original in Japanese). *Nippon Byori Gakkai Kaishi* 30:232–236.

Nozaki, M., M. Tsushima, Y. Mori. 1990. Diurnal changes in serum melatonin concentrations under indoor and outdoor environments and light suppression of nighttime melatonin secretion in the female Japanese monkey. *J. Pineal Res.* 9: 221–230.

Olcese, J.M. 1990. The neurobiology of magnetic field detection in rodents. *Prog. Neurobiol.* 35:325–330.

Olcese, J., S. Reuss. 1986. Magnetic field effects on pineal gland melatonin synthesis: Comparative studies on albino and pigmented rodents. *Brain Res.* 369:365–368.

Olcese, J., S. Reuss, L. Vollrath. 1985. Evidence for the involvement of the visual system in mediating magnetic field effects on pineal melatonin synthesis in the rat. *Brain Res.* 333:382–384.

Pévet, P. 1983. Anatomy of the pineal gland of mammals. In: *The Pineal Gland*, R. Relkin, ed., pp. 1-75. New York: Elsevier Biomedical.

Phillips, J.B., S.C. Borland. 1992. Behavioural evidence for use of a light-dependent magnetoreception mechanism by a vertebrate. *Nature* 359:142–144.

Raybourn, M.S. 1983. The effect of direct-current magnetic fields on turtle retinas in vitro. *Science* 220:715–717.

Reilly, J.P. 1992. *Electrical Stimulation and Electropathology.* Cambridge, Massachusetts: Cambridge University Press.

Reiter, R.J. 1980. The pineal and its hormones in the control of reproduction in mammals. *Endocrin. Rev.* 1:109–131.

Reiter, R.J., L.E. Anderson, R.L. Buschbom, B.W. Wilson. 1988. Reduction of the nocturnal rise in pineal melatonin levels in rats exposed to 60-Hz electric fields in utero and for 23 days after birth. *Life Sci.* 42:2203–2206.

Reiter, R.J., B. Poeggeler, L.D. Chen, L.C. Manchester, M. Hara, Y. Olatomiji-Bello. 1994. Nocturnal pineal serotonin metabolism in male rats subjected to short duration pulsed static magnetic fields.

In: Abstracts of Annual Review of Research on Biological Effects of Electric and Magnetic Fields from the Generation, Delivery, and Use of Electricity, Albuquerque, New Mexico, November 6–10, A-39, pp. 39–41. Frederick, Maryland: W/L Associates, Ltd.

Reuss, S., J. Olcese. 1986. Magnetic field effects on the rat pineal gland: Role of retinal activation by light. *Neurosci. Lett.* 64:97–101.

Rogers, W.R., J.L. Orr, R.J. Reiter. 1993. 60-Hz electric and magnetic fields and primate melatonin. In: *Electricity and Magnetism in Biology and Medicine*, M.Blank, ed., pp. 393–397. San Francisco: San Francisco Press.

Rogers, W.R., R.J. Reiter, H.D. Smith, L. Barlow-Walden. 1995a. Rapid onset/offset, variably scheduled 60-Hz electric and magnetic field exposure reduces nocturnal serum melatonin concentration in non-human primates. *Bioelectromagnetics* Suppl. 3:119–122.

Rogers, W.R., R.J. Reiter, L. Barlow-Walden, H.D. Smith, J.L. Orr. 1995b. Regularly scheduled, day-time, slow-onset 60-Hz electric and magnetic field exposure does not depress serum melatonin concentration in nonhuman primates. *Bioelectromagnetics* Suppl. 3:111–118.

Schneider, T., P. Semm. 1992. The biological and possible clinical significance of magnetic influences on the pineal melatonin synthesis. *Exp. Clin. Endocrinol.* 11:251–258.

Semm, P., T. Schneider, L. Vollrath. 1980. Effects of an earth-strength magnetic field on electrical activity of pineal cells. *Nature* 288:607–608.

Shigemitsu, T., K. Takeshita, Y. Shiga, M. Kato. 1993. A 50-Hz magnetic field exposure system for small animals. *Bioelectromagnetics* 14:107–116.

Stehle, J., S. Reuss, H. Schroder, M. Henschel, L. Vollrath. 1988. Magnetic field effects on pineal N-acetyltransferase activity and melatonin content in the gerbil—role of pigmentation and sex. *Physiol. & Behav.* 44:91–94.

Welker, H.A., P. Semm, R.P. Willing, J.C. Commentz, W. Wiltschko, L. Vollrath. 1983. Effects of an artificial magnetic field on serotonin N-acetyltransferase activity and melatonin content of the rat pineal gland. *Exp. Brain Res.* 50:426–432.

Wiesenfeld, K., F. Moss. 1995. Stochastic resonance and the benefits of noise: From ice ages to crayfish and squids. *Nature* 373:33–36.

Wilson, B.W., L.E. Anderson. 1990. ELF electromagnetic field effects on the pineal gland. In: *Extremely Low Frequency Electromagnetic Fields: The Question of Cancer*, B.W. Wilson, R.G. Stevens, L.E. Anderson, eds., pp. 159-186. Columbus, Ohio: Battelle Press.

Wilson, B.W., L.E. Anderson, D.I. Hilton, R.D. Phillips. 1981. Chronic exposure to 60-Hz electric fields: Effects on pineal function in the rat. *Bioelectromagnetics* 2:371–380.

Wilson, B.W., E.K. Chess, L.E. Anderson. 1986. 60-Hz electric-field effects on pineal melatonin rhythms: Time course for onset and recovery. *Bioelectromagnetics* 7:239–242.

Wilson, B.W., C.W. Wright, J.E. Morris, R.L. Buschbom, D.P. Brown, D.L. Miller, R. Sommers-Flannigan, L.E. Anderson. 1990. Evidence for an effect of ELF electromagnetic fields on human pineal gland function. *J. Pineal Res.* 9:259–269.

Wurtman, R.J., J. Axelrod. 1965. The pineal gland. *Sci. Am.* 213:50–60.

Yamazaki, K., T. Kawamoto, T. Shigemitsu. 1996. Fundamental study of induced current distribution inside living body caused by ELF magnetic fields (Japanese text). *Trans. Inst. Elect. Eng. Japan* 116-c:193–199.

Yellon, S.M. 1994. Acute 60 Hz magnetic field exposure effects on the melatonin rhythm in the pineal gland and circulation of the adult Djungarian hamster. *J. Pineal Res.* 16:136–144.

14 In Search of a Direct Effect of Weak (50-Hz) Magnetic Fields on the Pineal Gland of Djungarian Hamsters

ALEXANDER LERCHL
MICHAEL NIEHAUS
PETRA NIKLOWITZ
Institute of Reproductive Medicine of the
University, Münster, Germany

CONTENTS

INTRODUCTION
MATERIALS AND METHODS
  Animals
  Exposure System
  Experimental Procedure
RESULTS
DISCUSSION
CONCLUSION
REFERENCES

INTRODUCTION

An increasing number of epidemiologic studies indicate a possible connection between exposure to weak, power-frequency (50/60-Hz) magnetic fields and health risks (Chernoff et al. 1992; Sagan 1992;

Armstrong et al. 1994; Lundsberg et al. 1995; Savitz and Loomis 1995; Reif et al. 1995). However, a plausible explanation for these data is still lacking (for example, see Grundler et al. 1992; Kruglikov and Dertinger 1994; Blank 1995; Bowman et al. 1995; Goodman et al. 1995; Pickard 1995; Prato et al. 1995). Much attention has been given to the study performed by Semm et al. (1980), in which the neural activity of pineal cells was shown to be affected by magnetic fields of the same magnitude as the Earth's magnetic field. Subsequent studies in different rodent species have shown that the synthesis of melatonin, the principal hormone of the pineal gland, is suppressed by magnetic fields (Semm 1983; Welker et al. 1983; Olcese et al. 1988a; Rudolph et al. 1988). These observations led to the hypothesis that the possible health risks by power-frequency magnetic fields are mediated through an effect on the pineal gland. (For reviews, see Reiter 1993a, b, 1994; Reiter and Lerchl 1993; Reiter, Chapter 3 in this volume.) Although this hypothesis is very sound, there is yet no definitive explanation for how the pineal gland itself may be influenced by such fields. There are at least two possibilities to investigate.

First, the eyes may be a prime target for power-frequency magnetic fields because the eyes are also the target for light, which plays a critical role in melatonin synthesis under normal circumstances. Light suppresses melatonin; therefore, a similar effect of magnetic fields on the photoreceptors may result in a diminished melatonin production. There is evidence for such a possibility in several reports indicating that the pigmentation of the eyes is a critical factor in melatonin suppression, as is the mere presence of the eyes (Olcese et al. 1985, 1988b; Stehle et al. 1988; Olcese and Hurlbut 1989; Kato et al. 1994). Likewise, the exposure of the eyes of rats to dim red light reportedly affected their pineals' responses to magnetic fields (Reuss and Olcese 1986).

Second, the pineal gland itself may be the major target of power-frequency magnetic fields. So far, only few investigations have addressed this possibility. Lerchl et al. (1991a) discovered that the combination of a static and an alternating magnetic field at a frequency of 33.7 Hz can significantly suppress melatonin in a static culture of isolated rat pineal glands. To further address the possibility of direct effects of magnetic fields on melatonin synthesis in the pineal gland, we developed an exposure system by which isolated pineal glands can be exposed to various magnetic fields of defined character-istics. The fast rise time of the amplifiers used in this system allows exposure to magnetic fields with high dB/dt ratios. Previous in vivo studies have indicated that such high dB/dt ratios may be an essential parameter for their biological effects (Lerchl et al. 1990, 1991b).

In an investigation of how Djungarian hamsters respond to 60-Hz magnetic fields, Yellon (1994) found that acute exposure before the onset of night caused a significant reduction of melatonin in the pineals when animals were sacrificed during the night. Thus, this animal species seems to belong to the "responders" with respect to magnetic field effects on the pineal.

With this evidence at hand, we decided to perform experiments addressing the possibility of direct effects of magnetic fields on the pineal gland of Djungarian hamsters. The experimental set-up as well as the first results are presented in this chapter.

MATERIALS AND METHODS

Animals

Female Djungarian hamsters were bred and raised in our own colony (for details, see Lerchl 1995). They were maintained on a 16:8 hours light:dark cycle. Fresh water and standard food was available *ad libitum*. During morning (lights on at 0400 hours), groups of age-matched animals were sacrificed by decapitation. The pineal glands were removed immediately, together with a small piece of attached skull.[1]

Exposure System

The pineal–skull pieces were placed in glass cylinders of 0.5 cm diameter and 1 cm length, perfused with oxygenated Krebs-Ringer buffer at a pH of 7.2. For each of three experimental groups, eight identical

---

[1] Previous experiments with isolated pineal glands without skull have resulted in an undesirable instability of the organ, which was easily damaged either by the removal of the organ, or by later procedures throughout the superfusion period. The pineal–skull complex was mechanically much more stable, and the time for preparation was minimized.

cylinders were used. They were closed with rubber stoppers and connected to a 24-channel peristaltic pump (flow rate 0.4 mL/minute; Ismatech, Germany) by Teflon tubing. The perfusates were collected in standard plastic tubes (Fig. 1). Pineals were placed in the cylinders in an alternating order (e.g., group 1, group 2, group 3, group 1, etc.)

The groups of eight cylinders were placed within Helmholtz coils of 5 cm diameter. These coils were made of double copper wire to allow antiparallel wiring for true sham exposure. Three identical coil pairs, connected to the generators by a black box, were used. The three groups of glass cylinders, the Helmholtz coils, and the Krebs-Ringer buffer were located in an incubator at 37°C.

Before each experiment started, the switches of the black box were set by a person not involved in the experiments, and only after all experimental data were obtained was the code broken. Within the black box, three switches allocated the three sources (one DC power supply and two generators; see below) to the Helmholtz coil pairs, while another set of three switches enabled or disabled the antiparallel wiring. Thus, neither the identity of the active coils nor that of the sham coil was known to the person performing the experiment. Each

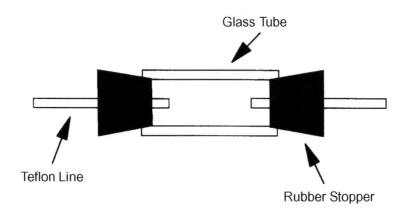

FIG. 1. Diagram of a chamber for exposing individual pineal glands of Djungarian hamsters. After decapitation, each pineal gland, still attached to a small fraction of the skull, was placed in a chamber. During the entire experiment, oxygenated buffer was pumped through each chamber.

coil was calibrated with a Bell Gaussmeter at static magnetic fields. To monitor varying magnetic fields, a shunt resistor was connected in series to the coils, and an oscilloscope picked up the current flowing through the coils, providing an indirect but precise measure of the magnetic fields. A thermoprinter attached to the oscilloscope (both from Hameg; Frankfurt, Germany) allowed a documentation of the field parameters. Of course, this oscilloscope was not used when an experiment was performed.

To generate the time-varying magnetic fields, two programmable generators were used (FG 9000, ELV; Leer, Germany). These generators are able to produce different wave forms as well as white noise, together with a broad spectrum of DC to 20 MHz. For our purposes, however, the most important feature of these generators was the main amplifying unit's remarkable rise time of approximately 7 nanoseconds. Although the inductivity of the coils prevented an exact rectangular shape of magnetic fields, the excellent control of the voltage was an important condition for precise experimental conditions.

Experimental Procedure

The magnetic fields and the sham "field" were activated for the entire experimental period. After the pineals had been transferred to the glass cylinders, they were perfused at a constant flow rate, and their perfusates were collected for 2 minutes every hour. After collection, the perfusates were immediately frozen. To stimulate the pineal glands for melatonin synthesis, they were superfused with buffer together with 10^{-7} M isoproterenol, a relatively pure beta-adrenergic agonist, for 30 minutes.[2] In addition, we discovered that the supplementation of the buffer with tryptophan at 10^{-4} M was necessary to obtain a marked increase of melatonin production due to the adrenergic agonist.

In the perfusates, melatonin was measured by an established radioimmunoassay (see Lerchl and Schlatt 1992 for details). The assay was validated for the experimental conditions, and the cross-reaction with tryptophan was negligible. Intra-assay variations were less than 8%,

---

[2] This treatment was necessary because the pineal glands of mammals neither respond to light nor produce melatonin during daytime hours.

while interassay variations were less than 14% (controlled by pooled sera at three different concentrations). Melatonin antiserum was obtained from Stockgrand Ltd. (Surrey, United Kingdom); melatonin tracer was obtained from Amersham (Braunschweig, Germany).

Melatonin concentrations at different time points were statistically compared with analysis of variance. Level of significance was set at $p < 0.05$.

RESULTS

The results obtained so far are given in Figure 2. The dimension of the Helmholtz coils and the maximal current of the power supplies (300 mA) limited the flux densities to 86 μT. At both 86 μT and 8.6 μT, no effects were seen in terms of any measurable decline or increase in melatonin production. In each case, both sinusoid wave forms and rectangular field forms were tested. Although in all cases the adrenergic stimulation resulted in a marked increase in melatonin production, magnetic fields of the tested frequency (50 Hz) and intensities had no significant influence.

An additional test (data not shown) revealed no significant difference between pineal glands exposed to white noise (86 μT) compared to controls.

DISCUSSION

Under the experimental conditions described, we could not identify any direct effect of 50-Hz magnetic fields up to 86 μT on the synthesis of melatonin by pineal glands of Djungarian hamsters. Any possible personal biases or influences by heat were excluded by means of the black box and the coils with antiparallel wiring, respectively. Thus, the experiments performed were done in a truly blind fashion.

When comparing our data with those of previous investigations, we could not identify any suppressing effects of magnetic fields on melatonin synthesis. However, as outlined in the introduction, our results showed that there was no direct effect of such fields on the pineal gland, at least with respect to Djungarian hamsters. Again, the results of these experiments must be interpreted with caution before general conclusions are drawn. Furthermore, thus far we have tested frequen-

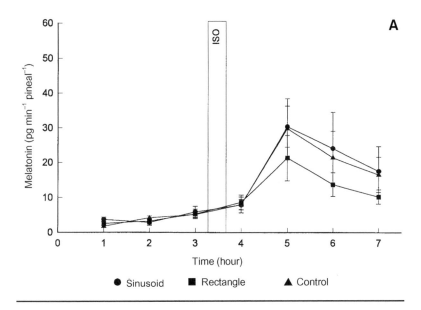

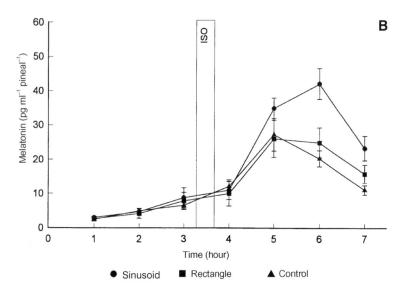

FIG. 2. Results of the experiments performed with pure beta-adrenergic stimulation. At both flux densities tested, 86 μT (Fig. 2A) and 8.6 μT (Fig. 2B), no significant changes were observed. n=8 glands per group; differences were tested for significant differences with analysis of variance.

cies of only 50-Hz, because this is the frequency of power lines in Europe. At other frequencies, effects may occur; however, our experiment with white noise also indicated no effects. Therefore, it appears rather unlikely that other frequencies may be able to suppress melatonin synthesis.

In an experiment with rat pineal glands kept in constant culture conditions (Lerchl et al. 1991a), a significant suppression of melatonin synthesis was observed at a frequency of 33.7 Hz together with a static magnetic field, theoretically fulfilling the conditions for ion cyclotron resonance (see Reiter and Lerchl 1993 for details). Although this theory is not generally accepted, it appears too early to definitely exclude that suppression may occur at these frequencies. Further studies are required to address this possibility. These special magnetic field configurations also can be tested using the exposure system described herein. Such experiments will be performed in the near future.

When comparing our hamster data with our results in rats and mice (Lerchl et al. 1991 a, b), we could not identify a reduction in melatonin synthesis, although rather high values for dB/dt were applied. In an in vivo experiment, we have demonstrated that rapidly changing magnetic fields cause reductions in pineal melatonin levels, while slowly changing fields have no such effects (Lerchl et al. 1991b). Hence it was postulated that the rise time of magnetic fields is an important parameter, probably by inducing currents which are proportional to the change of the magnetic field per time unit. Our present data do not support this idea with respect to the isolated pineal organ, at least as far as the experiments have been performed.

The discussion about possible health risks of power-frequency magnetic fields is primarily based on epidemiologic studies. However, the possible biological mechanism by which such magnetic fields may act is still unresolved. Notwithstanding open theoretical problems, a reliable and simple biological system is desirable for performing studies addressing these effects. When performing mechanistic experiments, whole animal studies have a number of disadvantages: First, the room required by animals may be a limiting factor (Lee et al. 1993). Second, the reactions of a whole organism are known to be influenced by many other physiological, chemical, and social stimuli that may interfere with the physical stimulus tested (e.g., magnetic fields). A well-defined organ system may be preferable, because all other influences are excluded in such a system. Because the melatonin hypothesis is still at the center of interest with respect to possible health risks of magnetic fields, the pineal gland itself may be the ideal object to study this hypothesis. Even if such experiments produce negative results (such as indicated by our data) in the end, these results could be useful for decisions regarding future research directions.

CONCLUSIONS

The exposure system for testing the direct effects of power-frequency magnetic fields on pineal gland function has been validated and shown to be useful for the questions addressed. The glands' responses to the adrenergic stimulation by isoproterenol were sufficient, which is an important precondition for testing a stimulated pineal gland. So far, no significant differences were identified between the three groups of glands exposed to, respectively, two different kinds of magnetic fields of the same intensity or the control condition. The relatively small variations within the groups indicated that the variability of the test system was acceptable. Under these circumstances, even a weak response of the pineal glands to the magnetic fields should be identifiable.

As pointed out before, our "negative" results do not mean that there is no adverse effect of magnetic fields of other frequencies and/or intensities. Likewise, if the system is used to test the responses of pineal glands of different species, results may well indicate species variations with respect to the stimulation by both isoproterenol and magnetic fields. Finally, we have tested so far only beta-adrenergic stimulation by isoproterenol, which is a relatively pure beta-adrenergic agonist. If an alpha-adrenergic agonist is used for stimulation of the glands, either alone or combined with isoproterenol, a different situation may evolve as well. It has been argued, for example, that calcium (Ca^{2+}) may play a central role in the biological response of cells to magnetic fields (Kavaliers and Ossenkopp 1987; Garcia-Sancho et al. 1994; Lindström et al. 1995). Because the stimulation of pineal cells by beta-adrenergic agonists alone will not cause an increase in intracellular Ca^{2+} concentrations, the use of alpha-adrenergic substances may be of additional significance.

The central question of how power-frequency magnetic or electric and magnetic fields (EMF) may adversely influence organisms is not yet answered (Stevens and Savitz 1992). The growing evidence by epidemiologic studies, however, supports the view that such influences do exist. Furthermore, the studies performed by Löscher and colleagues have used an animal model with a partial induction of cancer by 7,12-dimethylbenz(a)anthracene (DMBA). In their experiments, the authors demonstrated that magnetic fields are able to promote the chemically induced cancer significantly, together with a significant reduction of melatonin levels (Löscher et al. 1993a, b; Mevissen et al. 1994). Thus, the possible link between EMF exposure and disease is still a valid point to be discussed (Wilson et al. 1989).

From our point of view, and based on the data obtained so far, the pineal gland does not appear to be the prime target for nonthermal magnetic field effects in Djungarian hamsters. Hence, the biological effects observed are probably mediated through structures other than the pineal itself.

ACKNOWLEDGMENTS

This work was supported by a grant from the *Berufsgenossenschaft der Feinmechanik und Elektrotechnik*, Köln, Germany. The experiments performed were part of a diploma thesis at the Zoological Institute at the University of Münster (M.N.).

REFERENCES

Armstrong, B., G. Thériault, P. Guénel, J. Deadman, M. Goldberg, P. Heroux. 1994. Association between exposure to pulsed electromagnetic fields and cancer in electric utility workers in Quebec, Canada, and France. *Am. J. Epidemiol.* 140:805–820.

Blank, M. 1995. Biological effects of environmental electromagnetic fields: Molecular mechanisms. *Biosystems* 35:175–178.

Bowman, J.D., D.C. Thomas, S.J. London, J.M. Peters. 1995. Hypothesis: The risk of childhood leukemia is related to combinations of power-frequency and static magnetic fields. *Bioelectromagnetics* 16:48–59.

Chernoff, N., J.M. Rogers, R. Kavet. 1992. A review of the literature on potential reproductive and developmental toxicity of electric and magnetic fields. *Toxicology* 74:91–126.

Goodman, E.M., B. Greenebaum, M.T. Marron. 1995. Effects of electromagnetic fields on molecules and cells. *Int. Rev. Cytol.* 158:279–337.

Garcia-Sancho, J., M. Montero, J. Alvarez, R.I. Fonteriz, A. Sanchez. 1994. Effects of extremely-low-frequency electromagnetic fields on ion transport in several mammalian cells. *Bioelectromagnetics* 15:579–588.

Grundler, W., F. Kaiser, F. Keilmann, J. Walleczek. 1992. Mechanisms of electromagnetic interaction with cellular systems. *Naturwissenschaften* 79:551–559.

Kato, M., K. Honma, T. Shigemitsu, Y. Shiga. 1994. Horizontal or vertical 50-Hz, 1-μT magnetic fields have no effect on pineal gland or plasma melatonin concentration of albino rats. *Neurosci. Lett.* 168:205–208.

Kavaliers, M., K.P. Ossenkopp. 1987. Calcium channel involvement in magnetic field inhibition of morphine-induced analgesia. *Naunyn-Schmiedeberg's Arch. Pharmacol.* 336:308–315.

Kruglikov, I.L., H. Dertinger. 1994. Stochastic resonance as a possible mechanism of amplification of weak electric signals in living cells. *Bioelectromagnetics* 15:539–547.

Lee, J.M., F. Stormshak, J.M. Thompson, P. Thinesen, L.J. Painter, E.G. Olenchek, D.L. Hess, R. Forbes, D.L. Foster. 1993. Melatonin secretion and puberty in female lambs exposed to environmental electric and magnetic fields. *Biol. Reprod.* 49:857–864.

Lerchl, A. 1995. Breeding of Djungarian hamsters (*Phodopus sungorus*): Influence of parity and litter size on weaning success and offspring sex ratio. *Lab. Anim.* 29:172–176.

Lerchl, A., S. Schlatt. 1992. Serotonin content and melatonin production in the pineal gland of the Djungarian hamster (*Phodopus sungorus*). *J. Pineal Res.* 12:128–134.

Lerchl, A., K.O. Nonaka, K.A. Stokkan, R.J. Reiter. 1990. Marked rapid alterations in nocturnal pineal serotonin metabolism in mice and rats exposed to weak intermittent magnetic fields. *Biochem. Biophys. Res. Commun.* 169:102–108.

Lerchl, A., R.J. Reiter, K.A. Howes, K.O. Nonaka, K.-A. Stokkan. 1991a. Evidence that extremely low frequency Ca^{2+}-cyclotron resonance depresses pineal melatonin synthesis in vitro. *Neurosci. Lett.* 124:213–215.

Lerchl, A., K.O. Nonaka, R.J. Reiter. 1991b. Pineal gland "magnetosensitivity" to static magnetic fields is a consequence of induced electric currents (eddy currents). *J. Pineal. Res.* 10:109–116.

Lindström, E., P. Lindström, A. Berglund, E. Lundgren, K.H. Mild. 1995. Intracellular calcium oscillation in a T-cell line after exposure to extremely-low-frequency magnetic fields with variable frequencies and flux densities. *Bioelectromagnetics* 16:41–47.

Löscher, W., U. Wahnschaffe, M. Mevissen, A. Lerchl, A. Stamm. 1993a. The effect of 50-Hz low-energy magnetic fields on nocturnal melatonin production and the development of mammary tumors induced by 7,12-dimethylbenz(a)anthracene in rats. *Oncology* 51:288–295.

Löscher, W., M. Mevissen, W. Lehmacher, A. Stamm. 1993b. Tumor promotion in a breast cancer model by exposure to a weak alternating magnetic field. *Cancer Lett.* 71:75–81.

Lundsberg, L.S., M.B. Bracken, K. Belanger. 1995. Occupationally related magnetic field exposure and male subfertility. *Fertil. Steril.* 63:384–391.

Mevissen, M., S. Buntenkötter, W. Löscher. 1994. Effects of static and time-varying (50-Hz) magnetic fields on reproduction and fetal development in rats. *Teratology* 50:229–237.

Olcese, J., E. Hurlbut. 1989. Comparative studies on the retinal dopamine response to altered magnetic fields in rodents. *Brain Res.* 498:145–148.

Olcese, J., S. Reuss, L. Vollrath. 1985. Evidence for the involvement of the visual system in mediating magnetic field effects on pineal melatonin synthesis in the rat. *Brain Res.* 333:382–384.

Olcese, J., S. Reuss, P. Semm. 1988a. Geomagnetic field detection in rodents. *Life Sci.* 42:605–613.

Olcese, J., S. Reuss, J. Stehle, S. Steinlechner, L. Vollrath. 1988b. Responses of the mammalian retina to experimental alteration of the ambient magnetic field. *Brain Res.* 448:325–330.

Pickard, W.F. 1995. Trivial influences: A doubly stochastic poisson process model permits the detection of arbitrarily small electromagnetic signals. *Bioelectromagnetics* 16:2–8.

Prato, F.S., J.J.L. Carson, K.P. Ossenkopp, M. Kavaliers. 1995. Possible mechanisms by which extremely low frequency magnetic fields affect opioid function. *FASEB J.* 9:807–814.

Reif, J.S., K.S. Lower, G.K. Ogilvie. 1995. Residential exposure to magnetic fields and risk of canine lymphoma. *Am. J. Epidemiol.* 141:352–359.

Reiter, R.J. 1993a. A review of neuroendocrine and neurochemical changes associated with static and extremely low frequency electromagnetic field exposure. *Integr. Physiol. Behav. Sci.* 28:57–75.

Reiter, R.J. 1993b. Static and extremely low frequency electromagnetic field exposure: Reported effects on the circadian production of melatonin. *J. Cell. Biochem.* 51:394–403.

Reiter, R.J. 1994. Melatonin suppression by static and extremely low frequency electromagnetic fields: Relationship to the reported increased incidence of cancer. *Rev. Environ. Health* 10:171–186.

Reiter, R.J., A. Lerchl. 1993. Regulation of mammalian pineal melatonin production by the electromagnetic spectrum. In: *Melatonin: Biosynthesis, Physiological Effects, and Clinical Applications*, H.S. Yu and R.J. Reiter, eds., pp. 107–128. Boca Raton, Florida: CRC Press.

Reuss, S., J. Olcese. 1986. Magnetic field effects on the rat pineal gland: Role of retinal activation by light. *Neurosci. Lett.* 64:97–101.

Rudolph, K., A. Wirz-Justice, K. Kräuchi, H. Feer. 1988. Static magnetic fields decrease nocturnal pineal cAMP in the rat. *Brain Res.* 446:159–160.

Sagan, L.A. 1992. Epidemiological and laboratory studies of power frequency electric and magnetic fields. *J. Am. Med. Assoc.* 268:625–629.

Savitz, D.A., D.P. Loomis. 1995. Magnetic field exposure in relation to leukemia and brain cancer mortality among electric utility workers. *Am. J. Epidemiol.* 141:123–134.

Semm, P. 1983. Neurobiological investigations on the magnetic sensitivity of the pineal gland in rodents and pigeons. *Comp. Biochem. Physiol.* 76A:683–689.

Semm, P., T. Schneider, L. Vollrath. 1980. Effects of an Earth-strength magnetic field on electrical activity of pineal cells. *Nature* 288:607–608.

Stehle, J., S. Reuss, H. Schröder, M. Henschel, L. Vollrath. 1988. Magnetic field effects on pineal N-acetyltransferase activity and melatonin content in the gerbil—role of pigmentation and sex. *Physiol. Behav.* 44:91–94.

Stevens, R.G., D.A. Savitz. 1992. Is electromagnetic fields and cancer an issue worthy of study? *Cancer* 69:603–606.

Welker, H.A., P. Semm, R.P. Willig, J.C. Commentz, W. Wiltschko, L. Vollrath. 1983. Effects of an artificial magnetic field on serotonin N-acetyltransferase activity and melatonin content of the rat pineal gland. *Exp. Brain Res.* 50:426–432.

Wilson, B.W., R.G. Stevens, L.E. Anderson. 1989. Neuroendocrine mediated effects of electromagnetic-field exposure: Possible role of the pineal gland. *Life Sci.* 45:1319–1332.

Yellon, S.M. 1994. Acute 60 Hz magnetic field exposure effects on the melatonin rhythm in the pineal gland and circulation of the adult Djungarian hamster. *J. Pineal Res.* 16:136–144.

15 Studies of Melatonin, Cortisol, Progesterone, and Interleukin-1 in Sheep Exposed to EMF from a 500-kV Transmission Line

JACK M. LEE, JR.
  Bonneville Power Administration, Portland, Oregon
FRED STORMSHAK
JAMES THOMPSON
  Department of Animal Sciences, Oregon State
  University, Corvallis, Oregon
DAVID L. HESS
  Oregon Regional Primate Research Center,
  Beaverton, Oregon
STEVE HEFENEIDER
  Portland Veterans Affairs Medical Center and
  Oregon Health Sciences University, Portland,
  Oregon

CONTENTS

BACKGROUND
  Power-Frequency EMF and Melatonin in Animals
  EMF and Stress Responses
  EMF and the Immune System
MATERIALS AND METHODS
  Study Facilities and Animals
  Blood Samples

(continued)

CONTENTS (continued)

Assays
EMF, Noise, and Light Levels
Data Analyses
RESULTS
Melatonin
Progesterone and Puberty
Cortisol
Interleukin-1 Activity
EMF, Noise, and Light Levels
DISCUSSION
Melatonin
Cortisol
Interleukin-1 Activity
ACKNOWLEDGMENTS
REFERENCES

Most studies of the potential effects of electric and magnetic fields (EMF) on melatonin secretion have been conducted under laboratory conditions. This chapter describes studies of melatonin secretion conducted with sheep exposed to 60-Hz EMF from a 500-kV transmission line under natural environmental conditions. This is one of the few studies of melatonin secretion in which animals were exposed simultaneously to both electric and magnetic fields. Because of the essential role melatonin plays in regulating seasonal breeding in sheep, we also examined the onset of puberty as defined by progesterone secretion. Stress has been reported to affect melatonin secretion (Reiter 1990); therefore, cortisol secretion was included in the initial study as a measure of stress. Because melatonin interacts with the immune system (Maestroni et al. 1986), our later studies included measurement of changes in activity of the cytokine interleukin-1 (IL-1) from leukocytes of sheep exposed to EMF. The studies described in this chapter involved three separate experiments conducted during a 4-year period at a site in western Oregon.

Background

Power-Frequency EMF and Melatonin in Animals

Most concerns about possible health effects caused by transmission lines began in the early 1970s and involved power-frequency (50/60-Hz) electric fields, because reported health effects in Soviet substation workers were attributed to these fields (Asanova and Rakov 1966). The Soviet report, along with results of some early studies of laboratory animals (e.g., Marino et al. 1976) prompted further research on electric fields in several countries. One of the most dramatic effects reported in early laboratory studies was a large depression in nocturnal pineal melatonin in male laboratory rats exposed for 30 days to 60-Hz vertical electric fields of about 2 kV/m (Wilson et al. 1981, 1983). Nocturnal pineal melatonin concentrations were also reduced and the phase delayed 1.4 hours in young male rats exposed to 60-Hz electric fields of 10, 65, or 130 kV/m in utero and for the first 23 days after birth (Reiter et al. 1988). The effects on melatonin reported in the two latter studies occurred from exposures to 60-Hz electric field strengths that approximate the range of electric field strength found on the rights-of-way of extra-high-voltage transmission lines (2–10 kV/m). Another study, however, found that 30-day exposure to a 60-Hz, 65-kV/m, vertical electric field did not affect pineal melatonin in male rats, although a small depression in serum melatonin was detected (Grota et al. 1994).

If the reported effects on melatonin are associated with body currents induced by the electric field, then effects on larger animals such as livestock might occur with even lower field strengths because of scaling considerations. For example, the axial current density induced across the neck of a rat by 60-Hz electric fields of 2–10 kV/m is roughly comparable to the current induced across the neck of a pig in fields of about 1.4–7 kV/m (Kaune and Phillips 1980).

A more recent study reported that male rats exposed 6 weeks to circularly polarized, 50-Hz magnetic fields as low as 1 μT (a level produced by both transmission and distribution lines) exhibited statistically significant reductions in serum and pineal melatonin levels, during both day and night (Kato et al. 1993). These effects were not found by the same laboratory when 50-Hz horizontal or vertical magnetic fields were used (Kato et al. 1994). Another study of 50-Hz magnetic fields, comparable in strength to those from power lines, found that nocturnal serum melatonin amplitude was decreased in female rats exposed for 8–9 weeks to a field of 0.3–1 μT (Löscher et al. 1994).

Exposure of Djungarian hamsters of both sexes to a 60-Hz magnetic field of 100 μT for 15 minutes before lights out reduced nocturnal pineal and serum melatonin, and caused a phase delay (Yellon 1994a). However, no effects were detected after this exposure was applied daily for 3 weeks (Yellon 1994b). Nocturnal pineal melatonin was also not affected in rats and mice exposed for 10 weeks to 60-Hz magnetic fields ranging from 2 μT to 1 mT (McCormick et al. 1994). The study included both continuous and intermittent (1 hour on, 1 hour off) field exposures.

In addition to the studies of sheep described in this chapter, we are aware of only one other published study of melatonin secretion in which animals were exposed simultaneously to both electric and magnetic power-frequency fields. The study involved three experiments with baboons that were exposed for 6 weeks to 60-Hz EMF during daytime only, in a specially constructed indoor facility (Rogers et al. 1995a, b). In two experiments, three baboons were exposed to 60-Hz fields of either 6 kV/m and 50 μT, or 30 kV/m and 100 μT, and the fields were ramped on and off slowly to avoid producing field transients (Rogers et al. 1995b). These exposure conditions produced no changes in nocturnal serum melatonin concentrations. In a third experiment, two baboons were exposed to the same field strengths but with the fields switched on and off rapidly. This experiment resulted in significantly reduced nocturnal melatonin concentrations (Rogers et al. 1995a).

An important role of the pattern of melatonin secretion is that it provides information about day length. In seasonal breeding species such as sheep, melatonin plays a critical role in regulating the timing of the breeding season (Karsch et al. 1984). Treatments that alter key aspects of the melatonin signal in sheep can significantly affect the seasonal onset of reproductive activity, and the timing of puberty (see Foster 1994 for a review). For example, puberty was delayed about 13 weeks in female lambs in which the pineal gland was removed (Kennaway et al. 1985). When the pineal in female lambs was denervated by superior cervical ganglionectomy, puberty was delayed about 32 weeks (Yellon and Foster 1986).

EMF and Stress Responses

Several reports have suggested that power-frequency EMF affect various biological measures used to characterize a stress response. However, the issue remains unresolved because several other studies did not indicate an association between stress and EMF. Stress is one of the factors that has been reported to affect melatonin secretion patterns (Reiter 1990), so it is possible that this could be one mechanism to explain some EMF-related effects on melatonin. Exposure of rats to 60-Hz electric fields of 25 kV/m or 50 kV/m resulted in increased levels of serum corticosterone during the first few minutes of exposure (Hackman and Graves 1981). However, corticosterone levels were not affected in the study after 6 weeks of exposure. Similarly, when rats were exposed to 60-Hz, 100-kV/m electric fields for 1 or 3 hours, no effects were seen on corticosterone levels (Quinlan et al. 1985). In contrast, Free et al. (1981) found that corticosterone levels were significantly lower in rats exposed for 120 days to a 60-Hz electric field of 64 kV/m than in control rats. However, no effect was found in a replicate experiment, and the authors suggested that differences in sampling times may partly explain the inconsistency. In a study of mice, the median daytime level of corticosterone was elevated significantly by long-term exposure to a 50-Hz, 10 kV/m electric field (De Bruyn and De Jager 1994).

Wilson and Anderson (1990) suggested that effects of electric fields on pineal melatonin reported in some studies of laboratory rats are manifestations of stress. They cited studies by Leung et al. (1990) in which secretion of porphyrin from the Harderian gland was found in rats exposed to 60-Hz, 40- to 130-kV/m electric fields. This finding, along with changes found in serum prolactin levels, were reportedly similar to stress effects associated with the restraining of animals.

EMF and the Immune System

Although there are many reports of studies investigating the effects of EMF on various components of the immune system, this body of research is very difficult to evaluate (Chiabrera et al. 1994). The difficulty arises in part because the studies have used widely differing EMF exposures, with varying frequencies, wave shapes, magnitudes, and exposure durations. Some studies used in vitro EMF exposures; in others, animals were first exposed to EMF, and then immune system parameters were examined in vitro. Finally, a variety of mitogens and assays were used, which adds to the large number of experimental combinations that have been reported.

Morris et al. (1988) studied the immune response in rats exposed to 60-Hz electric fields of 10–130 kV/m. No major changes in in vitro and in vivo measurements of cell-mediated immunity were found. Exposure of lymphocytes in vitro for 48 hours to a 60-Hz electric field (1 V/m in the medium) resulted in a 25% inhibition in the cytotoxicity of T-cells (Lyle et al. 1988); cell numbers were not affected by the field exposure. Morris et al. (1990) exposed rats to 60-Hz, 1-mT magnetic fields applied either continuously or intermittently. Natural immunity measurements suggested that exposed animals exhibited an increased immune response, but the finding was not statistically significant. The mobilization of calcium is an important step in the immune response, and several studies have reported that EMF can affect calcium fluxes (Walleczek 1991).

Murthy et al. (1991) reported that expression of interleukin-2 (IL-2) receptors was depressed in a 5-week pilot study of six baboons exposed to combined 60-Hz fields of 6 kV/m and 50 μT. Exposure of human T-cells to a 15-Hz, 0.1-mT (peak) magnetic field, with the direct current (DC) field canceled to 0.5 μT, resulted in an increase in secretion and receptor binding of IL-1β (Mehta et al. 1992). In more recent studies, Mehta et al. (1994) reported that secretion of IL-1β by lipopolysaccharide (LPS)-stimulated human monocytes was reduced 38% by exposure to a 15-Hz magnetic field of 86 μT (peak). (LPS is a complex molecule consisting of fats and sugars). In contrast, IL-2 secretion increased three- to fourfold in the study. Morandi et al. (1994) found no differences in IL-1 production by murine thioglycollate-elicited peritoneal exudate cells when exposed for 24 hours to a 60-Hz electric field (11.8 kV/m), a 60-Hz magnetic field (0.3 mT), or to the combined EMF.

MATERIALS AND METHODS

During a period of 4 years we conducted three separate experiments to test hypotheses about possible effects of chronic exposure to 60-Hz EMF on female sheep (Lee et al. 1993, 1995; Hefeneider 1994; Thompson et al. 1995). The primary hypothesis for experiments 1 and 2 was that chronic exposure to EMF would significantly alter the melatonin pattern, resulting in an effect on the time of puberty in female lambs. A secondary hypothesis in these experiments was that exposure to EMF would represent a stressor on developing lambs. Experiment 3 tested the hypothesis that exposure to EMF results in a decrease in the in vitro activity of IL-1. For each of the three experiments, different groups of sheep were used. The EMF exposure duration for each of the experiments lasted about 10 months. Pre- and postexposure periods of various durations were also included; these and other details of the experiments are described below.

Study Facilities and Animals

Experiment 1
The study was conducted at a site 40 km southeast of Portland, Oregon (45° 24´ north latitude). A treatment (line) pen was located at the edge of a corridor containing three 500-kV transmission lines, and two 230-kV transmission lines. The line pen was beneath the outer conductors of the outermost 500-kV line, within the area of maximum field strength. A control pen was located 229 m from the 500-kV line. Both line and control pens were identical in size and construction. Pens were constructed of elevated, slatted metal floors with plastic (nonconducting) sides. The metal floor was grounded to prevent sheep from receiving shocks from voltages induced by the electric field. Plastic material was used above the pen floor to minimize shielding of the electric field. Each pen had a floor area of 24 m^2, which is about 2.5 times greater than recommended minimum floor space for sheep on slatted floor pens (Johnson et al. 1988).

Part of each pen was covered with plastic netting to act as a sunscreen. During inclement weather, plastic tarps were placed over the netting. Two 15-watt, red-coated, incandescent lights (Sylvania) were installed in each pen to facilitate collection of blood samples during nighttime.

From April 2–6, 1990, 20 female Suffolk lambs for experiment 1 were maintained in the control pen while pre-exposure data were collected. The lambs were assigned randomly in equal numbers to a control and a treatment group. Mean (± SEM) initial ages for control and line groups were $8.0 ± 0.1$ and $8.1 ± 0.1$ weeks, respectively. Initial weights (mean ± SEM) for the control and line groups were $27.4 ± 1.4$ and $27.6 ± 0.8$ kg, respectively. The line group was moved to the line pen on April 6, 1990 where the group remained until February 2, 1991. All the sheep were maintained in the control pen February 2–15, 1991, while post-exposure data were collected.

Sheep were fed a diet consisting of pelleted alfalfa, grass hay, and a commercial pellet (Lamb Creep & Finisher, Land O'Lakes, Inc., Seattle, Washington). The quantity was commensurate with weight and stage of growth based on National Research Council requirements (National Research Council 1985) for growth of replacement ewe lambs. Water and mineral supplement were fed ad libitum.

Experiment 2

Experiment 2 employed 30 female Suffolk lambs. To allow for the increased number of animals, the floor area was increased to 58.5 m^2 in both the control and line pens. Other details of facilities, feeding, and care were basically the same as in experiment 1. From April 1–6, 1991, all lambs were maintained in the control pen during collection of pre-exposure data. The animals were assigned randomly into two groups of 15 each. Mean (± SEM) ages for the control and line groups were $8.6 ± 0.2$ and $8.5 ± 0.2$ weeks, respectively. Mean weights (± SEM) for the control and line groups were $26.8 ± 1.3$ and $25.9 ± 1.0$ kg, respectively. The line group was maintained in the line pen from April 6, 1991–February 2, 1992. Post-exposure data were collected during February 2–8, 1992, while all sheep were again maintained in the control pen.

Experiment 3

The pen sizes were the same as used in experiment 2; the care and management of the animals were basically the same as in the previous experiments. Thirty-five female Suffolk lambs with a mean initial age of 7 weeks were maintained in the control pen while pre-exposure data were collected from April 1–May 8, 1992. Thirty of the lambs were selected for the experiment based on their serum chemistry, overall good health, complete blood counts, normal body weight, and normal levels of IL-1 activity and selenium. The 30 lambs were assigned randomly into two groups of 15 each. The mean (± SEM) weights of the control and line groups on May 6 were 40.2 ± 4.0 and 40.5 ± 5.4 kg, respectively. The line group was moved to the line pen on May 8, 1992, where the group remained until March 22, 1993. All sheep were transported 160 km to a pasture at Oregon State University in Corvallis, Oregon, where post-exposure data were collected until April 1994.

Blood Samples

Experiment 1
Blood samples (5–6 mL) used to monitor serum concentrations of melatonin and cortisol were collected during eight 48-hour periods from indwelling catheters placed in a jugular vein. During each 48-hour period, sampling began at 1200 hours on a Thursday and continued until 1200 hours on the following Saturday. Blood samples were taken at 3-hour intervals during daylight, at 30-minute intervals during 2-hour periods before sunrise and after sunset, and at 1-hour intervals during the remainder of the night. The first 48-hour sampling period was immediately prior to the start of EMF exposure, and the last sample was 5 days after the end of exposure. During the pre- and post-exposure samples, all lambs were housed in the control pen. The sample dates were chosen to provide data for representative day lengths throughout the year, and for different stages of development of the lambs. Samples were collected over two consecutive 24-hour periods so that variability in melatonin secretory patterns could be assessed.

To determine serum concentrations of progesterone, 10-mL blood samples were collected by jugular venipuncture during the morning, twice weekly (Monday and Thursday), beginning when the lambs were 19 weeks old.

Experiment 2
Methods for collecting blood samples to determine serum hormone

concentrations were basically the same as in experiment 1. During experiment 2, a pilot study was added to examine possible effects of EMF on IL-1 activity, and on some other components of the immune system (Stormshak 1993). This chapter describes only the IL-1 study. To analyze IL-1 activity, 10-mL blood samples were collected from all lambs by jugular venipuncture at approximately 2-week intervals during the 10-month EMF exposure period. Blood samples were also taken at 2, 3, and 5 months post-exposure. No pre-exposure data on IL-1 activity were obtained during the pilot study.

Experiment 3

To measure in vitro leukocyte production of IL-1, 10-mL blood samples were taken periodically during 1 month pre-exposure, 4 months of constant EMF exposure, 1.5 months of intermittent EMF exposure, 5 months of constant EMF exposure, and at 13 months post-exposure. The intermittent exposure was due to unscheduled maintenance which required that the 500-kV line crossing the line pen be turned off during the day on weekdays. The adjacent transmission lines remained in service during this intermittent period.

Assays

Experiment 1

Serum hormone concentrations were measured by radioimmunoassays (RIAs), and the 3_H-labeled hormones were obtained from NEN Research (Boston, Massachusetts). The melatonin RIA was described by English et al. (1986), and was later modified by Malpaux et al. (1987), then Foster et al. (1988). The antibody (Guildhay G/S/704-6483) has been shown to be specific for melatonin in sheep serum. Standard curves, percentage nonspecific binding, total binding, midpoints of standard curves, and melatonin concentrations were determined by the RIA AID computer program (Robert Marciel Associates, Arlington, Massachusetts). Mean intra- and interassay coefficients of variation were 8.9 and 12.4%, respectively. The limit of detection was 1 pg/mL.

Progesterone was analyzed by RIA after extracting 100-μL aliquots of sheep serum diluted with 100 μL of gelatin phosphate-buffered saline with diethyl ether (Hess et al. 1981). Progesterone antisera (R12) were obtained from Dr. A. Surve, Sandoz Pharmaceuticals (Summit,

New Jersey). The progesterone standard was assayed in duplicate, and calculations for standards, unknowns, and quality-control pools were performed using a logit-log transformation program. Intra- and interassay coefficients of variation were 4.7 and 9.6%, respectively.

Cortisol was analyzed by first extracting duplicate 20-μL serum aliquots diluted with 180 μL of 0.1% gelatin phosphate-buffered saline with a pH of 7.0. Cortisol antisera (R2P8) were obtained from ICN Biomedicals (Costa Mesa, California). Intra- and interassay coefficients of variation for the cortisol RIA were 5.8 and 13.7%, respectively.

Experiments 2 and 3

The melatonin and progesterone RIA methods in experiment 2 were the same as in experiment 1; cortisol was not assayed. For the IL-1 induction assays in experiments 2 and 3, leukocytes from whole blood samples were isolated by collecting buffy coats (a mixture of white blood cells), then stimulated with 20 μg/mL of the mitogen LPS per 2 x 10^6 cells. After incubation for 48 hours at 5% CO_2, cell-free supernatants were collected, and IL-1 activity was quantified using the IL-1 dependent D10.S cell line (Hefeneider et al. 1992). The assay for IL-1 activity consisted of measuring proliferation of D10.S (2 x 10^4 cells/well) exposed to a twofold dilution series of the cell-free supernatant (range 1:8 to 1:512) for 72 hours. Cell proliferation was assayed by adding 3_H-thymidine to the D10.S culture for an additional 6 hours. Incorporation of the 3_H-thymidine by the D10.S cells (determined by liquid scintillation counting) was correlated with the amount of IL-1 in the sample tested. IL-1 activity was quantified by comparison with a standard curve determined by titration of human recombinant IL-1.

EMF, Noise, and Light Levels

Electric and magnetic field levels were monitored for the line and control pens during all three experiments. The magnetic field is directly related to current on the transmission line, so it changes as loading on the line varies throughout the day. Because of this variability, the magnetic field was measured every 10 minutes with permanent monitors (Electric Research and Management, State College, Pennsylvania). During experiment 1, measurements were made of the Earth's DC magnetic field within the study area. The three orthogonal components of the DC field were measured 1 m above ground with a Rawson-Lush Instrument Company Model 906 Rotating Coil Gaussmeter (Acton, Massachusetts). The electric field, due to voltage on conductors, is relatively more stable than the magnetic field. Electric field strength in control and line pens was periodically measured with a hand-held meter (Electric Field Measurements Company Model 110, Stockbridge, Massachusetts). For the line pen, electric field strength was also periodically mapped with a hand-held meter at several locations throughout the pen.

A-weighted audible noise in the line and control pens was measured with Brüel & Kjaer 4921 (Nærum, Denmark) all-weather microphones. The "A" scale models how the human ear perceives sound. Measurements were also made of higher-frequency noise (6.5 kHz and above), which was believed to include the most sensitive hearing range of sheep. Measurements of nighttime light levels in the pens were made with a hand-held instrument (International Light, Model 710A, Newburyport, Maine). Measurements of the spectral response of the red lamps used for nighttime blood collection were made in a laboratory at Oregon State University.

Data Analyses

Melatonin
The circadian pattern of serum concentrations of melatonin during the 48-hour sampling periods in experiments 1 and 2 was characterized using three basic parameters to describe the nighttime elevation: (1) mean duration, (2) mean amplitude, and (3) mean phase. Prior to statistical analyses, melatonin concentration data were transformed to natural logarithms. Statistical tests on melatonin data were performed by analysis of variance (ANOVA) with repeated measures.

The beginning and end of the night elevation in serum melatonin were determined by first calculating the mean and standard deviation of the daytime melatonin concentration for each 48-hour period and each animal. Then, the onset of the night elevation was designated to be the first sample time after sunset when melatonin was equal to or exceeded the day mean plus two standard deviations. The end of the night elevation was designated to be the last night sample, before the first day sample after sunrise, that equaled or exceeded this daytime value. Duration of the night elevation for each animal was determined by calculating the time difference between the onset and ending times. Mean amplitude of the night elevation for each animal was the mean of all samples between these two times. Phase was determined by first calculating for each sample night the time midpoint between sunset and sunrise. Next, the midpoint of the night melatonin elevation was determined for each animal. The difference between these two midpoints represented the phase. For example, a phase advance means that the midpoint of the melatonin elevation occurs before the middle of the night.

Onset of the first normal ovarian cycle was defined as the time when a rise in serum progesterone above 0.3 ng/mL occurred in at least three consecutive samples collected twice weekly, one of which exceeded 1 ng/mL. Onset of puberty and number of estrous cycles were analyzed with one-tailed t-tests.

Cortisol

Cortisol measured in blood samples collected during the 48-hour periods in experiment 1 was divided into day and night components for analyses. Night was defined for each animal as all samples taken between sunset and sunrise, and day consisted of all remaining samples. Cortisol data were analyzed by ANOVA with repeated measures.

IL-1 Activity

Comparisons of relative IL-1 activity between control and line groups in cell-free supernatants were analyzed on an assay-by-assay basis, and for all assays combined. The IL-1 data, expressed as units/mL in all trials, were used to examine the difference in the absolute amount of IL-1 activity over time. Because the amount of IL-1 activity in response to LPS stimulation varied greatly from assay to assay, our analyses focused on the relative differences between line and control groups for each assay. IL-1 activity data for each assay were analyzed with two-tailed t-tests in experiment 2, and with one-tailed t-tests in experiment 3. Data for all IL-1 assays were also analyzed by ANOVA with repeated measures.

RESULTS

Melatonin

Experiment 1

Typically, serum melatonin concentrations in the lambs increased sharply after sundown and decreased sharply near sunrise. Combining all data, the nighttime melatonin concentration (mean ± SEM) was eight times higher than the daytime concentration (77.0 ± 5.8 versus 9.5 ± 2.0 pg/mL, respectively). During the night, considerable individual variation occurred in melatonin amplitude at various sample times. Mean day melatonin ± SEM for control and line lambs was 10.0 ± 2.4 versus 9.1 ± 1.6 pg/mL, respectively. Comparison of these levels showed that there was no statistically significant difference between groups (p = 0.59).

Duration of the melatonin elevation reflected the change in the duration of the dark period throughout the study (Fig. 1). For mean duration of the nighttime melatonin elevation, there was no signifi-

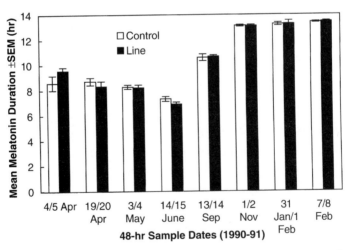

FIG. 1. Experiment 1 mean nighttime melatonin duration in serum collected in control and line lambs during eight 48-hour sample periods. The first sample period is pre-exposure; the last sample period is post-exposure. See text for sampling details.

cant difference between groups (p = 0.88), however, there was a highly significant effect of season (p < 0.001).

Analysis of group means for the amplitude of the nighttime melatonin elevation (Fig. 2) revealed no significant difference between control and line groups (p = 0.62). Mean amplitude did change during the study, with higher melatonin levels in the latter part of the period. This highly significant time effect (p < 0.001) corresponded with changes in photoperiod (longer nights) and with increasing age of the lambs.

The mean nocturnal melatonin for each lamb, combining data from all 16 sample nights, showed a similar distribution in control and line groups (data not shown). In each group, there was approximately a twofold difference in average melatonin between individual lambs with the highest and lowest mean melatonin values.

Data on the phase of the nighttime melatonin elevation suggested that means tended to be slightly phase-advanced (Fig. 3). However, there was no significant difference in phase between control and line groups (p = 0.56).

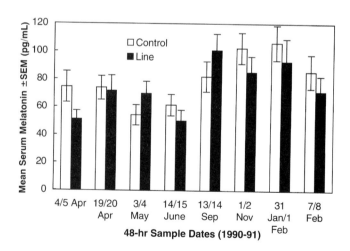

FIG. 2. Experiment 1 mean nighttime melatonin amplitude in serum collected in control and line lambs during eight 48-hour sample periods. The first sample period is pre-exposure; the last sample period is post-exposure. See text for sampling details (Lee et al. 1993).

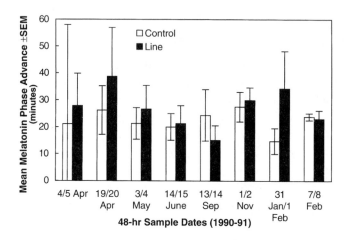

FIG. 3. Experiment 1 mean nighttime melatonin phase in serum collected in control and line lambs during eight 48-hour sample periods. The first sample period is pre-exposure; the last sample period is post-exposure. See text for sampling details (Lee et al. 1993).

Experiment 2

Melatonin in both groups of lambs again showed the normal pattern of low daytime and high nighttime serum concentrations. Daytime melatonin concentrations did not differ between groups (p = 0.18). The mean duration of nighttime melatonin is shown in Figure 4; there was no difference in duration between groups (p = 0.97). The duration corresponded with the changing day length throughout the year. This relationship resulted in an interaction between time of year and sample period that was statistically significant (p < 0.001).

The mean amplitude of the nighttime melatonin secretion (Fig. 5) also did not differ significantly between groups (p = 0.78). Mean nighttime melatonin did seem to change depending on the sample time (group × month interaction, p = 0.07). This response is attributed to seasonal changes in natural photoperiod, and to the increasing age of the lambs.

Data on the phase of the nighttime melatonin secretion is shown in Figure 6. Considering all sample periods, there was no difference in phase between the two groups (p = 0.19).

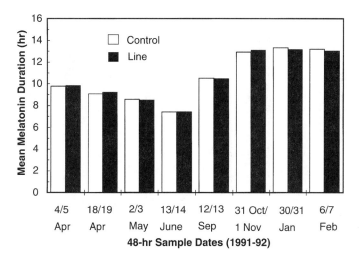

FIG. 4. Experiment 2 mean nighttime melatonin duration in serum collected in control and line lambs during eight 48-hour sample periods. The first sample period is pre-exposure; the last sample period is post-exposure. The common SEM for these data was 0.33. See text for sampling details (Lee et al. 1995).

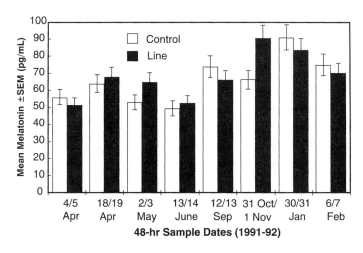

FIG. 5. Experiment 2 mean nighttime melatonin amplitude in serum collected in control and line lambs during eight 48-hour sample periods. The first sample period is pre-exposure; the last sample period is post-exposure. See text for sampling details (Lee et al. 1995).

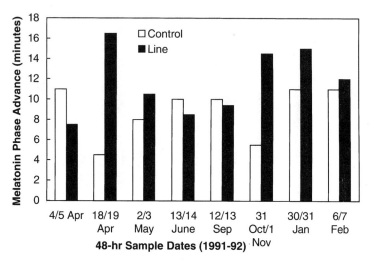

FIG. 6. Experiment 2 mean nighttime melatonin phase in serum collected in control and line lambs during eight 48-hour sample periods. The first sample period is pre-exposure; the last sample period is post-exposure. The common SEM for these data was 2.33. See text for sampling details.

Progesterone and Puberty

Experiments 1 and 2

Mean (± SEM) ages at puberty for experiment 1 control and line lambs were 34.5 ± 0.3 and 33.7 ± 0.5 weeks, respectively. These ages were not significantly different from each other (p = 0.11). The age-at-puberty distribution pattern among animals was also similar in both the control and line groups (data not shown). Mean (± SEM) number of estrous cycles following the onset of puberty was determined only for experiment 1, with the control and line groups exhibiting 8.8 ± 0.5 and 8.9 ± 0.4 cycles, respectively (p = 0.43).

For experiment 2, the mean (± SEM) ages at puberty for the control and line groups were 34.9 ± 0.5 and 35.0 ± 0.5 weeks, respectively; they were not statistically different from each other.

Cortisol

Mean serum cortisol for day and night for experiment 1 are shown in Figures 7 and 8, respectively. Daytime cortisol levels were significantly

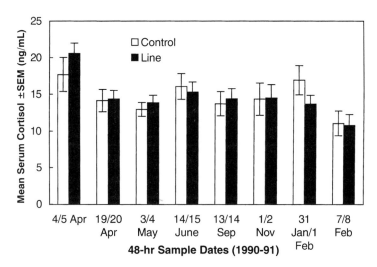

Fig. 7. Experiment 1 mean daytime cortisol in serum collected in control and line lambs during eight 48-hour sample periods. The first sample period is pre-exposure; the last sample period is post-exposure. See text for information on sampling details (Thompson et al. 1995).

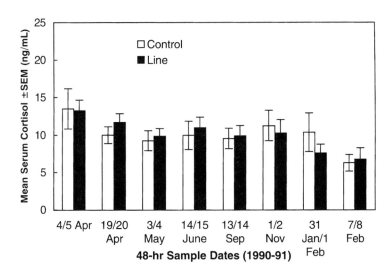

Fig. 8. Experiment 1 mean nighttime cortisol in serum collected in control and line lambs during eight 48-hour sample periods. The first sample period is pre-exposure; the last sample period is post-exposure. See text for sampling details (Thompson et al.1995).

higher than nighttime levels (p < 0.001), but there was no difference between the control and line groups in either category (p = 0.78). Mean cortisol levels for both groups were significantly higher in the pre-exposure sample than in the first exposure sample (control, p = 0.03; line, p = 0.001). This result most likely reflected the stress associated with the lambs being transported to the site, and with the recently weaned lambs being introduced into a new living environment. As a positive control, serum cortisol was measured in all sheep immediately before and after their transport from the site on February 15, 1991, at the conclusion of the EMF exposure part of the study. The sheep were transported in a stock trailer a distance of 160 km over hard-surface roads. Mean cortisol levels in both groups were more than twice as high after transport than before (p < 0.001); however, there was no difference in the levels between the two groups (p = 0.65; data not shown).

IL-1 Activity

Experiment 2

For the pilot study, IL-1 activity was measured in cell-free supernatants from LPS-stimulated leukocytes following 2, 5, and 6 months of EMF exposure (data not shown). At each of these times, IL-1 activity was less in the line group than the control group, and an ANOVA with repeated measures showed that the two groups were statistically different from each other (p = 0.01). At 2 and 3 months post-exposure, IL-1 activity was no longer different between the two groups. At the last post-exposure sample taken 5 months after exposure, IL-1 activity in the line group was significantly higher than in the control (p = 0.004).

Experiment 3

To determine whether differences in IL-1 activity existed between the two groups before the exposure period, three IL-1 assays were performed. These pre-exposure assays showed that there was no statistically significant difference between the two groups before the experiment began (p = 0.21; Fig. 9). Figures 9–13 show that the absolute amounts of IL-1 activity varied greatly from assay to assay. This variation is believed to reflect conditions existing during the induction phase of each IL-1 assay. As mentioned previously, our analyses

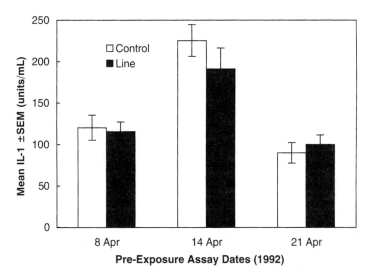

FIG. 9. Mean LPS-stimulated in vitro IL-1 activity in blood collected from control and line lambs during the 1-month pre-exposure period for experiment 3. All lambs were maintained in the control pen during pre-exposure. EMF exposure began on May 8. See text for details about sampling and assays.

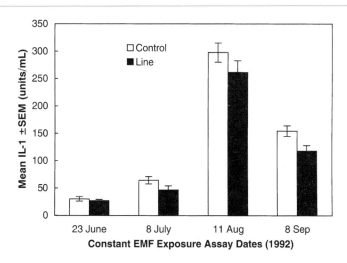

FIG. 10. Mean LPS-stimulated in vitro IL-1 activity in blood collected from control and line lambs during the first constant 4-month EMF exposure period for experiment 3. EMF exposure began on May 8. See text for additional details about sampling and assays.

focused on relative differences between groups. IL-1 activity during the first period of constant EMF exposure is shown in Figure 10. IL-1 activity was lower in the line group than the control in all four of the assays during this period; however, only in months 2 (assayed July 8) and 4 (assayed September 8) were the differences statistically significant ($p = 0.05$ and $p = 0.01$, respectively). During the 6-week intermittent exposure period, the six IL-1 assays showed no statistically significant differences between groups ($p = 0.44$; Fig. 11). The first three IL-1 assays during the second constant EMF exposure period showed no differences between the groups (Fig. 12). In the assays done after months 4 (assayed February 3) and 5 (assayed March 9) of the second constant exposure period, IL-1 activity was, again, significantly less in the line group ($p = 0.003$ and $p = 0.04$, respectively). When all nine IL-1 assays from the two constant exposure periods were analyzed by ANOVA with repeated measures, the reduction in IL-1 in the line group compared to the control was statistically significant ($p = 0.004$). The six assays done during a 13-month, post-exposure period showed no significant differences in IL-1 activity between the line and control groups ($p > 0.05$; Fig. 13).

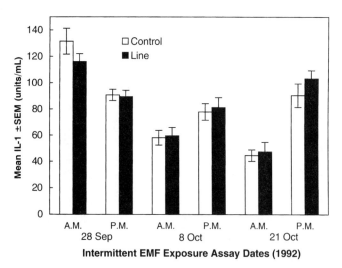

FIG. 11. Mean LPS-stimulated in vitro IL-1 activity in blood collected from control and line lambs during the 6-week intermittent EMF exposure period for experiment 3. During this period, the 500-kV transmission line crossing the line pen was turned off for maintenance during the day each weekday. The dates for the intermittent exposure period, and the EMF levels for the period are given in Table II. See text for additional details about sampling and assays.

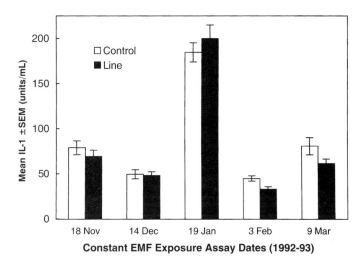

FIG. 12. Mean LPS-stimulated in vitro IL-1 activity in blood collected from control and line lambs during the second constant 5-month EMF exposure period for experiment 3. The dates for the second constant exposure period, and the EMF levels for the period are given in Table II. See text for additional details about sampling and assays.

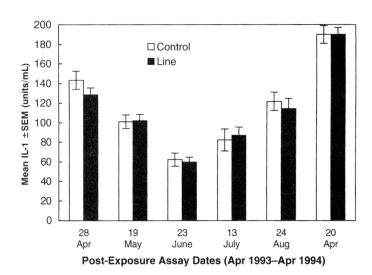

FIG. 13. Mean LPS-stimulated in vitro IL-1 activity in blood collected from control and line lambs during the 13-month, post-exposure period for experiment 3. The post-exposure period began on March 22, 1993. See text for additional details about sampling and assays.

EMF, Noise, and Light Levels

Comparative statistics for EMF and audible noise in the control and line pens for all three experiments are shown in Table 1. In general, EMF in the line pen were two orders of magnitude greater than the EMF in the control pen. The mean A-weighted audible noise in the line pen during the three experiments averaged only about 4.3% higher than in the control pen. For higher-frequency noise (> 6.5 kHz), the mean in the line pen averaged about 26% higher than in the control pen.

Table 2 summarizes 60-Hz EMF in the control and line pens during the intermittent exposure period, and during the two constant exposure periods in experiment 3. During the intermittent period, when the 500-kV line over the pen was off during the day, electric field strength was similar to the field in the control pen. During the same time, the magnetic field in the line pen averaged one order of magnitude stronger than the field in the control pen.

The Earth's total DC magnetic field in the study area was about 0.055 mT (0.019 mT horizontal, 0.051 mT vertical). The angle of inclination was about 70°, and the angle of declination was about 23°.

Typical illumination levels in the pens at night from the two, 15-watt red lamps were around 13 lux. The red lamps did not produce significant light below a wavelength of 600 nm.

Discussion

Melatonin

Circadian melatonin patterns in lambs in both experiments 1 and 2 were typical of those reported previously for lambs (Yellon and Foster 1986; Claypool et al. 1989), and for most other species studied (Reiter 1986). Daytime concentrations were very low and stable, with a very rapid increase shortly after sundown. Concentrations typically remained elevated throughout the night, although with high fluctuations, until declining rapidly around sunrise. Using artificial light shifts, Wood et al. (1989) determined that when lambs were at least 7 weeks of age, they could alter their pattern of melatonin secretion to match new light/dark cycles. Therefore, when our studies began, the

TABLE I
Comparison of 60-Hz EMF and Audible Noise During
Experiments 1, 2, and 3

Parameter	Index	Experiment 1		Experiment 2		Experiment 3	
		Line	Control	Line	Control	Line	Control
Electric field (kV/m)	Mean	5.9	< 0.01	5.3	< 0.01	5.8	< 0.01
Magnetic field (µT)	Mean	4.00	0.029	3.77	0.02	3.50	0.029
	L5[a]	6.16	0.052	5.06	0.031	5.06	0.052
Audible noise:							
dB(A)	Mean	44.7	41.5	49.3	47.1	50.2	49.6
>6.5 kHz (dB)	Mean	30.8	23.2	35.1	27.7	34.2	28.6

[a] The highest 5% of the measurements were above this level.

TABLE 2

60-Hz EMF in the Line Pen During Experiment 3

Period[a]	Electric field (kV/m)			Magnetic field (μT)		
	Mean	Median	SD	Mean	Median	SD
1	5.91	6.24	1.40	3.27	3.22	1.04
2 (all data)[b]	4.69	6.16	2.78	2.71	3.14	1.30
2 (line on)[b]	6.29	6.42	0.55	3.42	3.39	0.58
2 (line off)[b]	<0.01	<0.01		0.66	0.66	0.12
3	6.10	6.15	0.73	4.02	4.04	0.75

[a] Period 1 is the first constant EMF exposure period: May 8, 1992, to September 21, 1992; Period 2 is the intermittent exposure period: September 21 to November 4, 1992; Period 3 is the second constant EMF exposure period: November 4, 1992, to March 22, 1993.

[b] During the 6-week intermittent exposure period, the 500-kV line crossing the line pen was turned off during the day on weekdays for maintenance. The other adjacent lines in the corridor remained on during this period.

7- to 8-week-old lambs were readily capable of regulating the secretion of melatonin. We assumed that any deviations from the adult pattern of melatonin secretion in the lambs would be associated with exposure to the 500-kV line, and not to age-dependent development of the rhythm.

Melatonin amplitude at night tended to be higher during winter than during spring and summer. The winter pattern corresponds to periods of longer nights, and to increased age of the spring-born lambs. Although previously reviewed laboratory studies of rodents exposed to EMF generally reported decreases in melatonin amplitude, no such effects were found in our environmental studies of sheep.

Many investigators question the biological significance of the shape or amplitude of the nightly rise in melatonin secretion in regulating seasonal reproduction (Karsch et al. 1984), including timing of puberty in sheep (Foster et al. 1989). Our studies revealed large differences in the overall mean serum melatonin concentration among individual lambs; however, all lambs reached puberty at the expected time of year.

Duration of the nocturnal melatonin rise appears to be the critical factor in regulating reproductive cycles, because it closely reflected the length of the dark period in this and previous studies (Karsch et al. 1984). In our studies, exposure of lambs to EMF had no apparent effect on the duration of melatonin secretion.

Mean phase of the melatonin elevation tended to be advanced in both line and control groups, with no difference between groups. In another study, younger lambs were found to have phase delays in melatonin secretion at 1 and 6 weeks of age (Claypool et al. 1989), but by 27 weeks of age the lambs showed either no phase change or a slight phase advance. Exposure to EMF did not affect the phase of the melatonin secretion in lambs in our studies, as has been reported for laboratory rats (Reiter et al. 1988) and hamsters (Yellon 1994a).

Effects of EMF on melatonin amplitude and phase as reported for laboratory rodents were not observed in this environmental study of sheep either because of differences in study design, or because of differences in the mechanisms by which EMF interact with biological systems. Discussion of possible mechanisms must take into account possible interspecies differences in susceptibility to alteration of melatonin secretion by EMF. Considerable variability exists, for example, in regard to the intensity and wavelength of visible light required to suppress melatonin in various species (Reiter 1985).

Another general difference between our environmental study of sheep and studies of laboratory animals involves the type of electric and magnetic field exposures used. In our studies, lambs were exposed to the actual fields produced by three-phase transmission lines. In contrast, laboratory studies used a variety of AC or DC electric and/or magnetic fields of various intensities, none of which exactly duplicated actual power-line fields. There is some evidence that rapid field changes associated with switching fields on and off may be more significant in affecting melatonin than continuous field exposure (Lerchl et al. 1991; Rogers et al. 1995a). During our melatonin studies, very few line-switching operations occurred during the collection of 48-hour samples.

Unperturbed 60-Hz electric field strength in our study was well above the 2-kV/m level reported to affect melatonin in laboratory rats (Wilson et al. 1983). Mutual shielding of lambs by each other in our study reduced by an unknown amount the effective electric field exposure received by each animal. However, the same general effect occurs with laboratory animals in electric field studies. For example, young rats in the study by Reiter et al. (1988) presumably were significantly shielded at times while near their mother and littermates, yet their nighttime melatonin was still reduced by unperturbed 60-Hz electric fields as low as 10 kV/m.

Magnetic field strength in our study was also above the 1-μT level that was reported to affect melatonin secretion in laboratory rats (Kato et al. 1993). However, that study used 50-Hz, circularly polarized fields, whereas our study involved 60-Hz magnetic fields with elliptical polarization that was close to linear.

Because all characteristics (amplitude, duration, and phase) of the melatonin secretory patterns of lambs in this study appeared to be normal, and their body growth was normal (Thompson et al. 1995), puberty would be expected to occur at the usual age in the autumn. Indeed, progesterone concentrations indicative of corpus luteum activity after ovulation indicated that all lambs in both experiments reached puberty at the expected time of year.

Cortisol

As measured by serum cortisol, our study, overall, provided no indication that lambs experienced stress from chronic exposure to the environment of a high-voltage transmission line. The vehicle transport test conducted at the conclusion of EMF exposure in experiment 1 verified that the cortisol assay used in our study could detect effects of known stressors on sheep. In our study, the sheep were purposely placed on a grounded metal floor to minimize the potential for shocks from induced voltages. Different results might be expected if animals were frequently receiving shocks in an ungrounded facility. Possible stress effects reported in some studies of laboratory animals may have been related to shocks, or to perception effects from strong electric fields used in some studies.

The sheep in our study may have been responding to the metal slatted pen floor. In both line and control groups, cortisol levels were lowest in the post-exposure sample, when all the animals were taken out of the pens and placed on ground covered with sawdust.

IL-1 Activity

Results of our studies support the tentative conclusion that exposure of lambs to the environment beneath a 500-kV transmission line results in a reduction in the LPS-stimulated activity of leukocyte IL-1 by about 25%. This conclusion is strengthened by the fact that the depression in IL-1 activity closely matched the exposure periods; i.e., the only statistically significant depressions in the line group compared to the control occurred during constant EMF exposure periods. Also, the lack of a depression in the line group during the intermittent and post-exposure periods suggests that the effect on IL-1 activity is not permanent.

It is not possible to determine from our data whether the effect on IL-1 activity is caused by the electric field, the magnetic field, the two fields combined, or to audible noise produced by corona on the transmission-line conductors. A fourth experiment, begun in the spring of 1995, is designed to provide data to help answer this question.

We also do not know the mechanism(s) by which EMF might affect IL-1 activity. IL-1 is produced primarily by monocytes and macrophages, although other cells can also produce IL-1 after in vitro stimulation with LPS. The mechanism for the effect on IL-1 production could be at the cell level; i.e., less IL-1 produced per cell by all cells capable of IL-1 production. Alternatively, only the production of IL-1 in certain types of cells may be affected by EMF exposure. The decrease in IL-1 production could also be due to increased production of IL-1 inhibitors, which are molecules that are able to block the biological activity of IL-1.

Although we saw no effects of EMF on serum melatonin concentrations or on patterns of secretion in our studies, one could speculate that this hormone could be involved in the process leading to the observed effect on IL-1 activity. Human monocytes are activated by melatonin, including the secretion of IL-1 (Morrey et al. 1994), and a binding site for melatonin on T-helper-type 2 lymphocytes from human bone marrow has recently been described (Maestroni 1995). Activation of the receptor by melatonin resulted in enhanced production of the cytokine IL-4. Melatonin's natural oncostatic activity on human breast cancer cells was blocked at the cellular level by a 1.2-μT, 60-Hz magnetic field (Liburdy et al. 1993). Together, these studies suggest that exposure to EMF could affect the biological activity of melatonin, resulting in changes in production of cytokines, without measurably affecting the concentration of circulating melatonin. The biological importance, if any, of the reduction in IL-1 activity found in our studies needs to be examined. Over the course of the several months that sheep were exposed to EMF during the three experiments, there were no serious outbreaks of disease or infections in the animals. During experiment 2, there was an outbreak of a fungal infection that affected most of the line sheep, but none of the controls (Stormshak 1993; Ogden et al. 1993). The possible role of exposure to EMF in the development of the infection could not be determined.

ACKNOWLEDGMENTS

We are grateful to the following organizations for support of our studies: American Electric Power Service Corporation, Bonneville Power Administration, Houston Lighting and Power Company, Hydro-Quebec, Salt River Project, and Western Area Power Administration. David Hess was also supported by grants from the National Institutes of Health (HD18185, RR00163). We also want to acknowledge the assistance of many other people from several organizations who provided significant contributions to the studies of sheep and EMF described in this chapter. From Bonneville Power Administration: Phillip Havens, Vernon Chartier, Larry Dickson, Richard Stearns, and Gary Ihle. From Oregon State University: Beth Olenchek, Lucy Painter, Kenneth Rowe, Pamela Thinesen, and Diana Whitmore. From the Portland Veteran's Administration Medical Center: Alison Freed and Sharon McCoy. From Oregon Health Sciences University: Arthur Hall and Bryan Ogden. From Portland State University: Marc Carey, Richard Forbes, and Suzanne Krippaehne. Project science advisors: J. Richard Alldredge, Washington State University; Douglas Foster, University of Michigan; Russel Reiter, University of Texas; and Ellen Goldberg, University of New Mexico. The science advisors were sponsored by the Electric Power Research Institute. Additional quality-control support was provided by William Wisecup, Richard Phillips, and Fred Dietrich, all of whom were sponsored by Imre Gyuk, U.S. Department of Energy. Overall technical coordination for the project was provided by T. Dan Bracken, Inc. Portions of this chapter were previously published in *Biology of Reproduction* (Lee et al. 1993), *Bioelectromagnetics* (Lee et al. 1995), and in the *Journal of Animal Science* (Thompson et al. 1995).

REFERENCES

Asanova, T.P., A.I. Rakov. 1966. The state of health of persons working in electric field of outdoor 400-kV and 500-kV switchyards. *Hygiene of Labor and Professional Diseases* 5.

Chiabrera, A., R. Cadossi, F. Bersani, B. Bianco. 1994. Electric and magnetic field effects on the immune system. In: *Biological Effects of Electric and Magnetic Fields*, Volume 2, D.O. Carpenter, S. Ayrapetyan, eds., pp. 121–145. New York: Academic Press.

Claypool, L.E., R.I. Wood, S.M. Yellon, D.L. Foster. 1989. The ontogeny of melatonin secretion in the lamb. *Endocrinology* 124:2135–2143.

De Bruyn, L., L. De Jager. 1994. Electric field exposure and evidence of stress in mice. *Environ. Res.* 65:149–160.

English, J., A.L. Poulton, J. Arendt, A.M. Symons. 1986. A comparison of the efficiency of melatonin treatments in advancing oestrus in ewes. *J. Reprod. Fertil.* 77:321-327.

Foster, D.L. 1994. Puberty in the sheep. In: *The Physiology of Reproduction*, Second Edition, E. Knobil, J.D. Neill, eds., pp. 411–451. New York: Raven Press, Ltd.

Foster, D.L., F.J.P. Ebling, L.E. Claypool, C.J.I. Woodfill. 1988. Cessation of long day melatonin rhythms time puberty in a short day breeder. *Endocrinology* 123:1636–1641.

Foster, D.L., F.J.P. Ebling, L.E. Claypool, R.I. Wood. 1989. Photoperiodic timing of puberty in sheep. In: *Research in Perinatal Medicine (IX) Development of Circadian Rhythmicity and Photoperiodism in Mammals*, S.M. Reppert, ed., pp. 103–153. Ithaca, New York: Perinatology Press.

Free, M.J., W.T. Kaune, R.D. Phillips, H.C. Cheng. 1981. Endocrinological effects of strong 60-Hz electric fields on rats. *Bioelectromagnetics* 2:105–122.

Grota, L.J., R.J. Reiter, P. Keng, S. Michaelson. 1994. Electric field exposure alters serum melatonin but not pineal melatonin in male rats. *Bioelectromagnetics* 15:427–437.

Hackman, R.M., H.B. Graves. 1981. Corticosterone levels in mice exposed to high intensity electric fields. *Behav. Neural Biolog.* 32:201–213.

Hefeneider, S. (Principal Investigator). 1994. *Joint HVAC Transmission EMF Environmental Study Final Report on Experiment 3*. Portland, Oregon: Bonneville Power Administration.

Hefeneider, S.H., K.A. Cornell, L.E. Brown, A.C. Bakke, S.L. McCoy, R.M. Bennett. 1992. Nucleosomes and DNA bind to specific cell-surface molecules on murine cells and induce cytokine production. *Clin. Immunol. Immunopathol.* 63:245–251.

Hess, D.L., H.G. Spies, A.G. Hendrickx.1981. Diurnal steroid patterns during gestation in the rhesus macaque: Onset, daily variation, and the effects of dexamethasone treatment. *Biol. Reprod.* 24:609–616.

Johnson, D., D. Thomas, J. Leffel. 1988. *Sheep Barn Planning Extension Circular*. Corvallis, Oregon: Oregon State University.

Karsch, F.J., E.L. Bittman, D.L. Foster, R.L. Goodman, S.J. Legan, J.E. Robinson. 1984. Neuroendocrine basis of seasonal reproduction. *Recent Prog. Horm. Res.* 40:185–232.

Kato, M., K. Honma, T. Shigemitsu, Y. Shiga. 1993. Effects of exposure to a circularly polarized 50-Hz magnetic field on plasma and pineal melatonin in rats. *Bioelectromagnetics* 14:97–106.

Kato, M., K. Honma, T. Shigemitsu, Y. Shiga. 1994. Horizontal or vertical 50-Hz, 1-μT magnetic fields have no effect on pineal gland or plasma melatonin concentration of albino rats. *Neurosci. Lett.* 168:205–208.

Kaune, W.T., R.D. Phillips. 1980. Comparison of the coupling of grounded humans, swine and rats to vertical, 60-Hz electric fields. *Bioelectromagnetics* 1:117–129.

Kennaway, D.J., T.A. Gilmore, E.A. Dunstan. 1985. Pinealectomy delays puberty in ewe lambs. *J. Reprod. Fert.* 74:119–125.

Lee, J.M. Jr., F. Stormshak, J.M. Thompson, P. Thinesen, L.J. Painter, E.G. Olenchek, D.L. Hess, R. Forbes, D.L. Foster. 1993. Melatonin secretion and puberty in female lambs exposed to environmental electric and magnetic fields. *Biol. Reprod.* 49:857–864.

Lee, J.M. Jr., F. Stormshak, J.M. Thompson, D.L. Hess, D. L. Foster. 1995. Melatonin in female lambs exposed to EMF: A replicate study. *Bioelectromagnetics* 16:119–123.

Lerchl, A., K.O. Nonaka, R.J. Reiter. 1991. Pineal gland "magnetosensitivity" to static magnetic fields is a consequence of induced electric currents (eddy currents). *J. Pineal. Res.* 10:109–116.

Leung, F.C., D.N. Rommereim, R.A. Miller, L.E. Anderson. 1990. Brown-colored deposits on hair of female rats chronically exposed to 60-Hz electric fields. *Bioelectromagnetics* 11:257–259.

Liburdy, R.P., T.R. Sloma, R. Sokolic, P. Yaswen. 1993. ELF magnetic fields, breast cancer, and melatonin: 60 Hz fields block melatonin's oncostatic action on ER^+ breast cancer cell proliferation. *J. Pineal. Res.* 14:89–97.

Löscher, W., U. Wahnschaffe, M. Mevissen, A. Lerchl, A. Stamm. 1994. Effects of weak alternating magnetic fields on nocturnal melatonin production and mammary carcinogenesis in rats. *Oncology* 51:288–295.

Lyle, D.B., A.R. Ayotte, A.R. Sheppard, W.R. Adey. 1988. Suppression of T-lymphocyte cytotoxicity following exposure to 60-Hz sinusoidal electric fields. *Bioelectromagnetics* 9:303–313.

Maestroni, G.J.M. 1995. T-helper-2 lymphocytes as a peripheral target of melatonin. *J. Pineal Res.* 18:84–89.

Maestroni, G.J.M., A. Conti, W. Pierpaoli. 1986. Role of the pineal gland in immunity. *J. Neuroimmunol.* 13:19–30.

Malpaux, B., J.E. Robinson, M.B. Brown, F.J. Karsch. 1987. Reproductive refractoriness of the ewe to inductive photoperiod is not caused by inappropriate secretion of melatonin. *Biol. Reprod.* 36:1333–1341.

Marino, A.A., R.O. Becker, B. Ullrich. 1976. The effect of continuous exposure to low-frequency electric fields on three generations of mice. *Separatum Experientia* 32:565–566.

McCormick, D.L., M.A. Cahill, J.B. Harder, B.M. Ryan, J.C. Findlay, L.E. Pomerantz, R.R. Szymanski, G.A. Boorman. 1994. Pineal function assessment in F344 rats and B6C3F1 mice exposed to 60-Hz magnetic fields. In: Abstracts of the 16th Annual Bioelectromagnetics Society Meeting, Copenhagen, Denmark, June 12–17, p. 50. Frederick, Maryland: The Bioelectromagnetics Society.

Mehta, S., D. Blackinton, M. Lefebvre, D. Cherlin, H. Wanebo, C. Polk. 1992. Low frequency magnetic field effects on normal and neoplastic human lymphocytes. In: Abstracts of the Annual Review of Research on Biological Effects of Electric and Magnetic Fields From the Generation, Delivery, and Use of Electricity, San Diego, California, November 8–12, p. A-20. Frederick, Maryland: W/L Associates, Ltd.

Mehta, S., O. Chan, D. Blackinton, J. Pennucci, D. Cherlin, C. Polk. 1994. Low frequency magnetic field effects on cytokine production and human B-cell response. In: Abstracts of the 16th Annual Bioelectromagnetics Society Meeting, Copenhagen, Denmark, June 12–17, p. 135. Frederick, Maryland: The Bioelectromagnetics Society.

Morandi, M.A., J. Del Rio, R.P. Caren, L.D. Caren. 1994. Effects of short term exposure to 60-Hz electromagnetic fields on interleukin 1 and interleukin 6 production by peritoneal exudate cells. *Life Sci.* 54:731–738.

Morrey, K.M., J.A. McLachlan, C.D. Serkin, O. Bakouche. 1994. Activation of human monocytes by the pineal hormone melatonin. *J. Immunol.* 153:2671–2680.

Morris, J.E., M.E. Frazier, B.J. McClanahan, R.L. Buschbom, L.E. Anderson. 1988. Effects of 60-Hz electric fields on immune response in rats. In: Abstracts of the Annual Review of Research on Biological Effects from Electric and Magnetic Fields: Air Ions and Ion Currents Associated with High Voltage Transmission Lines, Phoenix, Arizona, October 30–November 3. Frederick, Maryland: W/L Associates, Ltd.

Morris, J.E., L.B. Sasser, R.L. Buschbom, L.E. Anderson. 1990. Natural immunity in rats exposed to 60-Hz magnetic fields. In: Abstracts of the Annual Review of Research on Biological Effects from Electric and Magnetic Fields, Denver, Colorado, November 5–8, A-23. Frederick, Maryland: W/L Associates, Ltd.

Murthy, K.K., W.R. Rogers, H.D. Smith, S. Singh. 1991. Studies on the effect of combined 60-Hz electric and magnetic field exposure on the immune system of nonhuman primates. In: Abstracts of the Annual Review of Research on Biological Effects from Electric and Magnetic Fields, Milwaukee, Wisconsin, November 3-7, A-17. Frederick, Maryland: W/L Associates, Ltd.

National Research Council. 1985. *Nutrient Requirements of Sheep*, 6th Edition. Washington, DC: National Academy Press.

Ogden, B.E., A.S. Hall, A.A. Padhye. 1993. Scopulariopsis brevicaulis dermatomycosis in electric and magnetic field-exposed sheep (abstract). *Contemp. Top. Lab. Anim. Sci.* 32:15.

Quinlan, W.J., D. Petrondas, N. Lebda, S. Pettit, S.M. Michaelson. 1985. Neuroendocrine parameters in the rat exposed to 60-Hz electric fields. *Bioelectromagnetics* 6:381–389.

Reiter, R.J. 1985. Action spectra, dose-response relationships, and temporal aspects of light's effects on the pineal gland. *Ann. N.Y. Acad. Sci.* 453:215–230.

Reiter, R.J. 1986. Normal patterns of melatonin levels in the pineal gland and body fluids of humans and experimental animals. *J. Neural. Trans.* 21(suppl):35–54.

Reiter, R.J. 1990. Effect of light and stress on pineal function, In: *Extremely Low Frequency Electromagnetic Fields: The Question of Cancer,*

B.W. Wilson, R.G. Stevens, L.E. Anderson, eds., pp. 87–107. Columbus, Ohio: Battelle Press.

Reiter, R.J., L.E. Anderson, R.L. Buschbom, B.W. Wilson. 1988. Reduction of the nocturnal rise in pineal melatonin levels in rats exposed to 60-Hz electric fields in utero and for 23 days after birth. *Life Sci.* 42:2203–2206.

Rogers, W.R., R.J. Reiter, H.D. Smith, L. Barlow-Walden. 1995a. Rapid onset/offset, variably scheduled 60-Hz electric and magnetic field exposure reduces nocturnal serum melatonin concentration in non-human primates. *Bioelectromagnetics* Suppl. 3:119–122.

Rogers, W.R., R.J. Reiter, L. Barlow-Walden, H.D. Smith, J.L. Orr. 1995b. Regularly scheduled, day-time, slow-onset 60-Hz electric and magnetic field exposure does not depress serum melatonin concentration in nonhuman primates. *Bioelectromagnetics* Suppl. 3:111–118.

Stormshak, F. (Principal Investigator). 1993. *Joint HVAC Transmission EMF Environmental Study Final Report on Experiment 2.* Portland, Oregon: Bonneville Power Administration.

Thompson, J.M., F. Stormshak, J.M. Lee, Jr., D.L. Hess, L. Painter. 1995. Cortisol secretion and growth in ewe lambs chronically exposed to electric and magnetic fields of a 60-Hertz 500-kilovolt transmission line. *J. Anim. Sci.* 73:3274–3280.

Walleczek, J. 1991. Electromagnetic field effects on cells of the immune system: The role of calcium signaling. *FASEB J.* 6:3177–3185.

Wilson, B.W., L.E. Anderson. 1990. ELF electromagnetic field effects on the pineal gland. In: *Extremely Low Frequency Electromagnetic Fields: The Question of Cancer*, B.W. Wilson, R.G. Stevens, L.E. Anderson, eds., pp. 159-186. Columbus, Ohio: Battelle Press.

Wilson, B.W., L.E. Anderson, D.I. Hilton, R.D. Phillips. 1981. Chronic exposure to 60-Hz electric fields: Effects on pineal function in the rat. *Bioelectromagnetics* 2:371–380.

Wilson, B.W., L.E. Anderson, D.J. Hilton, R.D. Phillips. 1983. Chronic exposure to 60-Hz electric fields: Effects on pineal function in the rat (erratum). *Bioelectromagnetics* 4:293.

Wood, R.I., L.E. Claypool, F.J.P. Ebling, D.L. Foster. 1989. Entrainment of the melatonin rhythms in early postnatal lambs and their mothers. *J. Biol. Rhyth.* 4:457–465.

Yellon, S.M. 1994a. Acute 60 Hz magnetic field exposure effects on the melatonin rhythm in the pineal gland and circulation of the adult Djungarian hamster. *J. Pineal Res.* 16:136–144.

Yellon, S.M. 1994b. Studies of acute and daily 60 Hz magnetic field exposures on the nighttime melatonin rhythm in adult Djungarian hamsters in short days. In: The Annual Review of Research on Biological Effects of Electric and Magnetic Fields From the Generation, Delivery & Use of Electricity, pp. 41–42. Albuquerque, New Mexico, November 6–10, 1994. Frederick, Maryland: W/L Associates, Ltd.

Yellon, S.M., D.L. Foster. 1986. Melatonin rhythms time photoperiod induced puberty in the female lamb. *Endocrinology* 119:44–49.

16 Effects of Exposure to 60-Hz EMF on Melatonin in Nonhuman Primates Might Depend on Specific Aspects of Field Exposure

WALTER R. ROGERS
Department of Biosciences and Bioengineering,
Southwest Research Institute, San Antonio, Texas
RUSSEL J. REITER
Department of Cellular and Structural Biology,
University of Texas Health Science Center,
San Antonio, Texas
JOHN L. ORR
Department of Biosciences and Bioengineering,
Southwest Research Institute, San Antonio, Texas

CONTENTS

INTRODUCTION
Field-Induced Melatonin Suppression in Rodents
Field-Induced Melatonin Suppression in Other Mammals
Nonhuman Primates as Models in Biomedical Research
Southwest Research Institute Primate Melatonin Experiments
Experimental Approach
METHODS OF EXPERIMENTS III, IIIA, AND IV
Experiment III

(continued)

Contents (continued)

Experiment IIIA
Experiment IV
Assay Performance
Data Review
RESULTS OF EXPERIMENTS III, IIIA, AND IV
Experiment III
Experiment IIIA
Experiment IV
Discussion
PROBE EXPERIMENT
Methods
Results
Discussion
DISCUSSION
Different Conditions and Different Outcomes
Suggestions for Additional Research
Nonhuman Primate Models for Other Problems in
      Bioelectromagnetics
CONCLUSIONS
ACKNOWLEDGMENTS
REFERENCES

INTRODUCTION

Field-Induced Melatonin Suppression in Rodents

Several reports indicate that subchronic exposure to power-frequency (50/60-Hz) electric or magnetic fields reduces nocturnal melatonin concentrations in pineal gland and blood of rodents. Wilson et al. (1981, 1983, 1986, 1989) and Wilson and Anderson (1990) described the melatonin-suppressing effects of 60-Hz electric fields. In these cases, maximum exposure duration was 4 weeks, with statistically significant differences occurring by the third week. One week after cessation of exposure, nocturnal melatonin was normal. Reiter et al. (1988)

described reductions in serum and pineal melatonin contents of rats exposed in utero and up to 23 days of age. Increasing electric field strength, tested at 10, 65, and 130 kV/m, appeared to produce a greater reduction and greater delay in the time of occurrence of peak nocturnal melatonin concentration.

Kato et al. (1993) reported that 6 weeks of exposure to circularly polarized, 50-Hz magnetic fields of 1.4 μT or greater suppressed melatonin in albino rats. Recovery of normal melatonin concentrations occurred within a week after cessation of exposure (Kato et al. 1994d). The depression effect also was observed in pigmented rats, at magnetic field intensities (0.02 μT) 70 times less those required in unpigmented rats (Kato et al. 1994a). Magnetic field orientation appears to be quite important: Horizontal or vertical 50-Hz magnetic fields of 1 mT had no effect on melatonin (Kato et al. 1994c), and exposure to a 4:1 ellipsoidal magnetic field also was without effect (Kato et al. 1994b). While completing this sequence of 18 experiments over a 4-year period, Kato et al. (Chapter 13, this volume) replicated their key finding of melatonin suppression at 1.4 μT with circularly polarized magnetic fields in each of the five experiments that examined this condition. In effect, 1.4 μT with circularly polarized magnetic fields served as a positive control condition while conducting their other experiments, some of which were negative when other exposure conditions were examined.

Yellon (1994) observed that, in two of three experiments, Djungarian hamsters receiving 15 minutes of exposure to a vertical, 60-Hz, 100-μT magnetic field late during the day showed an attenuated nocturnal increase in melatonin that night. Selmaoui and Touitou (1995) examined effects of exposure to 50-Hz magnetic fields of either 1, 10, or 100 μT for either 1 day (12 hours) or 30 days (18 hours per day). With chronic exposure, magnetic fields of either 10 or 100 μT produced reduced serum melatonin; with acute exposure, 100 μT was required to produce suppression. Löscher et al. (1994) found that exposure of rats to 50-Hz magnetic fields at a gradient of 0.3 to 1.0 μT produced depression of nocturnal melatonin in serum.

Field-Induced Melatonin Suppression in Other Mammals

The relevance of the rodent results to the human is not known. At the time of our experiments, little direct evidence had been presented to indicate that 60-Hz electric or magnetic field exposure reduces blood melatonin concentration in humans or other primates. Wilson et al. (1990) reported that 25% of the human subjects using electric blankets showed alterations in urinary excretion of melatonin. Graham et al. subsequently presented evidence from two experiments with humans exposed to circularly polarized magnetic fields of 1 or 20 μT: the first experiment (Graham et al.1996) indicated that some subjects, those with relatively low blood melatonin concentrations, showed melatonin suppression, but the second experiment (Graham et al. in press) did not indicate melatonin suppression. Schiffman et al. (1994) reported that humans exposed to magnetic resonance imaging at 1.5 T during the night had normal nocturnal plasma melatonin concentrations. Reiter (1993a, 1994) has reviewed the literature on effects of extremely low frequency (ELF) electric and magnetic fields (EMF) on melatonin production and secretion.

Nonhuman Primates as Models in Biomedical Research

Although rats have been used extensively and effectively in biomedical research, atherosclerosis, human immunodeficiency virus, and thalidomide are three examples which demonstrate that, for some processes, rodents cannot be used to model the human primate. Because it is not known if the effects of power-frequency EMF on melatonin are the same or different in rodents and primates, we thought it was important to conduct some experiments in nonhuman primates. Additionally, with respect to body-size scaling and the dosimetry of subject–field interactions, the relatively large size of the baboon makes it much more human-like than the rat. The large size also facilitates use of an indwelling cannula and allows collection of numerous, relatively large volume samples from the same subject, providing a within-subject assessment of longitudinal trends. To date, all rodent studies of electric or magnetic field effects on melatonin have involved killing the subject, meaning only one blood value is obtained from each subject.

There are well-recognized differences between the relative insensitivity of the pineal gland of the human to melatonin inhibition by light during the night, and the relative sensitivity of nocturnal rodents to the same phenomenon (Reiter 1985, 1991). (There also are large differences among various rodent species in melatonin sensitivity to light.) For example, Nozaki et al. (1990) show that the effects of light on melatonin in the monkey (*Macaca fuscata fuscata*) are much more like those in the human than are those of the rat. Although it is not known if visible light and energy at other portions of the electromagnetic spectrum act by the same or dissimilar mechanisms, such interspecies differences in pineal response to light raise the possibility that the nocturnally active laboratory rat might not be the most relevant model for studying the effects of power-frequency electric and/or magnetic fields on the pineal of the diurnally active (and electrically generated, artificial-illumination-using) human. For studies of electric and/or magnetic field effects on melatonin, a nonhuman primate might be a more appropriate surrogate for the human than is the rat. Additionally, a small set of primates can provide answers not obtainable from either humans or rodents. With human subjects, the environment (e.g., nocturnal light exposure) and behavior (e.g., drug usage) cannot be controlled fully, as they can be with nonhuman primates. Although large numbers of rats often are used, within-subject sampling can be used with primates to compensate for the relatively small numbers of subjects used.

Southwest Research Institute Primate Melatonin Experiments

The objective of our melatonin experiments at the Southwest Research Institute was to determine if daytime exposure to a 60-Hz EMF produced a 50% decrease in the nocturnal serum melatonin concentrations of nonhuman primates. This specification, which provides a benchmark for experimental design, is based on the assumption that an effect of this size would be considered robust.

Using an indwelling venous cannula to obtain multiple blood samples from tethered subjects, we completed a set of four experiments. The indwelling cannula approach allowed automatic sampling, without human presence, of all subjects simultaneously, at any time of day or night, without altering the exposure schedule to preclude human EMF exposure. The cannula and automatic blood sampling system used in these experiments was designed for use in EMF experiments conducted in an environmentally controlled Primate Electromagnetic Exposure Facility (PEEF). The PEEF included separate field- and sham-exposure areas, each capable of housing subjects in melatonin, operant-behavior, and social-behavior experiments (Fig. 1).

Combined electric and magnetic field exposure was used because it models the situation associated with a high-voltage power-transmission line. The EMF exposure was given only during the "lights-on" period. The exposure schedule for a series of behavioral experiments had been selected to simulate occupational daytime exposure. Because these melatonin experiments were conducted concurrently with some of these behavioral experiments, it was necessary to use the "daytime" exposure schedule in the melatonin experiments as well. The operant-behavior (Orr et al. 1995b) and social-behavior (Coelho et al. 1995) experiments were conducted using separate subjects housed in the same facility; the tethered subjects did not participate in the behavioral experiments.

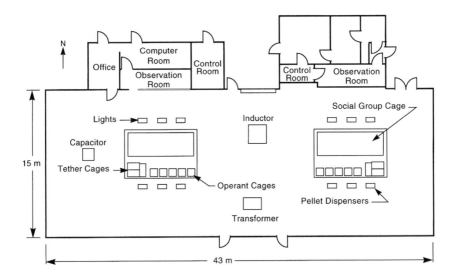

FIG. 1. Floor plan of the Primate Electromagnetic Exposure Facility, showing two equivalent areas housing operant, social, and tethered subjects. For the experiments reported here, the portion of the facility seen on the right in the figure served as the field-exposure area. (Reprinted from Rogers et al. 1995a by permission of John Wiley & Sons, Inc.)

Experimental Approach

Here we summarize two sets of experiments. The first involved a series of three "large" experiments including a common exposure protocol, use of simultaneous sham- and EMF-exposed groups, and extraordinary use of quality-control procedures with the melatonin assay. The second study was a single, small, "probe" experiment conducted without an independent control group and using only the quality-control procedures normally employed in a well-recognized laboratory specializing in melatonin. From a hazard/safety, decision-boundary perspective (Orr 1994), the former experiments individually and collectively count more heavily; i.e., they provide more information per experimental conclusion than does the latter effort. In the small experiment, which deliberately examined a set of exposure conditions quite different from those used in the large effort, all parameters were set at conditions which were assumed to be most likely to maximize occurrence of a melatonin-depression effect. Although the small experiment was completed first, the results of the series of the large experiments are presented first because they consistently support a clear conclusion.

The series of three experiments (Rogers et al. 1995d) was completed using a standardized exposure protocol emphasizing regularly scheduled, daytime exposure produced without the presence of transients. These experiments were referred to as Experiments III, IIIA, and IV; for the exposure conditions tested, these experiments detected no sign of an EMF-induced suppression of serum melatonin concentration in nonhuman primates.

The Probe Experiment (Rogers et al. 1995c) was conducted to examine a set of EMF exposure conditions different from those used in the series of three experiments. This experiment used an irregular, intermittent exposure schedule; electric field transients were present at field onset and offset; and exposure occurred during both daytime and nighttime. All of these conditions more closely simulate real-life exposure than do the artificial, well-regulated laboratory conditions used in Experiments III, IIIA, and IV. Although by no means definitive, this limited experiment showed a strong melatonin-suppressive effect, suggesting several possibilities of potential importance that require further research if they are to be fully understood.

It is important to note that the exposure protocol used in the Probe Experiment was different from that used consistently in the series of three experiments. Thus, the divergent results should be regarded as instructive, not inconsistent.

METHODS OF EXPERIMENTS III, IIA, AND IV

Experiment III

Subjects and Experimental Design
Six male baboons (*Papio cynocephalus*) with ages of 7–8 years and weights of 25–28 kg were used. The baboons were randomly assigned as three field-exposed ("exposed") and three sham-exposed ("control") subjects. This design allowed use of a within–between data-analysis approach. Each subject was implanted with a chronically indwelling venous cannula. The set of six automatic blood samplers was used to achieve simultaneous, undisturbed blood sampling from the subjects at regular intervals throughout the day and night, including during EMF exposure. Experiment III included 3-week pre-exposure and post-exposure periods; the exposure period was 6 weeks in duration.

Field Generation
Two transformers presented 60-Hz EMF concurrently (Rogers et al. 1995a). Homogeneous, vertical electric fields were generated between an overhead bus suspended 2.5 m above a large, grounded, nonferrous metal grate. Homogeneous, horizontal magnetic fields were generated by a series of conductors beneath the grate. EMF strength readings from multiple sensors in both exposure and control areas were logged at 15-minute intervals. The EMF within the fiber-glass cages were mapped before and after the experiment and were checked every 3 weeks during the experiment. In the control area, the stray magnetic fields from the exposure area averaged < one-fiftieth of the magnetic fields generated in the exposure area.

EMF Exposure
To avoid transients, the fields were turned on and off "slowly" by computer; it took 4 seconds for EMF strengths to linearly rise to, or fall from, the target values of 6 kV/m and 50 μT. Examination of the EMF

with a spectrum analyzer indicated there were no onset or offset transients in the EMF. The PEEF operated 7 days per week, providing 12 hours of EMF exposure in three 4-hour blocks (0830–1230 hours, 1300–1700 hours, and 1730–2130 hours). All EMF exposure occurred during the light phase of the photoperiod (light:dark = 15.5:8.5, with light onset at 0700 hours). The exposure schedule was regular, with field onsets and offsets occurring consistently at the same times every day for 3-week periods. A 2-day period without EMF exposure, to allow field mapping and facility maintenance, occurred every 3 weeks.

Sample Collection

A chronically indwelling venous cannula system designed for use in EMF experiments was used to automatically collect blood samples without the confounding effects of anesthesia or the stress of handling (Rogers et al. 1995b). Following 3 weeks of recovery from surgery, three "blood-sampling periods" were completed on all subjects at 1-week intervals during the 3-week, pre-exposure period. A blood-sampling period consisted of collection of 12 blood samples taken at 2-hour intervals, beginning at 0800 hours. Subjects then were sampled in the second, fourth, and sixth weeks of exposure. Blood-sampling periods also were completed in the first and third weeks of post-exposure. Each time a subject was sampled, two separately labeled, alphanumerically coded tubes of serum were produced and frozen for subsequent assay.

Overall, the sampler system was effective. For example, in Experiment III, 99.2% of the scheduled samples were acquired. If the automatic sampler did not obtain a blood sample, it automatically tried again 15 minutes later. In Experiment IV, 100% of the samples were acquired, 97.4% of them on the first attempt (Rogers et al. 1995b).

Melatonin Assay

Samples were delivered as separate batches, based on sequential blood-sampling periods, for "blind" analysis by a radioimmunoassay (RIA) laboratory. For each blood-sampling period, half the samples from a subject were in one batch, and the remainder were in a separate batch to provide back-up redundancy. Two log-logit standard curves were done in duplicate for each batch. Six blank (buffer) and six nonspecific binding (NSB) tubes were used, three per standard curve. One standard curve was constructed from samples placed at the beginning of the run, and the other was constructed from tubes counted at the end of the run. The 10-point standard curves included melatonin contents between 1.95 and 250 pg per tube.

Serum melatonin concentrations of pairs of independently coded tubes were measured in duplicate by RIA using the Guildhay antibody (Lerchl et al. 1990). Samples were analyzed in nine sequential batches. When analyzing each batch, eight samples from each of three reference serum pools, in the physiologically low, medium, and high range of melatonin concentrations for baboons, also were analyzed in duplicate. These multiple-pool samples within each batch provided data for assessment of both intra- and interassay variability for the assays completed during the experiments. Unless noted, all assay methods and practices in Experiments III, IIIA, and IV were identical.

Experiment IIIA

At the end of the post-exposure period of Experiment III, the same animals were used for Experiment IIIA, without changing exposed or control groups; the animals exposed in Experiment IIIA had also been exposed in Experiment III, but 8 weeks had elapsed between exposure periods. (The design of Experiment III had included a 6-week post-exposure period with melatonin sampling done only during the first 3 weeks of the post-exposure period). In Experiment IIIA, the subjects were sampled weekly during a new 2-week pre-exposure period followed immediately by a 3-week exposure period. Experiment IIIA used 30 kV/m and 100 μT. At 30 kV/m, it took 20 seconds for the EMF to be ramped slowly on or off at a linear rate. There were no transients, harmonics, or other irregularities associated with the EMF.

Experiment IV

A second set of six subjects, similar in age and weight to those used in Experiment III, was used in an independent experiment involving 30 kV/m and 100 μT. The exposure conditions and experimental design of Experiment IV were just like those of Experiment III, except that melatonin data were available from only the first week of post-exposure of Experiment IV.

Because the essential aspect of the experiment was within-subject comparison of melatonin scores of exposed subjects across periods, the batches in Experiment IV were formed by subject, rather than by blood-sampling period, to minimize any effects of interbatch variation on the scores. Half of the independently coded samples from a subject across pre-exposure, exposure, and post-exposure periods was analyzed in one batch, and the remaining samples from the subject were analyzed in a second batch. Assignment of sets of samples to batches was random, with the proscription that the first half of the set of batches include one tube from each sampling of all six subjects.

For each of the 12 batches of samples, the melatonin assay laboratory completed six standard curves, two each at the beginning, middle, and end of the set of samples in the scintillation counter; these curves were averaged to establish the standard curve for the assay. Nine buffer and nine NSB tubes were counted for each standard curve, and 12 samples were tested from each of the low, medium, and high serum pools.

Assay Performance

The RIA for melatonin performed as expected based on published data from RIAs of melatonin. For example, the standard curves for the nine batches of Experiment III were similar visually (Fig. 2). The intra-assay coefficient of variation for the three serum pools averaged 9.3%, and the interassay coefficient of variation averaged 13.0%. The least-squares linear regression terms "m" and "b" in the equation $Y = mX + b$ for the nine standard curves had coefficients of variation of 5.6% and 8.9%, respectively (Table 1). The square of the Pearson product moment correlation coefficient (r) gives the percentage of the variance accounted for by the linear regression. Substituting values of 32 or 16 pg/mL into the standard curves produced mean computed values of 33 and 16 pg/mL, with coefficients of variation of 8.5% and 10.0%, respectively.

Regression analyses showed good agreement among replicate tubes. For example, for Experiment IIIA, the mean r for the correlation between tubes was 0.972 (mean df = 111), and the coefficient of variation among the six subjects' r values was 1.8% (Table 2). The accuracy

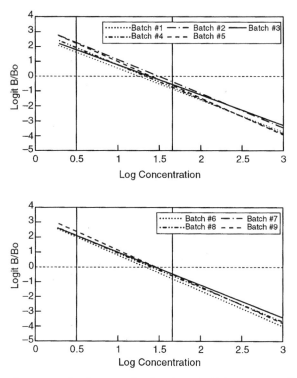

FIG. 2. Log-logit standard curves for batches 1–5 (upper panel) and batches 6–9 (lower panel) of Experiment III.

of three key parts of standard curves also was assessed. For Experiment IIIA, the coefficients of variation of the total, buffer, and NSB tube values across batches averaged 4.3% (Table 3).

Analysis of variance (ANOVA) can be used to partition the variance among the factors in an experiment and thus to discriminate between sampling errors, assay errors, and mixing errors. Using a method described by Box et al. (1978) on the data of Experiment IIIA, we found that the variation among the eight samples from each serum pool (mean = 2% of the total) is very small (Table 4), as is the variation between pairs of duplicate determinations (mean = 7% of the total). Variation among batches is clearly the predominant source of variability, averaging 91% of the total variance. A scatterplot for agreement

TABLE 1
Summary of Consistency of Standard Curves for Melatonin
Assays of Experiement III: Squared Correlation Coefficient (r^2),
Linear Slope (m) and Intercept (b) Terms, and Computed Scores
at High and Low Melatonin Concentrations

Batch	r^2	m	b	High (32 pg/mL)	Low 16 pg/mL
1	0.99	−2.18	2.64	32	16
2	1.00	−2.32	3.37	32	18
3	1.00	−2.08	2.77	34	15
4	1.00	−2.29	3.01	30	15
5	1.00	−2.48	3.42	30	17
6	0.98	−2.31	3.20	33	18
7	0.99	−2.46	3.54	37	16
8	0.99	−2.17	3.08	38	18
9	0.98	−2.40	3.14	30	13
Mean	0.99	−2.30	3.13	33	16
SD[a]	0.0079	0.13	0.28	2.81	1.62
% CV[b]	0.79	5.6	8.9	8.5	10

[a] Standard deviation
[b] Coefficient of variation

between duplicate tubes for Experiment IV (Fig. 3) shows the expected
degree of variation; r = 0.87 which is highly significant (p < 0.001)
with df = 106. Plots of means for the serum pools of Experiment IV
show the absence of systematic trends across batches (Fig. 4).

Data Review

To check for aberrant assay results, the four values for each blood sampling per subject were placed in an array with the data from the two
other subjects from the same group (exposed or control) at that time
(e.g., 0400 hours). The mean and standard deviation (SD) of the set of
12 values was determined; any value that was more than 2 SD larger

TABLE 2

Summary of Correlation Coefficients (r), with Linear Slope (m) and Intercept (b) Terms, for the Six Subjects of Experiment IIIA

Subject	r	m	b
23	0.936	0.947	−0.946
24	0.992	0.954	−0.518
26	0.973	0.935	−0.168
27	0.977	0.934	−0.432
933	0.983	0.941	−0.618
9063	0.970	0.934	−0.739
Mean	0.972	0.942	−0.570
SD[a]	0.018	0.0075	0.24
% CV[b]	1.8	0.80	43

[a] Standard deviation
[b] Coefficient of variation

TABLE 3

Principal Means, by Batch, for Key Components of Standard Curves Used in Experiement IIIA

Batch	Total	NSB	Buffer
1	1450.0[a]	74.4	650.0
2	1405.0	72.4	607.0
3	1368.0	85.1	605.0
4	1403.0	78.9	616.0
5	1358.0	79.3	659.0
Mean	1397.0	78.0	627.0
SD[b]	36.3	4.9	25.2
% CV[c]	2.6	6.3	4.0

[a] Mean dpm
[b] Standard deviation
[c] Coefficient of variation

TABLE 4
Partitioning of Error Variance for Assays of Serum Pools of Experiment IIIA

Source	Low Serum SS[a]	%	Medium Serum SS	%	High Serum SS	%	Mean %
Tubes	2.18	7.8	4.0	5.1	10.1	6.8	6.6
Samples	1.41	5.2	0.14	0.2	1.88	1.3	2.2
Batches	24.3	87.0	73.0	94.7	135.9	91.9	91.2
Total	27.86	100.0	77.46	100.0	146.9	100.0	100.0

[a] Sum of squares

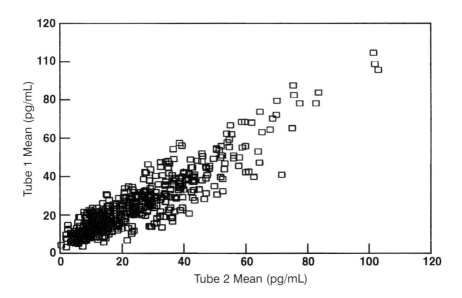

FIG. 3. Scatterplot showing good agreement between duplicate determinations for all melatonin samples measured in Experiment IV.

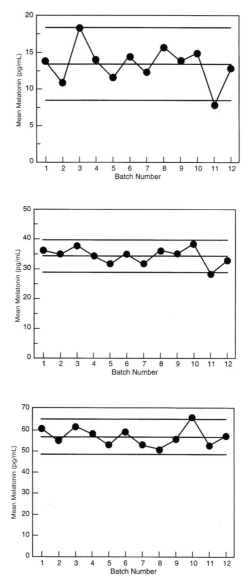

FIG. 4. Control charts showing successive mean melatonin results by batch in Experiment IV for standard lots of baboon serum containing melatonin at the low (upper panel), middle (middle panel), and high (lower panel) ranges of melatonin concentrations of baboons. The horizontal lines show the mean and the range of ± 2 SD.

or smaller than the mean was eliminated. If any values were eliminated, the mean for the remaining scores for each animal at that time
period was re-computed. This procedure required the elimination of
less than 2% of the measured melatonin concentration values.

RESULTS OF EXPERIMENTS III, IIIA, AND IV

Experiment III

During exposure, as in pre- and post-exposure, the patterns of serum
melatonin over time for control and exposed subjects were similar
(Fig. 5). An ANOVA was completed using a mixed, three-factor model
with the between-subjects factor of group (exposed or control) and the
within-subjects factors of period (pre-exposure, exposure, and post-
exposure) and time (day and night). The ANOVA indicated that only
the time melatonin concentration means differed significantly ($F =
9.61$; $df = 1,18$; $p < 0.02$); no other main effect or interaction terms
were significant. (The average of the values for 0800, 1000, 1200, 1400,
1600, 1800, and 2000 hours is the "day" value, and the average of values for 0000, 0200, 0040, and 0600 hours is the "night" value.) The day
and night means were 15.8 and 35.6 pg/mL, respectively (Table 5); the
exposed and control means were 25.7 and 25.8 pg/mL. The 12 hourly
means ranged from a low of 14 pg/mL at 1600 hours to a high of 40
pg/mL at 0600 hours (Fig. 6); the amplitude of the day–night difference
in the baboon is 2.9-fold.

Being able to sample each subject repeatedly, rather than terminally,
allows longitudinal description of melatonin patterns. The melatonin
rhythms of individual nonhuman primates have features previously
described for humans. For example, control subject 28 consistently
showed a pattern of nocturnal melatonin peak occurring early in the
evening (Fig. 7). Exposed subject 27 consistently showed the highest
nocturnal serum melatonin concentrations late in the evening (Fig. 8).
Although overall data analysis did not detect statistically significant
evidence for melatonin reduction across periods in Experiment III, this
particular subject appears to show a progressive reduction in
nocturnal melatonin across pre-exposure, exposure, and post-
exposure periods.

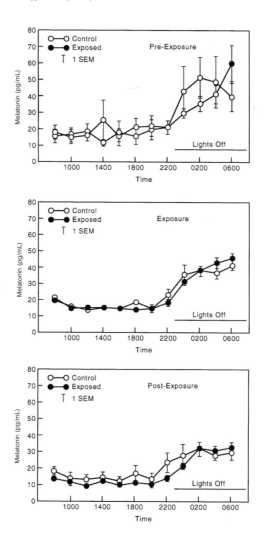

FIG. 5. Mean serum melatonin concentrations, with standard error of the mean (SEM), for three exposed and three control baboons during pre-exposure (n = 3 blood-sampling periods), exposure (n = 3), and post-exposure (n = 2) periods of Experiment III (6 kV/m and 50 μT). (Reprinted from Rogers et al. 1995d by permission of John Wiley & Sons, Inc.)

TABLE 5
Principal Melatonin Means (pg/mL) from Analysis of
Variance of Experiment III Melatonin Data

Group	Day	Night	Mean
Control	16.3	35.2	25.8
Exposed	15.3	36.0	25.7
Mean	15.8	35.6	25.75
E/C[a]	0.936	1.02	0.996

[a] Exposed divided by Control

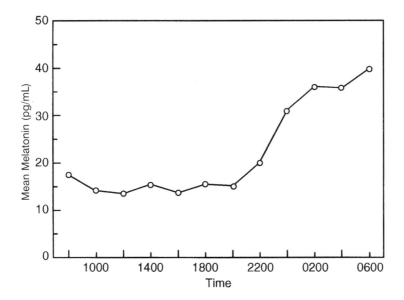

FIG. 6. Mean serum melatonin concentrations from the analysis of variance for the six subjects of Experiment III.

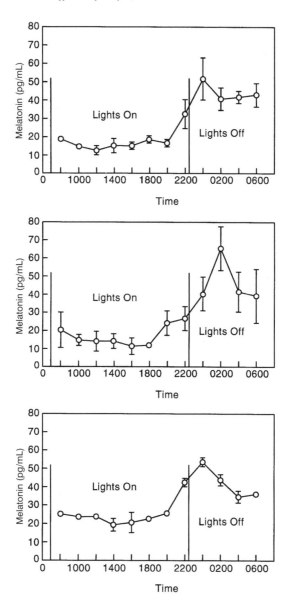

FIG. 7. Mean (SEM) serum melatonin concentrations for control subject 28 during the pre-exposure (top panel), exposure (middle panel), and post-exposure (bottom panel) periods of Experiment III. As indicated by the vertical lines, the lights were on from 0700–2230 hours.

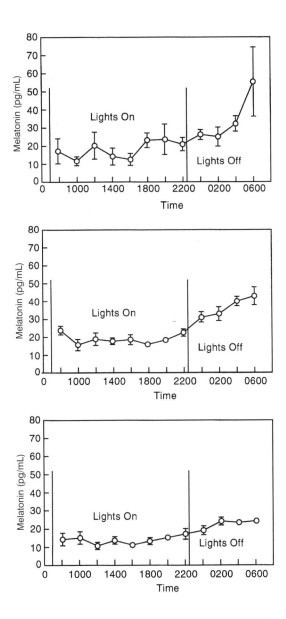

FIG. 8. Mean (SEM) serum melatonin concentrations for exposed subject 27 during the pre-exposure (sampled three times), exposure (sampled three times), and post-exposure (sampled twice) periods of Experiment III. The order of the panels and the meaning of the vertical lines are the same as in Figure 7.

Experiment IIIA

During both the pre-exposure and exposure periods of Experiment IIIA, the patterns of serum melatonin means across timepoints for control and exposed subjects were similar (Fig. 9). ANOVA confirmed presence of day–night differences and absence of differences between exposed and control groups. A three-factor, mixed ANOVA was completed with the between-subjects factor of group and the within-subjects factors of time and period. The F ratio for time was 12.7

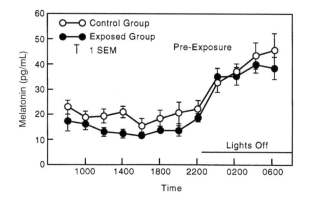

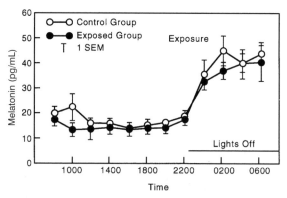

FIG. 9. Mean (SEM) serum melatonin concentrations for three exposed and three control baboons of Experiment IIIA (30 kV/m and 100 μT) during the pre-exposure (n = 2 blood-sampling periods) and exposure (n = 3) periods. (Reprinted from Rogers et al. 1995d by permission of John Wiley & Sons, Inc.)

(df = 1,5; P < 0.007). None of the other F-ratios was greater than 1. For all six subjects, the mean melatonin concentration during the pre-exposure period was 27.8 pg/mL; the exposure mean was 26.8 pg/mL. These mean values are very similar to those observed in Experiment III with the same subjects.

Experiment IV

In Experiment IV, mean melatonin concentrations of the control subjects were higher than those of the field-exposed group throughout the experiment (Fig. 10). When the nighttime means for the two groups during pre-exposure, exposure, and post-exposure periods were plotted (Fig. 11), the difference between control and exposed subjects remained nearly constant. Nighttime melatonin levels were rather consistent across the three periods, especially for the EMF-exposed subjects, indicating no EMF-induced melatonin suppression.

ANOVA using a mixed, three-factor model with the between-subject factor of group and the within-subject factors of period and time revealed that the only statistically significant effects were for time (F = 23.4; df = 1,5; p < 0.005) and period x time (F = 4.41; df = 2,10; p < 0.04). The day mean was 18 pg/mL, and the night mean was 28 pg/mL. The interaction, which does not involve differences between exposed and control groups, and therefore is uninteresting by itself, results from slight differences in the patterns of night- and daytime means across periods. The detection of this interaction shows that that very small effects can be statistically significant in experiments involving only three subjects per group.

Based on the methods given in Cohen (1988), the power of a t-test on the data of Experiment IV to detect a 50% drop in nocturnal melatonin at a single timepoint is 0.80, even with three subjects each in the exposed and control groups. (The conventional goal of experimental design is to have alpha = 0.05 and power = 0.80). The necessary parameters needed for the computation are M_1 = 30 pg/mL (mean nighttime level for all subjects during pre-exposure), M_2 = 15 pg/mL (a 50% reduction), mean SEM = 3.02, sigma = 7.35, and d = 2.04. Given their larger df, the power of the tests for main effects and interactions in the ANOVA is somewhat greater.

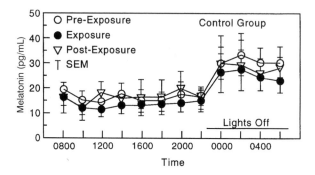

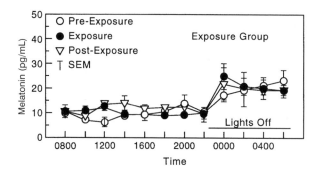

FIG. 10. Mean serum (SEM) melatonin concentrations of control (upper panel) and exposed (lower panel) baboons by period during Experiment IV (30 kV/m and 100 μT). The subjects were sampled three times during pre-exposure, three times during exposure, and twice during post-exposure. (Reprinted from Rogers et al. 1995d by permission of John Wiley & Sons, Inc.)

Discussion

Comments on Results

Collectively, Experiments III, IIIA, and IV establish that regularly scheduled exposure to EMF for three 4-hour periods (separated by 30 minutes without exposure) during the day for 6 weeks does not affect the 24-hour pattern of serum melatonin concentration in baboons. The data from all three experiments are quite clear and consistent.

Presumably as a result of normal intersubject differences in melatonin and random assignment of subjects to groups, melatonin con-

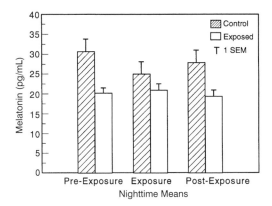

FIG. 11. Mean (SEM) serum melatonin concentrations of exposed and control baboons during the lights-off portion of the 24-hour cycle during pre-exposure, exposure, and post-exposure periods of Experiment IV (30 kV/m and 100 μT). (Reprinted from Rogers et al. 1995d by permission of John Wiley & Sons, Inc.)

centrations of the exposed group were greater than those of the control group throughout Experiment III. However, in Experiment IV, mean melatonin concentrations of the control subjects were higher than those of exposed subjects throughout the experiment. In future experiments with small groups of subjects, it would be appropriate to assign subjects to exposed and control groups as matched pairs to account for pre-existing differences in melatonin concentrations. Graham et al. (1996) reached the same conclusion, for similar reasons, in their studies with human subjects.

The control groups received a stray magnetic field exposure of less than 1 μT in Experiment III, and less than 2 μT in Experiments IIIA and IV. Kato et al. (1993, 1994d) reported that magnetic fields of 1.4 μT or greater suppressed melatonin equally in albino rats. If the stray magnetic fields had produced an effect in these baboon experiments, a reduction of melatonin would have appeared when the pre-exposure and exposure data for the control groups were examined. However, there was no sign of a melatonin suppression effect in either the exposed or control groups of these primate experiments with EMF.

Possible Reasons for Lack of Melatonin Effect

Previous experiments with rodents typically have involved exposure periods including most of the day and all of the night. Perhaps negative results occurred in Experiments III, IIIA, and IV with primates because EMF exposure did not occur at night, the time when active melatonin production by the pineal gland is high and therefore could be more easily inhibited. However, the results of Yellon (1994) demonstrate that concurrent nocturnal magnetic field exposure is not a necessary condition for reduced blood melatonin in Djungarian hamsters.

The results of these primate experiments also could differ from results of rodent experiments because a different magnetic field-exposure stimulus was used. Kato et al. (1994c) reported that although circularly polarized, 50-Hz magnetic fields depressed melatonin in rodents, vertical, elliptical, or horizontal 50-Hz magnetic fields did not. Our experiments used horizontal magnetic fields; the results of a primate experiment using circularly polarized magnetic fields, produced without transients, would be of interest. However, the melatonin suppression effect observed in the Probe Experiment (see p. 456), which also used horizontal magnetic fields, suggests that factors other than field orientation, such as transients, also might be involved in determining the effect.

An even more speculative possibility is that electric and magnetic fields interact so as to modify the effect on the pineal gland. This is one of only two melatonin research programs involving concurrent exposure to 60-Hz EMF. Sheep chronically exposed beneath a power line providing electric fields of about 6 kV/m and magnetic fields of about 3.3 μT also did not show melatonin suppression (Lee et al. 1993, 1995). Furthermore, in the behavioral experiments with baboons (Coelho et al. 1995; Orr et al. 1995b), there was a suggestion that with combined EMF exposure, the presence of the magnetic fields blocked the appearance of the transitory, excitatory effects produced by electric field exposure.

The absence of a melatonin suppression effect in Experiments III, IIIA, and IV could be attributed to differences between rodent and primates in pineal responsiveness to electric and/or magnetic fields. Although further study of this possibility is required, the demonstration of melatonin suppression in the Probe Experiment argues against the possibility that suppression of melatonin by exposure to power-frequency EMF is a unique response of rodents.

Efforts to confirm in rodents the melatonin-suppressing effects of 60-Hz electric or magnetic field exposure have reported mixed results. With electric field exposure, Sasser et al. (1991) did not detect plasma or pineal melatonin suppression in a series of experiments designed to replicate those of Wilson et al. (1981, 1983, 1986). In another effort to replicate the Wilson et al. observations, Grota et al. (1994) reported a drop in blood melatonin levels without statistically significant changes in pineal gland melatonin content. Kato (Chapter 13, this volume) reports such a "dissociation" between melatonin concentrations in gland and blood in some experiments.

McCormick et al. (1994, 1995) reported that 10 weeks of exposure to horizontal, 60-Hz, magnetic fields of 2, 100, or 1000 μT had no effect on melatonin concentrations of mice or rats. Bakos et al. (1995) reported that exposure to vertical, 50-Hz magnetic fields of 500 μT for 24 hours had no effect on urinary secretion of melatonin by rats. Perhaps if McCormick et al. and Bakos et al. had used circularly polarized magnetic fields, they would have seen melatonin reduction. Similarly, the effect reported by Yellon (1994) might have been clearer with circularly polarized magnetic fields. Interestingly, Jentsch et al. (1993) reported that rats exposed to vertical, 10-Hz, 100-μT magnetic fields during the day had elevated serum melatonin relative to controls. The magnetic field-exposed subjects also showed retarded extinction of an avoidance task. No such behavioral differences were observed when tested in the dark. Sasser et al. (1991) reported elevated melatonin in electric field-exposed female rats at one timepoint during the dark.

Although the conditions relating to electric or magnetic field exposure and melatonin depression in laboratory rodents are not fully understood (Reiter 1992, 1993b), electric or magnetic field-induced melatonin suppression has been reported by multiple investigators. Given the previously reported results of reduced melatonin in rodents exposed to power-frequency electric or magnetic fields, it is of interest to consider why melatonin depression did not occur in the rodent experiments just discussed. Presumably the most likely explanations involve details of exposure conditions.

PROBE EXPERIMENT

Methods

Subjects
Two young-adult, male baboons each were implanted with a chronically indwelling venous cannula. Three weeks were allowed for recovery from surgery before initiation of pre-exposure sampling.

Field Exposure
The subjects were exposed to 60-Hz EMF: the electric fields were vertical while the magnetic fields were horizontal; field-strength combinations were either 6 kV/m and 50 μT or 30 kV/m and 100 μT. The magnetic field was turned on quickly, by relay closure, reaching full intensity in one-half of a 60-Hz cycle (8.3 milliseconds). After a delay of about 2 minutes, the electric field was turned on by relay closure at either 6 kV/m (first 4 days) or 14 kV/m (remainder of experiment); the electric field then was ramped slowly to 30 kV/m over a period of about 10 seconds. Field offset was done in the reverse order. Measurements when the EMF were turned on or off by relay closure showed that sharp electric field irregularities occurred at onset/offset; there were no magnetic field irregularities (Rogers et al. 1995a). The electric field irregularity was characterized by nonharmonic, transient, transformer ringing with a frequency content primarily in the 300-Hz range; the amplitude was a random function of the power-frequency phase at the time of activation (Fig. 12).

Under the assumption that organisms rapidly adapt to constant conditions, a variable, intermittent exposure schedule was used. The possible role of sensory perception in electric field-induced melatonin suppression has received little attention. Behavioral experiments with baboons (Orr et al. 1995a) have indicated a mean electric field-detection threshold of 12 kV/m. Thus, an electric field of 6 kV/m is likely to be undetectable while an electric field of 30 kV/m would be highly salient. Magnetic fields of either 50 or 100 μT are presumed to be undetectable.

On the first day, subjects underwent daytime exposure to 6-kV/m electric fields and 50-μT magnetic fields for 0.5 hour. On the next 3 days, exposure occurred for 4 hours daily; onset and offset times were varied deliberately. After a day without exposure, use of 30 kV/m and

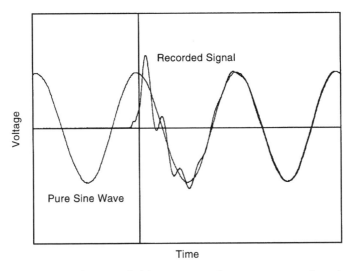

Time

FIG. 12. Example of electric field onset irregularity occurring when the electric field transformer was turned on, at 2 kV/m, by relay closure. For visual contrast, the measured signal is overlayed on a 60 Hz sine wave.

100 μT was initiated: The first day included 0.5 hours of exposure, and the next day 5.5 hours. After another day without exposure, the baboons were given 4–6 hours of exposure daily for 4 days to 30 kV/m and 100 μT. The first blood collection during the EMF exposure period occurred during the third night of this 4-day period.

After 2 days without field exposure, there were 5 more days of exposure, with 9.8–12.7 hours per day to 30 kV/m and 100 μT. After 2 more days without exposure, 6 additional days of exposure were given. The first consisted of 8.8 hours of daytime exposure. Thereafter, exposure continued into the night, giving total exposures of 19.1–23.5 hours per day. The second blood collection occurred on the last night of this 5-day period. On many exposure days, the EMF were turned on and off at least once or twice, and often more frequently, at irregular intervals. Additionally, on the day after the first nocturnal blood sampling, the EMF were turned on or off at 30-minute intervals. As in Experiments III, IIIA, and IV, the subjects were maintained on a 15.5:8.5 light:dark cycle, with lights on from 0700–2230 hours.

Blood-Sampling Procedures

Because the apparatus was being used before its operating software was complete, samples were collected by manual operation of the blood samplers. The EMF were turned off when personnel entered the facility to collect blood samples. To collect samples during the night, the same dim red illumination was used in the pre-exposure and exposure portions of the experiment. Personnel also entered the facility occasionally on some days to check operation of the facility and blood samplers; on some of these occasions, the EMF were left on. The baboons, which were accustomed to the personnel (and vice versa), displayed normal, calm behavior during sample collection. Pre-exposure (baseline) blood samplings were completed three times at weekly intervals before initiation of EMF exposure. Each time a subject was sampled, two separately labeled, alphanumerically coded tubes of serum were produced and frozen for subsequent assay.

Blood-Sampling Schedule

The first nocturnal blood sampling during exposure began on exposure day 9. By the end of this day, the baboons had received a total 60-Hz EMF exposure of 36 hours (including 12.5 hours at 6 kV/m and 0.50 μT) and had experienced 19 field onsets/offsets. All EMF exposure had been during the daytime ("lights on"). On this sampling, all six samples were obtained as planned from one subject, but only two were collected from the other (Rogers et al. 1995b).

On the second nocturnal sampling during exposure, beginning on exposure day 21, we successfully completed blood sampling with both baboons. At the end of this blood collection, each of the two baboons had received 193 hours of total EMF exposure, with 53 field onsets/offsets. When this set of samples was collected, EMF exposure was occurring during both day and night.

Additionally, to examine the acute effects of EMF exposure, blood samples were collected at 0800 on the first day of exposure to 6 kV/m and 50 μT, and on the first 2 days of exposure to 30 kV/m and 100 μT.

Melatonin Assay

Coded serum samples were sequentially extracted with chloroform, carbonate buffer, and petroleum ether. Melatonin was measured using an iodinated-tracer, double-antibody RIA technique (Rollag and Nieswender 1976) which detects as little as 10 pmol of melatonin and produces intra- and interassay coefficients of variation of less than 10% and 15%, respectively (Champney et al. 1984). Log-logit standard curves were used to estimate melatonin in duplicate. The samples from pre-exposure were analyzed as one batch, and the samples from exposure were analyzed subsequently as a second batch. Typical standard curves were obtained with each of the two batches.

Results

For baboon 1078, nocturnal serum melatonin concentrations after 21 days of exposure were between 4% and 17% of the mean concentrations observed at the same timepoints during pre-exposure (Fig. 13). For subject 9063, nocturnal serum melatonin concentrations were only 10–25% of baseline levels when sampled after 9 days of exposure, and the levels were only 8–12% of normal for the respective timepoints after 21 days of exposure (Fig. 14). With the Rollag assay, nocturnal melatonin concentrations were between 40 and 80 pg/mL. In this Probe

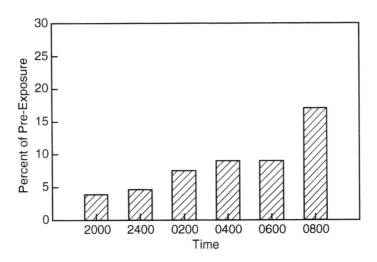

FIG. 13. Nocturnal serum melatonin concentrations for baboon 1078, expressed as percent of the mean of three pre-exposure control values at each timepoint, after 21 days of exposure to 60-Hz EMF.

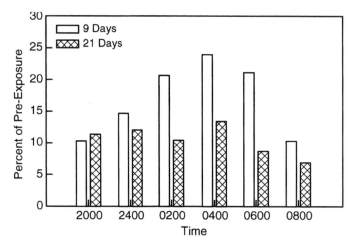

FIG. 14. Nocturnal serum melatonin concentrations for baboon 9063, expressed as percent of the mean of three pre-exposure control values at each timepoint, after 9 and after 21 days of exposure to 60-Hz EMF.

Experiment, it appeared that EMF exposure produced a near-complete blockage of the normal nocturnal melatonin rise in blood (Fig. 15).

The mean of the two early morning, lights-on (at 0800) samples from the first day of exposure to 6 kV/m and 50 μT was less than 40% of what had been observed during pre-exposure (Fig. 16). Furthermore, the degree of early morning melatonin depression appeared greatest at the first exposure. The means for the first and second days of exposure to 30 kV/m and 100 μT also were reduced, to less than 60% and then to 85%, respectively, but successively were closer to the mean values shown by the subjects previously during the pre-exposure baseline.

Discussion

It seems unlikely that aspects of sample collection and facility operation, including presence of humans, differentially affected the outcome of this Probe Experiment: Normal melatonin patterns were observed during the 3-week pre-exposure period. However, with the completely within-subjects design used in the Probe Experiment,

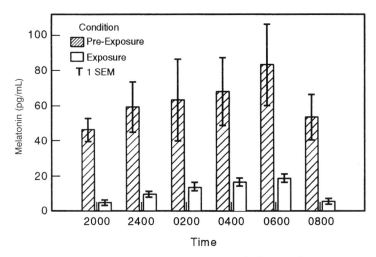

FIG. 15. Mean melatonin concentrations in two baboons during pre-exposure and after 21 days of exposure to 60-Hz EMF. The error bars show the SEM. (Reprinted from Rogers et al. 1995c by permission of John Wiley & Sons, Inc.)

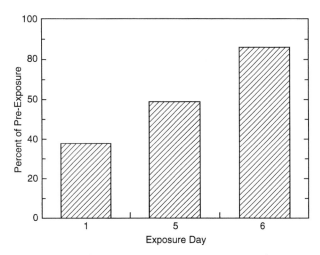

FIG. 16. Mean serum melatonin concentrations, expressed as percent of three pre-exposure control values, at 0800 on the first, fifth, and sixth days of exposure to 60-Hz EMF. The exposure conditions were 6 kV/m and 50 μT on the first day. The fifth day was the first of exposure to 30 kV/m and 100 μT, which continued until the end of the experiment.

there is no way to prove that the uniformly "low" melatonin scores from the second batch were not artificially low for some reason unrelated to EMF exposure. Furthermore, no other samples expected to be "high" in melatonin concentration were included in the sets of samples assayed. The authors do not believe that potential confounders, such as assay problems or nocturnal light leaks, affected the results of the Probe Experiment.

Rapid Onset of Effects

The large-magnitude reduction of serum melatonin concentration was present after only 9 days of exposure and despite the fact that all 60-Hz EMF exposure up to that time had occurred only during the day. Wilson et al. (1986) had reported that it takes 3 weeks of exposure for the suppression effect to develop with electric field exposure in the rat. Previous 60-Hz electric field experiments in rodents typically used nearly continuous exposure, with fields off for only a few hours each day during the light phase; exposure was occurring during most of the day as well as during all of the night, the period when the pineal gland actively produces melatonin.

Given the possibility that the time course for production of reduced blood melatonin differs with exposure to electric or magnetic fields, the rapid appearance of melatonin suppression in this experiment is less surprising. With inversion or rotation of the Earth's DC magnetic field, acute (15–60 minutes) effects on melatonin and/or its biosynthetic pathway have been reported (Welker et al. 1983; Olcese and Ruess 1986; Lerchl et al. 1990; Richardson et al. 1993). Furthermore, Yellon (1994) demonstrated that hamsters exposed to a 60-Hz magnetic field exhibited an acute depression of melatonin on the night of the first day of exposure. In the baboon experiments reported here, the exposure included both electric and magnetic fields; thus the rapid onset of effects could have been stimulated by the magnetic field.

The observation of reductions at 2000 hours, shortly before lights off, and at 0800 hours, shortly after lights on, suggests that EMF exposure can suppress daytime as well as nighttime melatonin. The detection of daytime differences in melatonin was a relatively surprising result first published by Kato et al. (1993) for rats exposed to circularly polarized, 50-Hz magnetic fields. Detection of such small differences requires considerable statistical power. This can be achieved with small variability, produced either by the use of one sample from each of a large number of subjects (e.g., Kato et al.) or by averaging of the multiple samples from each of the same few subjects (e.g., Rogers et al.).

The observation of an acute melatonin depression on the morning of the first day of exposure was unexpected from the perspective of an electric field orientation. From the magnetic field perspective, this observation is more predictable, but a daytime reduction was not expected. The additional possibility, that the acute daytime effect produced by magnetic field exposure might be followed by a partial return to normal, also was unexpected. However, Welker et al. (1983) provide one example suggesting rapid adaptation to magnetic field exposure: They reported that the pineal gland seemed to become refractory to magnetic field inversion after about 120 minutes of exposure. The "early adaptation" in 0800-hour melatonin levels stands in sharp contrast to the depression of nocturnal melatonin concentrations, which showed slight evidence of being progressive in baboon 9063, which was apparent when nocturnal sampling was completed after 9 and 21 days of exposure. These observations on the temporal patterns of melatonin response to EMF exposure were made possible largely by the ability to serially sample blood within the same subjects.

Transients

The results of the Probe Experiment are consistent with other indications suggesting that transients produced by rapid electric and/or magnetic field onset/offset might be a critical feature producing melatonin suppression. Lerchl et al. (1991) reported that "rapid" reversal of the Earth's magnetic field orientation during the dark produced melatonin suppression, but "slow" reversal did not. Presumably the fast rise-time signal induced internal electric currents expected to be an effective biological stimulus. Richardson et al. (1993) suggested that the eddy currents associated with rapid magnetic fields inversion were the cause of melatonin suppression in rodents. In addition, Wilson et al. (1990) reported that an electric blanket which produced transients, and which turned on/off relatively frequently, was more likely to influence urinary melatonin concentrations of humans than did electric blankets which did not produce transients and which turned on/off relatively infrequently. Wilson et al. (1994) described the transients associated with electrically powered personal appliances.

Irregularity and Intermittency

In the Probe Experiment, the onsets/offsets were relatively numerous, irregular in occurrence, and variable in duration. Randomness of exposure could be an important feature in EMF experiments because organisms usually adapt rapidly to regular stimuli; use of a variable exposure regimen might augment or prolong biological effects. From the perspective of adaptation, an exposure schedule of "X" on and "Y" off (a duty cycle) that is regularly followed for some time probably might be regarded as intermittent, but should not be regarded as irregular. Based on the concept of "coherence" (Litovitz et al. 1991), in vitro experiments (Nordenson et al. 1994) are beginning to assess the effects of various, rather short, duty cycles.

In summary, these limited data are consistent with the hypothesis that, under some circumstances, 60-Hz EMF exposure can produce a profound suppression of nocturnal melatonin production in a nonhuman primate.

DISCUSSION

Different Conditions and Different Outcomes

The apparent suppression of nocturnal serum melatonin concentration observed in the Probe Experiment stands in marked contrast to the absence of such an effect in Experiments III, IIIA, and IV. The exposure conditions of the two sets of experiments were not the same, and thus the results should not be regarded as inconsistent. Salient difference between the Probe Experiment and Experiments III, IIIA, and IV involve the number of field onsets/offsets, the presence or absence of transients at onset/offset, the degree of schedule regularity, and the time of exposure (daytime versus day and night).

Suggestions for Additional Research

Other than the demonstration that, under some circumstances, power-frequency electric or magnetic field exposure can reduce melatonin in rodents, little is known about EMF and melatonin. The negative studies in sheep and the negative-to-suggestive studies in nonhuman and human primates are too few to reach definitive conclusions about possible human effects, especially given the array of unanswered questions about exposure attributes.

Species Differences

Without additional data, it is not possible to evaluate the possibility that interspecies differences exist between rodent and primate with respect to pineal response to power-frequency EMF. Completion of a "Species Matrix" including various aspects of electric field, magnetic field, and/or EMF exposure in several species—including rat, primate, and human—is required to assess the hypothesis that there are species differences in pineal response to electric and/or magnetic field exposure.

Complex Temporal Patterns

Kato (personal communication) recently offered the suggestion that the effects of magnetic field exposure on the pineal involve dual processes (Fig. 17): (1) an acute process (dynamic response) occurring with "short" (circa minutes to days) exposures, and (2) a chronic process (integrated response) occurring with "long" (circa 1000 hours) exposures.[1] Kato notes that other processes besides exposure duration probably are involved; furthermore, the interaction site—be it retina, synaptic connections from retina to pineal gland, pinealocytes, or some other site or process—is not known.

To help illustrate and evaluate Kato's suggestion, the exposure durations in the melatonin experiments cited here were tabulated (Table 6). For magnetic fields, the positive results of Yellon (1994) and Selmaoui and Touitou (1995) could be cases of acute effects involving exposures of a few minutes to a few days, and the results of Kato et al.

---

[1] Perhaps this might be stated alternatively as an example of the General Adaptation Syndrome (Selye 1960) consisting of acute response, adaptation, and exhaustion. Additionally, the possibility of changing effects of EMF exposure on melatonin during the first few days of the Probe Experiment also suggests the occurrence of dynamic events with a relatively short time span.

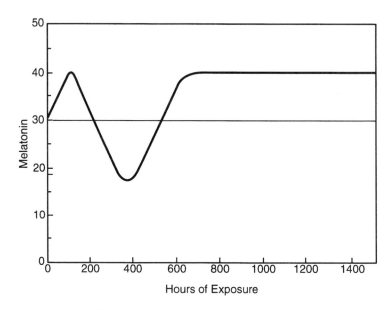

FIG. 17. Conceptual drawing suggesting how total exposure time might have a complex relationship to suprathreshold appearance of reduced blood melatonin following exposure to a power-frequency magnetic field. The data available is insufficient to plot a function; the shape of the indicated curve is arbitrary.

(1993) and Löscher et al. (1994) could be cases of chronic effects. However, the negative results of Graham et al. (1996, in press), Jentsch et al. (1993), and McCormick et al. (1994, 1995) represent possible exceptions to the "total-time-of-exposure" concept. Inversions of the Earth's magnetic field usually produce positive effects with very "short" exposure durations; long durations have not been tested. However, the negative results of Welker et al. (1983) after 24 hours of exposure suggest additional short-term complexity. If studies with EMF are regarded as magnetic fields studies, the results of Rogers et al. (1995c) could represent positive acute effects, and the results of Rogers et al. (1995d) could represent the absence of detectable effects during the intermediate phase. The negative results of Lee et al. (1993, 1995), which included interim samplings, do not fit the proposed temporal

TABLE 6

Total Exposure Duration and Occurrence of Melatonin Reduction Effect

Authors (et al.)	Ref.	Exper.	Hours/ day	# Days	Total hours	Fields off[a]	Exposed hours	Effect	Note
					I. Sinusoidal Magnetic Field Exposure				
Yellon	1994	1	0.25	1	0.25	0	0.25	Yes	
Yellon	1994	2	0.25	1	0.25	0	0.25	No	Possible effect?
Yellon	1994	3	0.25	1	0.25	0	0.25	Yes	
Graham	in press(b)	1	8.0	1	8.0	x 0.5	4.0	No	Low subjects?
Graham	in press(a)	2	8.0	1	8.0	0	8.0	No	No interaction
Selmaoui	1995	1	12.0	1	12.0	0	12.0	Yes	100 μT, not less
Selmaoui	1995	2	18.0	30	540.0	0	540.0	Yes	10 μT, not less
McCormick	1994	1	18.5	70	1295.0	x 0.5	648.0	No	
Kato	1993	1	24.0	42	1008.0	24	984.0	Yes	Circ. polarized
Kato	1994d	1	24.0	42	1008.0	24	984.0	Yes	Circ. polarized
Kato	1994a	1	24.0	42	1008.0	24	984.0	Yes	Circ. polarized
Kato	1994c	1	24.0	42	1008.0	24	984.0	Yes	Circ. polarized
Kato	1994b	1	24.0	42	1008.0	24	984.0	No	Not circular
McCormick	1994	2	18.5	70	1295.0	0	1295.0	No	
McCormick	1995	1	18.5	84	1554.0	0	1554.0	No	
Löscher	1994	1	24.0	91	2184.0	0	2184.0	Yes	

continued

TABLE 6 (continued)

Total Exposure Duration and Occurrence of Melatonin Reduction Effect

Authors (et al.)	Ref.	Exper.	Hours/day	# Days	Total hours	Fields off[a]	Exposed hours	Effect	Note
II. Inversions of Earth's Magnetic Field									
Welker	1983	1	0.25	1	0.25	0	0.25	Yes	NAT
Lerchl	1990	1	1.0	1	1.0	x 0.5	0.5	Yes	Fast
Olcese	1986	1	0.5	1	0.5	0	0.5	Yes	Slow
Lerchl	1991	1	1.0	1	1.0	0	1.0	No	NAT
Welker	1983	2b	2.0	1	2.0	0	2.0	Yes	NAT
Jentsch	1993	1	4.0	5	20.0	0	20.0	Rise	Day
Jentsch	1993	1	4.0	5	20.0	0	20.0	No	Night
Welker	1983	2a	24.0	1	24.0	0	24.0	No	NAT
III. Power-Frequency EMF									
Rogers	1995c	1	--	1	0.25	0	0.25	Yes	Daytime
Rogers	1995c	2	--	9	36.0	0	36.0	Yes	Transients
Rogers	1995c	3	--	21	193.0	0	193.0	Yes	Transients
Rogers	1995d	IIIA	12.0	21	252.0	0	252.0	No	Regular
Rogers	1995d	III	12.0	42	504.0	48	456.0	No	No transients
Rogers	1995d	IV	12.0	42	504.0	48	456.0	No	Daytime
Lee	1993	1	24.0	300	7200.0	0	7200.0	No	Powerline
Lee	1995	1	24.0	300	7200.0	0	7200.0	No	Powerline

continued

TABLE 6 (continued)

Total Exposure Duration and Occurrence of Melatonin Reduction Effect

IV. Power-Frequency Electric Fields

Authors (et al.)	Ref.	Exper.	Hours/day	# Days	Total hours	Fields off[a]	Exposed hours	Effect	Note
Wilson	1986	1	20	7	140	0	140	No	Not p < 0.05
Wilson	1986	2	20	14	280	0	280	No	Not p < 0.05
Wilson	1986	3	20	21	420	0	420	Yes	
Reiter	1986	1	19	23	437	0	437	Yes	In utero too
Wilson	1986	4	20	28	560	0	560	Yes	
Grota	1994	n = 4	20	30	600	1.5	599	Yes	Serum only
Wilson	1981	1	20	30	600	0	600	Yes	
Sasser	1991	1	20	30	600	0	600	No	Males
Sasser	1991	2	20	30	600	0	600	Rise?	Females

[a] In some experiments, fields were off half the time (x 0.5). In other experiments, fields were off some of the time for maintenance. In remaining experiments, the subtraction accounts for when the subjects were killed.

pattern. The limited database with electric field exposure suggests a temporally developing effect most effective in the range of 400–600 hours of total exposure. In summary, the observation by Kato is insightful, but the database available is too limited to assess the effects of exposure time without confounding by differences in factors such as species and field orientation. Collectively, these results and speculations suggest that further examination of the time course of electric and/or magnetic field exposure on effects relating to the synthesis, release, and metabolism of melatonin is required.

Complex Stimulus Space
It seems likely that no single-variate measure of exposure, such as total exposure time, will be able to provide a complete description of electric- and/or magnetic field-induced reductions in melatonin. It seems probable that many factors, including (1) field intensity, (2) duration of exposure, (3) presence of transients, (4) number of onsets/offsets, (5) regularity, (6) intermittency, (7) day and/or night exposure, (8) measurement during day or night, (9) species, and (10) type of photoperiod, will interact to produce a complex, but quite real, exposure function and resultant nonlinear response surface. Further discussions of these and related issues are provided by Morgan et al. (1995) and Valberg (1995).

Summary
Further research is required. First, the available database is very small, especially when it comes to nonhuman and human primates. Second, no one should take seriously an answer to the global question, "Does electric and/or magnetic field exposure reduce nocturnal melatonin?" based on the 50 (or so) available studies of this class. "EMF" is not a unitary entity, just as "chemical" is not a single entity. The effects of chemicals depend on the molecule, the dose, the route of delivery, the species, and so on. Similar complexity probably is true for the biological effects of EMF. Third, study of the "functional consequences" of melatonin reduction produced by electric and/or magnetic field exposure is required. Given the many functional roles of melatonin, alterations in behavior, endocrinology, and immunology—just to name a few important systems potentially affected—are to be expected if elec-

tric fields, magnetic fields, and/or EMF exposure does alter melatonin metabolism.

Nonhuman Primate Models for
Other Problems in Bioelectromagnetics

In recent years, some investigators have raised the possibility of unanticipated health effects from use of cellular phones, just as investigators did 20 years ago regarding ELF electric fields (and 20 years before that regarding microwaves). Once again, the nonhuman primate could provide an excellent model to examine the issue. For example, baboons could be fitted with cellular phones (Fig. 18) which then could be activated in patterns simulating those documented to be characteristic of human cellular telephone use. The tether also could be used to assess melatonin and immunology. For engineering reasons, the radio frequency (RF) signals (e.g., circa 900 MHz) of cellular

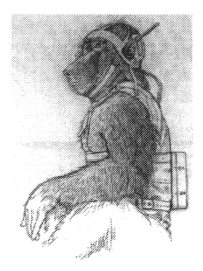

FIG. 18. Artist's sketch suggesting how a baboon could be fitted with a cellular phone to allow study of potential bioelectromagnetic effects in a model providing high dosimetric and phylogenetic equivalence to the human. The jacket for the tether used in the completed melatonin experiments also is indicated.

phones often are modulated at ELF (< 300 Hz). The work of Adey (1990) and others shows that ELF-modulated RF can be a very potent biological stimulus. Thus ELF-modulated cellular phone signals also might affect melatonin.

Because energy deposition into tissue is such a key concern, this arrangement with the relatively large head and brain of the baboon would provide far more realistic exposure, and accompanying dosimetry, than would be achieved by rodents in either waveguides or anechoic chambers. The use of an in vivo exposure and an in vitro assessment strategy, incorporating positive and negative controls, would be a very powerful approach. The spatially limited nature of exposure would allow use of within-subject designs with subjects the size of baboons. The dependent variables could be contemporary molecular biology processes measured in skin samples stimulated using conventional initiation–promotion approaches. (Other tissues or fluids also could be sampled.) In vitro assays might include, for example, assay of proliferating cell nuclear antigen and measurement of apoptosis by in situ end labeling or in situ hybridization.

CONCLUSIONS

The utility of primates in biological hazard assessment was demonstrated by a series of three experiments completed with sets of three field-exposed and three sham-exposed nonhuman primates. The study clearly established that 6 weeks of regularly scheduled, transient-free, daytime exposure to 60-Hz EMF does not affect nocturnal serum melatonin concentrations. Because conclusions reached with nonhuman primates generally extrapolate particularly well to humans, this observation strongly suggests that similar 60-Hz EMF exposure would not affect serum melatonin concentrations in humans.

However, it is premature to over-generalize these results and to conclude that 60-Hz EMF exposure, under any exposure condition, does not affect primate melatonin. With a different EMF exposure protocol, including both transients and an irregular and intermittent exposure schedule, the results of an experiment with two baboons were consistent with the hypothesis that profound suppression of nocturnal serum melatonin concentration can occur in nonhuman primates as a consequence of EMF exposure. Furthermore, the temporal dynamics of the melatonin response to EMF exposure might be far more complex than commonly assumed.

ACKNOWLEDGMENTS

This research was sponsored jointly by the Office of Energy Management of the U.S. Department of Energy (DOE) and the Central Research Institute of the Electric Power Industry (CRIEPI) of Japan, and was conducted as contract DE-AC02-80-RA50219 between DOE and the Southwest Research Institute. Masamichi Kato, of the Department of Physiology at Hokkaido University School of Medicine, generously shared his ideas.

REFERENCES

Adey W.R. 1990. Electromagnetic fields, cell membrane amplification, and cancer promotion. In: *Extremely Low Frequency Electromagnetic Fields: The Question of Cancer*, B.W. Wilson, R.G. Stevens, and L.E. Anderson, eds., pp. 211–249. Columbus, Ohio: Battelle Press.

Bakos, J., N. Nagy, G. Thuroczy, L. Szabo. 1995. Sinusoidal 50 Hz, 500 μT magnetic field has no effect on urinary 6-sulphatoxymelatonin in Wistar rats. *Bioelectromagnetics* 16:377–380.

Box, G.E.P., W.G. Hunter, J.S. Hunter. 1978. Chapter 17: Study of variations. *Statistics for Experimenters: An Introduction to Design, Data Analysis, and Model Building*, pp. 570–583. New York: Wiley & Sons.

Champney, T.H., A.P. Altdorf, R.P. Steger, R.J. Reiter. 1984. Concurrent determination of enzymatic activities and substrate concentrations in the melatonin synthetic pathway within the same rat pineal gland. *Neurosci. Res.* 11:59–66.

Coelho, A.M. Jr., W.R. Rogers, S.P. Easley. 1995. Effects of concurrent exposure to 60 Hz electric and magnetic fields on the social behavior of baboons. *Bioelectromagnetics* Suppl. 3:71–92.

Cohen, J. 1988. The t test for means. *Statistical Power Analysis for the Behavioral Sciences*, 2nd ed., pp. 19–74. Hillsdale, New Jersey: Lawrence Erlbaum.

Graham, C., M.R. Cook, D.W. Riffle, M.M. Gerkovich, H.D. Cohen. 1996. Nocturnal melatonin levels in human volunteers exposed to intermittent 60 Hz magnetic fields. *Bioelectromagnetics* 17(4):263–273.

Graham, C., M.R. Cook, D.W. Riffle. Human melatonin during continuous magnetic field exposure. *Bioelectromagnetics* (in press).

Grota, L.J., R.J. Reiter, P. Keng, S. Michaelson. 1994. Electric field exposure alters serum melatonin but not pineal melatonin synthesis in male rats. *Bioelectromagnetics* 15:427–437.

Jentsch, A., M. Lehman, E. Schone, F. Thoss, G. Zimmerman. 1993. Weak magnetic fields change extinction of a conditioned reaction and daytime melatonin levels in the rat. *Neurosci. Lett.* 157:79–82.

Kato, M., K. Honma, T. Shigemitsu, Y. Shiga. 1993. Effects of exposure to a circularly polarized 50-Hz magnetic field on plasma and pineal melatonin levels in rats. *Bioelectromagnetics* 14:97–106.

Kato, M., K. Honma, T. Shigemitsu, Y. Shiga. 1994a. Circularly polarized 50-Hz magnetic field exposure reduces pineal gland and blood melatonin concentrations of Long-Evans rats. *Neurosci. Lett.* 166:59–62.

Kato, M., K. Honma, T. Shigemitsu, M.Yasui, T. Kikuchi. 1994b. Ellipsoidal magnetic field exposure for 6 weeks has no effect on pineal or plasma melatonin concentration of the rat. In: Abstracts of the 16th Annual Bioelectromagnetics Society Meeting, Copenhagen, Denmark, June 12–17, pp. 98–99. Frederick, Maryland: The Bioelectromagnetics Society.

Kato, M., K. Honma, T. Shigemitsu, Y. Shiga. 1994c. Horizontal or vertical 50-Hz, 1-μT magnetic fields have no effect on pineal gland or plasma melatonin concentration of albino rats. *Neurosci. Lett.* 168:205–208.

Kato, M., K. Honma, T. Shigemitsu, Y. Shiga. 1994d. Recovery of nocturnal melatonin concentration takes place within one week following cessation of 50 Hz circularly polarized magnetic field exposure for six weeks. *Bioelectromagnetics* 15:489–492.

Lee, J.M. Jr., F. Stormshak, J.M. Thompson, P. Thinesen, L.J. Painter, E.G. Olenchek, D.L. Hess, R. Forbes, D.L. Foster. 1993. Melatonin secretion and puberty in female lambs exposed to environmental electric and magnetic fields. *Biol. Reprod.* 49:857–864.

Lee, J.M. Jr., F. Stormshak, J.M. Thompson, D.L. Hess, D. L. Foster. 1995. Melatonin in female lambs exposed to EMF: A replicate study. *Bioelectromagnetics* 16:119–123.

Lerchl, A., K.O. Nonaka, K.-A. Stokkan, R.J. Reiter. 1990. Marked rapid alterations in nocturnal pineal serotonin metabolism in mice and rats exposed to weak intermittent magnetic fields. *Biochem. Biophys. Res. Commun.* 169:102–108.

Lerchl, A., K.O. Nonaka, R.J. Reiter. 1991. Pineal gland "magnetosensitivity" to static magnetic fields is a consequence of induced electric currents (eddy currents). *J. Pineal. Res.* 10:109–116.

Litovitz, T.A., D. Krause, J.M. Mullins. 1991. Effect of coherence time of the applied magnetic field on ornithine decarboxylase activity. *Biochem. Biophys. Res. Commun.* 178:862–865.

Löscher, W., U. Wahnschaffe, M. Mevissen, A. Lerchl, A. Stamm. 1994. Effects of weak alternating magnetic fields on nocturnal melatonin production and mammary carcinogenesis in rats. *Oncology* 51:288–295.

McCormick, D.L., M.A. Cahill, J.B. Harder, B.M. Ryan, J.C. Findlay, L.E. Pomerantz, R.R. Szymanski, G.A. Boorman. 1994. Pineal function assessment in F344 rats and B6C3F1 mice exposed to 60 Hz magnetic fields. In: Abstracts of the 16th Annual Bioelectromagnetics Society Meeting, Copenhagen, Denmark, June 12–17, p. 50. Frederick, Maryland: The Bioelectromagnetics Society.

McCormick, D.L., M.A. Cahill, J.B. Harder, B.M. Ryan, G.A. Boorman. 1995. Pineal function in B6C3F1 mice exposed to 60 Hz magnetic fields: Time course studies. In: Abstracts of the 17th Annual Bioelectromagnetics Society Meeting, Boston, Massachusetts. Frederick, Maryland: Biolectromagnetics Society.

Morgan, M.G., I. Nair, J. Zhang. 1995. A method for assessing alternative effects functions that uses simulation with EMDEX data. *Bioelectromagnetics* 16:172–177.

Nordenson, I., K.H. Mild, G. Andersson, M. Sandstrom. 1994. Chromosomal aberrations in human amniotic cells after intermittent exposure to 50-Hz magnetic fields. *Bioelectromagnetics* 15:293–301.

Nozaki, M., M. Tsushima, Y. Mori. 1990. Diurnal changes in serum melatonin concentrations under indoor and outdoor environments and light suppression of nighttime melatonin secretion in the female Japanese monkey. *J. Pineal Res.* 9: 221–230.

Olcese, J., S. Reuss. 1986. Magnetic field effects on pineal gland melatonin synthesis: Comparative studies on albino and pigmented rodents. *Brain Res.* 369:365–368.

Orr, J.L. 1994. A graphic model for discussing activity and observational data. In: *Neurobehavioral Toxicity: Analysis and Interpretation*, B. Weiss and J. O'Donoghue, eds., pp. 159–172. New York: Raven Press.

Orr, J.L., W.R. Rogers, H.D. Smith. 1995a. Detection thresholds for 60 Hz electric fields by nonhuman primates. *Bioelectromagnetics* Suppl. 3:23–34.

Orr, J.L., W.R. Rogers, H.D. Smith. 1995b. Exposure of baboons to combined 60 Hz electric and magnetic fields does not produce work stoppage or affect operant performance on a match-to-sample task. *Bioelectromagnetics* Suppl. 3:61–70.

Reiter, R.J. 1985. Action spectra, dose-response relationships, and temporal aspects of light's effects on the pineal gland. *Ann. N.Y. Acad. Sci.* 453:215–230.

Reiter, R.J. 1991. Pineal melatonin: Cell biology of its synthesis and of its physiological interactions. *Endocrine Rev.* 12:151–180.

Reiter, R.J. 1992. Alterations of the circadian melatonin rhythm by the electromagnetic spectrum: A study in environmental toxicology. *Regul. Toxicol. Pharmacol.* 15:226–244.

Reiter, R.J. 1993a. Electric and magnetic fields and melatonin production. *Biomed. & Pharmacother.* 47:439–444.

Reiter, R.J. 1993b. Static and extremely low frequency electromagnetic field exposure: Reported effects on the circadian production of melatonin. *J. Cell. Biochem.* 51:394–403.

Reiter, R.J. 1994. Melatonin suppression by static and extremely low frequency electromagnetic fields: Relationship to the reported increased incidence of cancer. *Rev. Environ. Health* 10:171–186.

Reiter, R.J., L.E. Anderson, R.L. Buschbom, B.W. Wilson. 1988. Reduction of the nocturnal rise in pineal melatonin levels in rats exposed to 60-Hz electric fields *in utero* and for 23 days after birth. *Life Sci.* 42:2203–2206.

Richardson, B.A., K. Yaga, R.J. Reiter, P. Hoover. 1993. Suppression of nocturnal pineal N-acetyltransferase activity and melatonin content by inverted magnetic fields and induced eddy currents. *Int. J. Neurosci.* 69:149–155.

Rogers, W.R., J.H. Lucas, W.E. Cory, J.L. Orr, H.D. Smith. 1995a. A 60 Hz electric and magnetic field exposure facility for nonhuman primates: design and operational data during experiments. *Bioelectromagnetics* Suppl. 3:2–22.

Rogers, W.R., J.H. Lucas, B.C. Mikiten, H.D. Smith, J.L. Orr. 1995b. Chronically indwelling venous cannula and automatic blood sampling system for use with nonhuman primates exposed to 60 Hz electric and magnetic fields. *Bioelectromagnetics* Suppl. 3:103–110.

Rogers, W.R., R.J. Reiter, H.D. Smith, L. Barlow-Walden, L. 1995c. Rapid onset/offset, variably scheduled 60-Hz electric and magnetic field exposure reduces nocturnal serum melatonin concentration in nonhuman primates. *Bioelectromagnetics* Suppl. 3:119–122.

Rogers, W.R., R.J. Reiter, L. Barlow-Walden, H.D. Smith, J.L. Orr. 1995d. Regularly scheduled, daytime, slow-onset 60-Hz electric and magnetic field exposure does not depress serum melatonin concentration in nonhuman primates. *Bioelectromagnetics* Suppl. 3:111–118.

Rollag, M.D., G.D. Nieswender. 1976. Radioimmunoassay of serum concentrations of melatonin in sheep exposed to different lighting regimens. *Endocrinology* 98:482–489.

Sasser, L.B., J.E. Morris, R.L. Buschbom, D.L. Miller, L.E. Anderson. 1991. Effects of 60-Hz electric fields on pineal melatonin during various times of the dark period. In: Abstracts of the Annual Review of Research on Biological Effects of Electric and Magnetic Fields, Milwaukee, Wisconsin, November 3–7. Frederick, Maryland: W/L Associates, Ltd.

Schiffman, J.C., H.M. Lasch, M.D. Rollag, A.E. Flanders, G.C. Brainard, D.L. Burk, Jr. 1994. Effect of MR imaging on the normal human pineal body: Measurement of plasma melatonin levels. *J. Magnet. Res. Imag.* 4:7–11.

Selmaoui, B., Y. Touitou. 1995. Sinusoidal 50-Hz magnetic fields depress rat pineal NAT activity and serum melatonin. Role of duration and intensity of exposure. *Life Sci.* 57:1351–1358.

Selye, H. 1960. *The Physiology and Pathology of Exposure to Stress.* Montreal: Acta Inc.

Valberg, P.A. 1995. Designing EMF experiments: What is required to characterize "exposure"? *Bioelectromagnetics* 16:396–401.

Welker, H.A., P. Semm, R.P. Willig, J.C. Commentz, W. Wiltschko, L. Vollrath. 1983. Effects of an artificial magnetic field on serotonin N-acetyltransferase activity and melatonin content of the rat pineal gland. *Exp. Brain Res.* 50:426–432.

Wilson, B.W., L.E. Anderson. 1990. ELF electromagnetic field effects on the pineal gland. In: *Extremely Low Frequency Electromagnetic Fields: The Question of Cancer*, B.W. Wilson, R.G. Stevens, L.E. Anderson, eds., pp. 159-186. Columbus, Ohio: Battelle Press.

Wilson, B.W., L.E. Anderson, D.I. Hilton, R.D. Phillips. 1981. Chronic exposure to 60-Hz electric fields: Effects on pineal function in the rat. *Bioelectromagnetics* 2:371–380.

Wilson, B.W., L.E. Anderson, D.J. Hilton, R.D. Phillips. 1983. Chronic exposure to 60-Hz electric fields: Effects on pineal function in the rat (erratum). *Bioelectromagnetics* 4:293.

Wilson, B.W., E.K. Chess, L.E. Anderson. 1986. 60 Hz electric field effects on pineal melatonin rhythms: Time course of onset and recovery. *Bioelectromagnetics* 7:239–242.

Wilson, B.W., R.G. Stevens, L.E. Anderson. 1989. Neuroendocrine mediated effects of electromagnetic-field exposure: Possible role of the pineal gland. *Life Sci.* 45:1319–1332.

Wilson, B.W., C.W. Wright, J.E. Morris, R.L. Buschbom, D.P. Brown, D.L. Miller, R. Sommers-Flannigan, L.E. Anderson. 1990. Evidence for an effect of ELF electromagnetic fields on human pineal gland function. *J. Pineal Res.* 9:259–269.

Wilson, B.W., N.H. Hansen, K.C. Davis. 1994. Magnetic-field flux density and spectral characteristics of motor-driven personal appliances. *Bioelectromagnetics* 15:439–446.

Yellon, S.M. 1994. Acute 60 Hz magnetic field exposure effects on the melatonin rhythm in the pineal gland and circulation of the adult Djungarian hamster. *J. Pineal Res.* 16:136–144.

17 Human Exposure to Magnetic Fields: Effects on Melatonin, Hormones, and Immunity

Charles Graham
Michael Gibertini
  Midwest Research Institute, Kansas City, Missouri

Contents

Parsimonious Proposition: The Melatonin Hypothesis
Heterogeneity of Melatonin's Expression
  and Function
Current Research Program
Studies of Magnetic Field Exposure Effects
  on Melatonin
    Study 1
    Study 2
Discussion
Acknowledgments
References

Parsimonious Proposition: The Melatonin Hypothesis

The pineal neurohormone melatonin has been a focal point of research on the biological effects of electric and magnetic fields (EMF) since Stevens' (1987) proposition of the "melatonin hypothesis." In the past five years, this seminal paper has been cited over 50 times in the peer-reviewed literature. The hypothesis posits that EMF decreases pineal secretion of melatonin, a reduction that subsequently leads to a cascade of hormonal and immune-system changes relevant to the body's cancer-surveillance capacity. This hypothesis continues to capture the attention of researchers, because focus on a single hormone promises a parsimonious explanation of a variety of biological responses to EMF. In addition, the idea that pineal and retino-cortical systems are plausible sites of EMF action is consistent with many comparative studies on geomagnetic sensitivity in animals. Thus, the hypothesis represents a genuine synthesis of findings and proposals from many areas of biology. Its currency has increased in the past decade, as several of the chapters in this volume indicate.

The melatonin hypothesis assumes that melatonin influences the rhythms of reproductive hormones, especially estrogen and progesterone. Although data for this assumption are clear in lower animals, no such clarity exists in studies of humans. Studies have examined possible sex differences in melatonin secretion (e.g., Waldhauser et al. 1988 report no differences). Others have examined the relationship between melatonin, prolactin, and estrogen throughout the menstrual cycle (e.g., Brzezinski et al. 1988; Fernandez et al. 1990). Results have been conflicting. In the follicular phase, melatonin levels were positively correlated with both follicle-stimulating hormone and estradiol; in the luteal phase, melatonin levels were negatively correlated with progesterone and estradiol. Patterns for post-menopausal women were similar to those of women in the follicular phase.

Subsequent studies have involved either administering exogenous melatonin, or observing the correlations between melatonin and hormones. Exogenous melatonin increases prolactin in women (Cagnacci et al. 1991; Okatani et al. 1992; Terzolo et al. 1991, 1993), and there is some evidence that it does so in men as well (Waldhauser et al. 1987). In contrast, exogenous melatonin in rats decreases both prolactin and estradiol (Shah et al. 1984). The doses used in humans, however, provide serum concentrations above the physiological range. The role of endogenous melatonin in prolactin release in healthy men and women also is unclear. McIntyre et al. (1992) reported no changes in either prolactin or cortisol when melatonin was suppressed by bright light; however, the subjects were sleep-deprived, and prolactin is known to have both a sleep-dependent and a sleep-independent component to its circadian rhythm (Desir et al. 1982; Sassin et al. 1972). Melatonin may influence the sleep-independent component (Bispink et al. 1990; Okatani and Sagara 1993). In men, exogenous melatonin was associated with significant changes in the pattern of testosterone concentration (Terzolo et al. 1990).

The melatonin hypothesis also assumes that one effect of decreased melatonin secretion will be a change in the cancer-surveillance components of the immune system. Although direct evidence for this connection in humans is lacking, many studies converge to suggest that melatonin influences immunity both directly and through the mediation (to the extent such mediation is physiologically operational) of reproductive hormones. At physiological levels, melatonin stimulates the immune system (Maestroni 1993), and either surgical or functional pinealectomy affects major components of the immune system. Removal of the pineal gland causes involution of the thymus, decreased interleukin-2 (IL-2) production in spleen cells, and a concomitant down-regulation of natural killer cells (Del Gobbo et al. 1989). The circadian rhythm for activity of natural killer cells appears to follow melatonin, with an acrophase approximately 2 hours past that of melatonin (Angeli et al. 1988). Mice exposed to constant light or to the β-adrenergic blocker propranolol to reduce melatonin showed a depressed ability to mount a primary antibody response to sheep red blood cells, as well as decreased numbers of spleen cells (Maestroni and Pierpaoli 1981). Melatonin reversed a propranolol-induced decrease in spleen weight and reduced spleen cell blastogenesis in hamsters (Champney and McMurray 1991). Hansson et al. (1992) have demonstrated that exogenous melatonin exaggerates collagen-induced arthritis in mice, which involves T-cell-dependent autoimmunity. Interferon gamma (a cytokine released during expansion of T-cell clones) appears to increase pineal production of melatonin, providing a possible positive feedback link (Guerrero and Reiter 1992; Maestroni 1993; Withyachumnarnkul et al. 1990). The experimental evidence suggests that melatonin also may stimulate IL-2 production in activated T-helper cells. Release of this cytokine may be a first step in a cascade of melatonin-induced immune-system effects (Caroleo et al.

1992; Champney and McMurray 1991; Del Gobbo et al. 1989; Hansson et al. 1992; Maestroni and Conti 1990; Maestroni 1993).

It also should be noted that changes in reproductive hormones affect certain components of the immune system. Estrogen, for example, is a potent immunomodulator, with receptors expressed in many immune tissues. This may explain why, compared to men, women have heightened humoral immunity, greater graft rejection, and more susceptibility to autoimmune diseases. Some of these diseases (e.g., rheumatoid arthritis) are improved during the luteal phase of the menstrual cycle and during pregnancy (periods of high estrogens); other diseases (e.g., lupus) are made worse during this phase. Estrogen administration tends to decrease most components of cell-mediated immunity; antibody production in response to T-dependent antigens is enhanced, however. Estrogens also are potent stimulators of prolactin release. Prolactin itself is immuno-enhancing; it can restore the stress-induced decreases in lymphocyte proliferation. Chronically low levels of prolactin are associated with immunosuppression. Prolactin and cortisol tend to be inversely related, and it is well-established that cortisol tends to suppress nearly all immune components. These lines of evidence converge to suggest that one premise of the melatonin hypothesis—that melatonin may take part in the in vivo regulation of reproductive hormones and immunity—is valid and relevant to the EMF–cancer controversy.

As this discussion illustrates, Stevens' hypothesis suffers some ambiguity precisely because melatonin's role in important physiological systems is not well-described. The original hypothesis (Stevens 1987) and its subsequent elaboration (e.g., Wilson et al. 1989; Stevens 1992; Stevens 1995) are based on endocrine and immune-system interactions involving melatonin that have not been proved in humans. Further, the capacity of magnetic fields, especially power-frequency (50/60-Hz) magnetic fields, to have significant impact on the melatonin rhythm in humans is difficult to demonstrate. Field studies are plagued with problems of inadequate exposure characterization, sparse sampling of melatonin production, and the presence of confounders not easily dissociable from EMF exposure variables. Laboratory studies with human volunteers solve each of these problems through the use of specially designed exposure facilities that can deliver precisely characterized EMF in a controlled environment where physiological data can be frequently collected. But, laboratory studies are limited by the very intensity of their focus. Exposures are typically short-term (one to several nights), subjects are typically the least vulnerable in the population (healthy young males), and EMF exposure parameters must be worked out and verified empirically over separate experiments, each of which may take months to complete. Human-subject studies examining Stevens' hypothesis are, therefore, slow to accumulate and difficult to replicate.

Our research program at Midwest Research Institute ("Midwest") is designed to test several of the components of the melatonin hypothesis. Specifically, we have research in progress that will examine the melatonin rhythm in adult men and women during exposure to environmentally relevant levels of power-frequency magnetic fields. Our goal is to test Stevens' hypothesis and extend it by asking questions about exposure effects on physiology that do not involve melatonin, or do so only indirectly. Thus, direct exposure effects on reproductive hormone levels and rhythms is a second major focus of our program. The effect of field exposure on the circadian rhythm and overall functioning of the immune system is a third aim of this program. In pursuit of Stevens' hypothesis, we have designed studies to allow the examination of statistical models that posit an effect of EMF on hormones and immunity through the mediation of melatonin disturbance. Thus the research program will eventually illuminate many aspects of this important hypothesis.

It should be noted that the Midwest program is aimed at documenting the effects of short-term EMF exposures on the in vivo functioning of human hormonal and immune systems. Thus, in the experiments to date, subjects have spent one night in our facilities under EMF exposure (and, depending on the experiment, one more night under ambient conditions). Data from these studies represent a first and essential approach to testing the melatonin hypothesis in humans. If this minimal-impact but environmentally relevant EMF exposure proves potent in affecting any of the three physiological systems under investigation, then we will have a basis for describing the in vivo mechanisms by which chronic exposures may lead to health effects, such as cancer. If, on the other hand, short-term exposures are benign with respect to the levels or rhythms of melatonin, reproductive hormones, or immunity, then we will have demonstrated that the potency of EMF is well below that of known melatonin modulators (e.g., light-at-night, beta-blockers) that cause measurable changes in these systems.

HETEROGENEITY OF MELATONIN'S EXPRESSION AND FUNCTION

Melatonin's role in physiology changes across the phylogenetic scale (Arendt 1995). At the lower end of the scale, melatonin appears to control many physiological processes. Thus, basic events such as the timing of haircoat thickness, the timing of sexual activity, and the weight and size of the testes all depend on the melatonin signal. At the human level, however, melatonin has a more subtle role to play. It appears to function as a coordinator or facilitator, or as an interactive participant in multiple physiological processes.

Several interesting and potentially important differences exist between humans and the rodent, the most widely studied animal model. The anatomical location of the rodent pineal gland is peripheral in the brain just beneath the dura and skull; in the human, the gland is positioned deep inside the brain. It has been suggested that this difference may expose the rodent to eddy currents or to different and possibly stronger induced fields during exposure to power-frequency magnetic fields (Kato et al. 1993).

Bright light during the night suppresses melatonin. Rodents are more sensitive to light exposure than humans. In the nocturnally active rodent, a brief exposure at very low light levels will completely suppress melatonin (Reiter 1989). In humans, however, suppression typically requires a much longer duration exposure at significantly higher light levels (Lewy et al. 1980). But as can be seen in Figure 1, when light-induced suppression does occur in humans, it is neither complete nor very long-lasting. Figure 1 presents data for three volunteers who slept through the night in our laboratory on two occasions, once under dim-light (< 10 lux) control conditions, and once after exposure to very bright light (> 8000 lux) from 0200–0300 hours. Concentrations of melatonin measured in hourly plasma samples showed the expected circadian curve, with clear peaks during the

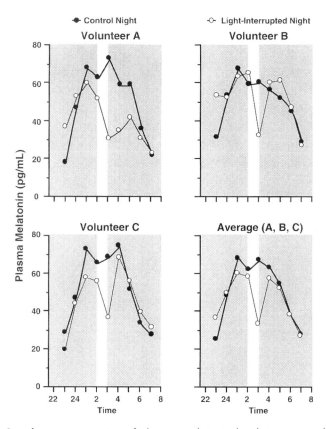

FIG. 1. Significant suppression of plasma melatonin levels is seen in these volunteers as a result of exposure to bright light (> 8000 lux) between 0200 and 0300 hours (open circles) compared to dim-light (< 10 lux) control conditions (dark circles). Within 2 hours, however, blood levels of melatonin return to control values.

dim-light control night. Exposure to bright light resulted in a significant suppression of melatonin with evidence of a rebound effect: Within 2 hours following exposure, melatonin concentrations soon approached and then began to track the dim-light control levels. More complex control mechanisms may be involved in light suppression in the human compared to the rodent. In this context, Monteleone et al. (1995) recently reported finding sex differences in the sensitivity of the human pineal gland to the suppressant effects of light. Women showed significantly greater reduction in plasma melatonin levels than men after equivalent exposure to bright light. Thus, important components of melatonin's secretion rhythm may be gender-dependent in humans. Finally, it should be recognized that there is a large degree of heterogeneity of melatonin secretion patterns, responsiveness to light, and role in reproduction and immunity across species and within humans. This heterogeneity complicates extrapolation of EMF results obtained in lower animals to the physiology of humans.

Perhaps the most striking distinction is not that humans differ from rodents, but that we differ so greatly from one another. People show very large individual differences in their typical nighttime peak melatonin levels, whereas rodents bred for laboratory studies do not (Reiter 1989). Figure 2 illustrates the broad range of individual peak melatonin levels (i.e., operationally defined as the level in blood at 0200 hours)

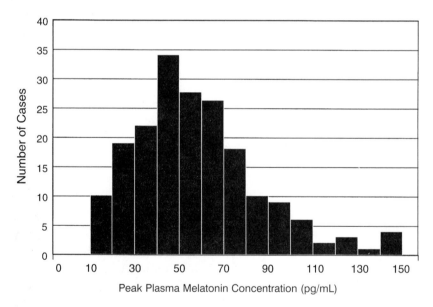

FIG. 2. Peak plasma melatonin concentrations vary widely in this sample of 192 healthy, young men. Peak levels in some volunteers are 15-fold greater than in other volunteers.

recently obtained on a sample of almost 200 healthy young men after each had been kept in the dark in our laboratory for 4 hours. As can be seen, peak levels in some of the volunteers are more than 15-fold greater than in other volunteers. Wetterberg (1993) has observed a genetic component to this phenomenon, with melatonin levels being more similar within than across families. Little is known about how such large differences in levels of this hormone affect individual health and well being.

Human melatonin levels also vary as a function of age. In general, levels are reported to be highest between 1 and 3 years old, decrease sharply until adolescence, remain fairly stable through adulthood, and finally begin a further decline after about age 50 (Waldhauser et al. 1988). There may be a much closer relationship, however, between age and melatonin level in adulthood than previously thought. In a recent study (Graham et al. 1994b), age proved to be the most powerful predictor of an individual's morning (0700 hours) melatonin level in a sample of male volunteers aged 18–35 years. Even within this limited range, age correlated negatively and significantly ($r = -52$, $p < 0.01$) with blood melatonin level (the older the volunteer, the lower the melatonin level). Several reports also suggest that peak melatonin levels in people may vary between the sexes, being relatively lower in women at the time of ovulation (Reiter 1989). If one is interested in determining whether EMF exposure reduces nocturnal levels of melatonin in the human, there is an obvious need to take into account these and other differences when designing human exposure studies.

CURRENT RESEARCH PROGRAM

A crucial link in the melatonin hypothesis, of course, is to determine if blood levels of melatonin are suppressed in people when they are exposed to power-frequency magnetic fields at night. Until recently, little data were available concerning the effects of exposure to 50- or 60-Hz magnetic fields on nocturnal melatonin levels in humans. In 1992, we began a series of human exposure studies to address the clear need for controlled, double-blind, laboratory-based research in this area. Our research to date has focused on evaluation of magnetic field effects on nocturnal melatonin in men; ongoing studies are now examining possible "downstream" influences of exposure on selected hormonal and immune measures in both male and female volunteers.

The work on melatonin is incorporated into and builds upon the capabilities of a larger EMF research program ongoing in our laboratory since 1982. Because environmental risk is often a function of effects that accumulate over time and interact with dose level, the goal of the larger program has been to determine if acute exposure to 60-Hz EMF has specific and reliable effects on well-established measures of human physiology, biochemistry, and performance. Studies are performed in the unique exposure test facility in our laboratory complex at Midwest. This is the only facility in the United States specifically designed for exposure research with human volunteers. Characteristics and control systems of this facility have been documented and are described in Cohen et al. (1992), Graham et al. (1994a), and Dietrich et al. (1995). The facility is designed to present uniform, 60-Hz electric (0–16 kV/m) and magnetic (0–400 mG) fields under controlled conditions of ambient temperature and relative humidity. Horizontal, vertical, and rotating magnetic fields can be presented separately or in conjunction with the electric field. Electric, magnetic, and combined fields can be presented either continuously or in a variety of intermittent patterns. Recent measurements indicate the geomagnetic field density in the facility is 380 mG at an inclination of 78.7° north.

The facility has two capabilities that make it unique. The first is a double-blind control system that allows volunteers to be exposed to real or sham fields without either the volunteers or experimenters being aware of which condition is in effect at any given time. Thus, effects due to field exposure can be distinguished from effects due to an individual's expectations about exposure. The facility also is capable of recording human physiological activity during, as well as before and after, exposure to high-voltage fields. This capability aids in tracking the time course of any effects observed. Multiple double-blind studies have now been performed in the facility under the larger research program. These studies have evaluated exposure effects at different levels of combined electric and magnetic field strength, and under both constant and intermittent exposure conditions. Field exposure has repeatedly resulted in statistically significant changes in measures of cardiovascular and central nervous system activity, and in performance decrements on tests of reaction time and time perception. Effects have been seen more clearly at certain combinations or "windows" of field strength, and individuals appear to differ in their sensitivity to the fields. (For details of this research, see Cook et al. 1992; Graham et al. 1987, 1990, 1994a.)

STUDIES OF MAGNETIC FIELD EXPOSURE EFFECTS ON MELATONIN

This section describes our first two double-blind, laboratory-based investigations of magnetic field exposure effects on nocturnal melatonin levels in human volunteers. Additional information on these studies can be found in Graham et al. 1994b, 1995, 1996, in press.

Study 1

In the first melatonin study conducted at Midwest, the effects of intermittent exposure to circularly polarized magnetic fields at 10 and 200 mG were compared to sham control. Previous work had indicated that intermittent exposure was an effective exposure condition in altering measures of human brain and heart activity (Graham et al. 1990). A field strength of 200 mG was selected because we have repeatedly found effects on a variety of endpoints at this level (Cook et al. 1992; Graham et al. 1994a). The comparison field strength of 10 mG was selected because it is a level often found in homes and workplaces. Comparison across field strengths is important, because it addresses a major concern people have about exposure to power-frequency magnetic fields.

The participation of volunteers in this study, as in all of our research with human volunteers, was reviewed and approved beforehand by the appropriate Institutional Review Board, and the study was conducting in accordance with Federal guidelines and regulations (Federal Register 1991). All subjects provided written informed consent. Because melatonin levels vary widely across people, the subjects were first screened to determine their basal peak melatonin level prior to exposure, and to measure their sensitivity to bright light, the known suppressor of melatonin. After screening, subjects were matched in triads on normal peak melatonin levels, and the members of each triad were randomly assigned to the 10-mG, 200-mG, or sham-control conditions. On the test night, each subject slept in the exposure facility from 2300–0700 hours. Blood samples were obtained every hour for determination of melatonin concentration.

Forty-two healthy young men participated in the screening sessions. Groups of two to four men came to the laboratory at 2200 hours. They slept in the dark from 2230–0200 hours. On one night, they were exposed under controlled test conditions to bright light (5500 lux) between 0200 and 0300 hours. On the other night, they remained awake in dim light (10 lux) from 0200–0300 hours. Blood samples were obtained at 0200 and 0300 hours. Half of the men were exposed to light on the first night, and half were exposed to light on the second night. The 0200-hour blood samples provided a measure of normal peak melatonin level prior to exposure, and the 0300-hour samples obtained after light exposure provided information about each individual's sensitivity to the known suppressor of melatonin.

Statistical analysis revealed that across the two sessions, melatonin levels at 0200 were very stable within an individual ($r = 0.92$, $p < 0.001$). No difference in 0200-hour melatonin levels was found between the sessions. Thus, while melatonin levels may vary between people, there is a high degree of consistency within a person. Melatonin level at 0300 hours was significantly suppressed by light exposure, as expected ($F = 93.34$, df 3,90, $p < 0.001$). Suppression by light, however, was not equal across the sample. Over these 42 men, suppression ranged from 20–90%. The distribution was normal, with most people showing suppression in the order of 50–70%. Further analysis provided evidence of an interesting relationship between basal melatonin level and percent melatonin suppression by light. Men with pre-existing low levels of melatonin at 0200 hours showed significantly greater melatonin suppression when exposed to light compared to men with high 0200-hour melatonin levels ($r = -0.36$, $p < 0.01$). We were, of course, interested in determining whether such a relationship also existed between basal melatonin level and suppression when the men were exposed to the magnetic field.

Thirty-three of the men who completed the screening sessions also participated in the experimental sessions; the mean age of the subjects was 23 years. They were predominantly white (97%), nonsmoking (88%) men of average height (70.7 in; 179.6 cm) and weight (171.5 lb;

77.8 kg). None of the subjects had irregular sleep habits, and they slept, on the average, 7 hours/night. The 11 men in the sham-control condition slept under ambient field conditions (< 2 mG); 11 men were exposed to an intermittent magnetic field at 10 mG, and 11 men were exposed to an intermittent, 200-mG field. The magnetic field was presented in alternating, 1-hour "field-on" and "field-off" periods. During field-on periods, the magnetic field cycled on and off every 15 seconds. During field-off periods, the exposure system was not energized. When intermittent exposure was used, gating circuits switched on when the AC voltage was at zero and switched off when the AC current was at zero. This type of zero-crossing characteristic produced field changes relatively free of transients. The study was performed double-blind, and neither subjects nor experimenters were able to judge at better-than-chance levels whether fields had or had not been activated during the night.

Analysis of variance revealed no significant difference (F = 0.25, df 2,30, p = 0.78) in melatonin levels between the sham control and the two exposure test groups. Because men in the pre-exposure screening sessions with low 0200-hour melatonin levels showed greater suppression to light, the study sample was divided at the median into "High" and "Low" melatonin groups based on the 0200-hour melatonin values from the screening nights. Analysis of variance incorporating this split as a between-subjects variable was performed. A significant interaction involving exposure group by time and peak melatonin level was found (F = 2.71, df 14,189, p = 0.035), indicating that magnetic field exposure had differential effects on the High and Low subgroups. Further analyses of variance were performed on the High and Low groups separately. No significant effects involving field exposure were found for the High group. For the Low group, changes in melatonin over the night were significantly different for the sham and the two exposure groups (F = 2.54, df 14,91, p = 0.043). Figure 3 illustrates the results observed. Further analyses of variance were performed to compare the 200-mG group directly with the sham group, and directly with the 10-mG group. These analyses revealed that, within the Low melatonin subjects, those exposed to the 200-mG magnetic field showed significantly lower levels of nocturnal melatonin compared to either sham (F = 3.53, df 7,56, p = 0.018) or 10-mG

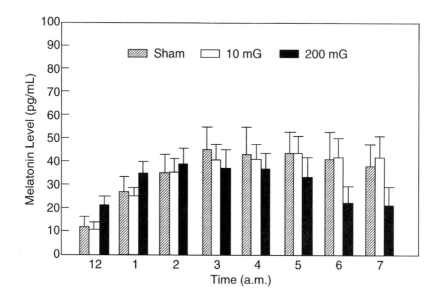

FIG. 3. Magnetic field exposure effects in healthy, young men with pre-existing low levels of melatonin. Mean melatonin level and SE are plotted from midnight to 0700 hours for control and test conditions. Low-melatonin volunteers exposed to the 200-mG magnetic field showed significantly lower levels of nocturnal melatonin compared to either sham-control (p = 0.018) or 10-mG exposure conditions (p = 0.03). Peak levels of melatonin were reduced during 200-mG exposure, as were levels in the latter portion of the exposure night.

subjects (F = 3.81, df 7,63, p = 0.03). Peak levels of melatonin were reduced during exposure, as were levels in the latter portion of the exposure night. The 10-mG group did not differ from the sham-control group (F = 0.155, df 7,63, p = 0.89).

The finding that men with low melatonin levels showed both greater suppression to light and greater suppression in response to 200-mG field exposure than those with high levels could have important implications for epidemiologic and occupational research on effects of magnetic field exposure, as well as for future studies of the biological mechanisms of EMF effects. The results provide partial support for the melatonin hypothesis, and they extend the focus of research from the rodent to the intact, functioning human being. Since the results were based on analysis of subsets of subjects, and the major finding had not been predicted in advance, it was also quite possible that the results were simply due to chance alone. Therefore, it was important to perform another study to directly test the hypothesis that men with pre-existing low melatonin levels are more sensitive to both light and magnetic field exposure than those with high pre-existing melatonin levels.

Study 2

Study 2 used a more powerful experimental design in which each subject served as his own control in addition to a larger control sample of volunteers. When suppression of melatonin has been observed in animal exposure studies, it is typically a 25–30% reduction. Statistical power analysis indicated that a sample of 40 volunteers would provide statistical power greater than 0.80 of detecting a similar degree of suppression in melatonin in humans at the 0.05 level of significance. Fifty-two healthy young men initially were screened to determine melatonin level at 0200 hours and light sensitivity prior to magnetic field exposure. As in Study 1, a broad range of individual melatonin levels at 0200 hours was observed (15–122 pg/mL). Exposure to bright light (5500 lux) had the expected effect of markedly suppressing melatonin. At 0200 hours, the mean melatonin concentration was 50.9 pg/mL; after light exposure, the mean was 22.3 pg/mL (t = 12.16, df 51, p < 0.0001). Again, individual differences in suppression of melatonin by light were observed. Percent suppression ranged from 20–80%. The observation in Study 1 that men with low 0200-hour melatonin concentration showed greater suppression, however, was not replicated. In fact, there was a significant positive correlation between 0200-hour levels and suppression (r = 0.32, p < 0.02), indicating that those individuals with higher levels of melatonin at 0200 hours had greater suppression than those with lower levels.

Forty of the volunteers participated in the experimental sessions. The mean age was 22 years. They were predominantly white (95%), nonsmoking (90%) men of average height (70.8 in; 179.8 cm) and weight (175.8 lb; 79.7 kg). They reported regular sleep patterns of 7–8 hours/night. Each man slept in the facility twice. One night was a sham-control night; on the other night, subjects were exposed to the same 200-mG, circularly polarized, intermittent magnetic field used in Study 1. On both nights, blood samples were drawn every hour for quantification of melatonin concentration. Order of sham control and exposure was counterbalanced, and the study was performed double-blind. Neither subjects nor experimenters could judge at better-than-chance levels which night was the exposure night.

Figure 4 shows mean levels and standard errors of melatonin concentration for both sham control and exposure nights. As in the first study, sham-control and field-exposure nights were not significantly different from one another. To test the hypothesis that men with low levels of melatonin showed reduced melatonin as a function of exposure to the 200-mG field, subjects were split into Low and High groups

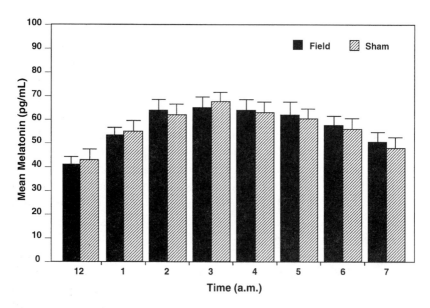

FIG. 4. Repeated measurements of plasma melatonin in 40 healthy, young men under sham-control conditions and again under magnetic field exposure conditions at 200 mG. Mean melatonin level and SE are plotted for each hour from midnight to 0700 hours. Blood levels of melatonin on sham-control and field-exposure nights were not significantly different.

based on the 0200-hour melatonin level on the screening night. The hypothesis was not supported. Neither the High nor the Low group showed significant effects of exposure to the magnetic field. Even when subjects were divided into extreme groups (0200-hour values > 60 pg/mL versus those < 41 pg/mL), no effects of field exposure were identified.

DISCUSSION

Field-related suppression of nocturnal levels of the hormone melatonin has been hypothesized to be a possible biological mechanism linking occupational and residential exposure to magnetic fields and increased cancer risk. Results of the two studies reported here do not support this hypothesis; under the field conditions used, no significant differences between sham control and field exposure were found. Results also failed to support the hypothesis derived from Study 1 that men with pre-existing low levels of melatonin show significantly greater suppression of melatonin when exposed to light and to the 200-mG magnetic field condition. Study 2 may not have provided the best situation in which to examine the interaction between basal melatonin level and sensitivity. The volunteers were young and the age distributions were restricted (e.g., 80% of the men in Study 2 were 18–22 years of age). This factor, together with differences across studies in the level and distribution of pre-exposure melatonin values, may have masked the possibility of observing a relationship.

Clarification of the concept of dose has come to be recognized as a central issue of general importance to researchers, risk analysts, and engineers. These initial studies used exposure conditions shown in earlier work to produce biological responses (Graham et al. 1990). Given the paucity of research in this area, however, arguments could as easily have been made for the selection of other exposure conditions. To fully understand the effects of magnetic field exposure on melatonin levels in humans, it is necessary to examine the effects of exposure to fields with other characteristics. In an industrialized society, magnetic field exposures from power-distribution systems consist of several components: the 50- or 60-Hz fundamental power frequency that is present at all times; harmonics; and "transient" events that result from normal utility operations, such as switching events, opening or closing of capacitor banks, etc. Transients also can result from the switching on and off of loads, whether residential or industrial. Recently, transients with a high-frequency content (ranging from several kHz to 10 MHz) have been measured in homes (Guttman et al. 1994). Biophysical calculations using realistic models of cells have shown that some of these transient events can induce transmembrane voltage changes in model cells that exceed thermal noise (Sastre et al. 1994; Vaughan and Weaver 1994). Therefore, these events can, in principal, affect biological systems. Reports by Lerchl et al. (1991), and more recently by Rogers et al. (1995), suggest that exposures involving transients produced by rapid field on/off conditions may reduce melatonin concentrations in the rat and the baboon. It should be noted that the zero-crossing technique used in our first two studies was designed to produce intermittent exposure conditions while specifically minimizing the presence of transients. Thus, the effects of transient fields, which are relevant both to power-distribution systems and to the use of common electrical appliances, need to be examined in humans. Similarly, brief daytime exposure has been reported to produce alterations in nocturnal melatonin levels in rodents (Yellon 1993). It is important to determine if daytime exposure has a similar influence on nocturnal levels of melatonin in humans.

The melatonin hypothesis is particularly relevant to women, and the initial studies summarized here were carried out in men. Ongoing research in our laboratory is now examining exposure effects on melatonin and other hormones in women as well as men. Few published studies in either rodents or humans directly address the relationship between EMF-related suppression of melatonin and changes in reproductive hormones. In 1978, Cohen et al. reported that melatonin inhibits ovarian estrogen production, and Stevens' (1987) hypothesis was based partly on this observation. We will be examining this relationship in detail in forthcoming experiments.

The present studies have helped us begin to understand what happens to melatonin in people exposed to magnetic fields at night. Further research is needed in several areas. It is important to obtain data on the interactions between specific magnetic field exposure parameters, melatonin, reproductive hormones, and immune function to identify the most plausible mechanisms by which exposure may increase the risk of cancer. Studies now ongoing in our laboratory are examining these relationships in both men and women. An important goal of these studies is to explore the possibility that EMF exposure affects the immune system, and thereby lowers the body's defense against cancer, either through melatonin or through some more direct route. To date, our research program has focused on short-term nocturnal exposures to environmentally relevant levels of EMF exposure. Effects of EMF exposure in vivo, however, may depend on when in the 24-hour day exposure occurs. Future studies will examine longer-term and daytime exposures, as well. We are still very much intrigued by the possibility that individual differences in peak melatonin level may be related to enhanced sensitivity or to differential immune responsivity. Further exploration is warranted.

We recently completed construction of new laboratory facilities capable of housing human volunteers over multiple days and presenting a variety of EMF exposure conditions at different frequencies and amplitudes. Multiple physiological, biochemical, and behavioral endpoints can be collected under controlled environmental test conditions. With these tools and the benefit of several recent studies with human volunteers from our laboratory and others, we hope to be able to better understand the possible interaction of EMF with human physiological systems in the near future.

ACKNOWLEDGMENTS

The research studies described in this chapter were supported by the Electric Power Research Institute under Contract No. WO4307, Dr. Robert Kavet, Project Officer. Manuscript preparation and additional research was supported by National Institute of Environmental Health Sciences Grant No. ES07053 to the senior author, and by Midwest Research Institute. The authors wish to thank members of the Biobehavioral Sciences Section who help make this research possible: Dr. Mary R. Cook, Section Head; Harvey D. Cohen, Biomedical Engineer; Donald W. Riffle, Night Supervisor; Nancy E. Phelps, Research Nurse; Deb Smith, Bioassays; Steve Hoffman, Programmer; and Mary M. Gerkovich, Biostatistics.

REFERENCES

Angeli, A., G. Gatti, D. Sartori, D. Del Ponte, R. Carignola. 1988. Effects of exogenous melatonin on human natural killer (NK) cell activity. An approach to the immunomodulatory role of the pineal gland. In: *The Pineal Gland and Cancer*, D. Gupta, A. Attanasio, and R.J. Reiter, eds., pp. 145–156. London: Brain Research Promotion.

Arendt, J. 1995. *Melatonin and the Mammalian Pineal Gland*. London: Chapman and Hall.

Bispink, G., R. Zimmermann, H.C. Weise, F. Leidenberger. 1990. Influence of melatonin on the sleep-independent component of prolactin secretion. *J. Pineal Res.* 8:97–106.

Brzezinski, A., H.J. Lynch, M.M. Seibel, M.H. Deng, T.M. Nader, R.J. Wurtman. 1988. The circadian rhythm of plasma melatonin during the normal menstrual cycle and in amenorrheic women. *J. Clin. Endocrinol. & Metab.* 66:891–895.

Cagnacci, A., J.A. Elliott, S.S. Yen. 1991. Amplification of pulsatile LH secretion by exogenous melatonin in women. *J. Clin. Endocrinol. & Metab.* 73:210–212.

Caroleo, M.C., G. Nistico, G. Doria. 1992. Effect of melatonin on the immune system. *Pharmacol. Res.* 26(2):34–37.

Champney, T.H., D.N. McMurray. 1991. Spleen morphology and lymphoproliferative activity in short photoperiod exposed hamsters. In: *Role of Melatonin and Pineal Peptides in Neuroimmunomodulation*, F. Fraschini and R.J. Reiter, eds., pp. 219–223. New York: Plenum Press.

Cohen M., M. Lippman, B. Chabner. 1978. Role of pineal gland in aetiology and treatment of breast cancer. *Lancet* 2(8094):814–816.

Cohen, H.D., C. Graham, M.R. Cook, J.W. Phelps. 1992. ELF exposure facility for human testing. *Bioelectromagnetics* 13:169–182.

Cook, M.R., C. Graham, H.D. Cohen, M.M. Gerkovich. 1992. A replication study of human exposure to 60-Hz Fields. 1. Effects on neurobehavioral measures. *Bioelectromagnetics* 13:261–285.

Deitrich, F., A. Sastre, H.D. Cohen, P. Doinov, C. Graham. 1995. Evaluation of high frequency magnetic field transients in the MRI human exposure facilities. In: Abstracts of the Annual Review of Research on Biological Effects of Electric and Magnetic Fields from the Generation, Delivery, and Use of Electricity, November 12–16, Palm Springs, California, pp. 83–84.

Del Gobbo, V., V. Libri, N. Villani, R. Calio, G. Nistico. 1989. Pinealectomy inhibits interleukin-2 production and natural killer activity in mice. *Int. J. Immunopharmacol.* 11:567–573.

Desir, D., E.Van Cauter, M. L'Hermite, S. Refetoff, C. Jadot, A. Caufriez, G. Copinschi, C. Robyn. 1982. Effects of "jet lag" on hormonal patterns. III. Demonstration of an intrinsic circadian rhythmicity in plasma prolactin. *J. Clin. Endocrinol. & Metab.* 55:849–857.

Federal Register. 1991. Federal policy for the protection of human subjects: Notices and rules. 56:(117).

Fernandez, B., J.L. Malde, A. Montero, D. Acuna. 1990. Relationship between adenohypophyseal and steroid hormones and variations in serum and urinary melatonin levels during the ovarian cycle, perimenopause and menopause in healthy women. *J. Steroid Biochem.* 35:257–262.

Graham, C., H.D. Cohen, M.R. Cook, J.W. Phelps, M.M. Gerkovich, S.S. Fotopoulos. 1987. *A Double-Blind Evaluation of 60-Hz Field Effects on Human Performance, Physiology, and Subjective State.* CONF-841041. Springfield, Virginia: NTIS.

Graham, C., M.R. Cook, H.D. Cohen. 1990. *Final Report: Immunological and Biochemical Effects of 60-Hz Electric and Magnetic Fields in Humans.* Report No. DE90006671. Springfield, Virginia: NTIS.

Graham, C., M.R. Cook, H.D. Cohen, M.M. Gerkovich. 1994a. A dose response study of human exposure to 60-Hz electric and magnetic fields. *Bioelectromagnetics* 15:447–463.

Graham, C., M.R. Cook, H.D. Cohen. 1994b. *Investigation of the Effects of Magnetic Field Exposure on Human Melatonin.* Report No. TR-104278, Palo Alto, California: Electric Power Research Institute (EPRI).

Graham, C., M.R. Cook, H.D. Cohen. 1995. *Human Melatonin in Magnetic Fields: Second Study.* Report No. TR-105766, Palo Alto, California: Electric Power Research Institute (EPRI).

Graham, C., M.R. Cook, D.W. Riffle, M.M. Gerkovich, H.D. Cohen. 1996. Nocturnal melatonin levels in human volunteers exposed to intermittent 60-Hz magnetic fields. *Bioelectromagnetics* 17(4):263–273.

Graham, C., M.R. Cook, D.W. Riffle. Human melatonin during continuous magnetic field exposure. *Bioelectromagnetics* (in press).

Guerrero, J.M., R. Reiter. 1992. A brief survey of pineal gland–immune system interrelationships. *Endocrine Res.* 18:91–113.

Guttman, J.L., J.C. Niple, J.M. Silva. 1994. Transient data acquisition system used in the California pilot study: A series of 24-hour measurements of transient magnetic fields performed in 21 residences. In: Abstracts of the Annual Review of Research on Biological Effects of Electric and Magnetic Fields from the Generation, Delivery and Use of Electricity, Albuquerque, New Mexico, November 6–10, A-51, pp. 57–58. Frederick, Maryland: W/L Associates, Ltd.

Hansson, I., R. Holmdahl, R. Mattsson. 1992. The pineal hormone melatonin exaggerates development of collagen-induced arthritis in mice. *J. Neuroimmunol.* 39:23–30.

Kato, M., K. Honma, T. Shigemitsu, Y. Shiga. 1993. Effects of exposure to a circularly polarized 50-Hz magnetic field on plasma and pineal melatonin levels in rats. *Bioelectromagnetics* 14:97–106.

Lerchl, A., K.O. Nonaka, R.J. Reiter. 1991. Pineal gland "magnetosensitivity" to static magnetic fields is a consequence of induced electric currents (eddy currents). *J. Pineal. Res.* 10:109–116.

Lewy, A.J., T.A. Wehr, F.K. Goodwin, D.A. Newsome, S.P. Markey. 1980. Light suppresses melatonin secretion in humans. *Science* 210:1267–1269.

Maestroni, G.J.M. 1993. The immunoneuroendocrine role of melatonin. *J. Pineal Res.* 14:1–10.

Maestroni, G.J., A. Conti. 1990. The pineal neurohormone melatonin stimulates activated CD4+, Thy-1+ cells to release opioid agonist(s) with immunoenhancing and anti-stress properties. *J. Neuroimmunol.* 28:167–176.

Maestroni, G.J.M., W. Pierpaoli. 1981. Pharmacological control of the hormonally mediated immune response. In: *Psychoneuroimmunology*, R. Ader, ed., pp. 405–425. New York: Academic Press.

McIntyre, I.M., T.R. Norman, G.D. Burrows, S.M. Armstrong. 1992. Melatonin, cortisol, and prolactin response to acute nocturnal light exposure in healthy volunteers. *Psychoneuroendocrinology* 17:243–248.

Montelone, P., G. Esposito, A. La Rocca, M. Maj. 1995. Does bright light suppress nocturnal melatonin secretion more in women than men? *J. Neural Transm. Gen. Sect.* 102:75–80.

Okatani, Y., Y. Sagara. 1993. Role of melatonin in nocturnal prolactin secretion in women with normoprolactinemia and mild hyperprolactinemia. *Am. J. Obstet. Gynecol.* 168:854–861.

Okatani, Y., M. Okada, Y. Sagara. 1992. Amplification of nocturnal melatonin secretion in women with nocturnal hyperprolactinemia. *Asia Oceania J. Obstet. Gynaecol.* 18:289–297.

Reiter, R.J. 1989. The pineal gland. In: *Endocrinology*, 2nd Ed. Vol. 1, L.J. DeGroot, ed., Chapter 20. Philadelphia: Saunders.

Rogers, W.R., R.J. Reiter, H.D. Smith, L. Barlow-Walden. 1995. Rapid onset/offset, variably-scheduled 60-Hz electric and magnetic field exposure reduces nocturnal serum melatonin concentration in non-human primates. *Bioelectromagnetics* Suppl. 3:119–122.

Sassin, J.F., A.G. Franz, E.D. Weitzman, S. Kapen. 1972. Human prolactin: 24-hour pattern with increased release during sleep. *Science* 177:1205–1207.

Sastre, A.R., R. Kavet, J.L. Guttman, J.C. Weaver. 1994. Residential magnetic field transients: How do their induced transmembrane voltages compare to thermal noise? In: Abstracts of the Annual Review of Research on Biological Effects of Electric and Magnetic Fields from the Generation, Delivery and Use of Electricity, Albuquerque, New Mexico, November 6–10, A-51, pp. 33–34. Frederick, Maryland: W/L Associates, Ltd.

Shah, P.N., M.C. Mhatre, L.S. Kothari. 1984. Effect of melatonin on mammary carcinogenesis in intact and pinealectomized rats in varying photoperiods. *Cancer Res.* 44:3403–3407.

Stevens, R.G. 1987. Electric power use and breast cancer: A hypothesis. *Am. J. Epidemiol.* 125:556–561.

Stevens, R.G. 1992. Use of electric blankets and risk of postmenopausal breast cancer. *Am. J. Epidemiol.* 135(7):834–835.

Stevens, R.G. 1995. Risk of premenopausal breast cancer and use of electric blankets. *Am. J. Epidemiol.* 42(4):446–446.

Terzolo, M., A. Piovesan, B. Puligheddu, M. Torta, G. Osella, P. Paccotti, A. Angeli. 1990. Effects of long-term, low-dose, time-specified melatonin administration on endocrine and cardiovascular variables in adult men. *J. Pineal Res.* 9:113–124.

Terzolo, M., A. Piovesan, G. Osella, M. Torta, T. Buniva, P. Paccotti, T. Wierdis, A. Angeli. 1991. Exogenous melatonin enhances the

TRH-induced prolactin release in normally cycling women: A sex-specific effect. *Gynecol. Endocrinol.* 5:83–94.

Terzolo, M., A. Revelli, D. Guidetti, A. Piovesan, P. Cassoni, P. Paccotti, A. Angeli, M. Massobrio. 1993. Evening administration of melatonin enhances the pulsatile secretion of prolactin but not of LH and TSH in normally cycling women. *Clin. Endocrinol.* (Oxf.) 39:185–191.

Vaughan, T.E., J.C. Weaver. 1994. Magnetite-mediated pore creation: Rare magnetic field events may be able to cause biological effects. In: Abstracts of the Annual Review of Research on Biological Effects of Electric and Magnetic Fields from the Generation, Delivery and Use of Electricity, Albuquerque, New Mexico, November 6–10, A-51, pp. 84–85. Frederick, Maryland: W/L Associates, Ltd.

Waldhauser, F., H.R. Lieberman, H.J. Lynch, M. Waldhauser, K. Herkner, H. Frisch, H. Vierhapper, W. Waldhause, M. Schemper, R.J. Wurtman, W.F. Crowley. 1987. A pharmacological dose of melatonin increases PRL levels in males without altering those of GH, LH, FSH, TSH, testosterone, or cortisol. *Neuroendocrinology* 46:125–130.

Waldhauser, F., G. Weiszenbacher, E. Tatzer, B. Gisinger, M. Waldhauser, M. Schemper, H. Frisch. 1988. Alterations in nocturnal serum melatonin levels in humans with growth and aging. *J. Clin. Endocrinol. & Metab.* 66:648–652.

Wetterberg, L. 1993. *Light and Biological Rhythms in Man.* New York: Pergamon Press.

Wilson, B.W., R.G. Stevens, L.E. Anderson. 1989. Neuroendocrine mediated effects of electromagnetic-field exposure: Possible role of the pineal gland. *Life Sci.* 45:1319–1332.

Withyachumnarnkul, B., K.O. Nonaka, C. Santana, A.M. Attia, R.J. Reiter. 1990. Interferon-gamma modulates melatonin production in rat pineal glands in organ culture. *J Interferon Res.* 10:403–411.

Yellon, S.M. 1993. Replication studies of the effect of an acute 60 Hz magnetic field exposure on the nighttime melatonin rhythm in the adult Djungarian hamster. In: Abstracts of the Annual Review of Research on Biological Effects of Electric and Magnetic Fields from the Generation, Delivery, and Use of Electricity, Savannah, Georgia, October 31–November 4, A-29. Frederick, Maryland: W/L Associates, Ltd.

18 60-Hz Magnetic Field Exposure Effects on the Melatonin Rhythm in the Djungarian Hamster

STEVEN M. YELLON

Loma Linda University School of Medicine and
Center for Perinatal Biology, Loma Linda, California

CONTENTS

MELATONIN RHYTHMS: A CLOCK-CONTROLLED MEDIATOR
  OF SEASONAL REPRODUCTION
MAGNETIC FIELD EXPOSURE EFFECTS ON PINEAL MELATONIN
ANIMAL MODEL AND METHOD FOR STUDIES OF
  MAGNETIC FIELD EXPOSURE EFFECTS
REPLICATE STUDIES OF ACUTE MAGNETIC FIELD EXPOSURES
  ON THE MELATONIN RHYTHM IN LONG-DAY HAMSTERS
REPLICATE STUDIES OF ACUTE MAGNETIC FIELD EXPOSURES
  ON THE MELATONIN RHYTHM IN SHORT-DAY HAMSTERS
EFFECTS OF DAILY MAGNETIC FIELD EXPOSURES ON THE
  MELATONIN RHYTHM AND REPRODUCTIVE FUNCTION
  IN SHORT DAYS
OTHER STUDIES FAIL TO SUPPORT A MAGNETIC FIELD
  EXPOSURE
PROGRESS AND CONCLUSIONS
ACKNOWLEDGMENTS
REFERENCES

MELATONIN RHYTHMS: A CLOCK-CONTROLLED
MEDIATOR OF SEASONAL REPRODUCTION

The production of melatonin, a pineal gland hormone, is directly regulated by day length. Melatonin synthesis by the pineal gland, as well as its concentration in serum, dramatically increases at night and remains elevated for the duration of darkness. During the day, pineal melatonin content and serum concentrations are typically low or near the limits of detection. This rise and fall in pineal melatonin production and its appearance in peripheral blood also occur when animals are in constant darkness. For this reason, the melatonin pattern over the course of a 24-hour day is considered a circadian rhythm.

Duration of the nocturnal rise in melatonin is recognized as a physiologically significant feature of the rhythm. The nighttime increase in circulating melatonin is proportional to the hours of darkness (Goldman and Elliott 1988; Karsch et al. 1991); it is abbreviated during the short nights of summer (long days) but extended during the long nights of winter (short days). As Reiter (1993b) has specified, this rise in melatonin serves as a clock and a calendar to convey information about time of day and season, respectively. In many species, it is the duration of the nighttime melatonin rise in circulation, not necessarily the pineal gland content or a concentration in circulation at a particular time of day, that regulates seasonal physiological processes, especially those related to reproduction. Studies in sheep and rodents have clearly demonstrated that the melatonin rhythm mediates the effects of photoperiod to control annual cycles of reproduction and infertility (Karsch et al. 1991; Bartness et al. 1993). Thus, melatonin currently is the only known hormone whose physiological function depends on its circadian rhythm in circulation.

The neural mechanism that controls the circadian melatonin rhythm involves an endogenous clock. The rise and fall of the melatonin rhythm depends on the activity of a population of neurons in the suprachiasmatic nuclei of the anterior hypothalamus. This group of neurons is viewed as the master oscillator that generates circadian rhythms (Illnerová 1991). In a variety of species, this endogenous biological clock is directly influenced by only a limited number of factors in the environment. It is well-recognized that photoperiod is the predominant environmental stimulus that affects circadian rhythms. By way of a retinohypothalamic pathway, light suppresses and entrains the various functions of the clock, including the circadian melatonin rhythm (Card and Moore 1991). This ability of light to specifically influence the circadian pineal melatonin rhythm directly depends on neural input from the retina to suprachiasmatic nuclei. Other considerations are known to modulate the amplitude of the 24-hour pattern of melatonin in circulation, including diet (Anderson et al. 1990; Berga et al. 1993), exercise or reproductive status (Laughlin et al. 1991; Monteleone et al. 1990), mood (Claustrat et al. 1984), and age (Waldhauser et al. 1988). Whether influences on amplitude of the melatonin rhythm have physiological consequences remains to be determined. Currently, the duration of pineal melatonin production is the only characteristic of the melatonin rhythm that is both regulated by the endogenous biological clock and known to mediate seasonal physiological processes.

MAGNETIC FIELD EXPOSURE EFFECTS ON PINEAL MELATONIN

Photoperiod has already been mentioned as a potent influence on circadian rhythms, including its affect on regulating pineal melatonin rhythm. For more than a decade, evidence has suggested that another factor in the environment with potential health risks (Stevens et al. 1992) may suppress the nighttime rise in melatonin. In a number of rodent species, exposures to electric or magnetic fields are reported to attenuate the nighttime increase in pineal melatonin production (Wilson et al. 1981, 1983; Reiter et al. 1988, 1993). Near Earth-strength inversions of the magnetic field significantly depress the nocturnal production of pineal melatonin and the activity of N-acetyltransferase (NAT), the rate-limiting enzyme for melatonin synthesis (Welker et al. 1983; Lerchl et al. 1990; Selmaoui and Touitou 1995). Magnetic field-induced reduction in pineal NAT in rats has been duplicated in other species, including albino gerbils, and albino and hooded rats, but this result has not been replicated in pigmented gerbils or Syrian hamsters (Olcese and Reuss 1986; Stehle et al. 1988).

It is hard to reconcile the fact that evidence which suggests magnetic field exposures depress the nocturnal pineal melatonin rhythm and/or NAT activity has been found in some (Lerchl et al. 1990; Olcese and Reuss 1986; Stehle et al. 1988; Welker et al. 1983) but not in other (Khoory 1987; Lerchl et al. 1990; Reuss et al. 1985) studies. Effects on the pineal melatonin response to a magnetic field may depend on specific dose or field strength parameters, or on the vector of the applied field (vertical or horizontal components). Other significant differences exist among the studies cited, involving, for example, exposure systems, treatment parameters (e.g., type of field, dose, duration, time of day), and frequency of blood sampling to define the melatonin rhythm. Diversity in experimental animal models may confound interpretation of magnetic field exposure effects; comparisons among different ages and regarding responsiveness to photoperiod, as well as the lack of replication in these studies are likely to render generalizations about the biological effects of magnetic field exposure on the nighttime concentration of melatonin in the pineal gland too simplistic.

ANIMAL MODEL AND METHOD FOR STUDIES OF MAGNETIC FIELD EXPOSURE EFFECTS

In our effort to investigate whether magnetic field exposures produce physiologically relevant consequences, it was important to choose an animal model with clearly defined parameters of melatonin production, its rhythm in circulation, and its biological function. For most of the studies already mentioned, nonseasonal breeders were exposed to a variety of magnetic field treatments. In species with limited photoperiodic responses, the role of melatonin or its rhythm in circulation for normal endocrine physiology has not been well-established. However, for the seasonally breeding Djungarian hamster (*Phodopus sungorus*), much is known about the neural mechanism that generates the melatonin rhythm and regulates the duration of its nighttime rise, and about the role of melatonin in the control of reproduction. Therefore, we chose this species for the series of studies described next, in which the overall goal was to determine whether exposures to a 60-Hz magnetic field would influence pineal melatonin production or the duration of the nighttime rise in serum melatonin, and whether these effects would have physiological consequences for reproductive function. In the Djungarian hamster, also known as the Siberian hamster, the nocturnal increase in pineal melatonin production is a true circadian rhythm (Yellon et al. 1982). As in other rodents, nighttime pineal melatonin production is regulated by light (Hoffmann et al. 1981; Yellon et al. 1985; Yellon and Hilliker 1993). The effects of light to modulate pineal melatonin production are mediated by input from the retina to the suprachiasmatic nuclei (Bittman et al. 1991; Yellon et al. 1993). As in other species, the duration of the nighttime rise in pineal melatonin content is proportional to the hours of darkness (Darrow and Goldman 1985; Hoffmann et al. 1985). Other studies with this species that involved infusion or injection of melatonin have been at the foundation of support for the current working hypothesis that duration of the melatonin rhythm mediates both inhibitory and stimulatory effects of photoperiod on reproductive function, on the neuroendocrine system that controls reproduction, and on metabolic activity (Buchanan and Yellon 1991; Bartness et al. 1993).

For our studies, a magnetic field apparatus was constructed. Two modified Merritt coil systems were built with horizontal and vertical winds (three each). Activation of the horizontal coils applied a uniform vertical magnetic field within a 90-cm^3 area (Yellon 1994). For the actual exposure, groups of hamsters (housed in polycarbonate plastic cages with a metal top without water bottle; n = 2–8/cage) were placed in a coil system and the vertical field applied. Sham-exposed controls were simultaneously placed in the adjacent coil system but no current was applied. The experiments involved a 1-G magnetic field dose, because this exposure is within the maximum range that is normally produced by ordinary household appliances. In the facility, background was less than 0.6 mG.

REPLICATE STUDIES OF ACUTE MAGNETIC FIELD EXPOSURES ON MELATONIN RHYTHM IN LONG-DAY HAMSTERS

Initial empirical evidence demonstrated that acute exposure to a 1-G, 60-Hz magnetic field for 15 minutes beginning 2 hours before lights off blunts or delays the nighttime rise in melatonin rhythm in the pineal gland and in serum in adult Djungarian hamsters on long days (Fig. 1, top panel) (Yellon 1991; Reiter 1993a). Replication of this study indicated that the magnetic field exposure diminished the nighttime melatonin rise in the pineal gland and serum in the first but not second experiment (Fig. 1, panels 2 and 3) (Yellon 1994). Even in the two studies in which an acute magnetic field exposure effect was found, significant differences in amplitude of increased melatonin at specific clock times were evident. Not only were magnetic field effects not repeated at some clock times (e.g., at 3 hours after lights off for pineal content and at 7.5 hours for both pineal and serum), but differences were apparent in the concentration of melatonin among the same treatment group (the "a" statistic in the figure). Questions about this variability led us to repeat this same study two more times. Although no magnetic field exposure effect was found in one study (Fig. 1, panel 4), the nighttime melatonin rise was suppressed or delayed in the other (Fig. 1, panel 5). Even so, significant amplitude differences were evident among replicate experiments for magnetic field-exposed hamsters and sham groups.

One explanation for variations among replicate studies in pineal melatonin content or serum concentrations at specific times of night may be the dynamic nature of production and secretion of the hormone. When circadian samples are repeatedly obtained,

---

FIG. 1 (facing page). Melatonin rhythms in the pineal gland (left column) and in serum (right column) of adult, long-day, male and female Djungarian hamsters exposed to a 60-Hz magnetic field of 1 G for 15 minutes beginning 2 hours before lights off (closed symbol = magnetic field). Sham-exposed controls were simultaneously placed in an adjacent chamber but current was not applied (open symbols = control). This same study was repeated five times (Yellon 1994, 1996). Melatonin data are the mean ± SE of 4–6 hamsters in each group/clock time. For some time points, the SE bars are encompassed by the area of the symbol. The black bar signifies the hours of darkness. Asterisks indicate significant differences in the log melatonin data in the pineal gland or serum between field-exposed and sham-exposed groups at the same clock time (p < 0.05, analysis of variance and Duncan's test). Lowercase letters indicate a significant difference in the log melatonin data between the same treatment group and clock time in the initial study (top panel; "a") or subsequent studies (panels 2 and 3; "b" and "c," respectively).

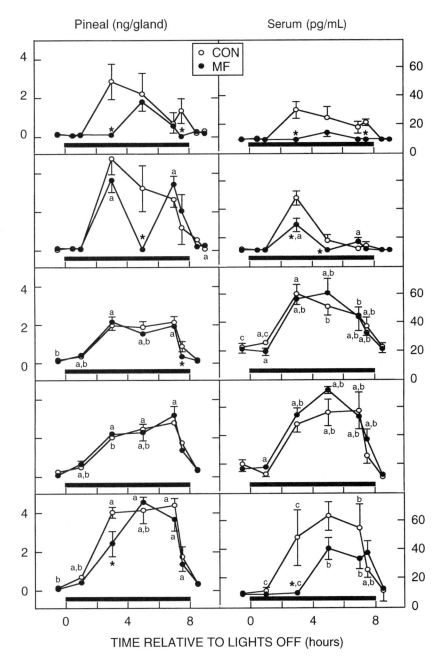

FIG. 1. (See caption on facing page.)

inherent variability in the amplitude of the melatonin rhythm has been reported in individual sheep (Lee et al. 1993). It is also conceivable that a magnetic field exposure effect on the melatonin rise could depend on a component of the experimental design or responsiveness of a subgroup, because distinct populations of adult male and female hamsters were used in these experiments. The time of year when the study was conducted, along with age and sex among experimental populations were considered as potential explanations for variability in the magnetic field effects on the melatonin rise in the long-day studies.

With these considerations in mind, all experiments presented in Figure 1 were planned to be conducted within a month of either the winter (panels 1, 3, and 5) or summer (panels 2 and 4) solstice. Differences in pineal or serum melatonin concentrations between sham- and magnetic field-exposed groups were not consistently found at either time of year. Another observation was that magnetic field effects were more prevalent in experiments with older subjects. Studies in which magnetic field effects were indicated (Fig. 1 panels 1, 2, and 5) involved hamsters that were 6 to 13 months of age; subjects ranged in age from 2 to 9 months in experiments that demonstrated no effect of treatment on the melatonin rhythm relative to that in sham controls (panels 3 and 4). This question of aged-related responsiveness of the mechanism controlling the melatonin rhythm to magnetic field exposure was recently addressed (Yellon 1995). In aged Djungarian hamsters on long days (10–22 months age range), acute exposure to the same magnetic field as that already described (1 G for 15 minutes beginning 2 hours before lights off) failed to influence the melatonin rhythm compared to that in sham controls. Thus, age is unlikely to be a significant consideration for understanding variations in melatonin rhythms among magnetic field studies.

Because adult male and female hamsters were used in these experiments, whether there were sex differences in melatonin rhythms or in the response to magnetic field exposure could be answered by further analysis of the data in Figure 1. In magnetic field-exposed hamsters, melatonin rhythms in male and female hamsters were the same across the five replicate studies (Fig. 2). A

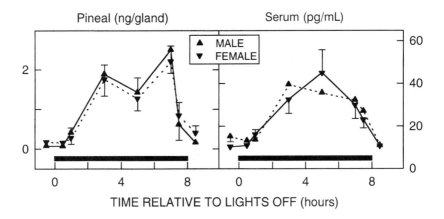

Pineal (ng/gland) Serum (pg/mL)

TIME RELATIVE TO LIGHTS OFF (hours)

FIG. 2. Absence of a sex difference in melatonin rhythms of magnetic field-exposed hamsters. Melatonin data from Figure 1 were segregated based on sex across replicate studies. At each respective clock time, melatonin concentrations are the mean ± SE of 7–23 hamsters/group. The melatonin rise from baseline was significant (p < 0.00001; df=15, F_{pineal} = 4.553 and F_{serum} = 4.62) but no statistical differences were evident between male and female hamsters at any clock time (p > 0.05). Black bar indicates hours of darkness.

comparison of the data in the three experiments in which an exposure effect was found (Fig. 1 panels 1, 2, and 5) and the two no-effect studies (panels 3 and 4) revealed no sex differences in melatonin concentrations at the same clock time. Among sham-control groups as well, melatonin rhythms in male compared to female hamsters were not statistically different (data not shown).

Thus, a variety of considerations fail to explain the significant variability in melatonin concentrations at some clock times and in some studies of hamsters exposed to the magnetic field. Of key importance is the observation that significant differences in the amplitude of the nighttime melatonin rhythm were also found in groups of sham-exposed hamsters at the same clock time in replicate studies. Thus, rather than a magnetic field effect on a circadian pattern of hormone production or secretion, the findings may be related to variability in repetitive melatonin rhythms among individual or groups of hamsters. Variability in nighttime amplitude, most commonly during the rising phase of the rhythm, contrasts with the fact that another parameter of the rhythm steadfastly reflected day length. Increased melatonin was extended for the duration of the night in four of the five long-day studies of hamsters (Fig. 1, panels 2–5). Because duration of the melatonin rhythm has been shown to convey day-length information and reflect circadian clock activity, the relevance of amplitude variability in the melatonin rise for this hamster model is difficult to appreciate. Moreover, even when duration of the melatonin rise was suggested to be abbreviated (panel 1), there is little basis to ascribe physiological meaning for the reproductive system to a truncated long-day melatonin rhythm.

While the importance of a reduced duration of the melatonin rise in the Djungarian hamster in long days is uncertain, abbreviating a short-day melatonin rhythm has clear implications to convey misinformation about ambient photoperiod. If exposure to a magnetic field could truncate the nighttime melatonin rise, then information about long days would be conveyed to the neuroendocrine mechanism that regulates reproductive function in this species. In the following series of studies, hamsters on short days were exposed to an acute magnetic field to assess effects on melatonin rhythm.

REPLICATE STUDIES OF ACUTE MAGNETIC FIELD EXPOSURES ON THE MELATONIN RHYTHM IN SHORT-DAY HAMSTERS

After 6 weeks in short days, during which gonadal function was completely inhibited, male and female hamsters were exposed to a 1-G, 60-Hz magnetic field for 15 minutes, beginning 2 hours before lights off. The nighttime melatonin rise in magnetic field-exposed hamsters was suppressed or delayed by 2 hours or more compared to that in sham-exposed controls (Fig. 3; Yellon 1996). In magnetic field-exposed hamsters, nighttime melatonin concentrations in the pineal and in serum at 3 hours after lights off (i.e., during the rising phase of the rhythm) were similarly reduced in both replicate studies. Although duration of the nighttime melatonin rise appeared to be abbreviated by acute magnetic field exposure in the two studies to less than 8 hours com-

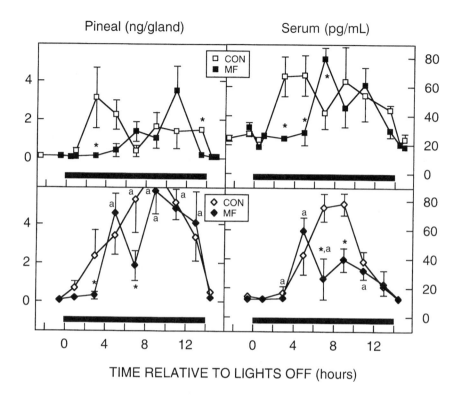

FIG. 3. Two replicate studies of melatonin rhythms in the pineal gland (left column) and in serum (right column) of adult, short-day Djungarian hamsters exposed to a 1-G, 60-Hz magnetic field for 15 minutes beginning 2 hours before lights off (from Yellon 1996). Significant differences in melatonin concentrations (mean ± SE, n = 6 hamsters/group/time) between magnetic field-exposed groups (closed symbols) and sham controls (open symbols) at the same clock time are indicated by the asterisk. The "a" indicates a statistical difference between the replicate study (bottom panel; conducted in June) compared to the same treatment group and clock time in the original experiment (top panel; conducted in January). Black bar indicates hours of darkness.

pared to about 12.5 hours in the control groups, amplitude differences at some clock times were not necessarily replicated; for example, pineal melatonin content at 5, 9, and 13 hours after lights off and serum concentrations at 5, 7, and 9 hours. Differences were also found between sham-exposed groups in short days; for example, pineal content at 7, 9, and 11 hours after darkness and serum concentration at 3 hours after lights off. These amplitude variations in the melatonin rhythm in short-day hamsters parallel findings in replicate long-day studies. As in the previous photoperiod study, comparison of melatonin concentrations between male and female hamsters at specific clock times did not indicate a sex difference in the melatonin rhythm on short days.

Among replicate studies, amplitude differences in the nighttime melatonin rise were evident at specific clock times in both magnetic field-treated and sham-exposed hamsters. As in long-day hamsters, this amplitude variability may be typical of differences in the daily melatonin rhythm in individuals or groups. The physiological significance of amplitude of the nighttime melatonin rise has yet to be fully appreciated, but a consistent delay in onset of pineal melatonin production following magnetic field exposure suggests that duration of the melatonin rise could be reduced each day with daily magnetic field exposure treatments. A chronically abbreviated nighttime melatonin rise that is mediated by magnetic field exposures would have clear physiological implications providing stimulatory, long-day misinformation to hamsters in which reproductive function is normally suppressed by the extended duration of the melatonin rhythm in short days (Bartness and Goldman 1988; Bartness et al. 1993). This concept was the foundation for the next study, in which we expected that daily exposures of hamsters in short days to the magnetic field would truncate the melatonin rise each night and stimulate reproductive development.

EFFECTS OF DAILY MAGNETIC FIELD EXPOSURES ON THE MELATONIN RHYTHM AND REPRODUCTIVE FUNCTION IN SHORT DAYS

The next study investigated the effects of daily exposure; the design of the study was the same as that already described for the acute short-day experiments, except that after 6 weeks in short days, adult male and female hamsters were placed each day in a coil system and exposed to the 1-G, 60-Hz magnetic field for 15 minutes (beginning 2 hours before lights off). Simultaneously, matched controls were placed in another set of coils but were without current (sham). After 21 days of this daily treatment, blood samples were obtained from six hamsters/clock time at 0.5- to 2.5-hour intervals over the course of the night. Analyses of pineal and serum melatonin rhythms indicated that concentrations were not significantly different in sham- and magnetic field-exposed hamsters throughout the night (Fig. 4) (Yellon 1996). Daytime melatonin concentrations in the pineal gland and circulation of both groups were at baseline or below the limit of detection. Within 3 hours of darkness, melatonin concentrations were significantly increased compared to daytime concentrations at 1 hour before lights off. Thus, duration of the nighttime melatonin rise extended for up to 12 hours in both groups and, contrary to expectations, was not abbreviated by the daily magnetic field treatment. Comparison of data from

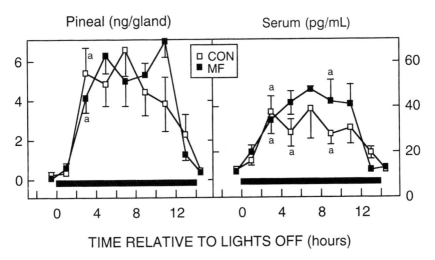

TIME RELATIVE TO LIGHTS OFF (hours)

FIG. 4. Pineal and serum melatonin rhythms of adult, short-day Djungarian hamsters sham-treated or exposed daily to a 1-G magnetic field (for 15 minutes beginning 2 hours before lights off). Although there was a significant circadian variation, the melatonin rhythm in hamsters exposed to this magnetic field (closed symbol) each day was no different than that in sham-exposed controls (open symbol; from Yellon 1996); both duration and amplitude were appropriate for the short daylength. The "a" indicates significant differences in the log melatonin data between the same treatment group and clock time in Figure 3 (Fig.3, top panel).

this daily magnetic field study with the previous acute exposure experiment indicated that melatonin rhythms were significantly different between the same treatment group ("a" = $p < 0.05$; data in Fig. 4 versus Fig. 3, top panel).

Consistent with the absence of an effect on the melatonin rhythm from daily magnetic field exposure is that the reproductive response to the inhibitory short day length also was not altered by treatment. At autopsy, the testes from sham- and magnetic field-treated hamsters were completely regressed (< 100 mg) and associated with atrophic sex accessory organs; uteri were thin and devoid of fluid. These findings indicate that photoperiodic control of the melatonin rhythm and reproductive function was not disrupted by daily exposure to this magnetic field.

Answers to why acute magnetic field exposure effects on the nighttime melatonin rise did not persist with daily magnetic field treatments can be viewed in several distinct ways. It is conceivable that the clock mechanism regulating the circadian melatonin rhythm becomes insensitive to repeated magnetic field treatments. Adaptation to repetitive magnetic field exposures may result if the melatonin rhythm maintains synchrony with a stronger entraining influence—for example, the environmental light cycle. Over a few days, information provided by the prevailing photoperiod would override (mask) or minimize the effects of repetitive magnetic field treatment. Individual adaptations to magnetic field exposure may, to an extent, contribute to response differences between acute and daily exposure studies.

Another possibility for the difference in effects between acute and daily exposure is that magnetic field exposures could have variable effects on amplitude of the nighttime melatonin rhythm. In the acute study (Fig. 3), conveyance of a short-day melatonin signal could still be accomplished if pineal production of melatonin and serum concentrations remained elevated above the daytime baseline from 4–14 hours after lights off. Melatonin rhythm durations of 10 or more hours are known to inhibit reproduction (Bartness et al. 1993). However, variable effects of daily magnetic field exposures on duration of the melatonin rhythm are also possible. If the rise in melatonin between 2.5 and 4 hours after lights off varied in response to daily magnetic field exposures, then duration could be abbreviated on some days but not others. In adult hamsters, increased melatonin in circulation must be consistently reduced to an 8-hour duration or less for several days to reverse short-day inhibition of gonadal function (Bartness et al. 1993). Since the reproductive effects of short days were not reversed by treatment, a lack of consistent responsiveness to magnetic field exposures may contribute to the conclusion that the gonads remained regressed because long-day misinformation was not conveyed.

As a final consideration, differences among melatonin rhythms between replicate studies were not present in only magnetic field-treated hamsters. Even among sham controls, statistically significant variations in the amplitude of the melatonin rise at specific clock times occurred among repetitive studies of both long and short days. Such variability has already been suggested to be a normal characteristic of an entrained circadian rhythm in melatonin synthesis and secretion. Accordingly, this perspective supports the conclusion that the magnetic field exposures in the current series of studies do not consistently affect melatonin production by the pineal gland or its rhythm in circulation.

OTHER STUDIES FAIL TO SUPPORT A MAGNETIC FIELD EXPOSURE EFFECT ON THE MELATONIN RHYTHM

It is well-recognized that photoperiod, as mediated by the circadian melatonin rhythm, controls the neuroendocrine mechanism that regulates sexual maturation in the Djungarian hamster (Darrow and Goldman 1985; Buchanan and Yellon 1991). In parallel with the adult studies that have already been described, juvenile hamsters were exposed each day to the same magnetic field treatment during a critical time when photoperiod is known to regulate the onset of puberty. Neither acute nor daily magnetic field exposures disrupted the ability of long days to initiate reproductive development or of short days to arrest puberty (Truong et al. 1996). As in the adult hamster, differences in amplitude of the melatonin rhythm occurred in replicate studies. Although concentrations differed between magnetic field- and sham-exposed hamsters at some clock times, significant differences in the nighttime melatonin rise in pineal content or serum concentration at specific clock times also were found between the same treatment group in both long- and short-day replicate studies. With the end-points studied, these data suggest that magnetic field exposures do not have physiologically significant effects on the clock control of the melatonin rhythm (production or secretion). Rather, repetitive melatonin rhythms are characterized by an inherent variability in amplitude of the rise among experimental populations or between individuals. Because magnetic field exposures did not affect photoperiod control of reproductive maturation, these results further support the conclusion that a variety of magnetic field treatments fail to disrupt photoperiodic time measurement or the neuroendocrine mechanism regulating reproductive maturation in the juvenile Djungarian hamster.

Certainly, other magnetic field dose and treatment parameters must be studied to determine whether a consistent suppression of the nighttime melatonin rise results from a particular exposure paradigm. Recently, adult hamsters were exposed to a 1-G, intermittent magnetic field (1 minute on/1 minute off) for 15 or 60 minutes. As in previous experiments, these treatments failed to interfere with the normal nighttime rise in melatonin production by the pineal gland or in circulation (Truong and Yellon 1995). In addition, preliminary findings indicate no effect of an acute 0.1- or 1-G magnetic field on melatonin production or serum concentrations when exposures occurred continuously for 15 minutes during the night (2 and 4 hours after lights off) (unpublished data). Collectively, these studies discount a physiologically significant role for magnetic field exposures to affect the endogenous timekeeping mechanism that regulates the circadian melatonin rhythm.

PROGRESS AND CONCLUSIONS

Over the last 20 years, progress has been made in understanding that the circadian melatonin rhythm mediates the effects of photoperiod on reproductive function in seasonal breeders. Furthermore, the melatonin rhythm has been implicated to be a physiologically important signal that conveys information about time of day and season in a variety of species. Information provided by the melatonin rhythm is useful in facilitating the synchrony of such diverse physiological processes as neural activity and endocrine secretion to circadian activity cycles, as well as in successfully adapting to circadian and annual changes in the environment. Although duration of increased melatonin in circulation has become recognized as a physiologically significant feature of the rhythm, further study of such parameters as amplitude, onset, or phase of the rhythm is needed. In humans, implications are that the melatonin rhythm plays an important role in the sleep–wake cycle, as well as in adaptations related to neuroendocrine function, jet lag, and sleep disorders (Wetterberg 1993). It remains open for further investigation as to whether the melatonin rhythm serves as an endogenous timekeeper for the seasonal changes in normal physiology that seem to persist among human populations (Bronson 1995).

Progress also has been made in understanding the physiological consequences of magnetic field exposures. In species where magnetic field effects on melatonin production have been reported, the connection between observed effects and significant physiological consequences has not been established. Various magnetic field exposures appear as likely as not to suppress the nighttime increase in pineal melatonin production (Welker et al. 1983; Reuss et al. 1985; Olcese and Reuss 1986; Khoory 1987; Stehle et al. 1988; Lerchl et al. 1990). Although different exposure conditions and experimental paradigms may account for discrepant findings, exact replication of the biological effects of magnetic field exposure on pineal melatonin content have not been reported, nor have effects been linked to physiological functions of the pineal gland. In the Djungarian hamster, acute magnetic field exposure has delayed or blunted the nocturnal increase in pineal and serum melatonin rhythms in most long-day studies, as well as in acute, short-day studies (Yellon 1994, 1996). Pathophysiological consequences of magnetic field exposure treatments in this model, though, have not been realized, because daily magnetic field treatments do not alter the photoperiodic control of the melatonin rhythm or adult reproductive function. Based on these results, the apparent absence of a consistent, predictable, and physiologically relevant magnetic field exposure effect suggests that studies of the molecular mechanisms through which magnetic field treatments may influence pineal melatonin synthesis or its rhythm in circulation in this species seem premature. Thus, the data strongly indicate that the magnetic field treatments used in these studies do not disrupt photoperiodic time measurement or the clock mechanism that controls reproduction.

The prospects for understanding the relationship between melatonin and magnetic field effects in other physiological systems are promising. The current findings relate to a specific known function of the circadian melatonin rhythm and do not discount the potential role melatonin may play as a link between electromagnetic field exposures and increased breast cancer risk (Stevens et al. 1992). Melatonin has been suggested to enhance immune function and to have considerable oncostatic properties as a potent free-radical scavenger (Reiter et al. 1993). 60-Hz magnetic field exposures at low environmental levels have been found to block the natural growth-inhibitory action of melatonin on human mammary cells in vitro (Blask 1993; Liburdy et al. 1993; Liburdy and Harland, Chapter 22 of this volume). Therefore, electric and magnetic field exposures may affect aspects of melatonin production or its rhythm in circulation, and may influence the normal physiological function of this hormone (Reiter and Richardson 1992). At this time, further studies with appropriate controls and peer review are necessary to address legitimate questions about the health risks of electric and magnetic field exposure, and the role of melatonin in the pathophysiology of disease.

In conclusion, it is well-understood that in seasonal breeders the melatonin rhythm functions to convey information about environmental photoperiod to regulate the annual cycle of reproductive activity. Studies of magnetic field exposures in the seasonally breeding Djungarian hamster indicate that acute effects of magnetic field treatment on the melatonin rhythm are variable, and daily exposures fail to affect the photoperiod control of reproduction.

ACKNOWLEDGMENTS

This work was supported by the U.S. Department of Energy, Office of Energy Management (Contract DE-A101-90CE35035, Dr. W.R. Adey,

Principal Investigator) and the National Institute of Environmental Health Sciences (ES06137). Animal studies were performed at the Pettis Veterans Affairs Medical Center, Loma Linda, California. Technical expertise provided by Mr. Darren Dong is appreciated. Huy Truong assisted in the graphics and statistical analysis of data.

REFERENCES

Anderson, I.M., S.E. Gartside, P.J. Cowan. 1990. The effect of moderate weight loss on overnight melatonin secretion. *Br. J. Psych.* 156:875–877.

Bartness, T.J., B.D. Goldman. 1988. Peak duration of serum melatonin and short day responses in adult Siberian hamsters. *Am J. Physiol.* 255:R812–R822.

Bartness, T.J., J.B. Powers, M.H. Hastings, E.L. Bittman, B.D. Goldman. 1993. Timed infusion paradigm for melatonin delivery: What has it taught us about the melatonin signal, its reception and the photoperiodic control of seasonal responses? *J. Pineal Res.* 15:161–190.

Berga, S.L., T.L. Daniels, J.L. Cameron. 1993. Fasting causes a phase advance and increased duration of nocturnal melatonin secretion in women. In: Abstracts of the 75th Endocrine Society Meeting, Las Vegas, Nevada, 237A, #748.

Bittman E.L., T.J. Bartness, B.D. Goldman, G.J. DeVries. 1991. Suprachiasmatic and paraventricular control of photoperiodism in Siberian hamsters. *Am. J. Physiol.* 260: R90–R101.

Blask, D.E. 1993. Melatonin in oncology. In: *Melatonin. Biosynthesis, Physiological Effects, and Clinical Applications*, H.-S. Yu and R.J. Reiter, eds., pp. 448–475. Boca Raton, Florida: CRC Press.

Bronson, F.H. 1995. Seasonal variation in human reproduction: Environmental factors. *Quarterly Rev. Biol.* 70:141–164.

Buchanan K.L., S.M. Yellon. 1991. Delayed puberty in the male Djungarian hamster: Effect of short photoperiod or melatonin treatment on the GNRH neuronal system. *Neuroendocrinology* 54:96–102.

Card, J.P., R.Y. Moore. 1991. The organization of visual circuits influencing the circadian activity of the suprachiasmatic nucleus. In: *Suprachiasmatic Nucleus: The Mind's Clock*, D.C. Klein, R.Y. Moore, and S.M. Reppert, eds., pp. 51–76. New York: Oxford University Press.

Claustrat B., G. Chazot, J. Brun, D. Jordan, G. Sassolas. 1984. A chronobiological study of melatonin and cortisol secretion in depressed subjects: Plasma melatonin, a biochemical marker of major depression. *Biol. Psychol.* 19:1215A.

Darrow, J.M., B.D. Goldman. 1985. Circadian regulation of pineal melatonin and reproduction in the Djungarian hamster. *J. Biol. Rhythms* 1:39–54.

Goldman, B.D., J.A. Elliott. 1988. Photoperiodism and seasonality in hamsters: Role of the pineal gland. In: *Processing of Environmental Information in Vertebrates*, M.H. Stetson, ed., pp. 203–218. New York: Springer-Verlag.

Hoffmann, K., H. Illnerová, J. Vaněček. 1981. Effect of photoperiod and of one minute light at nighttime on the pineal rhythm of N-acetyltransferase activity in the Djungarian hamster *Phodopus sungorus. Biol. Reprod.* 24:551–556.

Hoffmann, K., H. Illnerová, J. Vaněček. 1985. Comparison of pineal melatonin rhythms in young adult and old Djungarian hamsters (*Phodopus sungorus*) under long and short photoperiod. *Neurosci. Lett.* 56:39–43.

Illnerová, H. 1991. The suprachiasmatic nucleus and rhythmic pineal melatonin production. In: *Suprachiasmatic Nucleus: The Mind's Clock*, D.C. Klein, R.Y. Moore, and S.M. Reppert eds., pp. 197–216. New York: Oxford University Press.

Karsch, F.J., C.J.I. Woodfill, B. Malpaux, J.E. Robinson, N.L. Wayne. 1991. Melatonin and mammalian photoperiodism: Synchronization of annual reproductive cycles. In: *Suprachiasmatic Nucleus: The Mind's Clock*, D.C. Klein, R.Y. Moore, and S.M. Reppert eds., pp. 217–232. New York: Oxford University Press.

Khoory, R. 1987. Compensation of the natural magnetic field does not alter N-acetyltransferase activity and melatonin content of rat pineal gland. *Neurosci. Lett.* 76:215–220.

Laughlin, G.A., A.B. Loucks, S.S. Yen. 1991. Marked augmentation of nocturnal melatonin secretion in amenorrheic athletes, but not in cyclic athletes: Unaltered by opiodergic or dopaminergic blockade. *J. Clin. Endocrinol. & Metab.* 73:1321–1326.

Lee, J.M. Jr., F. Stormshak, J.M. Thompson, P. Thinesen, L.J. Painter, E.G. Olenchek, D.L. Hess, R. Forbes, D.L. Foster. 1993. Melatonin secretion and puberty in female lambs exposed to environmental electric and magnetic fields. *Biol. Reprod.* 49:857–864.

Lerchl, A., K.O. Nonaka, K.-A. Stokkan, R.J. Reiter. 1990. Marked rapid alterations in nocturnal pineal serotonin metabolism in mice and rats exposed to weak intermittent magnetic fields. *Biochem. Biophys. Res. Commun.* 169:102–108.

Liburdy, R.P., T.R. Sloma, R. Sokolic, P. Yaswen. 1993. ELF magnetic fields, breast cancer, and melatonin: 60 Hz fields block melatonin's oncostatic action on ER^+ breast cancer cell proliferation. *J. Pineal. Res.* 14:89–97.

Monteleone, P., M. Maj, M. Fusco, C. Orazzo, D. Kemali. 1990. Physical exercise at night blunts the nocturnal increase of plasma melatonin levels in healthy humans. *Life Sci.* 47:1989–1995.

Olcese, J., S. Reuss. 1986. Magnetic field effects on pineal gland melatonin synthesis: Comparative studies on albino and pigmented rodents. *Brain Res.* 369:365–368.

Reiter, R.J. 1993a. A review of neuroendocrine and neurochemical changes associated with static and extremely low frequency electromagnetic field exposure. *Integr. Physiol. Behav. Sci.* 28:57–75.

Reiter, R.J. 1993b. The melatonin rhythm: Both a clock and a calendar. *Experientia* 49:654–664.

Reiter, R.J., B.A. Richardson. 1992. Magnetic field effects on pineal indoleamine metabolism and possible biological consequences. *FASEB J.* 6:2283–2287.

Reiter, R.J., L.E. Anderson, R.L. Buschbom, B.W. Wilson. 1988. Reduction of the nocturnal rise in pineal melatonin levels in rats exposed to 60 Hz electric fields in utero and for 23 days after birth. *Life Sci.* 42:2203–2206.

Reiter, R.J., B. Poeggeler, D.-X. Tan, L.-D. Chen, L.C. Manchester. 1993. Antioxidant capacity of melatonin: A novel function not requiring a receptor. *Neuroendocr. Lett.* 15: 103–116.

Reuss, S., J. Olcese, L. Vollrath, M. Skalej, M. Meves. 1985. Lack of effect of NMR-strength magnetic fields on rat pineal melatonin synthesis. *IRCS Med. Sci.* 13:471.

Selmaoui, B., Y. Touitou. 1995. Sinusoidal 50-Hz magnetic fields depress rat pineal NAT activity and serum melatonin. Role of duration and intensity of exposure. *Life Sci.* 57:1351–1358.

Stehle, J., S. Reuss, H. Schröder, M. Henschel, L. Vollrath. 1988. Magnetic field effects on pineal N-acetyltransferase activity and melatonin content in the gerbil—role of pigmentation and sex. *Physiol. Behav.* 44:91–94.

Stevens, R.G., S. Davis, D.B. Thomas, L.E. Anderson, B.W. Wilson. 1992. Electric power, pineal function, and the risk of cancer. *FASEB J.* 6:853–860.

Truong, H., S.M. Yellon. 1995. Continuous or intemittent magnetic field exposures fail to affect the nightime rise in melatonin in the adult Djungarian hamster. In: Abstracts of the 28th Annual Society for the Study of Reproduction Meeting, Davis, California, #172.

Truong, H., J.C. Smith, S.M. Yellon. 1996. Photoperiod control of the melatonin rhythm and reproductive maturation in the juvenile Djungarian hamster: 60-Hz magnetic field exposure effects. *Biol. Reprod.* 55:455–460.

Waldhauser, F., G. Weiszenbacher, E. Tatzer, B. Gisinger, M. Waldhauser, M. Schemper, H. Frisch. 1988. Alterations in nocturnal serum melatonin levels in humans with growth and aging. *J. Clin. Endocrinol. & Metab.* 66:648–652.

Welker, H.A., P. Semm, R.P. Willig, J.C. Commentz, W. Wiltschko, L. Vollrath. 1983. Effects of an artificial magnetic field on serotonin N-acetyltransferase activity and melatonin content in the rat pineal gland. *Exp. Brain Res.* 50:426–432.

Wetterberg, L. 1993. *Light and Biological Rhythms in Man.* New York: Pergamon Press.

Wilson, B.W., L.E. Anderson, D.I. Hilton, R.D. Phillips. 1981. Chronic exposure to 60-Hz electric fields: Effects on pineal function in the rat. *Bioelectromagnetics* 2:371–380.

Wilson, B.W., L.E. Anderson, D.J. Hilton, R.D. Phillips. 1983. Chronic exposure to 60-Hz electric fields: Effects on pineal function in the rat (erratum). *Bioelectromagnetics* 4:293.

Yellon, S.M. 1991. An acute 60 Hz magnetic field exposure suppresses the nighttime melatonin rise in the pineal and circulation of the adult Djungarian hamster. In: Abstracts of the Annual Review of Research on Biological Effects of Electric and Magnetic Fields, Milwaukee, Wisconsin, November 3–7, A-25. Frederick, Maryland. W/L Associates, Ltd.

Yellon, S.M. 1994. Acute 60 Hz magnetic field exposure effects on the melatonin rhythm in the pineal gland and circulation of the adult Djungarian hamster. *J. Pineal Res.* 16:136–144.

Yellon, S.M. 1995. Melatonin rhythms in aged Djungarian hamsters: Magnetic field effects and photoperiod control of reproduction. *Society for Neurosciences Abstracts* 21:184, #78.15.

Yellon, S.M. 1996. Acute and daily 60 Hz magnetic field exposure effects on photoperiod control of the melatonin rhythm in adult Djungarian hamsters. *Amer. J. Physiol.* 33:E816–E821

Yellon, S.M., S.J. Hilliker. 1994. Influence of acute melatonin treatment and light on the circadian melatonin rhythm in the Djungarian hamster. *J. Biol. Rhythms* 9:71–81.

Yellon, S.M., L. Tamarkin, B.L. Pratt, B.D. Goldman. 1982. Pineal melatonin in the Djungarian hamster: Photoperiodic regulation of a circadian rhythm. *Endocrinology* 111:488–92.

Yellon S.M., L. Tamarkin, B.D. Goldman. 1985. Maturation of the pineal melatonin rhythm in long- and short-day reared Djungarian hamsters. *Experientia* 4:651–652.

Yellon, S.M., K.J. Thorn, K.L. Buchanan, M.A. Kirby. 1993. Retinal input to the suprachiasmatic nucleus before and after puberty in Djungarian hamsters. *Brain Res. Bull.* 32:29–33.

19 Effect of EMF Exposure on the Neuroendocrine System

BARY W. WILSON
Pacific Northwest National Laboratory,
Richland, Washington
KATHLEEN S. MATT
Arizona State University, Tempe, Arizona

CONTENTS

BACKGROUND
PINEAL GLAND FUNCTION
EMF EXPOSURE AND HEALTH RISK:
  THE NEUROENDOCRINE HYPOTHESIS
EMF EFFECTS ON PINEAL AND HPG AXIS IN THE HAMSTER
EMF AND NEUROENDOCRINE FUNCTION DURING PREGNANCY
DISCUSSION
REFERENCES

BACKGROUND

Several epidemiologic studies support associations between exposure to electric and magnetic fields (EMF) and increased risk of human breast cancer (Loomis et al. 1994) as well as miscarriage (Lindbohm et al. 1992). This chapter deals with the evidence that one factor in increased risk for these, and possibly other disorders, may be exposure to EMF, and that these effects may be mediated by the neuroendocrine system. Of particular interest is the hypothesis that risk for these disorders may be affected by the influence of anthropogenic magnetic fields on the pineal gland and its principal hormone melatonin (Stevens 1987; Wilson et al. 1989).

As a component of the neuroendocrine system, the pineal gland influences a number of physiologic functions through periodic secretion of the indole hormone melatonin. Melatonin concentrations in the body are linked to the daily light–dark cycle through the visual system, and this hormone provides a timing signal that modulates a number of physiologic functions, including immunity (Maestroni et al. 1989) and reproduction (Reiter 1980). Melatonin also appears to protect against development of several types of cancer in animals that have either been treated with chemical carcinogens (Tamarkin et al. 1981), or received cell or tumor explants (Buzzell et al. 1988).

In laboratory animals, exposure to EMF can reduce or phase delay the nightly increase in synthesis and secretion of melatonin by the pineal gland (Wilson et al. 1980; Welker et al. 1983; Lerchl et al. 1990). There is evidence from laboratory experiments that such exposure can affect the hypothalamic–pituitary–gonadal (HPG) axis as well as other neuroendocrine parameters in animals (Matt et al. 1994).

In this chapter, we describe how EMF exposure can affect the neuroendocrine system in laboratory models, and specifically, the consequences of EMF exposure on the HPG axis of the dwarf Siberian hamster (*Phodopus sungorus*; also known as the Djungarian hamster). This animal model is highly photosensitive, has a robust melatonin rhythm, and has exhibited sensitivity to magnetic fields in at least three types of experiments in several laboratories. As described later, the Djungarian hamster appears well-suited for the study of EMF effects on the neuroendocrine system, especially as mediated by the pineal gland. Observed effects of melatonin on hamster physiology are compared with what is known about the role of this hormone in human neuroendocrine function. The hypothesis that EMF may affect endocrine cancer and miscarriage risk is discussed in this context.

The neuroendocrine system can influence a range of physiologic functions, and its disruption thus may be a factor in the etiology of a number of diseases and disorders, including endocrine cancers and miscarriage. Because of the ubiquitous nature of anthropogenic magnetic fields in modern environments, whether or not increased EMF exposure can increase risk for certain cancers or miscarriage in humans is an important public health question.

Possible EMF effects on the neuroendocrine system—especially as mediated by melatonin—and the potential consequences of these influences is a central theme of this volume. Several cancers of interest in this regard, including some types of breast and prostate cancers, are hormone-dependent, and knowledge about effects of pineal function and consequent endocrine changes under the influence of EMF exposure is important in determining the probability that EMF exposures could increase risk for these disorders.

PINEAL GLAND FUNCTION

From antiquity until the middle of the 20th century, pineal gland function remained a matter of speculation. In humans, the pineal is a pea-sized body, situated between brain hemispheres and outside the blood brain barrier. It has been variously reputed to be no less than the "seat of the soul" or no more than a functionless vestigial appendage. It was not until Aaron Lerner and colleagues (1959) utilized some 250,000 bovine pineals, a two-story chromatographic column, and mass spectrometry to isolate and identify the pineal hormone melatonin that the task of understanding the enigmatic organ made any real progress. Knowledge of the pineal gained in the last 37 years has shown the gland to be an important neuroendocrine organ that employs the hormone melatonin to help synchronize internal physiologic functions with the external environment.

Humans evolved in an external environment that was, and remains, highly periodic. Daily cycles of light and dark, monthly variations in tides, and annual changes in temperature, day length, and food availability are among the rhythms to which the vast majority of organisms on Earth must adapt. Most organisms, including humans, have adapted by developing powerful internal rhythms of their own. Survival has required the maintenance and adaptation of these internal rhythms to the changing external environment. This synchronicity is one of the primary roles of the pineal gland and melatonin. Most biological rhythms in the animal kingdom are synchronized to the 24-hour light–dark cycle, and to annual cycles. These rhythms are termed circadian (circa one day) and circannual (about one year). Rhythms in melatonin corresponding with the menstrual cycle also have been reported (Kivela et al. 1988)

In humans, failure to maintain synchronized internal rhythms can have serious consequences. Reduction in work productivity, decreased alertness, and fatigue are well-recognized short-term consequences of disruption in the daily sleep–wake cycle, for example. Longer-term consequences such as increases in occurrence and severity of mood disorders, changes in the reproductive system, and increased stress symptoms (e.g., ulcers) also have been documented but are not as widely recognized and appreciated. Possible effects of chronic disruption in the circadian rhythms such as increased risk of certain cancers and miscarriage have received little attention.

Nonetheless, factors in the environment that can alter circadian rhythms are now recognized as being of importance to overall health. Light exposure is one such well-recognized factor, and the possibility exists that exposure to anthropogenic EMF may also disrupt these rhythms in some individuals. The pineal rhythm in melatonin is robust, and save for light exposure, few environmental factors are known to exert a strong influence. In some laboratory animals, exposure to EMF is among these factors.

In humans, the daily rhythm in melatonin secretion is present at, or soon after, birth (Waldhauser and Steger 1986). Melatonin levels in the circulation are low during the day and increase soon after the onset of darkness, reaching a peak usually between 0200 and 0400 hours. Exposure to light rapidly (within minutes) suppresses melatonin concentrations in the circulation (Lewy et al. 1980). Around the time of puberty, nighttime secretions of the hormone are known to decrease to some extent. Based on melatonin's demonstrated antigonadal action in animals (Reiter 1980), some investigators have speculated that this reduction permits the rapid gonadal development that occurs during the teen years (Wurtman 1984). In healthy individuals, melatonin secretion is thereafter maintained at a fairly constant level until the fifth or sixth decade of life, when it again begins to decline (Waldhauser and Steger 1986). Although the amplitude of the nighttime melatonin peak is highly variable among individuals, for a given individual, the pattern of melatonin rhythm is remarkably consistent over daily and monthly cycles.

To what extent EMF exposure may affect pineal gland function in humans is not yet clear. Some studies have indicated EMF effects on melatonin in humans (e.g., Wilson et al. 1990; Reif et al. 1996); others have not (e.g., Graham et al. 1995). Given the wide range of melatonin responses to light in humans and the variation in baseline melatonin levels in humans (McIntyre et al. 1990), much more study will be required to clarify the issue. As discussed elsewhere in this volume, there exist a number of epidemiologic studies regarding associations between EMF exposure and endocrine cancers (see review by Stevens et al. 1992) as well as associations between EMF exposure and miscarriage (Juutilainen et al. 1993; Goldhaber et al. 1988; Lindbohm et al. 1992) that appear consistent with an effect of EMF exposure on pineal gland function.

EMF EXPOSURE AND HEALTH RISK: THE NEUROENDOCRINE HYPOTHESIS

Experiments in our laboratory in the late 1970s showed that weak, 60-Hz electric fields could reduce the production of melatonin in the nighttime pineal of the rat (Wilson et al. 1980). It was determined that this decrease was due to reduced activity in N-acetyltransferase (NAT), the rate-limiting enzyme for melatonin synthesis (Wilson et al. 1983). This conclusion has been confirmed by a number of investigators (e.g., Welker et al. 1983). The precise mechanism by which EMF exposure affects NAT activity remains unclear, although there is evidence that the function of the retina and the optical tract are involved. Olcese and colleagues (1988) have reported, for example, that an intact visual system is required to observe the pineal response to magnetic fields in rats.

Early observations on the effects of electric fields led to work by others (Lerchl et al. 1990; Kato et al. 1993) which showed that under some circumstances (Kato et al. 1994), magnetic fields also can affect pineal function. This work eventually led to what we now term the neuroendocrine (Wilson et al. 1989) or melatonin (Stevens et al. 1992) hypothesis of how EMF affects physiologic function and may thus be

an etiologic factor in endocrine cancers, melanoma, and other disorders, including miscarriage (Juutilainen et al. 1993) and depression
(Wilson 1988).

As described earlier in this volume in the chapters by Miller and
Hansen (Chapters 4 and 5) on field characteristics of extremely low frequency (ELF) EMF, these fields have energies insufficient to break
chemical bonds, and it is therefore unlikely that they would cause
such damage to tissue as does ionizing radiation. The neuroendocrine
hypothesis, depicted in Figure 1, addresses the question of how these
fields may, nonetheless, effect changes in biological function that can
result in neuroendocrine-mediated disorders, including increased
cancer risk. The hypothesis states that EMF-induced suppression
or phase-shifting of the nighttime peak in melatonin synthesis and

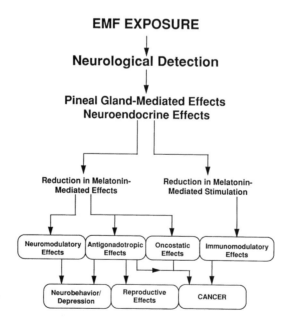

FIG. 1. Representation of the neuroendocrine, or melatonin, hypothesis suggesting how EMF, if detected by the neuroendocrine system, can influence risk for several groups of disorders through effects on melatonin.

subsequent release by the pineal gland may lead to the same kinds of biological changes that occur when pineal function is experimentally suppressed in laboratory animals by surgical or pharmacologic means, or by constant light exposure. Because of the diverse actions of melatonin in the neuroendocrine and immune systems, changes in the timing and rate of this hormone's synthesis in the pineal may affect cancer risk, reproduction, and other neuroendocrine-related physiologic functions.

The hypothesis is attractive because the proposed physiologic mechanisms do not require low-energy EMF exposure to cause chemical or thermal damage in biological tissue. These mechanisms require only that the fields be detected by the organism and subsequently affect neuroendocrine function. Because such exposure gives rise to changes in melatonin in some experiments, the involvement of the pineal in this response has been of central interest. As described in the chapter by Phillips in this volume (Chapter 6), detection of weak EMF is observed in a number of vertebrate species, and thus does not appear to be precluded by energetic considerations. The neuroendocrine hypothesis has been tested in a number of laboratory (e.g., Löscher et al. 1993, 1994; Wilson et al. 1988) and epidemiologic (e.g., Loomis et al. 1994; Tynes and Anderson 1990) studies.

EMF EFFECTS ON THE PINEAL AND THE HPG AXIS IN THE HAMSTER

For the reasons cited in the Background section, the Djungarian hamster is a useful model in which to study effects of magnetic field exposure on the neuroendocrine system, especially as mediated by melatonin. As reported by Yellon and described below, the animal exhibits a neuroendocrine response to changes in the magnetic field to which it is exposed.

Other preliminary experiments conducted to characterize the ability of this animal to detect magnetic fields also have yielded results consistent with the hypothesis that this animal is capable of sensing and responding to changes in the magentic sense. Experiments conducted by Deutschlander et al. (1996) have shown that the Djungarian hamster uses a magnetic sense in selecting nest-building sites in a round, featureless arena. In these experiments, the animal showed a clear preference for siting nests according to a specific magnetic orientation of the perceived geomagnetic field, and persisted in this preference when the magnetic field direction was altered with respect to the geographical orientation of the nest-building arena.

In addition to its apparent magnetic field sense and strong response to photoperiod, the animal is acutely sensitive to other environmental parameters, including social, dietary, and climatic changes (Matt 1990, 1993). It is known that the pineal gland is critical in the hamster's interpretation of the photoperiod (Illnerová et al. 1984). Pinealectomy abolishes the response of the animals to short photoperiod (Hoffman 1973).

In the hamster, the HPG axis responds rapidly to changes in the pattern of pineal melatonin secretions. In several species of the hamster, including *Phodopus*, both males and females are reproductively quiescent during the short days of winter. When day length is shorter than approximately 12 hours, the gonads in the males are regressed and the females are anestrous. When day length increases during the spring, the animals again become sexually competent and breeding resumes. This photoperiodic response is mediated by the pineal gland.

In selecting an animal model for these studies, we reasoned that if EMF exposure indeed alters pineal function, then such changes may be reflected in the HPG axis, and be measurable in such endpoints as changes in gonadal weights.

Specifically, Djungarian hamsters exhibit a pineal-mediated response to short-day photoperiod (6 hours of light, 18 hours of darkness) exposure, with testicular regression within 35–40 days (Hoffman 1973). Concomitant with these changes in testicular weight are decreases in body weight, seminal vesicle weight, and reproductive hormones, including luteinizing hormone (LH), follicle stimulating hormone (FSH), prolactin, and testosterone. During this period of testicular regression, there are decreases in the content of norepinephrine and dopamine within both the medial basal hypothalamus and the pre-optic area (Matt 1993).

EMF Effects on the Hamster Neuroendocrine System

We describe here a series of experiments designed primarily to determine consequential effects of one-time (acute) and repeated exposure to 60-Hz magnetic fields on the HPG axis of the hamster. Our objective in these three experiments was to determine if magnetic field-induced changes in pineal function could influence or be mediated by the HPG axis, and if longer-term changes in HPG function could be observed as a consequence of magnetic field exposure.

A magnetic field exposure of 0.1 mT was selected for these experiments because this flux density was earlier employed by Yellon (1994) in demonstrating that magnetic fields could affect melatonin in the hamster. It should be noted here that magnetic field exposure does not always result in decreased pineal melatonin in either the Djungarian hamster (Truong and Yellon 1995) or in the rat (Kato et al. 1994). It is likely that the effect of field exposure on the pineal (and the HPG axis) may depend on, among other things, the neuroendocrine status of the animal. Our experience indicates that animals may be more sensitive to effects of changing magnetic fields when they are in the process of adapting to an altered photoperiod. Animals used in this study were in the process of acclimating to a short-day photoperiod (8 hours of light, 16 hours of dark) after having been maintained in long days (16 hours light, 8 hours dark).

From the day of receipt at the laboratory, all animals were housed individually in clear polycarbonate cages maintained on the exposure systems. Cage floors were covered with wood chips, and food and water were available *ad libitum*. Once placed on the system, there was no moving or handling of the animals, nor were any other cues associated with exposure. Magnetic fields used for exposure in all experiments were linearly polarized in the horizontal plane at 60 Hz and at a flux density of 0.1 mT. Exposure fields were free of switching transients due to the tuned (LC) circuit design of the system. Sham-exposed animals were housed in an identical manner except that their systems were not energized during the exposure period. In the 42-day chronic experiment, a group of 28 unexposed cage control animals also were maintained in a long-day (16 hours light) photoperiod in a separate room within the same facility.

Acute Exposures

For the acute exposure experiment, 42 animals were exposed to a steady-state magnetic field for 15 minutes starting 2 hours before onset of darkness. Animals were killed during the following dark period. For the 16-day repeated-exposure experiment, approximately 40 animals were exposed daily to a 0.1-mT, 60-Hz magnetic field for 1 hour starting one-half hour before onset of darkness and continuing until one-half hour after darkness onset. Animals and their 40 sham controls were killed during the dark period after the last exposure. In the 42-day repeated-exposure experiment, approximately 48 animals were exposed daily to the field commencing 2 hours before dark onset. In this experiment, the field was turned on for 5 minutes and then off for 5 minutes over a period of 3 hours after onset of exposure. Field-exposed animals and their sham-exposed counterparts were killed during the night after the last exposure.

In the acute exposure experiment reported here, 41 short-day animals were divided into eight groups. Approximately half of the animals were exposed to a horizontally oriented, linearly polarized, 60-Hz magnetic field at a flux density of 0.1 mT, for 15 minutes starting 2 hours before the onset of darkness. Approximately half of the animals were sham exposed. Animals were killed immediately before exposure and at 1, 3, and 5 hours after the onset of darkness. Animals used in these experiments had been housed in their cages on the exposure system for approximately 16 days before the single 15-minute field exposure.

As shown in Figure 2, hypothalamic norepinephrine in the medial basal hypothalamus for short-day animals after a single exposure to a 60-Hz magnetic field for 15 minutes was increased in the hours after darkness. At 5 hours after dark onset, the hypothalamic norepinephrine in these animals was higher than that in both sham-exposed short-day animals and long-day controls. Norepinephrine levels also were reduced in the pre-optic area of the hypothalamus, but these reductions were not statistically significant.

The effect of day-length photoperiod on the Djungarian's metabolism was clearly demonstrated by the differences in the body weights of the animals during the 42-day repeated-exposure experiment. By the 40th day, there was a substantial and statistically significant ($p < 0.05$) difference in body weights between the short-day photoperiod and long-day photoperiod groups. Short-day groups (both sham and field exposed) lost body mass during the last 30 days of short-day pho-

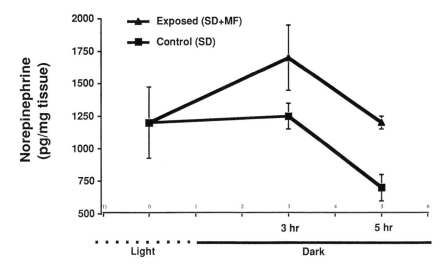

FIG. 2. Norepinephrine concentrations in the medial basal hypothalamus for short-day magnetic field-exposed (triangle) and short-day sham-exposed (square) hamsters at 3 and 5 hours after onset of darkness.

toperiod. Magnetic field exposure appeared to exacerbate this effect. Body weights for the magnetic field-exposed animals were lower than for the sham-exposed short-day animals starting approximately 4 weeks after onset of magnetic field exposure (Fig. 3).

In the 16-day repeated-exposure experiment, testes and seminal vesicle weights were lowest in the short-day group exposed to the magnetic field. As shown in Figure 4, the short-day sham-exposed animals in the 42-day experiment had substantially lower reproductive organ weights compared to the long-day animals. The effect of the repeated magnetic field exposure was to further reduce the reproductive organ weights. As in the 16-day experiment, testes and seminal vesicle weights were lowest in the group on short photoperiod that had been exposed to magnetic fields.

After 16 days of exposure to magnetic fields, prolactin levels in the short-day animals were significantly elevated at 5 hours after onset of darkness compared to both the sham-exposed short-day animals and

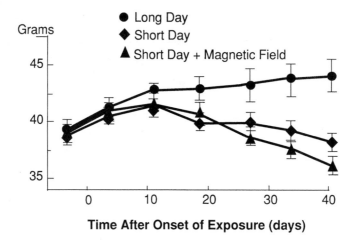

FIG. 3. Comparative body weights (in g) of hamsters exposed only to long days (circle), of short-day hamsters sham exposed to magnetic fields (diamond), and of short-day hamsters exposed to a 60-Hz magnetic field (triangle) as described in the text.

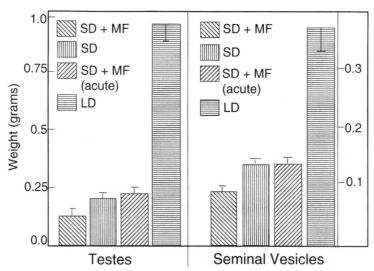

FIG. 4. Weights of the testes and seminal vesicles of long-day control (LD), short-day sham-exposed animals (SD), and short-day field-exposed animals after either 42 days (SD + MF) of repeated-field exposure or one-time field exposure on day 42 [SD + MF (acute)].

the long-day control animals. After 42 days of magnetic field exposure, there was no difference between prolactin levels of the short-day sham- and field-exposed animals.

In all three of the experiments described here (two repeated exposure and one acute), magnetic field exposure at 0.1 mT was associated with decreased pineal melatonin at 3, 4, or 5 hours after onset of darkness. In two of the three experiments (acute and 16-day repeated), the difference after 3 or 4 hours after dark onset was statistically significant ($p < 0.05$). Combined pineal melatonin concentrations from all of the experiments done in this series on the Djungarian hamster in this laboratory are shown in Figure 5.

Discussion

Although rare, exposures to fields of 0.1-mT flux density or higher may be encountered by humans in occupational environments (Hansen et al. 1995). When human-to-hamster dimensional scaling factors are

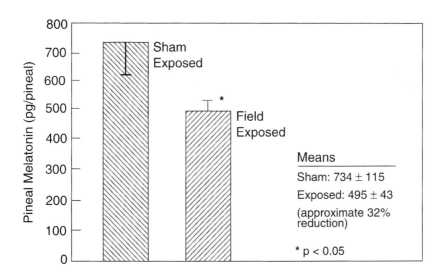

FIG. 5. Summary data for experiments wherein hamsters were exposed to magnetic fields, showing an approximate 32% reduction in pineal melatonin content for field-exposed animals compared to sham-exposed animals.

taken into account, it is apparent that the induced currents in several organs of interest, including the eyes, are on the same order of magnitude for hamsters exposed to 0.1 mT as in humans exposed to flux densities approximately 10-fold lower (in the 10-μT range). Exposure of humans to magnetic fields in the 10-μT range have been reported in both occupational (Hansen et al. 1995) and residential environments (Wilson et al. 1994).

In the 16-day repeated exposure study, we observed reduced pineal melatonin, consistent with an observed increase in blood prolactin levels. These responses would be expected if the animals had been exposed to light for an additional hour or so at a time corresponding to the normal beginning of the dark phase. These effects also are consistent with involvement of the visual system in the detection of the magnetic field and the transduction of that information to a neuroendocrine response. Results after 16 days of exposure, combined with those of our earlier acute studies, suggest that the acute effect of magnetic field exposure is stimulatory to the neuroendocrine system, as demonstrated by increases in hypothalamic norepinephrine content and increases in plasma prolactin.

Longer-term, subchronic effect (i.e., at 42 days) appears to be inhibitory to the HPG. This difference suggests that there might be a compensatory down-regulation of the system under longer-term subchronic exposure conditions. While the acute effects of magnetic fields appear to be mediated by changes in pineal melatonin, the mediation pathway of the signal during longer-term repeated exposures remains unclear. The pathway important in repeated exposures may still involve changes in melatonin, but it also may involve the classic "stress axis," the hypothalamic–pituitary–adrenal axis.

Repeated magnetic field exposure may mediate its effects on physiological systems in a manner similar to that of other environmental stressors, in which case it may provide an excellent model for the study of the physiological mechanisms responsible for the effects of environmental stressors on health and disease. These results show a pattern of neuroendocrine response to magnetic field exposure in the Djungarian hamster that is consistent with the earlier observed effects of magnetic fields on pineal gland function in this and other mammals.

EMF AND NEUROENDOCRINE FUNCTION DURING PREGNANCY

In several recent epidemiologic studies, increased time spent in close proximity to sources of time-varying magnetic fields was associated with increased risk of miscarriage. To date, attention in this area has been directed primarily toward two common sources of magnetic fields: electric bed-heating devices such as electric blankets (Wertheimer and Leeper 1986; Juutilainen et al. 1993) and personal-computer video-display terminals (VDT) (Goldhaber et al. 1988; Lindbohm et al. 1992). Each of these groups of investigators has reported an increased risk of miscarriage associated with increased use of these two electrical devices.

In a study of miscarriage and VDT exposure by Schnorr et al. (1991), as well as in a recent report by Savitz and Ananth (1994) on residential magnetic fields from external power lines, however, no association between estimated EMF exposure and increased miscarriage risk was observed. Several reported laboratory studies have failed to demonstrate adverse reproductive effects of EMF exposure in rats (Mevissen et al. 1994; Rommereim et al. 1996).

Maturation of the reproductive organs and maintenance of the menstrual cycle in females are regulated by periodic increases in circulating levels of pituitary gonadotropins, principally LH and FSH. LH is mainly responsible for ovulation and stimulates the production of estrogens as well as progesterone by ovarian cells. FSH stimulates maturation of the ovarian follicles and their secretion of estrogens. In addition, progesterone functions to prepare the uterine endometrium for implantation and to prevent rejection of the trophoblast.

The menstrual cycle itself reflects normal function of the HPG axis. Internal oscillators located in the hypothalamus generate periodic increases in the production and release of gonadotropin releasing hormone (GnRH). Release of FSH and LH from the pituitary is under the control of hypothalamic GnRH. Under normal conditions, these oscillators are synchronized to external environmental timing cues such as the daily photoperiod. Melatonin receptors are found in the human hypothalamus and pituitary (Weaver et al. 1993), and melatonin is thought to modulate release of GnRH from cells in the hypothalamus by helping to determine the firing rates of specific neurons in the arcuate nucleus (Sandyk 1992). GnRH release also is modulated by a number of other hormones and neurotransmitters, including serotonin, estradiol, and dopamine, as well as by prostaglandins and endogenous opioids.

In seasonally breeding animals, the pineal gland is a central regulator of reproduction timing (Reiter 1980). In several nonseasonal breeders such as the rat, melatonin has been shown to help maintain pregnancy. In the rat, melatonin decreased spontaneous uterine contractions (Herz-Eshel and Rahaminoff 1965), and in the same model, pinealectomy on the 11th day of gestation led to a significantly greater number of resorptions than were observed in sham controls (Guerra et al. 1993). Melatonin may help to maintain pregnancy directly by suppressing components of the immune system that may otherwise reject the fetus (Sandyk et al. 1992).

In humans, melatonin has been reported to exhibit a rhythm that is linked to the menstrual cycle. The characteristics of the reported monthly excretion pattern are consistent with what is observed in the rat and what is known about the interaction of melatonin with other hormones such as LH and estradiol. Melatonin tends to decrease levels of LH (Voordouw 1992); hence, the reported decrease in melatonin immediately prior to ovulation is thought by some to be permissive of the monthly LH surge that leads to ovulation. We have recently obtained evidence that supports the existence of the menstrual cycle-linked rhythms. Results were obtained in our laboratory from measurement of urinary melatonin metabolite excretion from 24 women over two or more menstrual cycles. Our results were based on a prospective study of several thousand women from the California Kaiser Permanente health system.

These data showed that melatonin excretion is highest during the luteal phase of the cycle and lowest just prior to ovulation. This pattern is illustrated in Figure 6. Not all women in the study exhibited this pattern, which was more pronounced during the long nights of winter than in the short nights of summer. However, as shown in Table 1, the increase in melatonin excretion during the luteal phase was statistically significant for the study group as a whole during the winter months. Also note from Table 1 that the lowest levels of melatonin excretion were observed around the time of ovulation. Although not

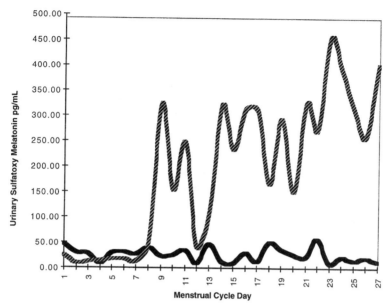

FIG. 6. Excreted sulfatoxymelatonin from one volunteer over two menstrual cycles, one in summer (solid line) and one in winter (stippled line), with the latter showing the luteal phase increase in melatonin excretion.

TABLE 1
Effect of Subject, Season, and Menstrual Cycle Phase on Urinary Excretion of Sulfatoxymelatonin

Condition (P > F)	Status	Number of samples	Mean sulfatoxymelatonin (pg/mL/urine)
Subject (0.0001)		1031	
Cycle season (0.0001)			
	Winter	534	88.2
	Summer	497	66.8
Cycle phase (0.007)			
	Follicular	512	67.3
	Mid-phase	38	65.0
	Luteal	481	90.1

statistically significant in the group as a whole, this dip in excretion was a clear feature in the pattern of many of the volunteers.

When administered over a period of several months, melatonin significantly decreased LH levels in circulation (Voordouw et al. 1992). Decreases in endogenous melatonin synthesis over extended periods may lead to an increase in LH levels, which may, in turn, increase the risk of miscarriage (Regan et al. 1990). From a study of 55 healthy pregnant women, Kivela (1991) showed that plasma levels of melatonin increased as pregnancy progressed. In a more detailed study, Pang et al. (1985) also observed increasing melatonin levels during the first 20 weeks of gestation. Melatonin levels decreased slightly between approximately 20 and 36 weeks, after which the levels again increased until the time of parturition. Thereafter, melatonin dropped quickly to levels lower than those observed in early pregnancy.

Figure 7 indicates many of the interactions of melatonin with reproductive function as reported in the literature. As shown in this illustration, the hormone has been reported to have some effect on every major component of the reproductive system. While these reports clearly indicate a neuroendocrine role in reproduction, the overall significance of melatonin in promoting and maintaining normal pregnancy and parturition in humans has yet to be determined.

Discussion

In this chapter, we have described the effects of EMF exposure on the pineal and HPG axis of a highly photoperiodic laboratory model. The precise pathways by which the magnetic field affects pineal function in the hamster are not yet understood. However, based on the literature, there are several reasonable possibilities.

As mentioned previously, the fields may mediate the sensing of light in the retina, as proposed by Schulten and colleagues (1978), and this altered signal along the optical tract may affect pineal function. A second possibility is that the pineal itself is sensitive to magnetic fields (Welker et al. 1983). Such appears to be the case in several avian species (Semm et al. 1980). A third proposed mechanism is one wherein the pineal receives input from magnetoreceptors elsewhere in the nervous system. For example, Kirschvink et al. (1992) have proposed that mag-

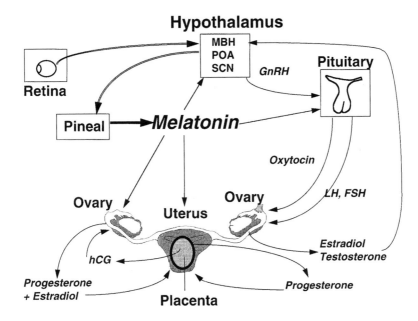

Hypothalamus

FIG. 7. Depiction of melatonin's interaction with the endocrine glands and tissue of the reproductive system.

netite may be present in the human brain in sufficient quantities to serve as a field transducer for fields in the low-millitesla range.

With regard to magnetic field detection in humans, it is unlikely that we can consciously sense 60-Hz magnetic fields, even at flux densities in the 1-mT range (Tucker and Schmitt 1978). However, there is evidence that magnetic fields can give rise to physiologic changes. This evidence includes careful, replicated studies showing EMF effects on neurobehavioral endpoints (Cook et al. 1992) and changes in electroencephalogram (ECG) (Bell et al. 1991; Lyskov et al. 1993). It is therefore not unreasonable to expect that EMF exposure conditions that alter ECG also may affect pineal function.

Humans exhibit wide variability in baseline melatonin levels, as well as in light flux density required to suppress melatonin production (McIntyre et al. 1990). If the response to EMF were dependent on signal transduction in the retina, as some investigators have proposed, then these wide variations would indicate that similar ranges may exist in the human response to EMF as reflected in pineal gland activity. If such is the case, then sufficient number and variety of subjects must be tested under a wide range of magnetic field exposure conditions before concluding that, unlike many animals, humans cannot detect and respond to weak magnetic fields.

Laboratory studies on EMF exposure and reproduction in rats have not provided much evidence to indicate that EMF is an etiologic factor in miscarriage. Some have suggested that in humans, EMF exposure tends to cause early pre-clinical miscarriage of fetuses that would eventually be nonviable. Before discounting the possibility of EMF-induced HPG effects in humans, additional appropriate human laboratory and epidemiologic studies need to be conducted, including as subjects a variety of populations, exposure conditions, and endpoints. Given the evidence that melatonin may play a role in maintenance of pregnancy, the possibility that EMF exposure may increase miscarriage risk in humans should not be dismissed out of hand.

References

Bell, G.B., A.A. Marino, A.L. Chesson, F.A. Struve. 1991. Human sensitivity to weak magnetic fields. *Lancet* 338:251.

Buzzell, G.R., H.M. Amerongen, J.G. Thoma. 1988. Melatonin in the growth of the Duning R3327 rat prostatic adenocarcinoma. In: *The Pineal Gland Cancer*, D. Gupta, A. Attanasio, and R. Reiter, eds., pp. 295–307. Brain Research Promotion, London: Tuebingen.

Cook, M.R., C. Graham, H.D. Cohen, M.M. Gerkovich. 1992. A replication study of human exposure to 60-Hz Fields. 1. Effects on neurobehavioral measures. *Bioelectromagnetics* 13:261–285.

Deutschlander, M.E., J.B. Phillips, S.C. Borland, L.E. Anderson, B.W. Wilson. 1996. Are in vivo effects of EMF in mammals mediated by a sensory system specialized for detection of the geomagnetic field? In: Abstracts of the 18th Annual Bioelectromagnetics Society Meeting, June 9–14, Victoria, British Columbia, Canada, p. 262.

Goldhaber, M.K., M.R. Polen, R.A. Hiatt. 1988. The risk of miscarriage and birth defects among women who use visual display terminals during pregnancy. *Am. J. Ind. Med.* 13:695–706.

Graham, C., M.R. Cook, D.W. Riffle. 1995. Human melatonin in 60-Hz magnetic fields: Continuous vs. intermittent exposure. In: Abstracts of the Annual Review of Research on Biological Effects of Electric and Magnetic Fields from the Generation, Delivery, and Use of Electricity, November 12–16, Palm Springs, California, A-43. Frederick, Maryland: W/L Associates, Ltd.

Guerra, M.O., N.O.G. Silva, C.S. Guimarges, J.P. Souza, A.T.L. Andrade. 1993. Pinealectomy and blindness during pregnancy in the rat. *Am. J. Obstet. Gynecol.* 62:574–581.

Hansen, N.H., L.M. Gillette, E. Sobel, Z. Davanipour, B.W. Wilson. 1995. Measurement and spectral characterization of magnetic fields in the garment industry. In: Abstracts of the Annual Review of Research on Biological Effects of Electric and Magnetic Fields from the Generation, Delivery, and Use of Electricity, November 12–16, Palm Springs, California, p. 38. Frederick, Maryland: W/L Associates, Ltd.

Herz-Eschel, M., R. Rahamimoff. 1965. Effect of melatonin on uterine contractility. *Life Sci.* 4:1367–1372.

Hoffman, K. 1973. The influence of photoperiod and melatonin on testes size, body weight, and pelage color in the Djungarian hamster (*Phodopus sungorus*). *J. Comp. Physiol.* 95:267–282.

Illnerová, H., K. Hoffmann, J. Vaněček. 1984. Adjustment of pineal melatonin and N-acetyltransferase rhythms to change from long to short photoperiod in the Djungarian hamster *Phodopus sungorus.* *Neuroendocrinology* 38:226–231.

Juutilainen, J., P. Matilainen, S. Saarikoski, E. Laara, S. Suonio. 1993. Early pregnancy loss and exposure to 50-Hz magnetic fields. *Bioelectromagnetics* 14:229–236.

Kato, M., K. Honma, T. Shigemitsu, Y. Shiga. 1993. Effects of exposure to a circularly polarized 50-Hz magnetic field on plasma and pineal melatonin levels in rats. *Bioelectromagnetics* 14:97–106.

Kato, M., K. Honma, T. Shigemitsu, Y. Shiga. 1994. Horizontal or vertical 50-Hz, 1-mT magnetic fields have no effect on pineal gland or plasma melatonin concentration of albino rats. *Neurosci. Lett.* 168:205–208.

Kirschvink, J.L., A.K. Kobayashi, B.J. Woodford. 1992. Magnetite bio-mineralization in the human brain. *Proc. Natl. Acad. Sci. USA* 89:7683–7687.

Kivela, A. 1991. Serum melatonin during human pregnancy. *Acta Endocrinol. Copen.* 124(3):233–237.

Kivela, A, A. Kauppila, P. Ylostalo, O. Vakkuri, J. Leppaluoto. 1988. Seasonal, menstrual and circadian secretions of melatonin, gonadotropins and prolactin in women. *Acta Physiol. Scand.* 132(3):321–327.

Lerchl, A., K.O. Nonaka, K.-A. Stokkan, R.J. Reiter. 1990. Marked rapid alterations in nocturnal pineal serotonin metabolism in mice and rats exposed to weak intermittent magnetic fields. *Biochem. Biophys. Res. Commun.* 169:102–108.

Lerner, A.B., J.D. Case, R.V. Heinzelman. 1959. Structure of melatonin. *J. Am. Chem. Soc.* 81:6085.

Lewy, A.J., T.A. Wehr, F.K. Goodwin, D.A. Newsome, S.P. Markey. 1980. Light suppresses melatonin secretion in humans. *Science* 210:1267–1269.

Lindbohm, M.-L., M. Hietanen, P. Kyyronen, M. Sallmen, P. von Nandelstadh, H. Taskinen, M. Pekkarinen, M. Ylikoski, K. Hemminki. 1992. Magnetic fields of video display terminals and spontaneous abortion. *Am. J. Epidemiol.* 136:1041–1051.

Loomis, D.P., D.A. Savitz, C.V. Ananth. 1994. Breast cancer mortality among female electrical workers in the United States. *J. Natl. Cancer Inst.* 86:921–925.

Löscher, W., M. Mevissen, W. Lehmacher, A. Stamm. 1993. Tumor promotion in a breast cancer model by exposure to a weak alternating magnetic field. *Cancer Lett.* 71:75–81.

Löscher, W., U. Wahnschaffe, M. Mevissen, A. Lerchl, A. Stamm. 1994. Effects of weak alternating magnetic fields on nocturnal melatonin production and mammary carcinogenesis in rats. *Oncology* 51:288–295.

Lyskov, E.B., J. Juutilainen, V. Jousmaki, J. Partanen, S. Medvedev, O. Haenninen. 1993. Effects of 45-Hz magnetic fields on the functional state of the human brain. *Bioelectromagnetics* 14:87–96.

Maestroni, G.J.M., A. Conti, W. Pierpoli. 1989. Melatonin, stress, and the immune system. *Pineal Res. Rev.* 7:203–226.

Matt, K.S. 1990. Neuroendocrine and endocrine correlates of pair bonds and parental care in the seasonal reproductive cycle of the Siberian hamster (*Phodopus sungorus*). In: *Proceedings of the XI International Symposium on Comparative Endocrinology*, A. Epple, ed., pp. 648–652.

Matt, K.S. 1993. Neuroendocrine mechanisms of environmental integration. *Am. Zool.* 33:266–274.

Matt, K.S., B.W. Wilson, J.E. Morris, L.B. Sasser, D.L. Miller, L.E. Anderson. 1994. The effect of EMF exposure on environmental integration. In: Abstracts of the 16th Annual Bioelectromagnetics Society Meeting, Copenhagen, Denmark, June 12–17, p. 49. Frederick, Maryland: The Bioelectromagnetics Society.

McIntyre, I.M., T.R. Norman, G.B. Burrows, S.M. Armstrong. 1990. Melatonin supersensitivity to dim light in seasonal affective disorder. *Lancet* 335:488.

Mevissen, M., S. Buntenkötter, W. Löscher. 1994. Effects of static and time-varying (50-Hz) magnetic fields on reproduction and fetal development in rats. *Teratology* 50:229–237.

Olcese, J., S. Reuss, P. Semm. 1988. Geomagnetic field detection in rodents. *Life Sci.* 42:605–613.

Pang, S.F., P.L. Tang, G.W.K. Tang, W.C. Yam. 1985. Melatonin and pregnancy. In: *The Pineal Gland: Endocrine Aspects*, G.M. Brown and S.D. Wainright, eds., pp. 157–162. Oxford: Pergamon Press.

Regan, L., E.J. Owen, H.S. Jacobs. 1990. Hypersecretion of luteinising hormone, infertility, and miscarriage. *Lancet* 336(8724):1141–1144.

Reif, J.S., J.B. Burch, C.A. Pitrat, T.J. Keefe, M.G. Yost. 1996. Melatonin levels in electrical utility workers. In: Abstracts of the 18th Annual Meeting of the Bioelectromagnetics Society, Victoria, British Columbia, Canada. June 9–14. Frederick, Maryland: W/L Associates, Ltd.

Reiter, R.J. 1980. The pineal and its hormones in the control of reproduction in mammals. *Endocrin. Rev.* 1:109–131.

Rommereim, D.N., R.L. Rommereim, D.L. Miller, R.L. Buschbom, L.E. Anderson. 1996. Developmental toxicology evaluation of 60-Hz horizontal magnetic fields in rats. *Appl. Occup. Environ. Hyg.* 4:313–323.

Sandyk, R. 1992. The pineal gland and the menstrual cycle. *Int. J. Neurosci.* 63(3–4):197–204.

Sandyk, R., P.G. Anastasiadis, P.A. Anninos, N. Tsagas. 1992. The pineal gland and spontaneous abortions: Implications for therapy with melatonin and magnetic field. *Int. J. Neurosci.* 62(3–4):243–50.

Savitz, D.A., C.V. Ananth. 1994. Residential magnetic fields, wire codes, and pregnancy outcome. *Bioelectromagnetics* 15:271.

Schnorr, T., B.A. Grajewski, W.E. Murray, R.W. Hornung. 1991. Video terminal displays and the risk of spontaneous abortion. *New England J. Med.* 324:727–733.

Schulten, K. C.E. Swenberg, A. Weller. 1978. A biomagnetic sensory mechanism based on magnetic field modulated coherent electron spin motion. *Zeitschrift fuer Chemie Neue Folge* 111:1–5

Semm, P., T. Schneider, L. Vollrath. (1980). Effects of an Earth-strength magnetic field on electrical activity of pineal cells. *Nature* 288:607–608.

Stevens, R.G. 1987. Electric power use and breast cancer: A hypothesis. *Am. J. Epidemiol.* 125:556–561.

Stevens, R.G., S. Davis, D.B. Thomas, L.E. Anderson, B.W. Wilson. 1992. Electric power, pineal function, and the risk of breast cancer. *FASEB J.* 6:853–860.

Tamarkin, L., M. Cohen, D. Roselle, C. Reichter, M. Lippman, B. Chabner. 1981. Melatonin inhibition and pinealectomy enhancement of 7-12-dimethylbenz(a)-anthracene-induced mammary tumors in rat. *Cancer Res.* 41:4432–4436.

Truong, H., S.M. Yellon. 1995. The rising phase of the melatonin rhythm in adult Djungarian hamster in long days is not altered by acute intermittent 60 Hz magnetic field exposure. In: Abstracts of the Annual Review of Research on Biological Effects of Electric and Magnetic Fields from the Generation, Delivery, and Use of Electricity, November 12–16, Palm Springs, California, p. 38. Frederick, Maryland: W/L Associates, Ltd.

Tucker, R.D., O.H. Schmitt. 1978. Tests for human perception of 60 Hz moderate strength magnetic fields. *IEEE Trans. Biomed. Eng.* BME-25:509–518.

Tynes, T., A. Andersen. 1990. Electromagnetic fields and male breast cancer. *Lancet* 336:1596.

Voordouw, B.C., R. Euser, R.E. Verdonk, B.T. Alberda, F.H. de Jong, A.C. Drogendijk, B.C. Fauser, M. Cohen. 1992. Melatonin and melatonin-progestin combinations alter pituitary-ovarian function in women and can inhibit ovulation. *J. Clin. Endocrinol. & Metab.*Jan. 74:108–117.

Waldhauser, F., H. Steger. 1986. Changes in melatonin secretion with age and pubesescence. *J. Neural Transm.* (Suppl.)21:183–197.

Weaver, D.R., J.H. Stehle, E.G. Stopa, S.M. Reppert. 1993. Melatonin receptors in human hypothalamus and pituitary: Implications for circadian and reproductive responses to melatonin. *J. Clin. Endocrinol. & Metab.* 76(2):295–301.

Welker, H.A., P. Semm, R.P. Willig, J.C. Commentz, W. Wiltschko, L. Vollrath. 1983. Effects of an artificial magnetic field a serotonin N-acetyltransferase activity and melatonin content in the rat pineal gland. *Exp. Brain Res.* 50:426–432.

Wertheimer, N., E. Leeper. 1986. Possible effects of electric blankets and heated water beds on fetal development. *Bioelectromagnetics* 1:13–22.

Wilson, B. 1988. Chronic exposure to ELF fields may induce depression. *Bioelectromagnetics* 9:195–205.

Wilson, B.W., L.E. Anderson, D.I. Hilton, S. Hewett. 1980. Pineal function in rats exposed to 60-Hz electric fields. *Bioelectromagnetics* 1:236.

Wilson, B.W., L.E. Anderson, D.I. Hilton, R.D. Phillips. 1983. Chronic exposure to 60 Hz electric fields: Effects on pineal function in the rat (erratum). *Bioelectromagnetics* 4:293.

Wilson, B.W., F. Leung, R. Buschbom, R.G. Stevens, L.E. Anderson, R.J. Reiter. 1988. Electric fields, the pineal gland, and cancer. In: *The Pineal Gland Cancer*, D. Gupta, A. Attanasio, and R. Reiter, eds., pp. 245–260. Brain Research Promotion, London: Tuebingen.

Wilson, B.W., R.G. Stevens, L.E. Anderson. 1989. Neuroendocrine mediated effects of electromagnetic-field exposure: Possible role of the pineal gland. *Life Sci.* 45:1319–1332.

Wilson, B.W., C.W. Wright, J.E. Morris, R.L. Buschbom, D.P. Brown, D.L. Miller, R. Sommers-Flannigan, L.E. Anderson. 1990. Evidence for an effect of ELF electromagnetic fields on human pineal gland function. *J. Pineal Res.* 9:259–269.

Wilson, B.W., N.H. Hansen, K.C. Davis. 1994. Magnetic-field flux density and spectral characteristics of motor-driven personal appliances. *Bioelectromagnetics* 15:439–446.

Wurtman, R.J. 1984. Fall of nocturnal melatonin during puberty and prepubsecence. *Lancet* 362:85.

Yellon, S.M. 1994. Acute 60 Hz magnetic field exposure effects on the melatonin rhythm in the pineal gland and circulation of the adult Djungarian hamster. *J. Pineal Res.* 16:136–144.

PART IV
Direct Evidence

20 Magnetic Fields and Breast Cancer: Experimental Studies on the Melatonin Hypothesis

Wolfgang Löscher
Meike Mevissen
Department of Pharmacology, Toxicology,
and Pharmacy, School of Veterinary Medicine,
Hannover, Germany

Contents

The Melatonin Hypothesis
Effect of ELF Magnetic Fields on Melatonin Levels
Effect of ELF Magnetic Fields on Breast Tissue Proliferation
Effect of ELF Magnetic Fields on Mammary Carcinogenesis
Effect of ELF Magnetic Fields on Immune Responses to
    Tumor Formation
Magnetic Field Exposure and Breast Cancer: Conclusions
Acknowledgments

In 1987, Stevens presented the hypothesis that use of electric power may increase the risk of breast cancer (Stevens 1987). This hypothesis was based on a number of experimental reports indicating an effect of light and extremely low frequency (ELF) electric fields on pineal melatonin production, and on the relationship of melatonin to mammary (breast) carcinogenesis. However, at the time when this hypothesis was presented, it was not known if ELF (50- or 60-Hz) magnetic fields affect pineal melatonin production in experimental animals and/or humans. Furthermore, there was no experimental evidence for increased breast cancer development or growth in response to magnetic field exposure. This lack of data prompted us to carry out a series of experiments designed expressly to test the "melatonin hypothesis" of magnetic field-promoted breast cancer development and growth in female rats.

THE MELATONIN HYPOTHESIS

Figure 1 illustrates the proposed mechanisms by which chronic exposure to an ELF magnetic field may increase mammary carcinogenesis in rats (modified from Stevens 1987). Based on this hypothesis, chronic exposure to an ELF magnetic field suppresses the normal nocturnal synthesis of pineal melatonin. Because melatonin physiologically suppresses estrogen production by the ovary and prolactin production by the pituitary (Reiter 1991), a melatonin reduction would in turn result in increased estrogen and prolactin production, and thereby induce increased turnover of the breast epithelial stem cells at risk for malignant transformation (Fig. 1). In other words, the likelihood that breast stem cells are affected by cancer-causing agents (e.g., chemical carcinogens) such as those occurring in the environment (cf., Huff 1993) would be increased by reduced production of melatonin. In addition, in view of the oncostatic effect of melatonin on breast cancer growth (Blask 1993), the development and growth of breast cancer, once initiated, would be facilitated by reduced melatonin levels. The risk of tumor formation could be further increased by the possible link between magnetic fields, melatonin, and the immune surveillance system (Fig. 1). Melatonin has been shown to stimulate various immune parameters involved in tumor defense mechanisms (Maestroni 1993; Maestroni and Conti 1993) so that magnetic field exposure, via reduction in melatonin, might impair the immune response to tumor cells. All these alterations in response to magnetic field exposure, and probably several additional magnetic field-induced effects not directly linked to melatonin (Stevens 1993), might ultimately increase the risk of breast cancer formation (Fig. 1).

Magnetic field exposure and breast cancer
Melatonin as a plausible biological link?
(modified from R.G. Stevens, American Journal of Epidemiology, vol. 125, 556-561, 1987)

50/60 Hz magnetic field exposure

↓

Pineal gland: Reduced nocturnal melatonin production

↓

Ovary: Increased estrogen production
Pituitary: Increased prolactin production

↓

Mammary gland: increased proliferation of breast epithelial stem cells

↓

Mammary gland: Increased susceptibility of breast epithelial stem cells to carcinogens such as DMBA

↑↓

Immune system: Suppressed immune response to tumor formation

↓

Consequence: Increased risk of breast cancer formation

FIG. 1. Proposed mechanisms by which chronic exposure to ELF (50- or 60-Hz) magnetic fields may increase development and growth of breast cancer.

This chapter describes how we experimentally examined the different steps of the melatonin hypothesis described above. In all experiments, female rats of the same strain and age were used under strictly controlled laboratory conditions. Most of the described experimental data have been published (Löscher et al. 1993, 1994, 1995; Baum et al. 1995; Mevissen et al. 1995, 1996a, b), but we will also include data from yet-unpublished experiments.

EFFECT OF ELF MAGNETIC FIELDS ON MELATONIN LEVELS

It is long known that weak, static magnetic fields induce pineal metabolic and physiologic changes (Semm et al. 1980), with the retinas considered as the site of magnetoreception (Reiter 1993). There is now general agreement that reduced pineal melatonin synthesis is a consequence of magnetic field exposure under certain conditions (Reiter 1993). More recently, it was demonstrated that exposure of male rats to 50-Hz magnetic field of low (μT) flux density for 6 weeks led to a drop in nighttime levels of both pineal and serum melatonin (Kato et al. 1993). In the female Sprague-Dawley rats at the age used for all experiments described in this paper, prolonged exposure to a 50-Hz magnetic field also significantly decreased nocturnal melatonin levels (Fig. 2). A significant decrease was observed already at a flux density of 0.3–1 μT; that is, in the range of flux densities associated with increased cancer risks in epidemiological studies on residential exposures in humans (Savitz and Ahlbom 1994). Increase of flux density to 10 μT appeared to be associated with a more marked suppression of melatonin levels (Fig. 2), although the difference could be due to the longer duration of magnetic field exposure (13 weeks for the experiment with 10 μT versus 8–9 weeks for the range of 0.3–1 μT).

These data in female rats thus confirm the initial step of the melatonin hypothesis—that ELF magnetic fields induce reduction in melatonin. Studies are under way to examine if this reduction in melatonin subsequently leads to increased estrogen and prolactin production in female rats. It is interesting to note that we obtained magnetic field-induced melatonin decreases in female rats using horizontally orientated fields, while Kato et al. (1994) reported that only circular—not horizontal or vertical—50-Hz, 1 μT magnetic fields have an effect on pineal gland or plasma melatonin in male rats. Our findings may thus point to the possibility that female rats are more sensitive than males to suppression of melatonin production in response to horizontal magnetic fields. Interestingly, a recent review of animal studies on the role of ELF magnetic fields in carcinogenesis indicated that sex might be a predisposing host susceptibility factor to tumor promoting or copromoting effects of magnetic field exposure (Löscher and Mevissen 1994). This important point deserves further investigation.

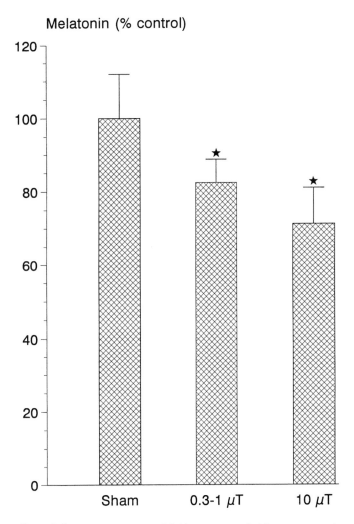

FIG. 2. Effect of chronic exposure to 50-Hz magnetic field on nocturnal melatonin in serum of female rats. Data are shown as percent control (± SE) of 12 rats (0.3–1 μT) or 20 rats (10 μT). In the experiment with a gradient field of 0.3–1 μT, blood was sampled at 11 p.m. in both sham controls and magnetic field-exposed rats after 8–9 weeks of exposure. In the experiment with magnetic field exposure at a flux density of 10 μT, blood was sampled at 11 p.m. following 13 weeks of exposure. In both experiments, the difference to sham control was significant (p < 0.05; indicated by asterisk). It should be noted that all rats (sham- and magnetic field-exposed) had been treated with DMBA. Data are from Löscher et al. (1994) and Mevissen et al. (1996b).

Effect of ELF Magnetic Fields on
Breast Tissue Proliferation

Melatonin is known to exert modulatory influences on the growth of certain tissues, such as the mammary gland (Reiter 1991; Mediavilli et al. 1992). For instance, suppression of pineal melatonin production in rats by continuous exposure to light was reported to increase mammary cell proliferation; however, such proliferation could be prevented by administering melatonin (Mhatre et al. 1984). In order to examine if ELF magnetic field exposure leads to increased breast tissue proliferation in vivo, we determined the activity of ornithine decarboxylase (ODC) in various tissues of female rats after prolonged magnetic field exposure. ODC is a key enzyme in the biosynthesis of polyamines; it promotes cell proliferation and has been suggested to play an important role in tumor promotion (O'Brien et al. 1975; O'Brien 1976; Russell 1980). First studies on the possibility of ODC alterations by exposure to electromagnetic fields used the electric component of such fields, showing that exposure of cell lines to a 60-Hz electric field produced changes in ODC levels similar to changes produced by exposure to the tumor promoter 12-O-tetradecanoylphorbol-13-acetate (TPA) (Byus et al. 1987; Cain et al. 1988). More recent experiments on the effects of ELF magnetic fields on ODC levels in mouse and human cell lines demonstrated that exposure at flux densities in the range of 10–100 μT significantly increased ODC, the increase differing in magnitude between cell lines from 50–500% (Litovitz et al. 1991; Mattsson et al. 1993a, b). To our knowledge, the possibility that 50/60-Hz magnetic fields increase ODC also in vivo has not been studied previously. In our in vivo experiments in female rats, ODC was determined in liver, spleen, intestine (duodenum), bone marrow, skin (epidermis) of the ears, and different parts of the mamma in order to examine if magnetic field exposure induces tissue-specific alterations in ODC. With respect to breast tissue, it should be noted that female rats possess six pairs of mammary gland complexes so that mammary tissue extends from the cervical to the inguinal part of the body (Fig. 3). Because of this extensive distribution of mammary tissue, we determined ODC separately in thoracic and inguinal mammary complexes in rats. If the melatonin hypothesis illustrated in Figure 1 is correct,

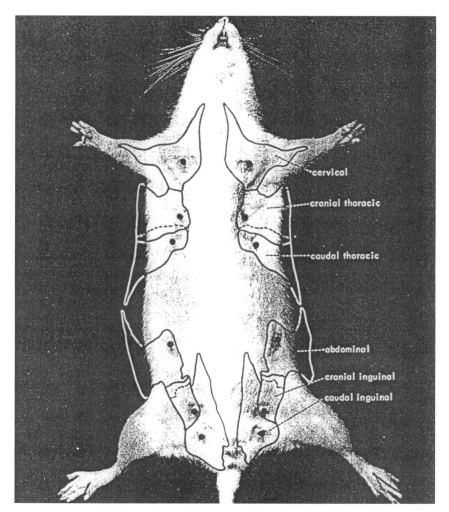

FIG. 3. Location and extension of the six pairs of mammary glands in female rats. (Reprinted from Van Zwieten 1984 with permission from Kluwer Academic Publishers.)

one would assume a regionally selective increase of ODC in all parts of the hormone-dependent mammary tissue, but not in various other, hormone-independent tissues. Indeed, as shown in Figure 4, after prolonged exposure of female rats in a 50-Hz, 50-μT magnetic field, a marked increase in ODC activity was found in mammary tissue, but

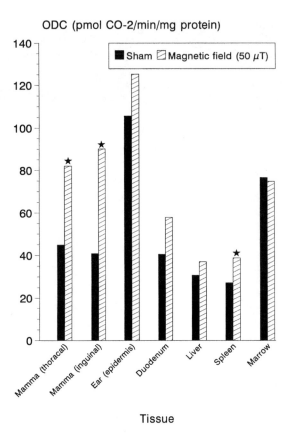

FIG. 4. Activity of ornithine decarboxylase (ODC) in different tissues of female rats. Animals were either sham-exposed or exposed in a 50-Hz, 50 μT magnetic field for 6 weeks. The animals were not treated with any carcinogen. Data are shown as means of six rats per group. Significant differences between sham controls and exposed rats is indicated by asterisk ($p < 0.05$). Data are from Mevissen et al. (1995).

not several other tissues examined in this respect. The only other significant, albeit much less marked, increase in ODC was seen in the spleen (Fig. 4). Thus, these data strongly indicated that in vivo exposure of female rats induced a pronounced increase in proliferation of breast epithelial stem cells, thereby substantiating the melatonin hypothesis.

EFFECT OF ELF MAGNETIC FIELDS ON MAMMARY CARCINOGENESIS

The next, most important question was, of course, whether the reduced melatonin levels and increased breast tissue proliferation in response to ELF magnetic field exposure result in increased susceptibility to carcinogens and enhanced mammary cancer development and growth. Beniashvili et al. (1991) performed a series of experiments in female Sprague-Dawley rats using the "complete" carcinogen N-nitroso-N-methylurea (NMU) to produce mammary tumors in female rats. They reported an increased tumor incidence and enhanced progression from benign to malignant tumor forms in animals exposed daily for 3 hours to 50-Hz, 20-μT magnetic fields over a period of up to 2 years. Furthermore, rats exposed without any carcinogen spontaneously developed significantly more mammary tumors than sham controls (Beniashvili et al. 1991; see statistical evaluation of data in Löscher and Mevissen 1994). In respect to these data from the NMU model, it should be noted that Blask (1993) reported that, while NMU-induced breast tumors are sensitive to alterations in melatonin, melatonin failed to reduce the circulating levels of either estradiol or prolactin. This result indicates that alterations in production of these hormones is not the mechanism by which melatonin affects tumor growth in this model.

In our studies, we used a well-established rat model of chemical carcinogenesis in which mammary tumors are induced by oral application of the polyaromatic hydrocarbon 7,12-dimethylbenz(a)anthracene (DMBA). Although the NMU system used by Beniashvili et al. (1991) appears to have some advantages over the DMBA approach (Blask 1993), we chose DMBA for the following reasons (Stevens et al. 1992; Blask 1993):

- DMBA is one of the most widely used and investigated chemical carcinogens used for induction of breast cancer in laboratory animals.

- Melatonin is obviously involved in DMBA-induced breast cancer, as suggested by the following observations.

–Melatonin levels decrease in DMBA-treated female rats. (Decreased melatonin levels have also been reported in patients with primary breast cancer.)

–Pinealectomy markedly facilitates the development and growth of DMBA-induced breast cancer in female rats.

–Suppression of melatonin synthesis by constant light facilitates the development and growth of DMBA-induced breast cancer in female rats.

–Administration of melatonin inhibits development and growth of DMBA-induced breast cancer in female rats.

Mammary adenocarcinoma induced by DMBA are estrogen- and prolactin-responsive, and would thus respond to any melatonin-induced alteration in circulating levels of either estradiol or prolactin (Welsch 1985). There is ample evidence that DMBA-induced breast cancer development and growth in female rats is sensitive to alterations of melatonin levels (cf., Stevens et al. 1992; Blask 1993). Thus, an enhanced cancer development and growth is seen in rats in which melatonin production has been suppressed by either exposure to constant light or removal of the pineal gland. Vice versa, DMBA-induced mammary carcinogenesis can be inhibited by administration of melatonin in rats, most likely by the melatonin-induced reduction in prolactin levels (cf., Blask 1993). All these data strongly indicate that a decrease of melatonin in response to magnetic field exposure should exert effects on DMBA-induced mammary carcinogenesis in rats.

Interestingly, in the absence of any other manipulation of melatonin production, it has been shown that levels of melatonin decrease during development and growth of DMBA-induced mammary tumors. It is not clear if this effect is the result of DMBA or, more likely, a result of tumor growth (Blask 1993). A similar observation of decreased melatonin levels has been reported in women with primary breast cancer, particularly in those with estrogen receptor positive tumors (cf., Blask 1993). Figure 5 demonstrates that a similar phenomenon of decreased melatonin during DMBA-induced mammary carcinogenesis also occurs under the experimental conditions of our studies. Thus, compared to rats without DMBA treatment, melatonin significantly decreased in both pineal and plasma of female rats after treatment

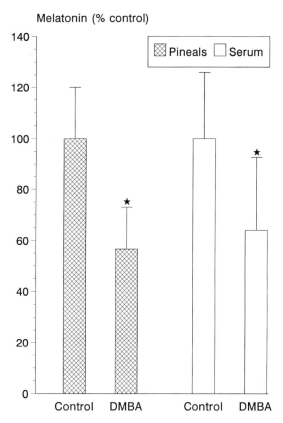

FIG. 5. Melatonin levels in pineal gland and serum of female rats 13 weeks after first DMBA application; i.e., at time of massive breast cancer growth and progression. Controls received vehicle. None of the animals was exposed to a magnetic field, because we wanted to examine how melatonin levels changed during DMBA-induced mammary carcinogenesis in the absence of magnetic field exposure. Data are shown as percent control (mean ± SE of 8–9 animals per group). Significant differences to control are marked by asterisk ($p < 0.05$). Data are from unpublished experiments.

with DMBA at time of massive cancer growth. It should be noted that the melatonin levels (both sham- and magnetic field-exposed) shown in Figure 2 were from DMBA-treated rats, demonstrating that magnetic field exposure led to a further decrease in melatonin in addition to that occurring in DMBA-treated rats in the absence of magnetic field exposure. All these data indicate that the rats used in our studies were sensitive to manipulations of melatonin production.

The experimental protocol used for our DMBA experiments is summarized in Figure 6. A detailed description of the exposure system and experimental protocol has been given elsewhere (Löscher et al. 1993; Baum et al. 1995). As illustrated in Figure 7, the DMBA administration and magnetic field exposure protocol allowed the magnetic field to interact with all processes of DMBA-induced mammary carcinogenesis. Because we did not know before if magnetic fields would affect the DMBA model and which process would be most sensitive, we developed a DMBA administration protocol with four oral DMBA applications over a period of 3 weeks in rats that were either magnetic field- or sham-exposed. By this protocol, about 40–60% of sham controls developed palpable and macroscopically visible mammary tumors over a period of 3 months, thus allowing us to study any effect (both inhibitory or stimulatory) of magnetic field exposure on development and growth of breast cancer.

After a series of preliminary experiments with relatively small numbers of rats (Mevissen et al. 1993), four experiments with larger sample sizes were undertaken. Each experiment comprised a sham control group and a group exposed to 1 magnetic field flux density. More groups not treated with DMBA were exposed or sham-exposed together with the DMBA-treated groups. Because of various factors, including season, which can affect mammary carcinogenesis even under strictly controlled laboratory environment (controlled temperature, light cycle, standardized food, etc.), all data obtained in magnetic field-exposed rats were compared to the concurrently processed sham control group. All experiments were done "blind"; that is, the experimenters involved in handling animals and collecting and evaluating data were not aware of which rat group was magnetic field-exposed and which was sham-exposed.

The four flux densities (all 50 Hz) studied were a gradient field of 0.3–1 μT, and three homogeneous fields of 10, 50, and 100 μT. Taken together, 333 rats were sham-exposed and 333 rats were magnetic field-exposed in these four experiments. The average incidence of mammary tumors (macroscopically visible at time of autopsy; i.e., after 3 months of exposure) was 51% in controls and 62% in magnetic field-

Experimental Methods

Model

Induction of breast cancer (mammary adenocarcinoma) by 7,12-dimethylbenz(a)anthracene (DMBA) in female rats (Sprague-Dawley; age at first DMBA application, 52 days)

Dose selection

Once-weekly oral doses of 5 mg DMBA/rat (total dose 20 mg). At this dosage about 40–60% of control animals develop mammary tumors within 3 months.

Size of groups

99 (or 36) magnetic field-exposed and 99 (or 36) sham-exposed rats. Additional groups (n = 9) are exposed or sham-exposed without DMBA.

MF exposure

50-Hz, linearly (horizontally) polarized, 0.3–100 mT r.m.s.; 24 hours/day, 7 days/week, for a total of 3 months

Observation and exposure period

3 months

Recordings (blind)

a) During exposure: body weight, general behavior, determination of tumor latency and growth by palpation of mammary tumors; determination of tissue ODC activity and serum melatonin levels

b) At autopsy: nocturnal melatonin levels in pineal gland and serum, blood chemistry and hematological values, pathological and histopathological examination of all organs, recording and classification of all preneoplastic and neoplastic lesions (including morphometry), immunohistological examination of tumor cell proliferation; cytogenetic studies on peripheral lymphocytes; evaluation of alterations within the immune system

FIG. 6. Summary of the experimental protocol used for the current studies on magnetic field exposure in the DMBA model of breast cancer.

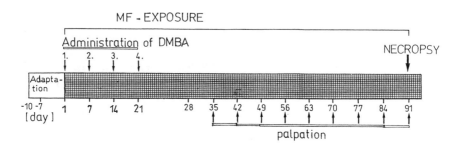

FIG. 7. Schematic presentation of the experimental protocol used for the current studies on magnetic field exposure in the DMBA model of breast cancer.

exposed rats, the difference being highly significant (Fig. 8). However, this type of data evaluation ignored the differences existing between different flux densities. As shown in Figure 9, exposure in a field of 0.3–1 μT did not lead to significant differences in tumor incidence at time of autopsy, but there was a tendency for enhanced tumor development or growth between 8 and 12 weeks of exposure. In this respect, it should be noted that the melatonin determinations carried out after 8–9 weeks of exposure in these animals had indicated a significant decrease in melatonin compared to controls (Fig. 2). Increase of flux density to 10 μT led to a similar time course of tumor development as in the experiment with 0.3–1 μT; exposed rats showed a tendency to enhanced tumor growth which, however, was again not significantly different from controls (not illustrated; Mevissen et al. 1996a). At time of autopsy, the incidence of rats with macroscopically visible mammary tumors in the magnetic field-exposed group was 10% higher than in the sham group.

Further increase of flux density to 100 μT induced several significant effects on mammary carcinogenesis in the DMBA model. As shown in Figure 10, significantly more rats developed palpable tumors during magnetic field exposure than during sham exposure. At the end of the exposure period, the difference to control was 50%. This result of palpation in animals before sacrifice was confirmed by autopsy; 51 of the magnetic field-exposed compared to 34 of the sham-exposed rats

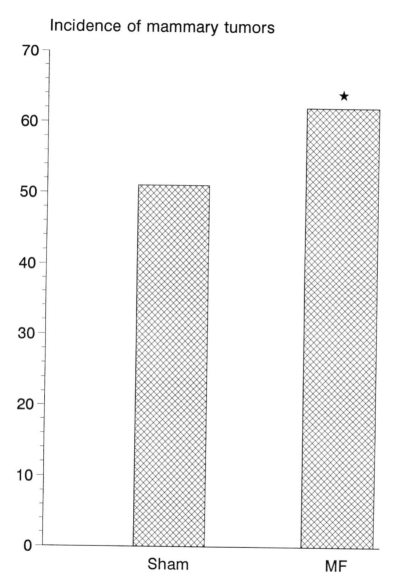

Incidence of mammary tumors

FIG. 8. Overall incidence of DMBA-induced mammary tumors in the four experiments on different flux densities. Data are from 333 sham controls and 333 magnetic field (50-Hz, 0.3–100-μT)-exposed rats. The incidence of mammary tumors refers to the number of rats with macroscopically visible mammary tumors at time of autopsy; i.e., 13 weeks after the first DMBA application (see Fig. 7). The difference between both groups was significant (p < 0.01; indicated by asterisk).

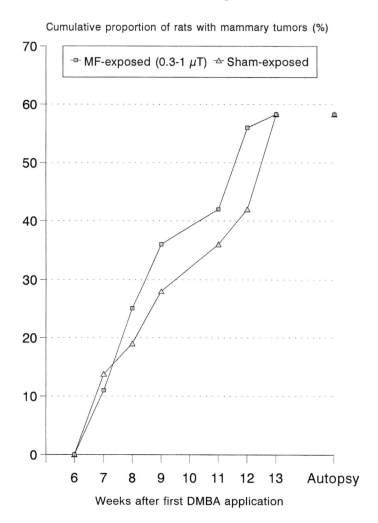

FIG. 9. Cumulative proportion of tumors as a function of time after the first DMBA application in the experiment with 50-Hz, 0.3–1-μT magnetic field exposure. Data shown for weeks 6–13 are from weekly palpation of the rats, whereas data shown for autopsy are from macroscopic examination of mammary tissue after dissection. Thirty-six rats were used per group; the differences between both groups were not significant. Data are from Löscher et al. (1994).

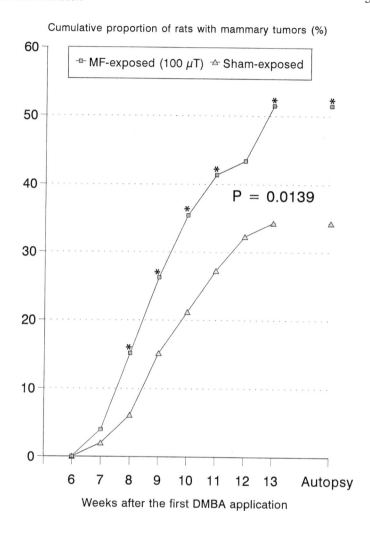

Cumulative proportion of rats with mammary tumors (%)

MF-exposed (100 µT) Sham-exposed

P = 0.0139

6   7   8   9   10   11   12   13   Autopsy

Weeks after the first DMBA application

FIG. 10. Cumulative proportion of tumors as a function of time after the first DMBA application in the experiment with 50-Hz, 100-µT magnetic field exposure. Data shown for weeks 6–13 are from weekly palpation of the rats, whereas data shown for autopsy are from macroscopic examination of mammary tissue after dissection. Ninety-nine rats were used per group. The differences between palpational data of both groups were significant (p = 0.0139) when compared by a log-rank test. Furthermore, several of the individual weekly data were significantly different (p < 0.05; indicated by asterisk). In addition, tumor incidence at time of autopsy was significantly different (p < 0.05). Data are from Löscher et al. (1993) and Baum et al. (1995).

exhibited macroscopically visible mammary tumors, the difference being statistically significant. The fourth experiment undertaken in this series used a flux density of 50 μT (Mevissen et al. 1996b). Again, a significantly higher number of rats with tumors was seen in the magnetic field-exposed compared to the sham-exposed group with a difference at time of autopsy of 25.5% (not illustrated). Linear regression analysis of the data from the four experiments indicated a highly significant ($p < 0.01$) linear relation between flux density and increase in incidence of macroscopically visible mammary tumors at time of autopsy (Fig. 11). To our knowledge, these data provide the first evidence of a linear relationship between flux density and effect of magnetic field exposure in a cancer model.

Interestingly, in all four experiments, the first indication of enhanced tumor growth was seen after 6–8 weeks; that is, at the time at which we had determined decreased melatonin and increased ODC in magnetic field-exposed rats. The increase in incidence of palpable tumors at 8 weeks of exposure (Fig. 12) is again consistent with enhanced tumor development and growth in response to magnetic fields. Similar to the data obtained after 3 months of exposure, flux densities exceeding 10 μT appeared to be associated with increased tumor incidence at 8 weeks. Although the effect of 50 and 100 μT appeared to be higher at 8 weeks compared to 13 weeks, it should be noted that at this time the tumor incidence in sham controls was much lower and variable than 3 months following the first DMBA application (see Figs. 9 and 10). Nevertheless, these data might indicate that magnetic field effects in the DMBA model might be much more marked if lower doses of DMBA (i.e., doses associated with lower tumor incidence in controls) would have been used.

In contrast to the increased number of rats with tumors in some of the magnetic field-exposed groups, the number of tumors per rat was not significantly altered. However, the median size of tumors in magnetic field-exposed rats was markedly enhanced in the experiment with 100 μT (Baum et al. 1995). In addition to increased incidence of rats with palpable and macroscopically visible tumors and increased size of the excised tumors in the experiment with 100 μT, histopathological examination of tumors indicated that significantly more rats of the magnetic field-exposed group developed malignant mammary tumors than rats of the control group, indicating that magnetic field

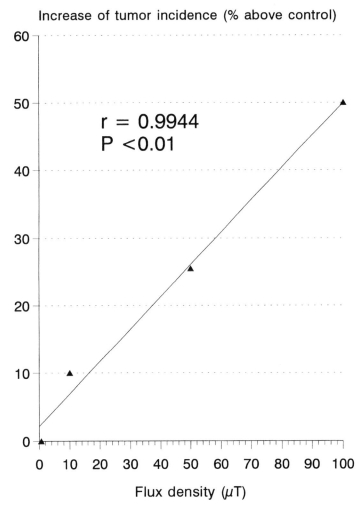

Increase of tumor incidence (% above control)

r = 0.9944
P <0.01

Flux density (μT)

FIG. 11. Increase in the incidence of DMBA-induced mammary tumors as a function of flux density of 50-Hz magnetic field exposure. The figure illustrates the incidence of macroscopically visible mammary tumors at autopsy relative to the tumor incidence in concurrent control groups for four flux density levels: 0.3–1 μT, 10 μT, 50 μT, and 100 μT. Duration of exposure was 3 months. Average tumor incidence in the four control groups from the four experiments with different flux densities was 51% (see Fig. 8). The line through the experimental values was calculated by linear regression analysis; the correlation coefficient (r) from this calculation is indicated in the figure. Data are based on experiments in a total of 666 female rats (333 exposed and 333 sham exposed). Data are from Löscher and Mevissen (1995).

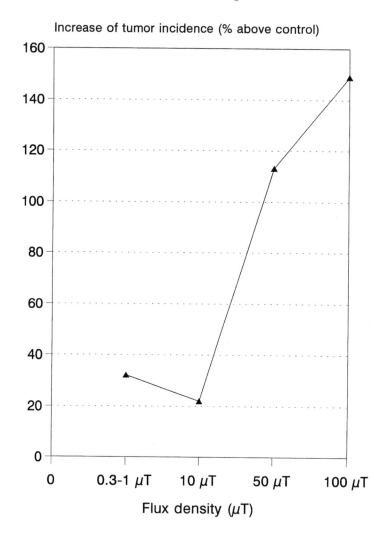

FIG. 12. Increase in the incidence of DMBA-induced mammary tumors as a function of flux density of 50-Hz magnetic field exposure. The figure illustrates the incidence of palpable mammary tumors relative to the tumor incidence in concurrent control groups for four flux density levels: 0.3–1 μT, 10 μT, 50 μT, and 100 T. Duration of exposure was 8 weeks. Average tumor incidence in the four control groups from the four experiments with different flux densities was 15%. Linear regression analysis of the dose–response data yielded a correlation coefficient of 0.9639 ($p < 0.05$). Data are based on experiments in a total of 666 female rats (333 exposed and 333 sham exposed). Data are from Löscher et al. (1993, 1994) and Mevissen et al. (1996a, b).

exposure had not only increased tumor growth but also progression to malignancy (Baum et al. 1995). However, in contrast to the findings from palpation and recording of macroscopically visible tumors at time of autopsy, histopathological examination of mammary tissue by serial sections of all six pairs of mammary glands (see Fig. 3) in each animal revealed that the incidence of mammary lesions was not significantly different between exposed rats and controls (Baum et al. 1995). These data thus strongly indicate that under the conditions of these studies, magnetic field exposure did not initiate cancers or increase the initiation of cancers by DMBA, but enhanced the growth and progression of the DMBA-induced lesions. These findings would be consistent with a copromoting effect of magnetic field exposure. In consequence, although magnetic field exposure did not lead to more tumors, tumors grew more rapidly and were thus diagnosed earlier by palpation or macroscopic examination at time of autopsy.

One may argue that the flux densities at which we found significant tumor copromoting effects (50 and 100 μT) of magnetic field exposure greatly exceed the range of flux densities occurring in human occupational or residential exposures. In this respect, two points can be made. First, if one assumes that biological effects of ELF magnetic fields are due to the induced electric fields or currents, the magnitude of the applied field may have to be adjusted to yield equivalent dosimetric exposure parameters in different species of different body shape and size (Bracken 1992). Respective scaling factors for rat:human are about 5–10:1; that is, a 100-μT field for a rat would correspond to a 10–20 μT field for humans (Bracken 1992). On the other hand, some experimental work suggests that time-varying magnetic field interactions with tissues and cells are related to the magnetic field itself rather than an induced electric field or current, in which case no scaling would be needed (Bracken 1992; Polk 1992). Even then, there may be marked species differences as known from cancer-causing or -promoting agents (Gold et al. 1992; Huff 1993; Vaino and Wilbourn 1993). Animal models used in identification of carcinogens are usually considered less susceptible than humans so that no direct extrapolation of dose from rodents to humans is possible; however, safety factors (i.e., factors by which a rodent carcinogenic dose is divided) are used in risk assessment that relates human exposures to carcinogenic potency of a given agent in rodents. In this respect, it is important to note that for many agents now known as causing or promoting cancers in humans, the first evidence of carcinogenicity was obtained in experimental animals. This knowledge, together with similarities in mechanisms of carcinogenesis across species, led to the scientific logic and public health strategy that chemical or other agents shown clearly to be carcinogenic (initiating, promoting, or copromoting) in animals should be considered as being likely and anticipated to present cancer risks in humans (Huff 1993).

Many factors relevant for development and growth of human breast cancer have been identified and characterized by the DMBA model (Huggins and Yang 1962; Russo and Russo 1978; Welsch 1985; Rogers et al. 1989; Cornélissen and Halberg 1992), so that findings such as the data presented here on magnetic field exposure cannot be ignored for reasons of "uncertainty." Furthermore, the similarities of our findings on magnetic field exposure in the DMBA rat model with the findings of Beniashvili et al. (1991) in the NMU rat model strongly suggest that these results are not restricted to one animal model system of breast cancer. Interestingly, as in humans, genetics play an important role in the susceptibility to cancer in models of mammary carcinogenesis such as the DMBA model in rats (Melhem et al. 1991); therefore, effects of ELF magnetic fields on gene expression, as suggested by some recent studies (e.g., Phillips et al. 1992), should be considered in addition to the melatonin hypothesis used to explain our findings in this study.

EFFECT OF ELF MAGNETIC FIELDS ON IMMUNE RESPONSES TO TUMOR FORMATION

We are currently carrying out a study to see if 50-Hz exposure of female rats in the μT range indeed affects the immune system as the body's main protective mechanism against tumor formation and growth. Resistance against the development of neoplasia depends on a variety of host immunologic and other factors (Welsch 1985; Cruse and Lewis 1988). For instance, chemical carcinogens such as DMBA have been shown to temporally suppress immune reactivity, and a positive correlation was found between the degree of immune-system depression and the individual rate of breast cancer growth in rats (e.g., Gallo et al. 1993). Thus, if magnetic field exposure depresses immune-system functions via reduced melatonin production or other mechanisms, this effect could be critically involved in enhanced tumor growth in response to magnetic fields. Although it has repeatedly been suggested that magnetic field exposure might affect the immune system, respective evidence is inconclusive, and the majority of data are from in vitro experiments without any direct relation to tumor formation (cf., Walleczek 1992).

In a first attempt to delineate in vivo effects of magnetic field exposure on the immune surveillance system in female rats as used in our studies, we examined mitogen-induced T-cell activation in female rats exposed to a 50-Hz, 50-μT magnetic field for 13 weeks. T cells (or T-lymphocytes) constitute the majority (65–85%) of lymphocytes in peripheral blood and appear to be important for antitumor activity and its immune regulation (Cruse and Lewis 1988). In magnetic field-exposed rats, activation (i.e., proliferation) of T-cells in response to a mitogen (concanavalin A; Con-A) was markedly suppressed compared to sham-exposed controls (not illustrated; Mevissen et al. 1996b). These data strongly suggest that immune-system depression is involved in the tumor copromoting effects of magnetic field exposure observed in rats. In this respect, it is interesting to note that a reduced stimulation of lymphocytes by the T-cell-selective mitogen, Con-A, has also been reported for 50-Hz magnetic field-exposed human lymphocytes (Conti et al. 1983). One can only speculate about the underlying cellular mechanisms of interaction between magnetic field exposure and the immune system. Both reduced melatonin level and function (Maestroni 1993) and altered Ca^{2+} signals (cf., Walleczek 1992) may play a key role in this respect. Experiments are under way to examine in detail how the observed alteration in T-cell reactivity depends on the duration and flux density of magnetic field exposure. Furthermore, levels of cytokines involved in T-cell growth and function will be determined in these studies, and intracellular Ca^{2+} concentration will be measured in lymphocytes isolated from magnetic field-exposed animals.

MAGNETIC FIELD EXPOSURE AND BREAST CANCER: CONCLUSIONS

The current data provide the first direct experimental evidence that the melatonin hypothesis first proposed by Stevens (1987) for chronic 60-Hz electric fields may explain carcinogenic effects of ELF magnetic fields, particularly facilitation of development and growth of breast cancer. Furthermore, the data from the DMBA model add to the accumulating evidence from laboratory studies that 50/60-Hz magnetic field exposure may exert a copromoting effect in carcinogenesis (reviewed in Löscher and Mevissen 1994). How relevant are the current data from the DMBA model of breast cancer with respect to human risk assessment? Wertheimer and Leeper (1982) were the first to see a magnetic field–breast cancer connection in their 1982 study of residential magnetic-field exposures of adults. They discovered a nearly threefold increase among women younger than 55 who lived near power lines, indicating that magnetic field exposure had accelerated development and growth of breast cancer. More recently, increased breast cancer risks were reported in both women and men in electrical occupations (for review see Gammon and John 1993; Thomas 1993; Tynes 1993; Loomis et al. 1994; Wertheimer and Leeper 1994). However, some reports that included women found no excess of breast cancer in an array of occupations related to enhanced magnetic field exposure as well as residential exposures. Such findings could be due to the various differences among studies and the uncertain exposure conditions in most studies. Therefore, prospective epidemiologic studies with more closely defined exposure conditions are needed to progress the understanding of breast cancer risk related to environmental and occupational magnetic field exposure.

One important question is whether ELF magnetic field exposure reduces melatonin in humans. The very few studies in this regard have used short-term magnetic field exposure in volunteers rather than prolonged or chronic exposure as occurring in residential and occupational magnetic field exposures. Both in the rat studies of Kato et al. (1993) and our studies, prolonged magnetic field exposure was shown to reduce melatonin, whereas effects of short-lasting ELF magnetic field exposure were not examined. We are currently investigating in rats the relation between duration of magnetic field exposure and alterations in melatonin levels in order to obtain more information in this respect. In hamsters, exposure to a 60-Hz, 100-μT magnetic field for only 15 minutes was shown to reduce nocturnal melatonin, but this finding was not strictly reproducible (Yellon 1994).

Independent of the effect of ELF magnetic fields on melatonin production, it is important to note that in vitro experiments indicate that the inhibitory effect of melatonin on human breast cancer growth is suppressed by ELF magnetic field exposure in the μT range (Liburdy et al. 1993). If interaction between magnetic fields and melatonin at the cellular level also occurs in vivo, it would add to any impairment of melatonin production so that even small decreases in circulating melatonin levels could have pronounced consequences. Such an effect of magnetic field exposure on melatonin level and function could not only increase breast cancer growth but also other types of cancer (cf., Blask 1993). However, it should also be considered that the effect of magnetic field exposure on carcinogenesis, if occurring in humans, will presumably be small compared to other known cancer promoters or copromoters. Therefore, it will be important to study experimentally if effects of magnetic field exposure on cancer growth are amplified in the presence of known cancer promoters or copromoters, because such interactions can be over-additive and thus markedly increase the risk of exposure (cf., Löscher and Mevissen 1995).

ACKNOWLEDGMENTS

We thank Dr. H. Kärner and colleagues (Department of High Voltage Engineering, Technical University of Braunschweig), Dr. U. Mohr and colleagues (Institute of Experimental Pathology, Medical School Hannover), Dr. M. Szamel and colleagues (Institute of Molecular Pharmacology, Medical School Hannover), Dr. A. Lerchl and colleagues (Institute for Reproductive Medicine, University of Münster), and Dr. W. Lehmacher and colleagues (Department of Biometrics and Epidemiology, School of Veterinary Medicine, Hannover) for collaboration and helpful discussions during the studies described in this paper. The studies were supported by equipment and grants from the *Forschungsverbund Elektromagnetische Verträglichkeit Biologischer Systeme* (Department of High Voltage Engineering, Technical University, Braunschweig, Germany) and the *Berufsgenossenschaft der Feinmechanik und Elektrotechnik* (Köln, Germany).

REFERENCES

Baum, A., M. Mevissen, K. Kamino, U. Mohr, W. Löscher. 1995. A histopathological study on alterations in DMBA-induced mammary carcinogenesis in rats with 50 Hz, 100 μT magnetic field exposure. *Carcinogenesis* 16:119–125.

Beniashvili, D.S., V.G. Bilanishvili, M.Z. Menabde. 1991. Low-frequency electromagnetic radiation enhances the induction of rat mammary tumors by nitrosomethyl urea. *Cancer Lett.* 61:75–79.

Blask, D.E. 1993. Melatonin in oncology. In: *Melatonin. Biosynthesis, Physiological Effects, and Clinical Applications*, H.-S. Yu and R.J. Reiter, eds., pp. 448–475. Boca Raton, Florida: CRC Press.

Bracken, T.D. 1992. Experimental macroscopic dosimetry for extremely-low-frequency electric and magnetic fields. *Bioelectromagnetics Suppl.* 1:15–26.

Byus, C.V., S.E. Pieper, W.R. Adey. 1987. The effects of low-energy 60-Hz environmental electromagnetic fields upon the growth-related enzyme ornithine decarboxylase. *Carcinogenesis* 8:1385–1389.

Cain, C.D., E.Q. Salvador, W.R. Adey. 1988. 60-Hz electric field prolongs ornithine decarboxylase activity response to 12-O-tetradecanoylphorbol-13-acetate (TPA) in C3H10T^1/$_2$ fibroblasts. In: Proceedings of the 10th Annual Bioelectromagnetics Society Meeting, p. 63. Stamford, Connecticut, June 19–23, 1988. Frederick, Maryland: The Bioelectromagnetics Society.

Conti, P., G.E. Giganti, M.G. Cifone, E. Alesse, G. Ianni, M. Reale, P.U. Angeletti. 1983. Reduced mitogenic stimulation of human lymphocytes by extremely low frequency electromagnetic fields. *FEBS Lett.* 162:156–160.

Cornélissen, G., F. Halberg. 1992. Chronobiologic response modifiers and breast cancer development: Classical background and chronobiologic tasks remaining. *In Vivo* 6:387–402.

Cruse, J.M., R.E.J. Lewis. 1988. Immunomodulation of neoplasia. In: *Progress in Experimental Tumor Research*, F. Homburger, J.M. Cruse, R.E.J. Lewis, eds., pp. 156–172. Basel:Karger.

Gallo, F., M.C. Morale, D. Sambatoro, Z. Farinella, U. Scapagnini, B. Marchetti. 1993. The immune system response during development and progression of carcinogen-induced rat mammary tumors:

Prevention of tumor growth and restoration of immune sytem responsiveness by thymopentin. *Breast Cancer Res. Treat.* 27:221–237.

Gammon, M.D., E.M. John. 1993. Recent etiologic hypotheses concerning breast cancer. *Epidemiol. Rev.* 15:163–168.

Gold, L.S., T.H. Slone, B.R. Stern, N.B. Manley, B.N. Ames. 1992. Rodent carcinogens: Setting priorities. *Science* 258:261–265.

Huff, J. 1993. Issues and controversies surrounding qualitative strategies for identifying and forecasting cancer causing agents in the human environment. *Pharmacol. & Toxicol. Suppl.* 1:12–27.

Huggins, C., N.C. Yang. 1962. Induction and extinction of mammary cancer. *Science* 137:257–262.

Kato, M., K.I. Honma, T. Shigemitsu, Y. Shiga. 1993. Effects of exposure to a circulatory polarized 50-Hz magnetic field on plasma and pineal melatonin levels in rats. *Bioelectromagnetics* 14:97–106.

Kato, M., K. Honma, T. Shigemitsu, Y. Shiga. 1994. Horizontal or vertical 50-Hz, 1-μT magnetic fields have no effect on pineal gland or plasma melatonin concentration of albino rats. *Neurosci. Lett.* 168:205–208.

Liburdy, R.P., T.R. Sloma, R. Sokolic, P. Yaswen. 1993. ELF magnetic fields, breast cancer, and melatonin: 60 Hz fields block melatonin's oncostatic action on ER$^+$ breast cancer cell proliferation. *J. Pineal Res.* 14:89–97.

Litovitz, T.A., D. Krause, J.M. Mullins. 1991. Effect of coherence time of the applied magnetic field on ornithine decarboxylase activity. *Biochem. Biophys. Res. Commun.* 178:862–865.

Loomis, D.P., D.A. Savitz, C.V. Ananth. 1994. Breast cancer mortality among female electrical workers in the United States. *J. Natl. Cancer Inst.* 86:921–925.

Löscher, W., M. Mevissen. 1994. Animal studies on the role of 50/60-Hertz magnetic fields in carcinogenesis. *Life Sci.* 54:1531–1543.

Löscher, W., M. Mevissen. 1995. Linear relationship between flux density and tumor copromoting effect of prolonged magnetic field exposure in a breast cancer model. *Cancer Lett.* 96:175–180.

Löscher, W., M. Mevissen, W. Lehmacher, A. Stamm. 1993. Tumor promotion in a breast cancer model by exposure to a weak alternating magnetic field. *Cancer Lett.* 71:75–81.

Löscher, W., U. Wahnschaffe, M. Mevissen, A. Lerchl, A. Stamm. 1994. Effects of weak alternating magnetic fields on nocturnal melatonin production and mammary carcinogenesis in rats. *Oncology* 51:288–295.

Maestroni, G.J.M. 1993. The immunoneuroendocrine role of melatonin. *J. Pineal Res.* 14:1–10.

Maestroni, G.J.M., A. Conti. 1993. Melatonin in relation to the immune system. In: *Melatonin. Biosynthesis, Physiological Effects, and Clinical Applications*, H.-S. Yu and R.J. Reiter, eds., pp. 289–309. Boca Raton, Florida:CRC Press.

Mattsson, M.-O., K.H. Mild, U. Rehnholm. 1993a. Ornithine decarboxylase activity and polyamine levels in cell lines exposed to a 50-Hz sine-wave magnetic field. In: Abstracts of the 15th Annual Bioelectromagnetics Society Meeting, Los Angeles, California, June 13–17, pp. 93–94. Frederick, Maryland: The Bioelectromagnetics Society.

Mattsson, M.-O., K.H. Mild, U. Rehnholm. 1993b. Ornithine decarboxylase activity in lymphoblastoid cell lines after 50 Hz sine-wave magnetic field exposure. In: Abstracts of the Annual Review of Research on Biological Effects of Electric and Magnetic Fields from the Generation, Delivery, and Use of Electricity, Savannah, Georgia, October 31–November 4, p. 3. Frederick, Maryland: W/L Associates, Ltd.

Mediavilla, M.D., S. San Martin, E.J. Sánchez-Barceló. 1992. Melatonin inhibits mammary gland development in female mice. *J. Pineal Res.* 13:13–19.

Melhem, M.F., H.W. Kunz, T.J. Gill. 1991. Genetic control of susceptibility to diethylnitrosamine and dimethylbenzanthracene carcinogenesis in rats. *Am. J. Pathol.* 139:45–51.

Mevissen, M., A. Stamm, S. Buntenkötter, R. Zwingelberg, U. Wahnschaffe, W. Löscher. 1993. Effects of magnetic fields on mammary tumor development induced by 7,12-dimethylbenz(a)-anthracene in rats. *Bioelectromagnetics* 14:131–143.

Mevissen, M., M. Kietzmann, W. Löscher. 1995. *In vivo* exposure of rats to a weak alternating magnetic field increases ornithine decarboxylase activity in the mammary gland by a similar extent as the carcinogen DMBA. *Cancer Lett.* 90:207–214.

Mevissen, M., A. Lerchl, W. Löscher. 1996a. A study on pineal function and DMBA-induced breast cancer formation in rats during exposure to a 100-mG, 50-Hz magnetic field. *J. Tox. Environment. Health* 48:101–117.

Mevissen, M., A. Lerchl, M. Szamel, W. Löscher. 1996b. Exposure of DMBA-treated rats in a 50-Hz, 50 μT magnetic field: Effects on mammary tumor growth, melatonin levels, and T lymphocyte activation. *Carcinogenesis* 17:903–910.

Mhatre, M.C., P.N. Shah, H.S. Juneja. 1984. Effects of varying photoperiods on mammary morphology, DNA synthesis, and hormone profile in female rats. *J. Natl. Cancer Inst.* 72:1411–1416.

O'Brien, T.G., R.C. Simsiman, R.K. Boutwell. 1975. Induction of polyamine-biosynthetic enzymes in mouse epidermis and their specificity for tumor promotion. *Cancer Res.* 35:2426–2433.

O'Brien, T.G. 1976. The induction of ornithine decarboxylase as an early, possibly obligatory, event in mouse skin carcinogenesis. *Cancer Res.* 36:2644–2653.

Phillips, J.L., W. Haggren, W.J. Thomas, T. Ishida-Jones, W.R. Adey. 1992. Magnetic field-induced changes in specific gene transcription. *Biochim. Biophys. Acta* 1132:140–144.

Polk, C. 1992. Dosimetry of extremely-low-frequency magnetic fields. *Bioelectromagnetics Suppl.* 1:209–235.

Reiter, R.J. 1991. Pineal melatonin: Cell biology of its synthesis and of its physiological interactions. *Endocrine Rev.* 12:151–180.

Reiter, R.J. 1993. Static and extremely low frequency electromagnetic field exposure—Reported effects on the circadian production of melatonin. *J. Cell. Biochem.* 51:394–403.

Rogers, A.E. 1989. Factors that modulate chemical carcinogenesis in the mammary gland of the female rat. In: *Integument and Mammary Glands*, T.C. Jones, U. Mohr, and R.D. Hunt, eds., pp. 304-314. Berlin:Springer-Verlag.

Russell, D.H. 1980. Ornithine decarboxylase as a biological and pharmacological tool. *Pharmacology* 20:117–129.

Russo, I.H., J. Russo. 1978. Developmental stage of the rat mammary gland as determinant of its susceptibility to 7,12-dimethylbenz(a)anthracene. *J. Natl. Cancer Inst.* 61:1439–1449.

Savitz, D.A., A. Ahlbom. 1994. Epidemiologic evidence on cancer in relation to residential and occupational exposures. In: *Biological Effects of Electric and Magnetic Fields*, D.O. Carpenter and S. Ayrapetyan, eds., pp. 233-261. San Diego, California:Academic Press.

Semm, P., T. Schneider, L. Vollrath. 1980. Effects of an earth-strength magnetic field on electrical activity of pineal cells. *Nature* 288:607–608.

Stevens, R.G. 1987. Electric power use and breast cancer: A hypothesis. *Am. J. Epidemiol.* 125:556–561.

Stevens, R.G. 1993. Biologically based epidemiological studies of electric power and cancer. *Environ. Health Perspect. Suppl.* 4:93–100.

Stevens, R.G., S. Davis, D.B. Thomas, L.E. Anderson, B.W. Wilson. 1992. Electric power, pineal function, and the risk of breast cancer. *FASEB J.* 6:853–860.

Thomas, D.B. 1993. Breast cancer in man. *Epidemiol. Rev.* 15:220–231.

Tynes, T. 1993. Electromagnetic fields and male breast cancer. *Biomed. & Pharmacother.* 47:425–427.

Vainio, H., J. Wilbourn. 1993. Cancer etiology: Agents causally associated with human cancer. *Pharmacol. & Toxicol. Suppl.* 1:4–11.

Van Zwieten, M.J. 1984. *The Rat as Animal Model in Breast Cancer Research.* Boston:Martinus Nijhoff.

Walleczek, J. 1992. Electromagnetic field effects on cells of the immune system: The role of calcium signaling. *FASEB J.* 6:3177–3185.

Welsch, C.W. 1985. Host factors affecting the growth of carcinogen-induced rat mammary carcinomas: A review and tribute to Charles Brenton Huggins. *Cancer Res.* 45:3415–3443.

Wertheimer, N., E. Leeper. 1982. Adult cancer related to electrical wires near the home. *Int. J. Epidemiol.* 11:345–355.

Wertheimer, N., E. Leeper. 1994. Re: Are electric or magnetic fields affecting mortality from breast cancer in women? *J. Nat. Cancer Inst.* 86:1797.

Yellon, S.M. 1994. Acute 60 Hz magnetic field exposure effects on the melatonin rhythm in the pineal gland and circulation of the adult Djungarian hamster. *J. Pineal Res.* 16:136–144.

21 Laboratory Studies on Extremely Low Frequency (50/60-Hz) Magnetic Fields and Carcinogenesis

ROBERT P. LIBURDY
Life Sciences Division, Lawrence Berkeley National
Laboratory, University of California, Berkeley
WOLFGANG LÖSCHER
Department of Pharmacology, Toxicology and Pharmacy,
School of Veterinary Medicine, Hannover, Germany

CONTENTS

INTRODUCTION
PROCESSES IN CARCINOGENESIS ON WHICH
  ELF MAGNETIC FIELDS MAY ACT
IN VITRO STUDIES ON THE ROLE OF ELF MAGNETIC FIELDS
  IN CARCINOGENESIS
  Signal Transduction: Receptor–Ligand Binding, Enzyme Activation,
    Calcium Mobilization
  Gene Induction, Gene Expression, and Protein Synthesis
  Ornithine Decarboxylase (ODC) and Promotion/Copromotion
  Cell Proliferation
  Gap Junctions and Intercellular Communication
  Free Radicals and Antioxidants in Biological Systems
ANIMAL STUDIES ON THE ROLE OF
  ELF MAGNETIC FIELDS IN CARCINOGENESIS
  Effects of Magnetic Field Exposure on Spontaneous Tumor
    Development

(continued)

CONTENTS (continued)

Effects of Magnetic Field Exposure on Implanted Tumor Cells
Effects of Magnetic Field Exposure in Cocarcinogenesis Models
In Vivo Studies on Mechanisms Potentially Linked to Carcinogenesis
Technical and Biological Factors Critically Involved in Laboratory
    Studies on Magnetic Field Effects
CONCLUSIONS
REFERENCES

INTRODUCTION

An unresolved issue in environmental toxicology is whether adverse human health effects, particularly cancer, could result from residential or occupational exposure to extremely low frequency (ELF) (i.e., 50- or 60-Hz) magnetic fields such as associated with electric power. In view of the methodological problems of epidemiologic studies on associations between exposures to ELF magnetic fields and increased incidence of cancers, laboratory studies are necessary to determine if any association exists. Most laboratory studies have indicated that nonionizing radiation has no mutagenic effect, i.e., does not initiate cancer (McCann et al. 1993; Murphy et al. 1993). Thus, if ELF magnetic fields are truly associated with an increased risk of cancer, then they must act as a promoter or copromoter of cancer in cells that have already been initiated. Many cellular studies support this view, because magnetic fields are observed to influence signal transduction, enzyme action, and protein synthesis/gene expression. These activities, discussed herein, play an important role in regulating cell growth and processes important to promotion. Furthermore, some studies have suggested that the genotoxic potential of certain chemical mutagens or ionizing radiation may be affected by co-exposure to magnetic fields (McCann et al. 1993).

In this chapter, the carcinogenic processes that magnetic fields may influence will be reviewed, as well as in vitro and in vivo laboratory studies on the question of whether ELF magnetic fields are cancer promoters or can progress cancers. Several caveats should be mentioned for the reader. Ideally, perfect scientific agreement would exist between all in vitro and in vivo experimentation, but this never happens in any field of science, particularly in a relatively new, multidisciplinary research area such as bioelectromagnetics. As in any developing research field, there is no universal consensus regarding the most appropriate laboratory model system; this review will discuss work carried out using many different biological endpoints and model systems. In addition, guidelines are currently evolving for developing standard approaches to magnetic field exposures, which, in the past, have made correlation of results across different laboratories difficult, if not impossible. Finally, given this "state of the science," it is premature to identify a specific interaction mechanism that is most relevant to carcinogenesis. However, this review presents some principles that have emerged which are important in understanding this relationship and in guiding future research.

PROCESSES IN CARCINOGENESIS ON WHICH ELF MAGNETIC FIELDS MAY ACT

Carcinogenesis is traditionally viewed as a two-stage, multistep (and multifactorial) process. In the first stage (initiation), a genotoxic carcinogen (initiator) interacts with cell DNA, resulting in cytogenetic (i.e., DNA) damage that leads to mutation (Fig. 1). In addition to initiation by chemical agents or ionizing radiation, the process of initiation is thought to encompass the actions of inherited mutations, cancer-causing viral genes, and altered cellular genes (oncogenes). The damaged DNA may revert to normal if DNA repair mechanisms operate successfully; if not, the transformed (initiated) cells may grow into a tumor that becomes apparent clinically. In the second stage (promotion) of carcinogenesis, a cell-division stimulus promotes tumor development. The initiated cells remain dormant or latent awaiting a promoting stimulus before a tumor results. Promotion by systemic (e.g., hormones and other growth-enhancing factors) or exogenous (environmental) factors involves facilitation of the growth and development of dormant or latent tumor cells. Thus, a promoter or cocarcinogen is not a carcinogen alone, but it potentiates the effects of a carcinogen. In addition to promoting factors, copromoting factors may

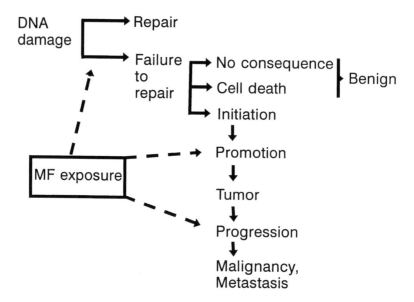

FIG. 1. Steps in classic carcinogenesis on which magnetic field exposure may act.

play a role in carcinogenesis by enhancing tumor development in response to promoters.

For many human tumors, the latent period from initiation to tumor development is 15–45 years, probably depending on the presence of tumor promoters and copromoters. It is important to note that a wide variety of promoting or enhancing agents has been identified in the human environment, including dietary, medicinal, industrial, or agricultural chemicals. After an overt tumor has been formed, the continued exposure to promoters or other selective forces may cause the further evolution or progression of the tumor to a more malignant character with less differentiation and increased invasive and metastatic properties. Numerous in vitro studies have indicated that ELF magnetic fields are not mutagenic, but may act to facilitate promotion and progression of tumors, and possibly also interfere with DNA repair (Fig. 1). Chemical agents or other factors that function as pure promoters do not themselves cause mutations but may alter gene expression or other processes, and thus change cellular metabolism and growth rates. Relevant experimental findings from magnetic field exposure will be reviewed in this chapter.

In addition to promotion or copromotion in the conventional genotoxic pathway of carcinogenesis, altering cellular metabolism and growth rates is an important concept in understanding how magnetic field exposure may influence the process of nongenotoxic carcinogenesis. This process is the epigenetic pathway to cancer and does not invoke any genotoxic or clastogenic initial events (Fig. 2). Chemicals or

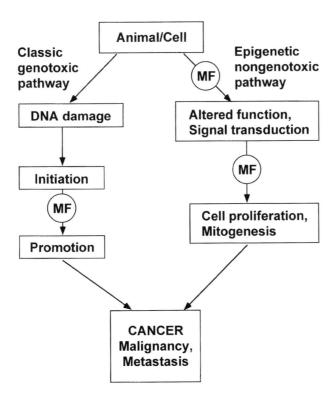

FIG. 2. In addition to the classic genotoxic pathway to cancer (see Fig. 1 and left part of Fig. 2), magnetic field exposure may act on nongenotoxic (epigenetic pathways (right part of Fig. 2).

other agents that induce this process are termed nongenotoxic carcinogens (Shaw and Jones 1994). The mechanism of nongenotoxic carcinogenesis is not fully understood, but is believed to involve stimulation of cell division with a consequent increased probability of a spontaneous mutation (Ames and Gold 1990a, b; Shaw and Jones 1994). Relevant in vitro findings from magnetic field exposure of cell cultures involve alterations in gene transcription and protein synthesis, increases in ornithine decarboxylase (ODC) activity, stimulated cell growth and proliferation, suppressed immune responses to tumor cells, alterations in intercellular communication, and effects on calcium (Ca^{2+}) homeostasis that may have implications for oncogene activation and immune responses.

Unfortunately, apparently conflicting results and the inability to replicate some of the experimental findings have complicated the interpretation of these in vitro experiments. One exception is the observation that μT-level magnetic fields block the oncostatic action of melatonin on MCF-7 breast cancer cell growth (Liburdy et al. 1993b; Blask et al. 1993; Blackman et al. 1996). In vivo animal experiments have indicated that ELF magnetic field exposure exerts suppressive effects on the immune system (e.g., McLean et al. 1991) and on melatonin synthesis (Kato et al. 1993; Löscher et al. 1994). Melatonin, a hormone secreted by the pineal gland, is known to exert oncostatic effects on various types of tumors, including leukemia, breast cancer, prostate cancer, and melanoma (Blask 1993). Although these findings may be accepted as evidence that ELF magnetic fields interact with biological systems, they provide no direct proof that in vivo exposure to such fields leads to cancer promotion or copromotion. Thus, studies on cancer in laboratory animals exposed to magnetic fields under well-defined laboratory exposure conditions are needed.

IN VITRO STUDIES ON THE ROLE OF ELF MAGNETIC FIELDS IN CARCINOGENESIS

Important to remember is that magnetic fields alter or influence cellular metabolism and mitogenesis through different pathways of carcinogenesis that do not involve direct damage to DNA (Fig. 2) (Scarfi et al. 1993; McCann et al. 1993). These interactions, reviewed herein, necessarily involve events that can profoundly effect the process of mitogenesis (cell proliferation), such as altered signal transduction, enzyme activity, and gene expression. Such effects on mitogenesis can and do lead to cancer via the epigenetic pathway (Ames and Gold 1990a, b); agents that increase levels of mitogenesis lead to an increased probability of carcinogenesis. Although the precise interaction mechanism(s) of magnetic fields is not fully elucidated, on balance, current in vitro laboratory observations are consistent with the idea that magnetic fields operate, at least in part, through such a nongenotoxic pathway.

This review will cover recent published research dealing with the question of magnetic field exposure that relates to carcinogenesis. The intent of this review is not to identify every published report nor to identify a consensus viewpoint regarding magnetic field effects, but, rather, to identify the major research topic areas being investigated and review representative papers. The areas of in vitro studies deemed most relevant to carcinogenesis fall into the following categories: signal transduction and calcium, gene expression and protein synthesis, ODC, cell proliferation and melatonin, intercellular (gap junction) communication, and free radicals. Arguably, all of these topics may be interrelated at the cellular and organism level, and the reader will appreciate the complexity in sorting out specific effects as isolated events. Several reviews on magnetic field interactions with cellular systems (no special emphasis on carcinogenesis) have been published, and these are recommended to the reader: Adey 1993; Cadossi et al. 1992, 1994; Cleary 1993; Frey 1993; Goodman and Henderson 1991, 1992; Liburdy 1992c, 1994, 1995; Luben 1991, 1993, 1994; Tenforde 1991, 1992, 1993; and Walleczek 1992. As in vitro research continues to evolve, this database will increase and replication studies will emerge to support or refute findings. This natural progression, which takes time, should lead ultimately to consensus.

Before a discussion of recent in vitro research, several comments should be made regarding exposure systems (Liburdy 1994, 1995) (Table 1). A large proportion of in vitro research is conducted using cultured cell lines, and commercial cell culture incubators are a known source of magnetic fields (Yost and Liburdy 1992; Berglund et al. 1991). This fact has two serious implications for in vitro studies: (1) cells may be pre-exposed to magnetic fields of undefined field strength and frequencies while they are being maintained in culture; and (2) if mag-

TABLE 1
Important Points in Planning and Interpretation
of Laboratory Studies of Magnetic Fields and Cancer

Prior Magnetic Field History
It is important to determine the past magnetic field exposure history of
the model system(s) to be used in the laboratory. For cell lines, the cell
culture incubator must be carefully evaluated for the presence of both
static and time-varying magnetic fields. Commercial incubators are
known to generate significant fields; these must be assessed and eliminated by engineering approaches such as mu-metal shielding. For
example, it is possible that cells to be used in magnetic field experiments
are continuously exposed to undefined AC and DC magnetic fields for
many passages over a long period of time in an incubator, and then
removed and used for low-level magnetic field experiments. These
assessments apply for animal studies as well; however, the physical
scale of the problem is larger. If at all possible, shielded rooms are advisable, but there are other approaches to "buck" out spurious, ambient
magnetic fields in the animal rooms using sensing coils.

Exposure Conditions
When conducting a magnetic field exposure, it is important to ensure the
generation of a spatially uniform flux density, and to monitor for quality
assurance such factors as the waveform and intensity over time. A complete description of magnetic field exposure should include: flux density,
waveform, AC and DC magnetic field, type of polarization [circular, linear
(vertical, horizontal)], intermittency/ transients, exposure duration, presence of electric fields. A complete description of the magnetic field environment should be given in publications to ensure that investigators can
reproduce these conditions in future studies. When mapping magnetic
fields, it is important to use calibrated probes for AC and DC measurements, in combination with calibrated oscilloscopes, if possible; probes
that measure flux density and waveform features are desirable. If the
Earth's magnetic field is not shielded, its direction and strength should
be described. In addition to field specifications, it should be described
how light, noise, vibration, and temperature were controlled.

Cell Lines
Cell lines to be used for in vitro research should be obtained from
sources that ensure the validity of the biological status of the cells.

continued

TABLE 1 (continued)
Important Points in Planning and Interpretation
of Laboratory Studies of Magnetic Fields and Cancer

Commercial sources are usually reliable; however, if a true replication experiment is to be undertaken, it is advisable to obtain cell lines, and protocols, from the laboratory investigator that published the original report. Cell lines derived from the same source but maintained in different laboratories can and do change phenotype over time due to factors such as the serum employed or other culture conditions. This is an important factor in any in vitro experiment and precautions should be taken to measure and follow standard biological markers for function or structure in a cell line used in experimentation.

Animal Species
May be important for biological mechanisms of electric and magnetic fields (EMF) in in vivo studies; e.g. melatonin suppression by EMF has been reported for rats but not mice.

Strain and Sex of Laboratory Species
May be important for interlaboratory differences in in vivo studies.

Protocol for Tumor Initiation and Promotion
(e.g., spontaneously developing vs. chemically induced vs. implanted tumors; dose of promoter in chemically induced tumors, etc.)

Type and Characteristics of Tumor
(e.g., hormone-dependent vs. non-hormone-dependent)

Consequences
Because of these various factors (and many more) which potentially affect results from in vivo studies investigating the relationship between EMF and cancer, data obtained with one type of experimental protocol should not be used to draw general conclusions on presence or absence of effects that might be relevant for carcinogenesis. *The same is true for in vitro studies.* Although standard approaches to biological model systems are not established with regard to magnetic field experimentation, the foregoing considerations are important to keep in mind in designing experiments. Engineering issues about how magnetic field exposures are to be conducted are perhaps better resolved now; the consensus approach to exposures is outlined above.

netic field exposures are conducted in incubators, the presence of endogenous, spurious magnetic fields will introduce confounding factors into the exposure. Although all commercial incubators generate magnetic and electric fields associated with operating the heating and gas exchange equipment of the incubator, considerable variation exists across manufacturers; therefore, the internal magnetic fields need to be carefully assessed in the laboratory. In most low-field exposure situations, it is advisable to shield the interior space of the incubator using 80% nickel mu-metal (e.g., see Maltin 1993). Liburdy and colleagues employ a mu-metal chamber that is ventilated at the upper and lower corners with 2.5-cm diameter holes that have 5-cm extension tubes to prevent entry of stray fields (Liburdy 1994, 1995). Exposing a large volume of space inside such a chamber to a uniform magnetic field can be accomplished using a Merritt four-coil exposure device that has been double-wound with wire so that a switch can be thrown to send current through the coils in an antiparallel or parallel fashion. The antiparallel operation mode will generate opposing magnetic fields that cancel and result in a true sham exposure (Liburdy et al. 1993b). This exposure coil can be placed inside of the mu-metal box and incubator for cell culture studies. In addition, it is important that a temperature probe be placed inside of the chamber to monitor temperature continuously in the vicinity of the cells.

Signal Transduction: Receptor–Ligand Binding, Enzyme Activation, Calcium Mobilization

A discussion of signal transduction (ST) merits introductory remarks because ST appears to be important for understanding cellular responses to magnetic fields, particularly with regard to carcinogenesis. As will be apparent in the following sections, ST most likely represents the underlying process through which a variety of magnetic field effects are mediated.

Signal transduction, one of the major, fundamental pathways for cell communication, is a general process in which a ligand molecule binds to its receptor site on the cell surface. This binding, in turn, triggers a cascade of biochemical events associated with the cell membrane that lead to, for example, calcium mobilization, enzyme activation, gene induction, protein synthesis, and, ultimately, mitogenesis and cell proliferation (Morgan 1989). The ST process is required for cell function, growth, and differentiation. (For a more detailed discussion of specific biochemical events in the ST cascade and their significance, see Berridge 1993.)

Within the architecture of the cell, it is important to remember that the cell membrane is responsible for the first event in ST—receptor–ligand binding. The ensuing ST cascade, which triggers enzyme activity (e.g., phosphatases and kinases), second-messenger mobilization involving calcium, gene induction, protein synthesis (gene expression), and, ultimately, cell proliferation, is a complex cellular process that links events at the cell surface to activities in the nucleus. One of the chief features of ST is that early signaling events at the cell surface, sometimes involving only several molecules, are, in turn, amplified many times in the ST cascade. Magnetic field effects that give rise to small alterations in early ST events have the potential to be amplified in this cascade. In addition, as discussed in the next subsection, the cell membrane appears to play a major role in magnetic field effects mediated through the ST cascade.

An important concept to emphasize, therefore, is that magnetic field alterations on elements of the ST cascade are not necessarily isolated, static events without the potential for biological consequences relating to cancer, because (1) small alterations in early events (e.g., extracellular calcium ions moving through channels into the cell and acting as second messengers) can be amplified by orders of magnitude in the ST cascade, and (2) such small alterations in ST ultimately lead to effects on cell proliferation and mitogenesis (Liburdy 1992a, 1994, 1995).

Receptor–Ligand Binding

Several investigators have studied whether magnetic fields alter the first event in ST—receptor–ligand binding. Luben has investigated whether magnetic fields alter beta-adrenergic receptor activity [cyclic AMP (cAMP) accumulation] of primary osteoblast-enriched bone cells from 5-day-old mice, and of pineal cells from pineal glands excised from 10-day-old mice (Luben 1991, 1993, 1994). Cells were cultured for 6 hours in the presence or absence of a 60-Hz, 100-μT, sinusoidal magnetic field, then treated with isoproterenol (an agonist that binds primarily to beta-adrenergic receptors) for 5 minutes, and finally, cAMP accumulation was measured. As isoproterenol concentration was increased in control cultures, cAMP accumulation increased in a standard sigmoidal fashion. In the exposed cells, there was a significant inhibition of cAMP activation in which the dose–response curve for isoproterenol was shifted to the right, without decreasing the maximum cAMP response at high doses of agonist. This shift was interpreted by Luben as indicating a desensitization or loss of affinity of the beta-adrenergic receptor to isoproterenol; more agonist would be required in the presence of the field to achieve the higher values of cAMP accumulation observed in the control cells. This data also demonstrated that the most effective concentrations for agonist in eliciting a field effect were in the suboptimal range, because no effect was seen at high doses of isoproterenol. The requirement for suboptimal dose is significant, particularly because suboptimal doses of the mitogen concanavalin A (Con-A) is also effective in eliciting a magnetic field effect on calcium influx in lymphocytes (see p. 599).

Luben hypothesized that the changes observed in the cAMP effector enzyme during ST were most likely mediated by a field-induced conformational change in the G-protein linked receptor, which links the cell surface receptor and the internal membrane effector molecule into a ternary complex. This hypothesis was suggested by his observation that binding of a highly specific ligand to the beta-adrenergic receptor, cyanopindolol, is inhibited during pulsed magnetic field exposures of mouse osteoblasts. This result makes sense, because a reduction in ligand binding to its receptor would be expected to result in a reduction in ST and a reduction in cAMP accumulation. The reduction in binding due to the field is perhaps most easily explained by a conformational change in the binding site, and it is known that the binding of cyanopindolol, a small molecule, takes place inside the membrane pocket formed by the seven transmembrane protein helices of the G-protein linked receptor.

Liburdy and colleagues recently investigated receptor–ligand binding in human lymphocytes exposed to magnetic fields (Liburdy et al. 1993e). In these studies, human peripheral blood lymphocytes that were prelabeled with fluorescently modified antibody markers directed against the CD20 (pan B-cell surface marker) or against the CD3 (T-cell receptor) determinant were exposed to 60-Hz, 22-mT, sinusoidal magnetic fields at 37°C for 60 minutes. Following field exposures, the cells were rapidly spun down and the release of antibody was assayed. T-lymphocytes were reported to exhibit significantly more anti-CD3 antibody released from cells compared to that for the sham-treated controls. Magnetic field-exposed B-lymphocytes exhibited a slight increase in CD20 release compared to controls; however, the result was not considered biologically meaningful. These data suggest that magnetic fields have the potential to alter receptor binding involving the CD3 receptor in T-lymphocytes. The CD3 molecule is physically integrated with the T-cell receptor in the lymphocyte cell membrane, and is the major complex responsible for T-cell activation and triggering of the ST cascade in this cell.

Following receptor–ligand binding, the next series of events triggered in the ST cascade is activation of membrane-bound enzymes. Several investigators have studied different membrane-associated enzymes during magnetic field exposures.

Enzyme Activation

Barbiroli and colleagues have investigated whether magnetic field exposure alters protein kinase C (PKC) activity (Monti et al. 1991, 1993). PKC is a key enzyme in the ST cascade and, with regard to cancer, it represents the cellular receptor for phorbol esters—a potent class of tumor promoters. Therefore, if the binding of phorbol esters to PKC is influenced by magnetic fields, one would expect cancer promotion to be altered. PKC associates with the cell membrane following the influx of extracellular calcium during early ST. Calcium mobilization, thus, plays an important role during activation of PKC. Membrane-associated PKC can be followed as an ST parameter using phorbol esters in binding experiments. Barbiroli and colleagues investigated the effect of magnetic field exposures on phorbol ester binding to membrane-associated PKC in a human leukemia cell line, HL-60. Exposure of cells at 37°C for up to 30 minutes to pulsed magnetic fields (50-Hz, 8-mT peak) resulted in significant activation of PKC (i.e., increased binding of phorbol ester) compared to control cells. The investigators performed Scatchard analyses and observed that the apparent dissociation constant, Kd, was not altered, but that there was a significant increase in the maximal number of specific binding sites

(PKC molecules) on the cell surface. The investigators hypothesized that the influx of calcium due to the magnetic field exposure was a plausible explanation for this response, because it is known that PKC is activated by an increase in intracellular calcium. To test this hypothesis, they repeated their experiments with a calcium chelator in the extracellular medium, ethylenediaminetetraacetic acid (EDTA), to complex free calcium outside the HL-60 cells. This culture medium significantly reduced the stimulatory effect of magnetic fields on PKC activation without showing any effect on the control cells. This result is consistent with magnetic fields increasing calcium influx (as opposed to release of intracellular calcium from internal stores), which in turn activates PKC. Here we see a magnetic field effect on PKC that is associated with calcium influx. As discussed below, influx of extra-cellular calcium appears to play a critical role in magnetic field effects on ST parameters.

With regard to PKC, it is of interest to mention that there is one in vivo study on the snail, *Cepaea nemoralis*, that implicates PKC in the magnetic field inhibition of opiate-induced analgesia (Kavaliers et al. 1991). Exposure of snails for 2 hours to a 0.1-μT, 60-Hz magnetic field reduced morphine-induced analgesia; when control snails were treated with the PKC activator SC-9, similar results were observed. In addition, the magnetic field effect was significantly reduced by treatment of snails with PKC inhibitors (H-7 and H-9), and enhanced when snails were treated with SC-9. The investigators concluded that the magnetic field effect involves or is mediated through alterations in PKC activity.

Calcium Mobilization

Calcium ions act as second messengers during ST, and they have been extensively studied (Gardner 1989; Putney 1993; Putney and Bird 1993, 1994). Calcium ion concentration is tightly regulated inside the cell, because they are toxic at high doses and trigger endogenous endonucleases that result in programmed cell death or apoptosis (Trump and Berezesky 1995). For this reason, calcium ion influx plays a critical role in the death of target cells by cytotoxic T-lymphocytes. During ST in nonexcitable cells (e.g., lymphocytes; see next paragraph), calcium enters cells via specialized calcium channels that open in response to receptor–ligand gating at the cell surface (T-cell receptor for the T-lymphocyte), and free calcium ion concentration rises rapidly within seconds. The influx of free calcium ions plus the release of some internal calcium from internal stores is referred to as the second-messenger event. As a result, calcium ions bind to proteins such as calmodulin and kinases (e.g., PKC); this binding sustains the ST cascade within the cell and ultimately leads to DNA, RNA, and protein synthesis; clonal expansion; or cell proliferation. In the lymphocyte, free intracellular calcium ion levels are sustained above baseline levels for several hours during the sequelae of early events in the ST cascade, and free calcium is eventually pumped out of the cell or sequestered in internal stores so that baseline levels are restored for the next round of ST.

Evidence for 60-Hz magnetic fields increasing the calcium-45 influx during ST in the lymphocyte has been reported (Liburdy and Walleczek 1989; Walleczek and Liburdy 1990; Liburdy 1992a–c; Liburdy et al. 1993a, d). A 60-minute exposure of rat thymic lymphocytes to a 22-mT magnetic field ($E_{induced}$ = 1.0 or 1.7 mV/cm) at 37°C was performed in the presence or absence of Con-A , a mitogen which is believed to interact with the T-cell receptor. Nonactivated cells (no mitogen) were unresponsive to the field; calcium-45 influx was not altered. When Con-A was present, the exposure led to a significant increase in calcium-45 influx. This variation depended on the level of calcium influx achieved by Con-A; weakly activated cells were associated with maximal response to the field. Follow-on studies investigated this observation further and they revealed that animal age is strictly correlated to this variation (Liburdy 1992a, c); cells from older animals displayed reduced calcium influx in the presence of Con-A but showed the greatest increase in calcium influx when the magnetic field was also present. This observation is consistent with existing reports indicating that lymphocytes from older animals display a reduced calcium influx to Con-A. Thus it appears that the level of mitogen activation (biological state of the cell) is critical for the magnetic field effect on calcium influx. Cells that are exposed in the absence of Con-A do not respond to the field. Cells maximally stimulated by Con-A alone also do not respond to the field, as they are at the upper limit of their dynamic range. In contrast, cells that are suboptimally activated by mitogen can respond to magnetic fields by exhibiting a further increase in calcium influx.

These studies provide examples of how a magnetic field interaction (1) is mediated by a ligand, the mitogen con-A; (2) is dependent on ST in the cell; and (3) is associated with suboptimal biological function. The latter is important and relevant to a recent tumor promotion study by M.A. Stuchly and colleagues, in which SENCAR mice were initiated with the genotoxic carcinogen 7,12-dimethylbenz(a)anthracene (DMBA) and promoted with a suboptimal dose of 12-0-tetradecanoylphorbol-13-acetate (TPA) during exposure to a 60-Hz, 0.1-mT magnetic field (Stuchly et al. 1992). The investigators found that the magnetic field significantly increased the rate of tumor development per animal, although overall yield was not affected. This finding is consistent with the idea that suboptimal dosing is important, and that the biological state of the target tissue is critical (but see McLean et al. 1995, and more detailed discussion later in this chapter).

Calcium influx has recently been followed in real time during field exposures using fluorescence spectroscopy in several laboratories. The great advantage of this approach is the ability to observe field effects as they occur. Liburdy first reported real-time changes in intracellular calcium in cells exposed to 60-Hz electric fields (Liburdy 1992a, b). Thymic lymphocytes were loaded with the calcium-sensitive dye FURA-2AM and the cells exposed to a 60-Hz electric field (1.7 mV/cm; to match the induced electric field associated with a magnetic field exposure at 22 mT) in a special electrode cuvette while fluorescence was monitored. Levels of intracellular calcium in resting cells (no mitogen) were not influenced by the field; this result corroborates the calcium-45 influx data for resting cells, mentioned previously. When Con-A was added to the cells during field exposure, levels of intracellular calcium immediately began rising to levels that were, by about 400 seconds later, significantly higher than that for unexposed, Con-A treated cells. In these studies the initial rise in calcium was not altered by the field over the first 100 seconds, but the levels of calcium influx sustained afterwards were enhanced. The finding that the initial rise in intracellular calcium during Con-A treatment was not influenced by the field suggests that the release of calcium from intracellular stores inside of the cell during ST was not disturbed by the field.

Other laboratories have studied calcium ion influx in lymphocyte cells exposed to electric or magnetic fields using fluorescence spectroscopy. Human T-cell leukemia cells (E6.1 Jurkat cell line) were used in fluorescence cuvette studies to investigate calcium influx during ST (Walleczek et al. 1993). The researchers reported an increase in calcium ion influx over about 1000 seconds, followed indirectly using manganese ion quenching of FURA-2, in Jurkat cells exposed to a 50-Hz electric field of 50 mV/cm, but not in field of 1 mV/cm. In magnetic field studies, they reported that exposures to 50-Hz, 1-mT fields resulted in reduced calcium influx after ST activation using anti-CD3 antibody; the effect was not observed at 5 and 10 mT. Lyle and colleagues (1993) also studied E6.1 Jurkat cells using fluorescence techniques with the dye INDO-1, and reported that exposure of these cells to an induced electric field of 1 mV/cm (23.8 mT, 60-Hz) during activation of ST with anti-CD3 antibody at 24°C or 37°C for up to 60 minutes did not alter intracellular calcium as measured by flow cytometry. These studies suggest that E6.1 Jurkat cells may not be sensitive to ELF electric fields (induced or applied directly to the cells) below about 1 mV/cm, or to ELF magnetic fields greater than 1 mT.

Lindström and colleagues have employed the E6.1 Jurkat cell, as well as human peripheral blood lymphocytes, and studied the calcium response to magnetic field exposures using single-cell fluorescence techniques (Lindström et al. 1993, 1995b). The use of fluorescence microscopy to investigate single-cell responses to magnetic fields, particularly calcium, is a relatively new development in bioelectromagnetics (Liburdy 1994, 1995), and the findings of Lindström are the first such published laboratory work in this area. In addition to being able to follow calcium in real-time in single cells, this approach permits the investigation of calcium oscillations that cannot be evaluated in fluorescence cuvette or flow cytometry studies unless the cells are synchronized, which is difficult, if not impossible, to accomplish. Calcium oscillations are observed in a wide variety of cells, including the lymphocyte, and the full biological significance of these periodic alterations in the temporal and spatial distribution of calcium within the cell is not yet understood (Putney and Bird 1994). It has been hypothesized that such calcium oscillations represent frequency encoded information that the cell utilizes in ST. The application of a time-varying magnetic field to the cell might influence such a periodic process; this idea is currently speculation, although Lindström and colleagues present evidence from their laboratory in several papers for such an interaction.

Lindström and coworkers applied a 50-Hz, 0.1-mT magnetic field to E6.1 Jurkat cells at 37°C and monitored intracellular calcium using FURA-2. Their first report (Lindström et al. 1993) indicated that when stable cells were viewed, with a relatively flat baseline not exhibiting oscillations, the application of the magnetic field triggered a pattern of calcium oscillations or spikes that was reversible. The patterns varied from cell to cell with differences in peak calcium and the duration of oscillation. When these cells were treated with anti-CD3 to trigger ST, similar types of calcium oscillation patterns were observed. The investigators also extended these observations to human peripheral blood lymphocytes and observed that magnetic field exposures led to calcium oscillations in resting cells, and in cells that were treated with phorbol ester and ionomycin to raise calcium levels. Jurkat cells were more responsive (85%) compared to the unactivated or activated blood lymphocytes (10%). The investigators interpreted their findings as indicating that magnetic field exposure of the Jurkat cells is comparable to that achieved by anti-CD3 antibody, which is known to act through the T-cell receptor. The magnetic field may trigger ST by interacting with the T-cell receptor or other early events in the ST cascade linked to calcium mobilization.

Lindström et al. (1995b) recently extended their studies by investigating the frequency and dose threshold for the magnetic field effect on intracellular calcium in Jurkat cells. Their original response (described previously) observed at 0.1 mT (at 50-Hz) was tested across the frequency range of 5 to 100 Hz; they observed a broad response having its maximum at about 50 Hz (92% responsive cells, 22/24 cells). The result of testing increasing flux densities at 50-Hz was linear with an apparent threshold above 0.025 mT and a maximal response at 0.1 mT or greater (~90% responding cells, 9–11/10–12 cells). The investigators state that because the responses to magnetic field exposures are similar to that observed for anti-CD3 (a biological stimulation of the ST cascade), magnetic field coupling to the cell may be mimicking early ST events at the cell surface receptor level. They recently tested this hypothesis by repeating their experiments using a somatic mutant of the Jurkat cell, the J45.01 clone, which has diminished CD45 phosphatase activity (Lindström et al. 1995a). CD45 phosphatase, the major membrane phosphatase in lymphocytes, is a 200-kD transmembrane protein involved in early ST events in the human lymphocyte. This phosphatase functions as a major dephosphorylation enzyme, and, along with kinases, coordinates early events associated with T-cell receptor activation in ST (Cahir-McFarland et al. 1993). Lindström et al. reported that magnetic field exposures of the J45.01 clone did not result in alterations of intracellular calcium. In contrast, clones with genetically restored CD45 phosphatase activity could respond to the magnetic field seen as an increase in intracellular calcium. They interpreted these findings to indicate that CD45 or molecules in the T-cell receptor signaling complex are involved in magnetic field interactions. A number of laboratories are involved in similar single-cell studies to confirm and extend these important findings.

Other laboratories have reported effects on calcium ion flux in cells including lymphocytes; these past studies are, in general, in agreement that magnetic fields have been observed to trigger calcium flux. The reader is directed to several recent reviews (Liburdy 1992c, 1994, 1995; Luben 1991, 1993, 1994; Tenforde 1991, 1992, 1993; Walleczek 1992). The conditions required for a magnetic field response varies across a range of exposure conditions and biological conditions that involve ST activation and the biological state of the cells (e.g., donor age). At this point it seems fair to say that calcium flux has been one of the most frequently reported alterations observed in cells in response to magnetic field exposures. Because the significance of alterations in calcium homeostasis is considerable, replication efforts are being pursued in a number of laboratories involving protocols, training, and exchange of cell lines.

Gene Induction, Gene Expression, and Protein Synthesis

Within the framework of ST, gene induction leading to gene expression and protein synthesis is triggered in the cell after binding of a ligand such as a hormone or growth factor to its receptor. Since magnetic field effects on early events in the ST cascade have been demonstrated in a number of laboratories, it is reasonable to consider that such effects will result in alterations in downstream events such as gene induction and expression within the ST framework. Direct support for this concept is derived from studies that do not provide evidence for a genotoxic effect of magnetic fields of environmental intensity on cells (Scarfi et al. 1993; McCann et al. 1993).

Goodman and Henderson first described an increase in mRNA transcript levels for selected chromosomes of salivary gland cells of *Drosophila* and *Sciara* (reviewed in Goodman and Henderson 1991). After brief exposures of up to 60 minutes, 37°C, to sinusoidal fields of 72 and 60 Hz, 5–11 G (1 G = 100 μT), and 0.3–5 x 10^{-4} V/m, some chromosomes showed loci with an increase in transcription of from 10- to 1000-fold over control-treated cells. When the data were analyzed, it was observed that field-induced transcription occurred at chromosome loci that were active in the control cells. Thus, the degree of transcriptional activity was critical to the field response, because resting or inactive loci did not respond to the field. The concept of activation appears as a common theme in the study of biological responses to magnetic fields.

Recently, Goodman and Henderson have reported studies in which increases in mRNA transcripts were induced in the human lymphocytic-derived HL-60 cell line by 60-Hz, sinusoidal magnetic fields (0.0057–5.7 G); 0.011–11 x 10^{-4} V/m) (Goodman and Henderson 1992) and by 60-Hz, sinusoidal electric fields (0.3 x 10^{-4} V/m) (Blank et al. 1993). These studies are of interest because they concern a human cell line. For the electric field exposures, mRNA transcripts for c-*myc* and histone H2B were significantly elevated over that observed in control-treated cells. These transcripts are normally expressed in this cell line, and a field-induced increase in normal transcription activity is consistent with the results using salivary gland cells discussed above. Interestingly, in the magnetic field studies they probed for the presence of mRNA transcripts for alpha-globin, which is not expressed in HL-60 cells, and they reported that field exposure did not increase transcripts. In these studies, two important features were noted: A field-induced increase in transcript levels was not proportional to increasing time of exposure (exposures longer than 20 minutes were not effective) or to increasing field strength. These findings support the idea of "window" effects (Adey 1992a, b), and they underscore the nonlinear, complex nature of the interaction.

Greene and colleagues (1991) have recently investigated transcriptional rates in HL-60 cells exposed to 60-Hz, sinusoidal magnetic fields. They measured transcription rates by pulse-labeling the cells with ^{3}H-uridine and, thus, reported on total transcriptional activity in the cells. They reported a maximal 50–60% increase in overall transcriptional rates in HL-60 cells exposed to a 60-Hz, 10-G, sinusoidal magnetic field. This increase was time-dependent and transient, with maximal enhancement occurring at 30–120 minutes of exposure and a decline to basal levels by 18 hours. The increase in transcription activity in HL-60 cells and the time dependence are in general agreement with the findings of Goodman and Henderson.

An important finding by Goodman and Henderson in their studies was that c-*myc* mRNA transcripts were elevated by magnetic fields. The oncogene *myc* belongs to a set of cellular messengers commonly referred to as "immediate early response" genes because their expression is activated by a variety of mitogenic stimuli—independent of de novo protein synthesis—early during the G_0 to G_1 transition of cells from a resting to a growing state (Marcu et al. 1992). The protein products of immediate response genes, such as *myc*, are thought to facilitate progression of the cell through the cell cycle, and to synthesize DNA in S phase. MYC polypeptides play roles in the transcriptional and post-transcriptional control of other cellular genes and in DNA replication. Strong evidence indicates that they mediate their function as site-specific, DNA-binding proteins (Marcu et al. 1992); cells keep *myc* under very tight regulation.

Given the importance of the oncogene *myc*, it is significant that J. Phillips and colleagues recently reported that magnetic field exposure of a T-lymphoblastoid cell line, CEM-CM3, also increased c-*myc* m-RNA (Phillips et al. 1992). Their study was the first to employ the nuclear run-off assay technique to assess alterations in specific gene transcription for *myc, jun, fos,* and PKC. Magnetic field exposures were performed at an intensity of 1 G and for times ranging from 15–120 minutes at 37°C, and at two different cell densities because transcription of the immediate early response genes has been shown to be sensitive to the density parameter. The investigators reported that the magnetic fields induced a time-dependent and a cell density-dependent change in specific gene transcription of these genes. It is of interest that the report by Phillips et al. is consistent with Goodman and Henderson's findings in that increases in c-*myc* mRNA transcripts were time-dependent, with a time "windowing" in the range of 20 minutes. The finding of Phillips et al. that cell density is an important parameter to control in cell culture studies underscores the importance of the biological state of the target cells. Replication studies are under way in several laboratories and such issues need to be carefully addressed. Some of the replication studies have been completed and contradict Goodman and Henderson (Saffer and Thurston 1995a, b; Lacy-Hulbert et al. 1995a, b). Further research is needed to identify the factor(s) that are critical for magnetic field interactions influencing gene induction.

In these gene expression studies, it was suggested that magnetic fields might trigger changes in gene transcription through an effect on some essential element in ST (Goodman and Henderson 1991, 1992; Phillips et al. 1992). Calcium has been recently suggested for this role, because experimental observations support the idea that magnetic fields alter calcium cycling in cells (Liburdy 1992a–c; Walleczek and Liburdy 1990; Yost and Liburdy 1992; Liburdy and Yost 1993). Several laboratories have addressed this link. Liburdy and colleagues correlated alterations in calcium influx and in c-*myc* mRNA gene induction in experiments that measured both parameters for in the same exposed cell population (Liburdy et al. 1993a, c, d). The hypothesis was that increases in calcium influx induced by a magnetic field would subsequently lead to increases in c-*myc* mRNA transcription via the ST cascade; this chain of events represents an attractive and plausible biological framework for understanding how a magnetic field effect at the cell surface (calcium ion influx) can influence subsequent events such as RNA, DNA, and protein synthesis.

In these experiments, rat thymocytes were placed in an annular ring Petri dish and exposed to an incident 60-Hz, 220-G magnetic field ($E_{induced}$ = 1.7 mV/cm) for 60 minutes, 37°C, as described (Liburdy 1992a–c), and the cell sample was split and assessed for calcium influx and for c-*myc* mRNA (Liburdy et al. 1993a, c, d). Before exposure, some cells were treated with a suboptimal dose of Con-A (1 μg/mL) and no significant increase in calcium uptake was detected. However, in the presence of the magnetic field, a 1.5-fold increase in calcium increase was observed for Con-A-treated cells. The same cell population was assessed for c-*myc* mRNA transcription via Northern analysis. Northerns were quantitated using a CCD camera and the digitized images of bands were integrated on a computed, pixel-by-pixel basis (total band gray-scale intensity $\times$ mm^2); this quantity was then linearized by conversion to (OD $\times$ mm^2). Finally, the results of each c-*myc* mRNA Northern band were normalized against the presence of m-RNA for the housekeeping gene glyceraldehyde-6-phosphate dehydrogenase (GAPDH), which is not altered during mitogen activation in the cell. (The latter step is important because it corrects for any generalized, nonspecific changes in total mRNA in the cells.) The findings correlate across treatment groups with that observed for calcium uptake. Suboptimal mitogen treatment by itself did not lead to increases in c-*myc* mRNA; however, the presence of magnetic fields resulted in an approximate fourfold increase in c-*myc* mRNA.

These data strongly suggest that the two events—mitogen activation and exposure—are linked. Based on the role of calcium in the ST cascade, the data provide evidence for an interaction mechanism in which the magnetic field triggers calcium influx at the level of the cell membrane, which leads to an increase in c-*myc* mRNA via the ST pathway.

This hypothesis was further tested by Goodman and Henderson using HL-60 cells (Karabakhtsian et al. 1994). Steady-state transcript levels for c-*fos* and c-*myc* were determined in cells exposed to a 60-Hz, 8-μT magnetic field for 20 minutes at 37°C. These cells were placed in either RPMI 1640 buffer with a normal level of calcium ($\sim$2 mM) or in calcium-depleted buffer with a calcium level adjusted to $\sim$10^{-6} M. Steady-state levels of transcripts were measured in two ways: by the reverse transcription–polymerase chain reaction technique and by dot blot hybridization. The results showed that the stimulatory effect magnetic fields have on these transcripts was significantly suppressed when cells were placed under conditions of calcium reduction. The authors concluded that calcium is needed for the magnetic field response. These results are consistent with magnetic fields triggering calcium influx, and, as a consequence of the ST cascade, triggering the subsequent induction of the early response genes c-*fos* and c-*myc*.

The ST cascade also predicts that magnetic fields have the potential to alter downstream cellular events such as protein synthesis. Goodman and Henderson (1991) have reported that exposure of human HL-60 cells to 60-Hz, 8-μT, sinusoidal magnetic fields for 45 minutes results in a significant increase in incorporation of ^{35}S-methionine, reflecting an increase in total protein synthesis. Similar magnetic fields employed by Goodman and Henderson were associated with increases in c-*myc* mRNA, discussed previously.

Summary

Taken together, findings across a number of laboratories report that magnetic fields can alter receptor–ligand binding, calcium ion flux, gene induction, and protein synthesis. These findings are consistent with magnetic fields interacting at cell membrane level and triggering changes in transcription and translation via the ST cascade. Such changes can have profound effects on end-stage ST (cell proliferation) and carcinogenesis. However, particularly the issue of magnetic field effects on gene expression continues to be debated because of equivocal laboratory studies.

Ornithine Decarboxylase (ODC) and Promotion/Copromotion

The enzyme ODC is necessary for progression of cells into S phase, and, thus, it is a critical enzyme in the regulation of DNA replication and cell proliferation (Bello-Fernandez et al. 1993). ODC is the controlling enzyme in the polyamine synthesis pathway and is regulated by a wide variety of growth factors and mitogens at the cell surface. This enzyme is unique in its ability to change rapidly and markedly in response to extracellular signals (Byus et al. 1987), a feature that makes ODC important to magnetic field studies, because it can interact with the field through the cell membrane. Virtually all rapidly growing cells, including transformed and cancer cells, exhibit elevated ODC activity; ODC activity is also markedly induced by phorbol ester tumor promoting compounds (Byus et al. 1987). Thus, ODC is relevant to early cellular events involved in growth, and, by extension, to aspects of carcinogenesis, which is a complex series of processes.

Because ODC activity is triggered by membrane-mediated signaling events and its activity is associated with important control processes in carcinogenesis, Byus and colleagues (1987) first studied ODC activity in cells exposed to 60-Hz, sinusoidal electric fields. Byus et al. reported that three different cell lines—human lymphoma CEM cells, mouse myeloma cells (P3), and Reuber H35 hepatoma cells—each experienced an increase in ODC activity in response to a 1-hour exposure to electric field strengths of 10 mV/cm (1 V/m); a dose–response study with Reuber H35 cells indicated that field-induced increases in ODC were detected as low as 0.1 mV/cm. Across these three cell lines, ODC always increased; the observed increase in activity varied from 30–500%. For comparison, phorbol ester activation, which stimulates tumor promotion, can increase ODC activity by more than 1000%. A second observation across cell lines was that the field-induced increase in ODC activity was transient; the increased activity remained for several hours post exposure and then declined. The kinetics of the rise and decline in activity varied among cells; CEM and H35 hepatoma cells showed increased ODC immediately after the 1-hour field exposure, whereas the P3 cells showed increased ODC at 1–2 hours post exposure.

Byus and colleagues (1987) state that their findings support the idea that the 60-Hz electric fields act at the level of the cell membrane, probably at a cell membrane receptor site analogous to a tumor-promoting stimulus. Their findings raise the important question of whether electric and magnetic fields (EMF) act as tumor-promoting agents in cellular systems.

Recently, a second laboratory has reported that ODC activity is increased by exposure to a 60-Hz magnetic field. Litovitz and colleagues (1991) exposed mouse L929 cells for up to 8 hours to magnetic field intensities of 1, 10, or 100 μT. A maximal enhancement of approximately twofold in ODC activity was produced by 4-hour exposure to a magnetic field of 10 μT. This group has extended their original findings in experiments using 55-, 60-, and 65-Hz, amplitude-modulated 915-MHz fields (SAR 2.5 W/kg). Interestingly, these ELF-modulated fields doubled ODC activity after 8 hours. The authors suggest that the ELF component may play an important factor in this cellular response. Further studies by this group with developing chick embryos have been reported (Farrel et al. 1993). ODC activity in the developing chick embryo is reported to peak twice within the first 53 hours of development: at 15 hours (gastrulation) and at 23 hours (the onset of neurulation and early organogenesis). Experiments were conducted in which developing chick embryos were exposed to 60-Hz magnetic fields (4 μT peak) for an incubation time of 15 hours; a 74% increase in the exposed group compared to the control group was observed. Interestingly, the magnetic field effect could be blocked by the superimposition of "noise" (randomly generated frequencies from 30–90 Hz with an RMS value of ~4 μT) on top of the magnetic field signal. The authors interpreted these findings as indicating that ODC activity was significantly increased by the field, and that this effect was associated with the waveform characteristic of the 60-Hz, sinusoidal magnetic field.

Mattsson et al. (1993) recently reported that three different mammalian cell lines—human promyelocytic leukemia HL-60, mouse ascites tumor ELD, and mouse teratocarcinoma F9—exhibited elevated levels of ODC in response to a 30-μT, 50-Hz magnetic field. The magnitude of ODC elevation varied across cell lines (20% for HL-60 cells, to 5- to 6-fold for ELD cells), and factors such as serum and protein (bovine serum albumin) appeared to play a role in ODC activity in the exposed cells.

The studies of these three laboratories, employing eight different model cellular systems and all reporting an ODC response to ELF EMF, raise the important question of whether 60-Hz fields act as promoters, which was first suggested by Byus et al. (1987). Given these results, it is reasonable to consider investigating promotion in a cell model system. The question of promotion has been recently addressed in experiments using a coculture model system by Cain and associates (1993). They studied whether the phorbol ester tumor promoter TPA and 60-Hz EMF are copromoters that enhance focus formation of transformed cells in coculture with normal cells. In this model system, parental 10T½ fibroblasts are cocultured with mutant daughter cells that can form foci; the parental cells suppress focus formation by the mutant daughter cells, but this suppression can be relieved by the addition of a tumor-promoter such as TPA. It is thought that focus formation is due in part to intercellular communication between parental and daughter cells via paracrine factors or direct cell-to-cell contact (Herschman and Brankow 1987).

Cain and colleagues (1993) reported that chronic, intermittent exposures to 60-Hz, 1-G magnetic fields increased, by approximately twofold, the total number of foci observed, the total area of foci per dish, and the number of cells in stained foci compared to sham-treated cells. Exposures were carried out over a 28-day period with four 1-hour exposures per day. Interestingly, magnetic fields alone (no TPA present) had no effect on the growth curves of parental or daughter cells, or when these cells were cocultured. A TPA dose response was evident, with focus formation detected for TPA at 3 ng/mL but no difference detected between field-exposed and sham-treated cocultures. The magnetic fields did increase focus formation by an average of 150% across TPA doses of 10, 20, 40, 50, and 100 ng/mL. These results indicate that the combination of a 60-Hz magnetic field plus a chemical tumor promoter can influence focus formation in a coculture assay. Cain and colleagues interpret their findings to suggest that membrane-related events associated with TPA binding and intercellular communication in copromotion were influenced by the magnetic fields.

For perspective, it is important to remember that TPA and other phorbol ester tumor promoters trigger calcium influx and PKC activity (as discussed on p. 597), as well as ODC activity. The ST pathway, as discussed previously, is involved in tumor promotion. TPA is a structural analog of diacylglycerol, which is present in the cell membrane, and TPA activates PKC involved in calcium recycling across the cell membrane. Thus, although these studies do not identify a specific molecular site of field interaction, the results are consistent with a membrane-receptor-associated interaction that involves the ST pathway to relay a magnetic field effect across the cell membrane.

Cell Proliferation

The final endpoint in the process of carcinogenesis is uncontrolled cell proliferation (Cohen and Ellwein 1990). For this reason, studies should be conducted to evaluate the effect of magnetic fields on cell proliferation and growth.

Recently, Liburdy and colleagues published a report that human breast cancer cell growth can be altered by a 60-Hz, 1.2-μT magnetic field in vitro (Liburdy et al. 1993b). In these studies, melatonin was employed to inhibit breast cancer cell growth and cells were exposed to magnetic fields. In a sense, this methodology is analogous to the studies discussed previously, in which a mitogen or a promoter such as TPA is used to elicit a biological response in cells subsequently exposed to magnetic fields. This approach appears to be an important feature in cellular studies.

The experiments conducted by Liburdy and colleagues employed a human breast cancer cell line, MCF-7, and tested whether the growth of MCF-7 cells is suppressed by melatonin in the presence of a 0.2- or 1.2-μT, 60-Hz, sinusoidal magnetic field (Liburdy et al. 1993b; Liburdy 1994, 1995; also see Chapter 22, this volume). Melatonin, a hormone and natural growth inhibitor of estrogen receptor-positive breast cancer cells, is normally released into the bloodstream at night. Melatonin is of interest in these studies because (1) it displays natural oncostatic action towards breast cancer cells (Blask 1990, 1993); (2) its release into the bloodstream in animals has been reported to be depressed by 60-Hz EMF (Wilson et al. 1990; Reiter and Richardson 1990; Lerchl et al. 1991; Haggren et al. 1992; Stevens et al. 1992; Reiter 1992); and (3) 60-Hz magnetic field exposures are postulated to be a risk factor in human breast cancer (Stevens 1987; Tynes and Andersen 1990; Demers at al. 1991; Matanoski et al. 1991; Guénel et al. 1993; Loomis et al. 1991, 1994). As discussed in the section on free radicals (p. 618), Reiter and colleagues have recently identified melatonin as a potent free radical scavenger (Reiter et al. 1995); this feature may play an important role in magnetic field biological effects (see pp. 618 and 623).

The 0.2- and 1.2-μT field strengths employed by Liburdy et al. are among the lowest reported in the literature for cell culture studies; special precautions were taken to ensure that these magnetic field exposures were not confounded. Exposing cultured cells to magnetic fields inside a commercial incubator has to be done carefully, taking into account several important considerations (see p. 591 and Table 1). Liburdy and colleagues have developed a mu-metal, shielded magnetic field exposure system that employs a four-coil, bifilar, Merritt design and generates a very uniform field free of artifacts (Liburdy

1994, 1995). In addition, these investigators used multiple, matched incubators outfitted with identical magnetic field exposure systems in simultaneous experiments so that results could be carefully compared across treatment groups using cells of the same passage. This approach was thought to help reduce biological variation and to contribute to the reproducibility of results.

The first question addressed was whether MCF-7 cell growth was altered by magnetic fields. In the absence of melatonin, MCF-7 cells grew identically in a 0.2 or 1.2 μT field. This result indicated that unregulated breast cancer cell growth was not significantly influenced by these fields. Second, the experiments were repeated with cells in the presence of physiological concentrations of melatonin and in the presence of 0.2-μT magnetic fields, which was employed as a "background" or baseline field that might be commonly encountered in the environment. In this experiment, MCF-7 cells showed a significant inhibition of growth during a 7-day growth cycle. These results confirmed the original observation of Blask (1990) that melatonin inhibits MCF-7 cell growth. When a 1.2-μT field was employed in simultaneous exposures in a second, matched incubator, the natural oncostatic action of melatonin was completely blocked. Thus, in the presence of the magnetic field, melatonin was ineffective in inhibiting MCF-7 cell growth. Conversely, when melatonin was absent in the cell culture media, the 1.2-μT field did not affect MCF-7 cell proliferation. These findings were interpreted as indicating that a 1.2-μT magnetic field can act to enhance breast cancer cell proliferation by blocking melatonin's action on cell growth.

Because these studies indicated that the magnetic field interaction depended on the presence of a hormone that regulates cell growth, identical studies were conducted in which tamoxifen, instead of melatonin, was used to inhibit MCF-7 cell growth (Harland and Liburdy 1994; also see Chapter 23, this volume). Tamoxifen is the most widely prescribed drug treatment for the control of breast cancer recurrence in humans. When MCF-7 cells were cultured in the presence of pharmacological doses of tamoxifen in a 0.2-μT magnetic field, tamoxifen was observed to significantly inhibit cell growth. Thus, the drug was able to display normal oncostatic action. In the presence of a 1.2-μT magnetic field, the action of tamoxifen was significantly blocked, but not completely. This blocking effect could be overcome at higher doses of tamoxifen, indicating that the magnetic field shifted the effective dose required for tamoxifen's oncostatic action by several log units. Because tamoxifen acts by binding to the estrogen receptor, this is a possible interaction site for magnetic fields.

The studies by Liburdy and colleagues are potentially significant with regard to cancer in several ways. First, the studies indicate that magnetic fields can modulate the action of a hormone/drug on tumor cell growth. No evidence is apparent for a direct effect of the field on MCF-7 cell growth in the absence of drug or hormone. Thus the magnetic field effect is one that enhances tumor cell growth in the presence of these two compounds. Second, a 1.2-μT magnetic field completely blocked melatonin's action and partially blocked tamoxifen's action in a dose–response manner; suprapharmacological doses of tamoxifen could overcome the magnetic field effect. These findings also indicate that an apparent magnetic field dose threshold exists between 0.2 and 1.2 μT. This very low range of field intensities falls well within values encountered in the work environment and in the home (Stuchly et al. 1983; Tenforde and Kaune 1987). Third, melatonin was employed at concentrations that approximate levels found in the bloodstream, and tamoxifen was employed at pharmacological levels similar to those in the clinical setting. Thus, these findings have some plausible relationship to drug/hormone dosages in situ. And finally, because tamoxifen has oncostatic action against a variety of breast cancer cells in vivo, any inhibition of its oncostatic action by magnetic fields has the potential to increase the likelihood of breast cancer tumor incidence in vivo.

Mikorey-Lechner and colleagues also have investigated the effect of magnetic fields on breast cancer cell growth in vitro (Mikorey-Lechner et al. 1993; Johann et al. 1993). These investigators exposed MCF-7 cells in culture to a 20-Hz, 5.3-mT magnetic field and followed cell growth in the absence or presence of a variety of cytostatic drugs. These fields are lower in frequency and approximately 4000-fold higher in intensity than the Liburdy studies; in addition, the exposures were intermittent, with a 6-hour on/off pattern. The investigators observed that such a magnetic field exposure led to an enhancement of mitochondrial activity [as measured by the methyltetrazolium (MTT) assay], which they used as an indicator of cell viability. This increase in cell viability was interpreted as reflecting either cell proliferation or differentiation; field-treated cells showed membrane ruffling and the formation of microvilli. When MCF-7 cells were grown in the presence of one of several cytostatic agents but without magnetic fields, the cells experienced reduced mitochondrial activity, a result consistent with the cytostatic activity of these drugs. The cytostatic agents employed were methotrexate, cisplatin, cyclophosphamide, doxorubin, mitoxantron, mitomycin, and 5-fluorouracil. In all cases in which the magnetic field exposure took place in the presence of a drug, the cells experienced a greater reduction in mitochondrial activity, suggesting that the drugs were more effective.

Although these studies employed MCF-7 cells, it is difficult to directly compare results, because there are significant differences in field intensity, field frequency, exposure duration, and drug treatment. This situation is typical of the difficulties inherent in assessing the literature on magnetic field studies—many experimental factors can differ across studies. However, in these MCF-7 cell studies, the common ground appears to be that magnetic fields are capable of altering the growth of this cancer cell in vitro by altering the action of drugs/hormones that regulate cell proliferation. Thus, cell and drug/hormone interactions should be considered as a potentially important factor in the relationship magnetic fields have to cancer and cell growth.

Our initial observation that 60-Hz magnetic field exposure in the μT range blocks the ability of melatonin to inhibit the growth of MCF-7 breast cancer cells (Liburdy et al. 1993b) was subsequently confirmed by Blask et al. (1993). Their study showed that melatonin's inhibitory effect on the growth of MCF-7 cells was blocked by exposure to a 1.5-μT magnetic field, but not a 0.2-μT field. More recently, Blackman et al. (1996) have replicated the original findings of Liburdy et al. (1993b) following identical protocols and using MCF-7 cells obtained from Liburdy (see Table 1).

In a recent study by Kwee and Raskmark (1995), a 50-Hz, 80 μT, sinusoidal magnetic field influenced the proliferation of human epithelial amnion cells, as measured by manual cell counting and by MTT assay. Cells were grown in monolayer culture at different exposure times and at different field intensities. The investigators observed distinct windowing effects; for example, when exposure times were varied from 15–60 minutes, a maximal increase of 70% in the proliferation rate was observed at 30 minutes, with no significant changes at 15 and 60 minutes. Interestingly, this effect was observed for cells at 50% confluency (log-phase growth) but not 100% confluency; this observation implicates a cell cycle dependence. When 30-minute exposures were performed at field strengths in the range of 25–175 μT, a maximal increase in cell proliferation was observed at 80 μT.

Two reports from Obe and colleagues (Rosenthal and Obe 1989; Antonopoulos et al. 1995) indicate that human peripheral lymphocytes exhibit enhancement of cell cycle progression when cultured in the presence of a 50-Hz, 5 mT, sinusoidal magnetic field. In their 1989 study, a significant increase in cell cycle progression (quantified as a proliferation index computed from cell cycle state) was observed for exposures of 48 and 72 hours. Exposure to the magnetic field did not result in changes in sister-chromatid exchanges (SCEs), consistent with the idea that magnetic fields are not genotoxic. However, when cells were cocultured in the presence of the magnetic field plus one of three known mutagens (trenimon, diepoxybutane, and methylnitrosourea), there was a significant increase in SCEs. This result is consistent with the idea that magnetic fields act as a promoter. The recent 1995 study by this group extended their original findings. They compared results from two different exposure systems: one similar in design to that used in their 1989 study, with the magnetic field parallel to the axis of the culture tube and the temperature controlled by air convection; and a second exposure system that generated a magnetic field perpendicular to the culture-tube long axis with better temperature control of ≤0.05°C. Both exposure systems gave essentially the same effect on cell cycle progression as previously reported. Because similar effects were obtained for control experiments at a temperature of 38°C, the authors made the important conclusion that the influence on cell cycle was an effect of the magnetic field, and not associated with any thermal loading.

Several laboratories have investigated the effects of pulsed magnetic fields on cell proliferation and reported an increase in cell proliferation. In most of these studies, cultured human peripheral blood lymphocytes (HPBL) were employed, as well as pulsed waveforms with similar physical characteristics: 50 Hz, 1.2-millisecond rise time, 2.5-mT peak intensity, ~1.0 dB/dt (T/s), ~0.1 duty cycle, and approximately triangular in shape. Cossarizza and colleagues (1989b) reported that phytohemagglutinin (PHA)-induced proliferation of HPBL was increased by continual exposure to pulsed magnetic fields for 72 hours. The same fields alone showed no evidence of genotoxic effects, as assessed by DNA repair tests (Cossarizza et al. 1989a) and by micronucleus formation (Scarfi et al. 1991, 1993). Other investigators also have reported that magnetic fields do not induce any genotoxic effects (Murphy et al. 1993). One group reported a decrease in HPBL cell proliferation index, as well as an increase in chromosome aberrations and SCEs (Khalil and Qassemm 1991). Scarfi and colleagues revisited their original study in light of this report and have recently reported that they confirm their original findings of an increase in HPBL proliferation with no genotoxic effects as assessed by the sensitive micronucleus assay (Scarfi et al. 1994). They state that the differences might be due to donor age and health, because Cossarizza et al. (1991) have reported that aged subjects and those suffering from Down's syndrome are higher responders to magnetic fields in cell proliferation assays.

In contrast to these HPBL studies, other studies of cell proliferation employing tumor or transformed cells have shown an association between magnetic fields and a decrease in cell proliferation. A 24-hour exposure of HeLa cells to a pulsed magnetic field (square waveform, 0.18-T peak intensity, 0.8 Hz) led to a 15% decrease in cell proliferation (Tuffet et al. 1993). When mouse fibroblasts (SV40-Swiss-3T3 cells) were exposed for 1 hour to a 50-Hz, 2-mT, sinusoidal magnetic field, the investigators observed a small but statistically significant decrease in DNA content and a slight but statistically significant accumulation of cells in G_1 phase. This observation was in accordance with the small decreases observed in mean DNA content.

It is difficult, based on the studies discussed, to generalize about how magnetic fields influence cell proliferation because both normal and tumor cells were used and different magnetic fields were employed. One common theme that emerges from these studies is that magnetic fields appear to influence processes critical to cell proliferation when the cells are biologically activated or modulated with chemicals, drugs, or hormones. This was the case with the human breast cancer studies in which melatonin and tamoxifen were required, and the HPBL studies in which activation by the mitogen PHA was required. This finding underscores the importance of the biological state of the cell or of the donor and the importance of the ST cascade.

Gap Junctions and Intercellular Communication

Regarding carcinogenesis, it is generally recognized that tumor cells do not exhibit normal intercellular communication, and that most tumor cells either do not express gap junction proteins or they possess abnormally functioning gap junctions. This is consistent with gap junction involvement in control of cell proliferation and differentiation (Trosko 1990).

It is therefore important that the function of gap junctions in cells be assessed, in both normal and transformed cells, during exposure to magnetic fields. Currently, there exists only one report that specifically deals with this issue. Ubeda and colleagues (1995) investigated the effect of a 50-Hz, sinusoidal magnetic field on gap junction communication in C3H10T½ mouse embryo fibroblasts. First, quiescent monolayers of cells were scrape-loaded with Lucifer yellow in the absence or presence of a range of melatonin concentrations. The investigators observed that a significant increase in intercellular communication occurred when melatonin was present. This observation is consistent with the concept that melatonin has an oncostatic effect on these mouse fibroblasts. When the melatonin-treated cells were exposed to a 50-Hz, 1.6-mT, sinusoidal field for 30 minutes before scrape-loading, this increase in intercellular communication was not observed. The authors hypothesized that the magnetic field effect of blocking gap junction intercellular communication might contribute to neoplastic processes in similar cells. These results are preliminary, and if confirmed, would shed light on how magnetic fields might influence carcinogenesis via alterations in intercellular communication.

Free Radicals and Antioxidants in Biological Systems

The topic of free radicals is included in this review because free radicals are (1) known to be an important factor in cell proliferation and in the process of carcinogenesis (Burdon and Rice-Evans 1989; Rose and Bode 1993), and (2) evidence based on physical theory indicates that magnetic fields have the potential to alter free radical recombination in chemical systems (Scaiano et al. 1994a, b; Grissom 1995). Although there currently exists only one report (Roy et al. 1995) demonstrating a direct effect of environmental-level magnetic fields on free radicals in a cellular system (see p. 621), the plausibility of such interactions is compelling enough to make such a discussion worthwhile (Frankel and Liburdy 1995).

Reactive free radical species are known to play a significant role in processes associated with tissue damage, aging, and carcinogen metabolism. Although free radical species are necessary, they are rather tightly regulated in biological systems via a redundancy of antioxidant systems. Thus, at the cellular level, any untoward increase in reactive free radical species will, in general, be mitigated by a variety of enzymatic or nonenzymatic antioxidant mechanisms. This balance is important to maintain.

A number of observations reported in the field of chemistry indicate that magnetic fields increase the yields of some types of free radicals formed by homolytic cleavage, photoinduced processes, or random encounters (Scaiano et al. 1994a, b; Canfield et al. 1994; Grissom 1995). Although currently no direct evidence exists in a biological system for such effects, it should be realized that magnetic fields have the potential to upset the balance between reactive free radical species and antioxidant action in biological systems.

A number of examples of the effects of magnetic fields on free radical chemistry exist in the literature; these reports indicate that geminate radical pairs in solutions and, in particular, in micellar environments, can be significantly modified by magnetic fields of ~100 mT (Evans et al. 1988; Scaiano et al. 1994a, b; Canfield et al. 1994; Grissom 1995). Several systems of triplet-derived neutral radical pairs have been studied in detail. Indeed, several mechanisms may give rise to magnetic field effects on radical pairs; at strengths of several hundred mT, Zeeman splitting of the triplet sublevels usually is the dominate interaction. This interaction will lead to a slow-down of intersystem crossing, which will permit other processes to proceed more favorably, such as a separation of radical pairs that can become available for reaction with nearby molecules (instead of the recombination of radical pairs, which yields inert products). Pertinent to biological systems, effects of this type are strongly favored in organized media such as micelles, lipid bilayers, and cell membranes.

With regard to this review of magnetic fields and their relationship to carcinogenesis, two questions arise. First, is there sufficient evidence to support the idea that such magnetic field effects on radical chemistry may be relevant to biological systems? Second, are such interactions plausible at environmental-level magnetic field strengths? We will address each of these questions separately.

Evidence that magnetic fields can influence the activity of a biologically relevant enzyme reaction in vitro (in contrast to a natural biological environment such as inside a living cell) was reported recently by Harkins and Grissom (1994). The application of a static magnetic field of 100 mT was observed to decrease the kinetic parameter Vmax/Km (where Km is the Michaelis-Menten constant) by 25% for the coenzyme B_{12}-dependent enzyme ethanolamine ammonia lyase (EAL). Currently, approximately two dozen enzymes are thought to incorporate radical chemistry in the conversion of substrates to products; the authors chose to study EAL in a reaction in which it initiated the homolysis of a Co-C bond to yield a radical pair; the Co-C bond represents one of the weakest organometalic bonds known (Kd ~31 kcal/mol). The report by Harkins and Grissom demonstrates that a 100-mT, static magnetic field can influence, in a dose-dependent fashion, the kinetics of this enzyme in a manner consistent with a decrease in intersystem crossing rates between the singlet and triplet spin-correlated states. Thus, this report provides evidence that a magnetic field can have an effect on an in vitro enzymatic reaction with known radical intermediates.

One feature of the Harkins and Grissom study, however, was that a ~100-mT, static magnetic field was required to influence this particular enzyme. This field intensity is certainly well above environmental levels. The result obtained in this study would also be expected with a time-varying, 60-Hz magnetic field, because the time course for radical pair recombination is on the order of 10^{-10} to 10^{-6} seconds; over this time period a static and 60-Hz magnetic field would appear indistinguishable. Scaiano et al. (1994b) has provided experimental evidence for the fact that free radical recombination events are indistinguishable regarding 60-Hz versus static magnetic fields. He has further predicted that no time-varying (AC) magnetic field effect would be anticipated for fields strengths significantly below that of the Earth's geomagnetic field. This suggests a lower threshold of approximately 20–50 μT (RMS) for ELF magnetic fields, although taking into account variations in the local geomagnetic (DC) field intensity, there is at present no experimental evidence to support this threshold.

Other investigators have provided arguments supporting lower thresholds. For example, Polk (1992) discusses the possibility of combinations of AC and DC magnetic fields to affect chemical reactions in biological systems that involve free radicals as intermediates. As Polk states, it is possible that a small-amplitude AC magnetic field could add to an existing DC magnetic field to periodically establish conditions for optimum interconversion between singlet and triplet states. This situation is interesting because it occurs in nature and in man-made environmental settings. Canfield and associates (1994) have recently reported a perturbation theory method that also supports the combination of a very weak (environmental-level) oscillating magnetic field and a steady magnetic field operating in the radical pair mechanism. McLauchlan and Steiner (1991) also argue that effects of magnetic fields will be important in biological systems at environmental field strengths. However plausible these predictions may seem, currently, little experimental evidence exists to support environmental-level thresholds.

In this regard, only one experimental study has tested the hypothesis that time-varying 60-Hz magnetic fields might influence free radical recombination events in a biological system such as a living cell (Roy et al. 1995). In these in vitro studies, primed neutrophils were harvested from rats and activated in vitro by the phorbol ester tumor promoter phorbol-12-myristate-13-acetate (PMA) to produce large quantities of free radicals corresponding to the respiratory burst. The generation of these free radical species was followed in real time using the fluorescent dye DCFH, which was loaded into the neutrophils. When the dye is oxidized by free radical species, it forms a highly fluorescent product, DCF; therefore, increases in fluorescence correspond to an increase in the relative concentration of free radical species. In the presence of a 60-Hz, 0.1-mT magnetic field, a 12.4% increase in the fluorescence signal was observed in PMA-stimulated neutrophils (n = 5, p < 0.02, 18 pairs of measurements). This report represents the first experimental observation of magnetic fields influencing events involving free radical species generated during ST in living cells. It should be emphasized that activated neutrophils represent a very specialized cell that undergoes a respiratory burst to generate a large quantity of free radical species; the respiratory burst is a major mechanism of bacterial killing in vivo. Whether other cell types that generate significantly fewer free radical species are influenced by magnetic fields remains to be seen.

Therefore, currently there does exist plausible experimental evidence to support the idea that magnetic fields of ~100 μT can influence radical-mediated enzyme reactions, and one experimental report to argue that environmental-level magnetic fields alter free radical biochemistry. This area of research is in its infancy, and additional studies will undoubtedly appear in the literature soon.

Some conservative speculation is provided here regarding free radicals, magnetic fields, and carcinogenesis. With the field strengths of the discussed magnetochemical studies in mind, it is plausible that occupational-level (in contrast to environmental-level) magnetic fields may influence free radical processes in biological systems. Several comments need to be added for perspective. First, within the complex environment inside a living cell, free radicals are aggressively scavenged; this activity should be considered as mitigating any damage to cellular function, including free radical-mediated initiation in carcinogenesis (Rose and Bode 1993). Second, it is not yet clear whether a magnetic field effect on free radicals would necessarily act to promote or inhibit carcinogenesis. For example, innate immunological responses mediated by macrophages and neutrophils depend heavily on reactive oxygen species—such as superoxide free radicals and the hydroxyl free radical (Rosen et al. 1993)—and may, in fact, be facilitated in magnetic fields via such an interaction. Regarding a magnetic field interaction at environmental-level field strengths, it currently seems that the weight of the experimental evidence on hand favors a magnetic field mechanism involving critical events in ST (e.g., receptor–ligand binding, calcium mobilization, and subsequent cellular reactions in the ST cascade), which bear directly on cellular differentiation and carcinogenesis.

A discussion of free radical scavenging in biological systems also should make special mention of melatonin. Reiter and colleagues have shown in a number of recent, important articles that melatonin is a very efficient free radical scavenger, and, indeed, may represent one of the most potent free radical scavengers in biology (Reiter 1995; Reiter et al. 1993, 1994, 1995; Hardeland et al. 1993; Vijayalaxmi et al. 1995). Given that melatonin blood concentrations undergo a biphasic rise in the nighttime and fall at the onset of daylight, we speculate that any interaction between magnetic fields and free radicals that occurs may be favored during the daytime, when levels of circulating melatonin in the bloodstream are at their lowest. We note that a number of animal studies have reported that melatonin levels at nighttime are reduced or time-shifted for animals maintained in magnetic fields (see discussion of in vivo studies, p. 643). Thus, a reduction in circulating melatonin at nighttime by magnetic fields would decrease the effective concentration of melatonin available for free radical scavenging, and this would enhance the probability of carcinogenesis (Reiter et al. 1994). In addition, melatonin has been shown to have an oncostatic activity against tumor cells in vitro, such as in human breast cancer cells, as discussed previously. Thus, regarding carcinogenesis, magnetic fields can block the oncostatic activity of melatonin at the cellular level possibly by reducing or neutralizing the ability of melatonin to act as a free radical scavenger (Reiter, personal communication).

In summary, a variety of cellular-level interactions with magnetic fields have been described in the literature. With specific regard to carcinogenesis, laboratory evidence exists that supports the concept that magnetic fields act through the classic pathway at the level of copromoter (Fig. 1), and through the nonclassic pathway at several levels involving alterations of the ST cascade and cell proliferation (Fig. 2). Information from several laboratories indicates that early events in the ST cascade, such as receptor–ligand binding and calcium mobilization, are involved in magnetic field coupling to cellular systems. In this regard, subtle alterations in these early events can be greatly amplified via the ST cascade to have potentially profound effects on downstream events such as gene induction, gene expression (e.g., protein synthesis), and cellular proliferation leading to alterations in mitogenesis. Tumor promoters such as phorbol esters, which are structural analogs for diacylglycerol and a critical element in early ST events in the cell membrane, act through this pathway at the cellular level.

ANIMAL STUDIES ON THE ROLE OF ELF MAGNETIC FIELDS IN CARCINOGENESIS

Animal studies are one of the principal ways of determining toxic and carcinogenic potential of various chemical or physical agents in the environment. In animal studies, the variables are rigorously controlled so that the only difference between control and exposure groups is the agent in question. Studies on magnetic field exposure in laboratory animals are helpful in estimating risks of cancer, yet until recently only few published reports on such studies existed. In the last 4–5 years, several animal studies on the role, if any, of ELF magnetic fields in carcinogenesis became available. These studies will be reviewed herein; papers that have been published in peer-reviewed journals are discussed, but in some instances data that have appeared only in conference abstracts are included.

Animal studies on carcinogenic effects of ELF magnetic field exposure can be subdivided into three categories: (1) long-term (often lifespan) studies that expose normal animals to magnetic fields and follow the spontaneous development of tumors; (2) studies that expose animals after implantation of tumor cells; and (3) studies using cocarcinogenesis models in which tumors are induced by known chemical carcinogens or ultraviolet (UV) radiation, and magnetic field exposure is used as a promoter or copromoter. Data from studies of these three categories are summarized in Tables 2–3.

Effects of Magnetic Field Exposure on Spontaneous Tumor Development

A series of studies on this subject was undertaken by two Canadian researchers, Mikhail and Fam (Fam and Mikhail 1990b; Mikhail and Fam 1991, 1993), using mice of both sexes exposed continuously for 23 hours/day to a 60-Hz, 25-mT magnetic field. In most experiments,

continued

TABLE 2
Laboratory in Vivo Studies on Carcinogenic Effects of Magnetic Fields:
Spontaneous Tumor Development or Models with Implantation of Tumor Cells

Model	Species (sex)	Animals per Group	Flux density/ frequency	Duration of exposure	Results	References
Spontaneous Tumor Development						
Spontaneous tumor development	Mice (male and female)	24–55	25 mT 60 Hz	23 hours/day up to 418 days	Increased incidence of malignant lymphoma at exposures > 133 days	Fam and Mikhail 1990b; Mikhail and Fam 1991, 1993
Spontaneous mammary tumor development	Rats (female)	25–50	20 µT 50 Hz	0.5–3 hours/day up to 2 years	Increase of tumor incidence at 3 hours/day	Beniashvili et al. 1991
Spontaneous tumor development	Mice (female)	36	50 or 500 µT 50 Hz	19–21 hours/day 103 weeks	Reduction of survival time at 500 µT; trend to increase of leukemia at 500 µT; no effects at 50 µT	Rannug et al. 1993b

TABLE 2 (continued)

Laboratory in Vivo Studies on Carcinogenic Effects of Magnetic Fields:
Spontaneous Tumor Development or Models with Implantation of Tumor Cells

Model	Species (sex)	Animals per Group	Flux density/ frequency	Duration of exposure	Results	References
Spontaneous tumor development	Rats (male and female)	96	0.5 or 5 mT 50 Hz	22.6 hours/day 104 weeks	No increase in tumor incidence	Yasui et al. 1993 a, b
Implantation of Tumor Cells						
Implantation of P388 leukemia cells	Mice (female)	20	1.4, 200, or 500 μT 60 Hz	6 hours/day 5 days/week until death (about 2 weeks)	No effect on survival time	Thomson et al. 1988
Implantation of murine mammary adenocarcinoma in the hind feet	Mice (female)	60	2 mT 50 Hz	60 hours in 2 weeks	No effect on growth trend	Marino et al. 1995

TABLE 3
Laboratory in Vivo Studies on Carcinogenic Effects of Magnetic Fields:
Cocarcinogenesis Models with Chemical or UV Initiation of Tumors

Model	Species (sex)	Animals per Group	Flux density/ frequency	Duration of exposure	Results	References
Chemical Initiation of Skin Tumors						
Induction of skin tumors by DMBA[a]/TPA[b]	Mice (female)	32	2 mT 60Hz	60 hours/day 5 days/week 21 weeks	Trend to more rapid development of tumors	McLean et al. 1991
Induction of skin tumors by DMBA/TPA	Mice (female)	48	2 mT 60Hz	6 hours/day 5 days/week 23 weeks	Decrease in latency and increase in incidence of tumors	Stuchly et al. 1992
Induction of skin tumors by DMBA/TPA	Mice (female)	60	2 mT 60Hz	8 hours/day 5 days/week > 40 weeks	Decrease in latency and increase in incidence or size of tumors	Byus et al. 1995
Induction of skin tumors by DMBA/PMA[c]	Mice (female)	60	2 mT 60Hz	8 hours/day 5 days/week 23 weeks	Significant increase in tumor incidence and yields in 1 experiment, but no effect in 2 subsequent experiments	McLean et al. 1995

continued

TABLE 3 (continued)
Laboratory in Vivo Studies on Carcinogenic Effects of Magnetic Fields:
Cocarcinogenesis Models with Chemical or UV Initiation of Tumors

Model	Species (sex)	Animals per Group	Flux density/ frequency	Duration of exposure	Results	References
Chemical Initiation of Skin Tumors (continued)						
Induction of skin tumors by DMBA	Mice (female)	36	50 or 500 μT 50 Hz	19–21 hours/day 103 weeks	No effect on latency and incidence of tumors	Rannug et al. 1993b
Induction of skin tumors by DMBA	Mice (female)	50	50 or 500 μT 50 Hz either continuously or 15 seconds on/off	19–21 hours/day 105 weeks	Significant increase in tumor incidence in intermittently exposed mice compared to continuously exposed	Rannug et al. 1994
Chemical Initiation of Mammary Tumors						
Induction of mammary tumors by NMU[d]	Rats (female)	50	20 μT 50 Hz	0.5—3 hours/day up to 160 hours total	Decrease in latency and increase in incidence of tumors at 3 hours exposure/ day; more malignant tumors	Beniashvili et al. 1991

continued

TABLE 3 (continued)

Laboratory in Vivo Studies on Carcinogenic Effects of Magnetic Fields: Cocarcinogenesis Models with Chemical or UV Initiation of Tumors

Model	Species (sex)	Animals per Group	Flux density/ frequency	Duration of exposure	Results	References
Chemical Initiation of Mammary Tumors (continued)						
Induction of mammary tumors by DMBA	Rats (female)	15–18	30 mT 50 Hz	24 hours/day 3 months	Increase of tumor number per animal but not reproducible upon repeat	Mevissen et al. 1993b
Induction of mammary tumors by DMBA	Rats (female)	36	0.3–1 μT (gradient field) 50 Hz	24 hours/day 3 months	Trend to decrease in tumor latency; decrease of nocturnal melatonin secretion	Mevissen et al. 1993a; Löscher et al. 1994
Induction of mammary tumors by DMBA	Rats (female)	99	100 μT 50 Hz	24 hours/day 3 months	Decrease in latency and increase in growth in tumors	Löscher et al. 1993; Baum et al. 1995
Chemical Induction of Liver Tumors						
Induction of liver tumors by DENA[e]	Rats (male)	9–10	0.5 or 500 μT 50 Hz	19–21 hours/day 12 weeks	No tumor promotion	Rannug et al. 1993c

continued

TABLE 3 (continued)

Laboratory in Vivo Studies on Carcinogenic Effects of Magnetic Fields: Cocarcinogenesis Models with Chemical or UV Initiation of Tumors

Model	Species (sex)	Animals per Group	Flux density/ frequency	Duration of exposure	Results	References
Chemical Induction of Thymic Lymphoma/Leukemia						
Induction of thymic lymphoma/leukemia by DMBA	Mice (male and female)	75–89	1 mT 50 Hz	3 hours/day 6 days/week 16 weeks	No significant difference to control	Shen et al. 1995
Induction of lymphoma in PIM transgenic mice by ENU[f]	PIM mice (male and female)	30 per sex	2,200 or 1000 μT 60 Hz	18.5 hours/day 175 days	No effect on incidence and latency of tumors or mortality	McCormick et al. 1994
UV Initiation of Skin Tumors						
Induction of skin tumors by UV irradiation	ODC transgenic mice (female)	22	100 μT 50 Hz	Continuous and intermittent exposure	Significantly enhanced tumor growth	Kumlin et al. 1995

[a] 7,12-dimethylbenz(a)anthracene
[b] 12-O-tetradecanoylphorbol-13-acetate
[c] phorbol-12-myristate-13 acetate
[d] nitrosomethylurea
[e] diethylnitrosamine (plus Phenobarbital as promoter)
[f] N-ethyl-N-nitrosourea

the animals were conceived, born, and raised in the field until they were sacrificed for pathological examination. Details of the exposure system were recently described (Fam and Mikhail 1990a; Mikhail and Fam 1993). Control groups were located in the same room as the exposed group, but sufficiently far from the exposure system to ensure segregation from stray magnetic fields exceeding 0.05 mT. After different periods of exposure, a complete autopsy was performed on all animals and tissue sections were taken from thymus, spleen, lymph nodes, liver, kidney, lung, and bowel.

In a first experiment, groups of 24 animals were continuously exposed for an average of 120 days (Fam and Mikhail 1990b). Examination of tissue sections from the exposed animals showed that 50% of the males and 92% of the females had enlarged lymph nodes. Some of the exposed animals showed peripheral and bone marrow leucocytosis but no evidence of leukemic transformation. In addition, splenic hyperplasia was noted in some of the exposed animals. There was no gross or histopathologic evidence of brain tumor or any other organ neoplastic transformation. In a subsequent study, a group of 55 mice was continuously exposed from conception until sacrifice at an age of 133–257 days (Mikhail and Fam 1991). Examination of tissue sections from these animals showed that 33–45% had developed malignant lymphoma, 13% had premalignant changes, and 31% had lymphoid hyperplasia. Thus, only 25% of the exposed animals did not show evidence of disease. In the control group, only 5% of the animals showed lymphoid hyperplasia; the remaining 95% exhibited no pathological changes. In a third study, which was published recently in more detailed form (Mikhail and Fam 1993), the duration of exposure was prolonged to 363–418 days. Malignant lymphoma was determined in 56% of the 41 exposed animals. Premalignant changes were seen in 22% and lymphoid hyperplasia in 17%; only 5% of the exposed animals were without pathological changes. In the control group (which was exposed to a stray field of 50 μT), 8% developed lymphoid hyperplasia and 6% early thymic lymphoma.

Although Mikhail and Fam did not evaluate their data by statistical methods, it can be easily demonstrated by Fisher's exact test or the chi-square test that the differences in incidence of lymphoma between exposed animals and controls were highly significant. Interestingly, female mice were clearly more susceptible to the carcinogenic effects of exposure than males. For example, in the last study 86% of females but only 25% of males developed malignant lymphoma. Overall, the studies may indicate a direct correlation between the duration of magnetic field exposure and the incidence of lymphoma in the exposed animals. Unfortunately, the exposure conditions were not fully described by the authors; although several studies suggested that interactions between the artificially generated ELF field and the static geomagnetic field might be important for bioeffects produced by the ELF magnetic field (Polk 1992), the direction and strength of the Earth's static magnetic field in the exposure room was not documented by Mikhail and Fam. Furthermore, the experimental data of these authors have not been published in any peer-reviewed forum.

A group from the Oncology Research Center in Tbilisi, Republic of Georgia, exposed groups of 25–50 female rats to 50-Hz, 20-μT magnetic fields for either 0.5 or 3 hours/day over a period of 2 years; total exposure time reached up to 425 hours (Beniashvili et al. 1991). Histopathologic examination of the mammary gland showed that 7 out of 25 animals exposed for 3 hours/day had developed mammary tumors (2 adenocarcinomas and 6 fibroadenomas) compared to 0 out of 50 controls; the difference was highly significant ($p < 0.001$ by chi-square test). In animals exposed for 0.5 hours/day, only 1 out of 25 rats developed mammary tumors. Similarly to the studies by Mikhail and Fam, the exposure and, particularly, sham-exposure conditions were not sufficiently described by Beniashvili et al. (1991).

In a recent study in Sweden, Rannug et al. (1993b) exposed groups of 36 female mice to 50-Hz magnetic fields of either 50 or 500 μT for up to 103 weeks. Six animals of each group were taken for skin hyperplasia analysis and were not included in the statistical calculations. Following death or termination of the maximum exposure period, all organs or tissues were carefully observed during necropsy for possible abnormalities, and all lesions underwent histopathologic diagnosis. Animals exposed at 500 μT had a significantly shorter survival (74 weeks) than animals exposed at 50 μT (87.5 weeks) or controls (94.5 weeks). Leukemia tended to be more frequent among animals exposed to 500 μT (8 out of 30 mice) compared to controls (4 out of 30 mice). The frequencies of other tumor types were similar in all groups. The small group sizes, however, made the experiment relatively unsensitive as a test for complete carcinogenesis. It should be noted that the primary purpose of this study was to test magnetic field effects on chemically induced skin tumors (see p. 636).

In a recent study from Japan (Yasui et al. 1993a, b), groups of 48 male and 48 female F344 rats per exposure level were exposed to 50-Hz magnetic fields at flux densities of 500 μT or 5 mT, or sham exposed for 5 to 109 weeks of age, according to the Organization for Economic Cooperation and Development test guideline 451. Following macroscopic examination, all organs and tissues suspected of tumoral lesion were histopathologically examined. No significant differences in incidence of tumors—including lymphoma, leukemia and brain tumors—were found between groups. Furthermore, survival time was not altered by magnetic field exposure.

Effects of Magnetic Field Exposure on Implanted Tumor Cells

Magnetic field exposure of mice in which leukemia rapidly develops from intraperitoneal implantation of P388 leukemia cells provides an approach to investigate if the "take" and progression of leukemia are modified by magnetic fields. Using survival time as the endpoint, Thomson et al. (1988) found no effect of 60-Hz magnetic field exposure at flux densities of 1.4, 200, or 500 μT compared to controls. However, because of the short survival time of this model, animals could be exposed only for about 2 weeks after implantation of leukemia cells (Table 2). Furthermore, studies with implantation of cells from tumor lines are of questionable relevance to carcinogenesis, representing rather a test of tumor progression and growth.

In an attempt to study tumor growth under 50-Hz magnetic field exposure, Marino et al. (1995) injected a suspension of murine mammary adenocarcinoma in the right hind feet of female mice and determined alteration in tumor volume at different times thereafter. Magnetic fields did not modify the tumor growth trend; however, only relatively short exposure periods (60 hours) were examined (Table 2).

Effects of Magnetic Field Exposure in Cocarcinogenesis Models

In these models, chemical carcinogens with well-characterized tumor initiating and/or promoting effects are administered alone (initiator) or in combination (initiator and promoter) in normal rodents. Depending on the type of carcinogen and its administered dosage and target organ(s), tumors develop within a range of latency periods of several weeks. Thus, promoting or copromoting effects of additional factors (e.g., magnetic field exposure) can be studied in much shorter time than in experiments with spontaneous tumor development. Because the genetic alterations (e.g., the activation of oncogenes) operatives in chemical carcinogenesis are thought to be comparable if not identical to respective alterations operatives in "spontaneous" tumor development (Anderson et al. 1992), data on factors that modulate chemical carcinogenesis in rodents are considered relevant for human risk exposures. Furthermore, it should be noted that the human diet contains several chemical carcinogens, which may play an important role in modulating carcinogenic risk (Gold et al. 1992). It has been estimated that at least 50% of the cancer incidence in human populations may be attributable to environmental factors, including exposure to chemical carcinogens in the occupational environment and intake of chemical carcinogens through food (Anttila et al. 1993; Moller 1993). Thus, any interaction of magnetic field exposure with chemical carcinogenesis would be important in terms of both basic mechanisms and risk assessment.

The carcinogenesis of three types of chemically induced tumors has been studied during ELF magnetic field exposure in mice or rats: skin tumors, mammary tumors, and liver tumors (Table 3).

Chemically Induced Skin Cancer

Using a well-designed magnetic field exposure system for in vivo studies (Stuchly et al. 1991), the Canadian group of M.A. Stuchly and coworkers used the mouse skin model of multistage tumorigenesis to investigate the effects of exposure to a 60-Hz, 2-mT magnetic field (McLean et al. 1991; Stuchly et al. 1992). The effect of magnetic fields on natural killer cell activity in spleen and blood was also examined, because these cells are part of the immune surveillance system known to be suppressed by tumor promoters such as TPA. In a first series of experiments (McLean et al. 1991), two groups of 32 juvenile female SENCAR mice were treated with a subthreshold dose of the carcinogen DMBA (applied to the dorsal skin) and sham- or magnetic field exposed for 6 hours/day, 5 days/week, for 21 weeks to test whether the field would act as a tumor promoter. No tumors developed in these two groups of mice. Two additional groups of mice were treated weekly with the tumor promoter TPA after the initial application of DMBA, and were then either sham or field exposed (McLean et al. 1991). The time to appearance of tumors was shorter (but not statistically so) in the group exposed to magnetic fields and TPA. Because almost all animals developed tumors under both sham and magnetic field conditions, the experimental design did not allow detection of differences in tumor incidence. However, magnetic field-exposed mice exhibited a significantly greater number of enlarged spleens and of mononuclear cells in spleen, which might indicate the possible development of leukemia due to suppression of the immune system (McLean et al., 1991). Consistent with this interpretation, natural killer cell activity was below detection limit in several of the magnetic field-exposed mice.

In a subsequent study by Stuchly et al. (1992), the experimental design of the skin tumor model was altered to allow examination of potential tumor copromoting effects of magnetic field exposure. The dorsal skin of SENCAR mice was treated with DMBA to initiate the carcinogenic process, and then tumor development was promoted, for 23 weeks, by weekly applications of suboptimal concentrations of TPA. Magnetic field exposure resulted in a significant increase in the rate of tumor development following 12 weeks of exposure and thereafter, demonstrating that magnetic fields acted as a copromoter. The authors concluded that their data represent the first indication of a modification of animal multistage carcinogenesis by magnetic field exposure (Stuchly et al. 1992).

In a collaboration between Stuchly and the group of C.V. Byus at the University of California, Riverside, the ability of a 60-Hz magnetic field to serve as a copromotional stimulus to the development of DMBA-induced skin cancer in SENCAR mice was further investigated. Two suboptimal doses of TPA (i.e., those not producing maximal numbers of tumors) were chosen from a dose–effect curve generated previously. In the animals receiving the higher of the two TPA doses, there was no difference between magnetic field-exposed (2 mT, 60-Hz) or sham-exposed subjects in terms of tumor incidence, total numbers of tumors, or the tumor burden (i.e., the number of tumors per animal) through a 35-week promotional period. However, tumor weights were significantly higher in magnetic field-exposed mice. In the animals receiving the lowest of the TPA promotion treatments, there was a significant increase in the percentage of mice with tumors in magnetic field-exposed mice compared to sham-exposed controls. These data demonstrate that there appears to be a differential effect upon the size of papillomas as well as the tumor incidence when the 60-Hz magnetic field is used as a copromotional stimulus with suboptimal or low doses of TPA (Byus et al. 1995).

In a study not yet available in fully published form, McLean et al. (1993) found that the light conditions of the exposure room significantly interacted with magnetic fields, which could be explained on the basis of the "melatonin hypothesis" (see p. 643). In contrast to previous studies with the skin tumor model, PMA was used instead of TPA. Animals exposed to 60-Hz, 2-mT magnetic fields in the dark developed markedly fewer tumors than animals exposed to magnetic fields in ambient light, suggesting that both PMA and light may be acting as tumor promoters in this mouse model (McLean et al. 1993).

More recently, McLean et al. (1995) compared the data from three subsequent studies on the effect of 60-Hz, 2-mT magnetic fields on copromotion of DMBA-induced skin tumors in SENCAR mice, using PMA for promotion. In the first experiment, tumor incidence and yields for weeks 16 through 18 were significantly higher in the magnetic field-exposed group. However, in the subsequent two experiments, no difference was found between sham- and field-exposed mice. Preliminary analysis of the combined results suggested that magnetic fields had no effect on tumor promotion.

The Swedish group of Holmberg published a detailed experiment with the DMBA skin tumor model using female NMRI mice (Rannug et al. 1993b). For tumor initiation, DMBA was applied to the dorsal skin, then the mice were exposed to a 50-Hz magnetic field at flux densities of 50 or 500 μT for 103 weeks, starting 1 week after the initiator treatment. The tumor promoter TPA was used in a separate group of mice as positive control for skin tumor promoting activity. The percentage of animals bearing skin tumors was 27% with DMBA alone,

20% with DMBA plus 50 μT, 37% with DMBA plus 500 μT, and 80% with DMBA plus TPA; the differences between DMBA with and without the magnetic field were not statistically significant. Similarly, tumor latencies were not significantly different in sham-exposed and magnetic field-exposed groups. The data substantiate that continuous magnetic fields at selected flux densities do not promote skin tumorigenesis per se.

In a subsequent study, Rannug et al. (1994) examined the effect of intermittent, 50-Hz magnetic field exposure on skin tumor promotion in SENCAR mice. In order to test if intermittent magnetic fields act as a tumor promoter, a long-term skin carcinogenicity study was performed starting 1 week after application of DMBA to the dorsal skin at a subcarcinogenic dose. The fields employed were 50-Hz, sinusoidal magnetic fields with flux densities of 50 μT and 500 μT continuous, as well as with an intermittency of 15 seconds on/off. Again, TPA was used in a separate group of mice as positive control for skin tumor promoting activity. The animals exposed to continuous fields showed no skin tumor. The on/off exposed groups differed significantly from the continuously exposed groups; 5 out of 50 mice exposed to 500 μT on/off had a total of 13 skin tumors and 4 out of 50 mice exposed to 50 μT on/off had a total of 4 skin tumors. These data thus indicate that, while continuous magnetic fields at selected flux densities do not promote skin tumorigenesis per se, intermittent magnetic fields do, suggesting that transients potentially associated with turn-on and turn-off may be involved in such an effect.

Chemically Induced Breast Cancer
Beniashvili et al. (1991) used the "complete" carcinogen nitrosomethylurea (NMU) to produce mammary tumors in female rats aged from 55 to 60 days. NMU was injected intravenously at a dose of 50 mg/kg; magnetic field exposure started 2 days after NMU administration. Groups of 50 rats were exposed at a 50-Hz, 20-μT field for 0.5 or 3 hours daily over a period of up to 2 years after the carcinogen injection. Whereas 59% of the nonexposed controls developed mammary tumors, tumor incidence was 67% with 0.5 hours and 93% with 3 hours daily exposure; the difference between 3 hours daily exposure and controls was statistically significant. The mean number of tumors

per rat with tumors was 1.2 in controls and in rats exposed 0.5 hours/day, but 1.7 in rats exposed 3 hours/day. Tumor latency was 74.4 days in controls, 64.8 days in rats exposed 0.5 hours/day, and 45.5 days in rats exposed 3 hours/day. Furthermore, in animals exposed daily to magnetic fields for 3 hours, the tumor progression from benign to malignant forms was accelerated in that more malignant mammary tumors were determined compared to the other groups. Thus, these data indicate that magnetic field exposure at relatively low flux density markedly copromotes cancer development in a mammary tumor model.

Löscher's group in Hannover, Germany, used the well-established DMBA rat model of mammary carcinogenesis (cf., Huggins and Yang 1962; Russo et al. 1977; Welsch 1985) to study the effects of magnetic field exposure. This model has a number of features that make it particularly attractive to the experimental oncologist; for example, tumor induction ease and reliability, organ site specificity, tumors of ductal origin, tumors of predominantly carcinomatous histopathological characteristics, tumors of varying growth factor and/or hormone responsiveness, and the potential to examine tumor initiation and promotion processes. Because of these advantages, this model is one of the standard laboratory animal models in the study of human breast cancer (Welsch 1985). In these experiments, DMBA (5 mg/rat) was administered by gastric intubation four times at intervals of 1 week. By this procedure, about 50% of the female Sprague-Dawley rats (age at first administration was 52 days) developed mammary cancer within 3 months. In a first series of experiments (Mevissen et al. 1993), groups of 15–18 rats were exposed to homogeneous, 50-Hz, 30-mT magnetic fields for 3 months, starting immediately after the first DMBA application. Concomitantly, groups of the same size were sham exposed in the same room (resulting in a stray field exposure of about 20–40 μT) or in another room with ambient ELF magnetic fields (0.015–0.15 μT). In the exposure room, the generated 50-Hz fields were parallel to the horizontal component of the Earth's north/south static magnetic field. Exposures of 50 Hz at 30 mT resulted in a 40% increase in tumor incidence and a significant increase in the number of tumors per tumor-bearing rat. However, these findings could be not be reproduced when the experiment was repeated. It should be noted that the two experiments with magnetic field exposure at 30 mT were done during different seasons, which might be important, because chronobiologic response modifiers, such as melatonin, have been implicated in breast cancer development (Cornélissen and Halberg 1992). In other words, in view of the circannual rhythm in melatonin production (Bartsch et al. 1994), the time of the year might influence the effect of magnetic fields on mammary carcinogenesis.

In a subsequent experiment, larger groups of rats (36 per group) were exposed to a 50-Hz, gradient magnetic field at a flux density of 0.3–1 μT, mimicking elevated domestic magnetic field exposure as arising from neighboring power lines (Mevissen et al. 1993; Löscher et al. 1994). After 3 months of continuous exposure, tumor incidence (as based on palpation of mammary tumors) was the same in sham-exposed and field-exposed groups (but see the next paragraph). There was a tendency to decreased tumor latency during magnetic field exposure, which was associated with a significantly decreased nocturnal secretion of melatonin in magnetic field-exposed rats (Löscher et al. 1994). A detailed histopathologic evaluation of preneoplastic and neoplastic mammary lesions demonstrated that the incidence of hyperplasias and tumors was 24% higher in field-exposed than in sham-exposed rats, which, however, was not statistically significant (Löscher et al. 1994). Examination of tumor size did not indicate significant differences in tumor burden between groups.

As shown in Table 3, most studies on magnetic field exposure and carcinogenesis used relatively small sample sizes. Thus, significant effects of magnetic field exposure on tumor development might have been missed in some of these studies, including the initial experiments of Löscher's group. For instance, by using 30 animals in a model which gives a tumor incidence of 50% in control animals, an increase of tumor incidence of 50% by magnetic field exposure would mean that 22–23 instead of 15 animals develop tumors; this difference would not be statistically significant. The same experiment with 100 animals, however, would yield a highly significant difference. In order to avoid this important bias of sample size, a new exposure system allowing the concurrent exposure of more than 100 rats was used for subsequent experiments by Löscher's group (Löscher et al. 1993; Baum et al. 1995). An identical second exposure system in the same room allowed simultaneous sham exposure under "blind" conditions, because both systems could be switched on independently in a blinded fashion. Using this exposure system with 99 rats per group, Löscher et al. studied the effects of a 50-Hz, 100 μT magnetic field in the DMBA mammary cancer model (Löscher et al. 1993; Baum et al. 1995). After 3 months of exposure, the incidence of palpable and, after autopsy, macroscopically visible mammary tumors in magnetic field-exposed rats was 50% higher than in sham-exposed rats, the difference being statistically significant. Furthermore, the size of mammary tumors excised from exposed rats was significantly larger compared to sham controls (Baum et al. 1995). Detailed histopathologic examination of the rats from these experiments showed that the number of neoplastic and non-neoplastic lesions of the mammary glands did not significantly differ between groups, indicating that magnetic field exposure did not alter the incidence of mammary lesions but accelerated tumor growth, consistent with a copromoting effect. Furthermore, in the field-exposed group, significantly more rats exhibited malignant mammary tumors than in controls, indicating that magnetic field exposure had affected the progression of DMBA-induced lesions. Subsequent experiments with 10 and 50 μT indicated that the copromotional effect of exposure to 50-Hz fields in the DMBA model of breast cancer in rats was dose-dependent in that flux density and tumor copromotion were linearly correlated in a highly positive fashion (Löscher and Mevissen 1995; see also Chapter 20, this volume).

Chemically Induced Liver Tumors

Rannug et al. (1993c) used the enzyme-altered rat liver model to study if 50-Hz magnetic fields influence the initiation event or the process of liver tumor development in response to known initiators or promoters of cancer. Groups of 9–10 male Sprague-Dawley rats were subjected to a 70% partial hepatectomy; 24 hours later, they received an intraperitoneal injection of diethylnitrosoamine (DENA) as a tumor initiator. Starting one week after the DENA treatment, Phenobarbital (PB) was given via the diet to promote growth of enzymatically altered foci of liver cells. The rats were exposed to homogeneous, horizontal, 50-Hz magnetic fields with flux densities of 0.5 μT or 500 μT immediately after the partial hepatectomy; exposure continued until sacrifice after

12 weeks of PB exposure. Compared to controls treated with DENA and PB alone, a slight inhibition of liver foci formation was found in the field-exposed groups. Rannug et al. (1993c) suggested that, due to the experimental protocol, magnetic field exposure might have interacted with the initiation phase of liver foci formation, so that a tumor promoting or copromoting effect of magnetic field exposure could not be excluded by the experiment. In another large study by the same group, the liver foci model was used without PB treatment and rats were exposed to 50-Hz field at flux densities of 0.5, 5, 50 or 500 μT starting 1 week after an initiating treatment with partial hepatectomy and DENA (Rannug et al. 1993a). That study did not suggest a tumor promoting activity of magnetic fields in this model.

Interestingly, recent in vitro data demonstrated that magnetic field exposure (60-Hz, 100 μT) alone did not promote focus formation in the absence of a promoter (TPA), but exposure significantly copromoted with TPA by producing 1.9-fold more foci than sham-exposed cultures treated with TPA alone (Cain et al. 1993; see detailed description on p. 610). Similarly, Balcer-Kubiczek and Harrison (1991) reported from in vitro experiments with cloned C3H10T mouse embryo cells that magnetic field exposure, while ineffective alone, induced neoplastic transformation in the presence of TPA, ranging up to a level equivalent to that produced by X-rays. These in vitro findings, which demonstrate synergistic interaction between magnetic fields and tumor promoters, might explain why magnetic field exposure exerted no effect in the in vivo studies of Rannug et al. (1993a), suggesting that any carcinogenic effects of magnetic field exposure critically depend on the experimental protocol.

Chemically Induced Lymphoma/Leukemia

In view of epidemiologic studies suggesting an association between magnetic field exposure and lymphoma or leukemia, some recent experimental studies examined if 50- or 60-Hz magnetic field exposure exerts tumor promoting effects in models of such cancers (Table 3). Shen et al. (1995) induced thymic lymphoma and granulocytic leukemia in mice by subcutaneous injection of DMBA within 24 hours after birth. Beginning 2 weeks after DMBA injection, the newborn mice were exposed to a 50-Hz, 1-mT magnetic field 3 hours/day, 6 days/week for successive 16 weeks. At the age of 32 weeks, all surviving mice were examined pathologically. In the sham-exposed group, 29.7% of animals had developed thymic lymphoma and 2.6% of animals granulocytic leukemia, compared to 30.3% and 3% in the magnetic field-exposed group, respectively, without significant difference between groups. Thus, under the conditions of this study, a 50-Hz magnetic field exposure did not affect the incidence of lymphoma/leukemia, or the life-span and metastatic rate of tumors. The data, however, do not rule out that such a field acts as a copromoter in this model.

McCormick et al. (1994) used PIM transgenic mice to evaluate the hypothesis that magnetic field exposure may enhance hematopoietic neoplasia. The PIM mouse, a transgenic mouse strain carrying the *pim* oncogene, develops lymphoma following a single injection of the nitrosamide, N-ethyl-N-nitrosourea (ENU). Beginning on the day after ENU injection, groups of 60 PIM mice (30 per sex) were exposed to pure 60-Hz magnetic fields at flux densities of 2, 200, or 1000 μT, or were sham exposed. An additional group of PIM mice was exposed intermittently (1 hour on, 1 hour off) to a 1000-μT field. The experiment was terminated after 175 days of magnetic field exposure. The field exposure had no effect on the incidence, latency, or infiltrative behavior of induced lymphoma in any group, or on the incidence or latency of tumor-related mortality. Similar to the report of Shen et al. (1995), these data of McCormick et al. (1994) suggest that exposure to magnetic fields does not promote lymphoid neoplasia. However, it is important to note that these animal models are far from being as well-characterized as conventional tumor models of skin or breast cancer. Thus, any conclusion on promoting or copromoting effects of magnetic field exposure on the development of hematopoietic neoplasia must await further experiments.

UV-Initiated Skin Tumors

In addition to cocarcinogenesis models with chemical initiation of tumors, a recent study used UV irradiation to initiate tumors (Kumlin et al. 1995). The study involved ODC-transgenic mice, which have been shown to be more prone than normal mice to develop skin tumors after topical application of chemical initiators and promoters.

Exposure of mice to a vertical, sinusoidal, 50-Hz magnetic field at a flux density of $100 \, \mu T$ led to a significant tumor promoting effect in this model (Kumlin et al. 1995).

In Vivo Studies on Mechanisms
Potentially Linked to Carcinogenesis

The most plausible evidence for an in vivo effect of magnetic field exposure that could be related to tumor promotion is reduction of circulating levels of melatonin, a hormone which is inhibitory to the growth of a wide range of cancers. Melatonin's mechanisms of oncostatic action involve complex interactions with hormones, growth factors, lymphokines, cytokines, and their receptors as well as with various ST pathways, cytoskeletal elements, and genomic components such as oncogenes (Blask 1993). So far, the most abundant data supporting a role for melatonin as an oncostatic hormone is in the realm of breast cancer (Blask 1993; Stevens et al. 1992). While melatonin administration has been shown to suppress mammary tumorigenesis in experimental animal models such as the DMBA model, decrease of melatonin levels by pinealectomy or bright light at night accelerated neoplastic growth in these models (Stevens et al. 1992; Blask 1993).

Static magnetic fields have long been known to suppress pineal melatonin synthesis and secretion (c.f., Stevens et al. 1992; Reiter and Lerchl 1993), but respective effects of ELF magnetic fields have been reported only recently. Kato et al. (1993) demonstrated that a 6-week, 50-Hz magnetic field exposure at flux densities as low as $1 \, \mu T$ significantly decreased nocturnal melatonin levels in plasma and pineal gland of male rats. Consistent with this finding, Löscher et al. reported that exposure to a 50-Hz gradient field at $0.3–1 \, \mu T$ significantly decreased nocturnal melatonin serum levels in female rats, associated with a trend towards accelerated development of mammary tumors (Löscher et al. 1994).

There are at least three possible mechanisms by which reduced circulating melatonin concentrations may enhance mammary carcinogenesis in rats (Stevens et al. 1992). Reduced melatonin may (1) increase proliferation of breast epithelial stem cells at risk, (2) facilitate proliferation of mammary cancer cells, and (3) impair immune tumor surveillance. First evidence for increased proliferation of mammary tissue in response to 50-Hz magnetic field exposure was recently provided by studies demonstrating that a 50-μT magnetic field significantly increases ODC activity in the mammary gland but not several other tissues of female rats (Mevissen et al. 1995), which would be consistent with the melatonin hypothesis. However, substantial species differences in the sensitivity of pineal gland function to light exist (Reiter and Lerchl 1993); therefore, in order to extrapolate animal data to humans, it is necessary to demonstrate that magnetic field exposure in the μT range can decrease nocturnal melatonin levels not only in laboratory animals but in humans. A previous study of Wilson et al. (1990) showed that the initiation and termination of field exposure from electric blankets changed the excretion of urinary 6-hydroxy melatonin sulfate (6-OHMS), a metabolite of melatonin. More direct data on magnetic field effects on human melatonin synthesis and secretion were recently presented by Graham et al. (1993), who found a significant reduction of nocturnal melatonin levels in plasma when male volunteers who had pre-existing low levels of melatonin were exposed during night to a circularly polarized, intermittent, 60-Hz, 20-μT magnetic field (cf., Graham et al. 1994).

An open question is whether long-term exposure to a 50/60-Hz magnetic field is more potent to reduce melatonin than the short-term exposures used in the human studies. It is important to note that a recent study by Selmaoui and Touitou (1995) demonstrated that both duration and intensity of exposure play an important role in this effect. Thus, in rats exposed to a 50-Hz magnetic field of either 1, 10 or 100 μT for 12 hours or 30 days, short-term exposure depressed pineal N-acetyltransferase (NAT), the rate-limiting enzyme for melatonin synthesis, and nocturnal serum melatonin concentration only at the highest flux density; long-term exposure significantly depressed pineal NAT and serum melatonin already at 10 μT, indicating a cumulative effect of magnetic fields on pineal function.

The mechanisms whereby nonvisible magnetic fields influence the melatonin-forming ability of the pineal gland remain unknown; however, it has been theorized that the retinas serve as magnetoreceptors (Olcese 1990; Reiter 1993). The disturbances in pineal melatonin production induced by either light exposure or nonvisible magnetic field exposure at night appear to be the same (Reiter 1993), so that it is conceivable that both light and magnetic field exposure could act synergistically to suppress pineal function. Although decrease of melatonin levels alone could explain tumor promoting or copromoting effects of magnetic field exposure, recent data from Liburdy's group indicate that exposure also impairs the effects of melatonin at the cellular level (see section on in vitro studies). All these data indicate that interactions between ELF magnetic field exposure and melatonin may be the key mechanism of any carcinogenic effects.

Technical and Biological Factors Critically Involved in Laboratory Studies on Magnetic Field Effects

It is often argued that data from laboratory studies on biological or carcinogenic effects of magnetic field exposure are equivocal or lack independent replication (e.g., Lacy-Hulbert et al. 1995a; Saffer and Thurston 1995a). It is important to note that any effect of magnetic field exposure depends on a variety of technical and biological factors, only few of which are known sufficiently (Table 1). Thus, variation in such technical and biological factors among laboratory studies on magnetic field effects may explain, at least in part, most apparent discrepancies between results of different reports. For instance, Kato et al. (1994) have recently shown that the field orientation may be important in magnetic field effects on melatonin levels in that pineal and plasma melatonin significantly decrease in response to 6 weeks of exposure to circularly, but not horizontally or vertically polarized, 50-Hz, 1-μT magnetic fields in male rats. Data from Löscher's group indicate that female rats may be more sensitive to reduction of melatonin levels than male rats, because a significant reduction was seen by exposure to a horizontally polarized, 50-Hz, 0.3- to 1-μT field in female Sprague-Dawley rats (Löscher et al. 1994), while such a field had no effect in male rats of the same strain (Kato et al. 1994). Indeed, the available animal studies on carcinogenic effects of magnetic field exposure indicate that sex is an important host susceptibility factor for magnetic field effects. All studies that found tumor promoting or copromoting actions used female animals. Furthermore, life-span magnetic field exposure of mice resulted in much higher incidences of cancers in females than in males.

Sex is long known to be a predisposing host susceptibility factor to certain carcinogens. For instance, women and girls are two to four times as susceptible as men and boys to thyroid cancer induction by ionizing radiation, and are many times more susceptible to breast cancer induction (Shore 1988). In addition to host susceptibility factors such as age and sex, a possible synergism of other environmental exposures with magnetic field effects is also a concern. The best studied human synergism is between radon exposures and smoking. Radon exposures produce roughly four to five times as much risk among smokers as among nonsmokers (Shore 1988). Little is known about such synergisms in humans exposed to nonionizing ELF magnetic fields.

CONCLUSIONS

As shown in this review, an increasing number of laboratory studies on ELF magnetic field exposure indicates that intermediate exposure exerts copromoting effects in different tumor models. Furthermore, there is some as-yet preliminary evidence that chronic (up to life-span) exposure to high flux density may exert promoting effects on "spontaneous" development of certain tumors. In view of the high tumor incidence found in some animal studies on life-span magnetic field exposure (Mikhail and Fam 1991, 1993), the possibility of tumor initiating or co-initiating effects at high flux densities cannot be ruled out. Although most of the available evidence does not suggest that magnetic fields cause genotoxic effects (Murphy et al. 1993), nongenotoxic carcinogens do exist (Butterworth and Slaga 1987; Shaw and Jones 1994); magnetic fields may belong to this category of carcinogens. In general, carcinogenicity findings from experiments in laboratory animals are logical and scientifically reasonable for identifying and predicting potential carcinogenic effects to humans (Huff 1993). For example, almost all chemicals known to cause or be strongly associated with cancer in humans, and that have been studied adequately in experimental animals, likewise are carcinogenic in animals, and in most cases exhibit target organ concordance (Huff 1993; Vainio and Wilbourn 1993). Many agents were first identified as carcinogens in experimental studies, and were only later confirmed to cause or promote cancer in humans by epidemiologic studies (Huff 1993; Vainio and Wilbourn 1993). With respect to magnetic field exposure, the first evidence of (co)carcinogenic effects came from various epidemiologic studies (c.f., Savitz and Ahlbom 1994). In this case, laboratory studies are needed to prove the cause–effect relationship and thus substantiate hazard identification. Indeed, both epidemiologic investigations and animal experimentation have been recognized as the two primary sources of evidence necessary to establish etiology of environmental cancers (Kraybill and Mehlmann 1977).

With respect to the flux densities used in the reviewed animal studies, one may raise the objection that most studies which found magnetic field effects used flux densities far exceeding those relevant for human exposure situations. For example, the guidelines of the International Radiation Protection Association (IRPA) and the International Non-Ionizing Radiation Committee (INIRC) for 50/60-Hz fields propose limits of exposure between 100 and 1000 μT for general public (e.g., residential) exposures, and 500 to 5000 μT for occupational exposures, the individual limit depending on the duration of exposure per day (Grandolfo and Repacholi 1993). Carcinogenic effects of magnetic field exposure found in animal experiments at, for instance, 25 mT (as in Fam and Mikhail 1990b, and Mikhail and Fam 1991, 1993) would then appear to be irrelevant to human risk assessment. However, most animal studies did not undertake "dose" (i.e., flux density)–effect experiments in order to determine "threshold doses" of ELF magnetic field exposure. Furthermore, magnetic field dosimetric parameters depend on body size and shape; different geometric coupling factors exist between external fields and different species (Bracken 1992). Thus, the magnitude of the applied field may have to be adjusted to yield equivalent dosimetric exposure parameters in different species and in animals of different size in the same species. Respective scaling factors for human versus rat are about 5; exposure of a rat to a field of 100 μT would be equivalent to exposure of a human to a 20-μT field (Bracken 1992). However, such scaling factors are only valid if one assumes that biological effects are due to the induction of electric fields or currents in response to magnetic fields (Polk 1992). Currently it is not known whether observed bioeffects of low-level

ELF magnetic fields are due to these fields themselves, or are a consequence of the electric fields that they induce (Polk 1992; Sagan 1992).

Another complicating factor in risk assessment of magnetic field exposure is the possibility that dose–response features of such exposure do not follow a simple linear function but exhibit "windows"— ranges in which the system displays enhanced sensitivity (Litovitz et al. 1992). Such windows have been reported for field amplitude, frequency, and exposure duration (Litovitz et al. 1992). Goodman et al. (1991) found a striking example of an amplitude window in a study in which the maximum enhancing effect of 60-Hz magnetic fields on the level of RNA transcripts in HL-60 cells occurred at a flux density of 10 μT, with a markedly decreasing effect at higher flux densities. If such window effects exist in vivo, the traditional way of using "high doses" to identify carcinogenic effects of a specific agent (Huff 1993) would not be adequate for studies on magnetic field exposure.

The tumor promoting or copromoting effects of ELF magnetic field exposure found in several animal studies could relate to actions of such fields on gene expression, immune surveillance, intercellular communication and Ca^{2+} homeostasis, as demonstrated by in vitro experiments in cell cultures. However, the most plausible evidence for an in vivo effect of magnetic field exposure that could be related to tumor promotion is reduction of circulating melatonin concentrations, possibly combined with an impairment of melatonin's oncostatic effect at the cellular level. With respect to the accumulating experimental data showing magnetic field effects on mammary carcinogenesis—possibly caused by impaired melatonin synthesis, secretion and/or function—it should be noted that it is unique in this area of research that such effects were predicted based on biological reasoning, before experiments were conducted (Stevens 1987). On the basis of the melatonin hypothesis and epidemiologic findings indicating an increased risk of breast cancer in workers occupationally exposed to magnetic fields, Stevens et al. (1992) recently proposed that the use of electrical power accounts, in part, for the higher risks of breast cancer in industrialized societies. Wertheimer and Leeper (1982) were the first to see a magnetic field–breast cancer connection in their 1982 study of residential magnetic field exposures of adults. They uncovered a nearly threefold increase among women younger than 55 years who lived near high-current power lines. More recently, the first evidence of increased breast cancer risk in women in electrical occupations was reported by Loomis et al. (1994). In this study, twice the expected number of breast cancer deaths was observed for female electrical workers aged 45 to 54 compared to women working at other jobs. In view of these epidemiologic and experimental data and the plausible biological hypothesis behind these findings, the possible role played by magnetic fields in breast cancer risks should be examined further.

Risk assessment of a particular agent must be considered in terms of the total background, with an additional consideration of the added risk from a specific component. Evaluating the impact of environmental effects such as magnetic field exposure on human health is a complex process; it requires the problem to be put in proper perspective, with an equitable assessment made in terms of benefits and possible risks to society. Whether exposure to ELF magnetic fields does in fact pose health risks is still an open question, but many concerned citizens and government officials are not willing to suspend all risk management activities until laboratory and epidemiologic research provides a definitive answer to this question. For this reason, issues of risk perception, communication, assessment, and management are of great and growing importance (Morgan 1993). With respect to exposure management options, "prudent avoidance" (removing people from certain exposure situations at low cost and with modest inconvenience) is considered the most viable current option (Morgan 1993).

The current controversy about health effects of magnetic field exposure resembles historical controversies about health effects of low levels of ionizing radiation, asbestos, or chronic use of tobacco at times when the scientific knowledge about the toxic effects of these agents was incomplete. In such periods, uncertain and incomplete scientific evidence may be interpreted differently by the various interested parties (Nair 1993). As shown by this review, evidence is accumulating that exposure of laboratory animals to power-frequency magnetic fields induces a carcinogenic response. Although the existing evidence is still insufficient for discerning a cause–effect relationship for magnetic field exposure and human disease or injury, it does suggest the need for further laboratory research under well-defined exposure conditions to allow for a realistic assessment of the possible health risks and their magnitude. In the end, it will be a combination of the results of epidemiologic, animal, and mechanistic studies that will provide data for a sound scientific judgment on the potential adverse human health effects of exposure to magnetic fields associated with the generation, transport, and use of electricity.

ACKNOWLEDGMENT

We thank Dr. Meike Mevissen for her help in the literature research. Support for Robert Liburdy was provided in part by the Office of Utility Technologies of the Office of Energy Efficiency and Renewable Energies. U.S. Department of Energy under contract AC03-76SF00098; the National Institutes of Health, National Institute of Environmental Health, through Project ES07279; and by the Department of the Army, U.S. Medical Research and Development Command, through Project 2198.

REFERENCES

Adey, W.R. 1992a. Collective properties of cell membranes. In: *Interaction Mechanisms of Low-Level Electromagnetic Fields in Living Systems*, B. Norden and C. Ramel, eds., pp. 47–77. New York: Oxford University Press.

Adey, W.R. 1992b. ELF magnetic fields and promotion of cancer: Experimental studies. In: *Interaction Mechanisms of Low-Level Electromagnetic Fields in Living Systems*, B. Norden and C. Ramel, eds., pp. 23–46. New York: Oxford University Press.

Adey, W.R. 1993. Biological effects of electromagnetic fields. *J. Cell. Biochem.* 51:410–416.

Ames, B.N., L.S. Gold. 1990a. Chemical carcinogenesis: Too many rodent carcinogens. *Proc. Natl. Acad. Sci. (USA)* 87:7772–7776.

Ames, B.N., L.S. Gold. 1990b. Too many rodent carcinogens: Mitogenesis increases mutagenesis. *Science* 249:970–971.

Anderson, M.W., S.H. Reynolds, M. You, R.M. Maronpot. 1992. Role of proto-oncogene activation in carcinogenesis. *Environ. Health Perspect.* 98:13–24.

Antonopoulos, A., B. Yang, A. Stamm, W.D. Heller, G. Obe. 1995. Cytological effects of 50 Hz electromagnetic fields on human lymphocytes in vitro. *Mutat. Res.* 346:151–157.

Anttila, A., M. Sallmén, K. Hemminki. 1993. Carcinogenic chemicals in the occupational environment. *Pharmacol. Toxicol.* 72 (Suppl. 1):69–76.

Balcer-Kubiczek, E.K., G.H. Harrison. 1991. Neoplastic transformation of C3H/10T½ cells following exposure to 120-Hz modulated 2.45-GHz microwaves and phorbol ester tumor promoter. *Radiat. Res.* 126:65–72.

Bartsch, H., C. Bartsch, D. Mecke, T.H. Lippert. 1994. Seasonality of pineal melatonin production in the rat—possible synchronization by the geomagnetic field. *Chronobiol. Int.* 11:21–26.

Baum, A., M. Mevissen, K. Kamino, U. Mohr, W. Löscher. 1995. A histopathological study on alterations in DMBA-induced mammary carcinogenesis in rats with 50 Hz, 100 μT magnetic field exposure. *Carcinogenesis* 16:119–125.

Bello-Fernandez, C., G. Packham, J.L. Cleveland. 1993. The ornithine decarboxylase gene is a transcriptional target of *c-myc*. *Proc. Natl. Acad. Sci. (USA)* 90:7804–7808.

Beniashvili, D.S., V.G. Bilanishvili, M.Z. Menabde. 1991. Low-frequency electromagnetic radiation enhances the induction of rat mammary tumors by nitrosomethyl urea. *Cancer Lett.* 61:75–79.

Berglund, A., K.H. Mild, M. Sandstrom, M.-O. Mattsson. 1991. Background ELF magnetic fields in incubators. In: Abstracts of the 13th Annual Bioelectromagnetics Society Meeting, Salt Lake City, Utah, June 22–27, p. A-2–8.

Berridge, M.J. 1993. Inositol triphosphate and calcium signaling. *Nature* 361:315–325.

Blackman, C.F., S.G. Benane, D.E. House, J.P. Blanchard. 1996. Independent replication of the 12 mG magnetic field effect on melatonin and MCF-7 cells in vitro. In: Abstracts of the 18th Annual Bioelectromagnetics Society Meeting, June 9–14, 1996, Victoria, Canada, #A-1-2, pp. 1–2.

Blank, M., L. Soo, H. Lin, R. Goodman. 1993. Stimulation of transcription in HL-60 cells by alternating currents from electric fields. In:

Electricity and Magnetism in Biology and Medicine, M. Blank, ed., pp. 516-519. San Francisco: San Francisco Press.

Blask, D.E. 1990. The emerging role of the pineal gland and melatonin in oncogenesis. In: *Extremely Low Frequency Electromagnetic Fields: The Question of Cancer,* B.W. Wilson, R.G. Stevens, and L.E. Anderson, eds., pp. 319–325. Columbus, Ohio: Battelle Press.

Blask, D.E. 1993. Melatonin in oncology. In: *Melatonin. Biosynthesis, Physiological Effects, and Clinical Applications,* H.-S. Yu and R.J. Reiter, eds., pp. 448–475. Boca Raton, Florida: CRC Press.

Blask, D.E., S.T. Wilson, J.D. Saffer, M.A. Wilson, L.E. Anderson, B.W. Wilson. 1993. Culture conditions influence the effects of weak magnetic fields on the growth-response of MCF-7 human breast cancer cells to melatonin *in vitro.* In: Abstracts of the Annual Review of Research on Biological Effects of Electric and Magnetic Fields from the Generation, Delivery, and Use of Electricity, Savannah, Georgia, October 31–November 4, Abstract P-45, p. 65. Frederick, Maryland: W/L Associates, Ltd.

Bracken, T.D. 1992. Experimental macroscopic dosimetry for extremely-low-frequency electric and magnetic fields. *Bioelectromagnetics Suppl.* 1:15–26.

Burdon, R.H., C. Rice-Evans. 1989. Free radicals and the regulation of mammalian cell proliferation. *Free Radical Res. Commun.* 6:345–358.

Butterworth, C.E., T.J. Slaga. 1987. *Nongenotoxic Mechanisms in Carcinogenesis.* New York: Wiley & Sons.

Byus, C.V., S.E. Pieper, W.R. Adey. 1987. The effects of low-energy 60-Hz environmental electromagnetic fields upon the growth-related enzyme ornithine decarboxylase. *Carcinogenesis* 8:1385–1389.

Byus, C.V., Y. Ma, M.A. Stuchly. 1995. The ability of magnetic fields to serve as a co-promotional stimulus to the development of papillomas on the skin of the mouse. In: Abstracts of the 17th Annual Bioelectromagnetics Society Meeting, Boston, Massachusetts, p. 79.

Cadossi, R., F. Bersani, A. Cossarizza, P. Zuchini, G. Emilia, G. Torelli, C. Franceschi. 1992. Lymphocytes and low-frequency electromagnetic fields. *FASEB J.* 6:2667–2674.

Cadossi, R., P. Zuchini, G. Emilia, G. Torelli, F. Bersani, L. Bolognani, A. Cossarizza, M. Petrini, C. Franceschi. 1994. In vitro and in vivo effects of low frequency energy pulsed electromagnetic fields in hematology and immunology. In: *On the Nature of Electromagnetic Field Interactions with Biological Systems*, A.H. Frey, ed., pp. 157–166. Austin: R.G. Landes Co.

Cahir-McFarland, E.D., T.R. Hurley, J.T. Pingel, B.M. Sefton, A. Shaw, M.L. Thomas. 1993. Correlation between Src family member regulation by the protein-tyrosine-phosphate CD45 and transmembrane signaling through the T-cell receptor. *Proc. Natl. Acad. Sci. (USA)* 90:1402–1406.

Cain, C.D., D.L. Thomas, W.R. Adey. 1993. 60 Hz magnetic field acts as co-promoter in focus formation of C3H/10T½ cells. *Carcinogenesis* 14:955–960.

Canfield, J.N., R.L. Belford, P.G. Debrunner, K.J. Schukten. 1994. A perturbation theory treatment of oscillating magnetic fields in the radical pair mechanism. *Chem. Phys.* 182:1–18.

Cleary, S.F. 1993. A review of in vitro studies: Low-frequency electromagnetic fields. *Am. Ind. Hyg. Assoc. J.* 54:178–185.

Cohen, S.M., L.B. Ellwein. 1990. Cell proliferation in carcinogenesis. *Science* 249:1007–1011.

Cornélissen, G., F. Halberg. 1992. Chronobiologic response modifiers and breast cancer development: Classical background and chronobiologic tasks remaining. *In Vivo* 6:387–402.

Cossarizza, A., D. Monti, P. Sola, G. Moschini, R. Cadossi, F. Bersani, C. Franceschi. 1989a. DNA repair after gamma irradiation in lymphocytes exposed to low-frequency electromagnetic fields. *Radiat. Res.* 118:161–168.

Cossarizza, A., D. Monti, F. Bersani, M. Cantini, R. Cadossi, A. Sacchi, C. Franceschi. 1989b. Extremely low frequency pulsed electromagnetic fields increase cell proliferation in lymphocytes from young and aged subjects. *Biochem. Biophysic. Res. Commun.* 160:692–698.

Cossarizza, A., D. Monti, F. Bersani, M.R. Scarfi, M. Zanotti, R. Cadossi, C. Franceschi. 1991. Exposure to low-frequency pulsed electromagnetic fields increases mitogen-induced lymphocyte proliferation in Down's syndrome. *Aging* 3:241–246.

Demers, P., D.B. Thomas, K.A. Rosenblatt, L.M. Jimenez, A. McTiernan, H. Stalsberg, A. Stemhagen, W.D. Thompson, M.G. McCrea-Curnen, W. Satariano, D.F. Austin, P. Isacson, R.S. Greenberg, C. Key, L.

Kolonel, D.W. Weat. 1991. Occupational exposure to electromagnetic fields and breast cancer in men. *Amer. J. Epidemiol.* 134:340–347.

Evans, C., K.U. Ingold, J.C. Scaiano. 1988. Magnetic field effects on the decay of ketyl-aryloxy radical pairs in micellar solution. *J. Phys. Chem.* 92:1257–1262.

Fam, W.Z., E.L. Mikhail. 1990a. A system for the exposure of small laboratory animals to a 25-mT 60-Hz alternating or travelling magnetic field. In: Abstracts of the 12th Annual Bioelectromagnetics Society Meeting, San Antonio, Texas, p. 62.

Fam, W.Z., E.L. Mikhail. 1990b. Biological effects in mice exposed to a 25-mT, 60-Hz magnetic field. In: Abstracts of the 12th Annual Bioelectromagnetics Society Meeting, San Antonio, Texas, pp. 17–18.

Farrel, J.M., M. Barber, P. Doinov, D. Krause, T. Litovitz. 1993. Superposition of a temporally incoherent magnetic field suppresses the change in ornithine decarboxylase activity in developing chick embryos induced by a 60 Hz sinusoidal field. In: *Electricity and Magnetism in Biology and Medicine,* M. Blank, ed., pp. 342–344. San Francisco: San Francisco Press.

Frankel, R.B., R.P. Liburdy. 1995. Biological effects of static magnetic fields. In: *Handbook of Biological Effects of Electromagnetic Fields 2nd Ed.,* C. Polk and E. Postow, eds., pp. 148–183. Boca Raton, Florida: CRC Press Inc.

Frey, A. 1993. Electromagnetic field interactions with biological systems. *FASEB J.* 7:272–281.

Gardner, P. 1989. Calcium and T-lymphocyte activation. *Cell* 59:15–20.

Gold, L.S., T.H. Slone, B.R. Stern, N.B. Manley, B.N. Ames. 1992. Rodent carcinogens: Setting priorities. *Science* 258:261–265.

Goodman, R., A.S. Henderson. 1991. Transcription and translation in cells exposed to extremely low frequency electromagnetic fields. *Bioelectrochem. Bioenerg.* 25:335–355.

Goodman, R., A.S. Henderson. 1992. Exposure of human cells to electromagnetic fields: Effect of time and field strength on transcript levels. *Electro- and Magnetobiol.* 11:11–28.

Goodman, R., L.X. Wei, J.C. Xu, A.S. Henderson. 1991. Exposure of human cells to electromagnetic fields: The amplitude affects the level of RNA transcripts. *Biochim. Biophys. Acta* 1009:216–224.

Graham, C., M.R. Cook, H.D. Cohen, D.W. Riffle, S.J. Hoffman, F.J., McClernon, D. Smith, M.M. Gerkovich. 1993. EMF suppression of nocturnal melatonin in human volunteers. In: Abstracts of the Annual Review of Research on Biological Effects of Electric and Magnetic Fields from the Generation, Delivery, and Use of Electricity, Savannah, Georgia, October 31–November 4, A-31. Frederick, Maryland: W/L Associates, Ltd.

Graham, C., M.R. Cook, H.D. Cohen, D.W. Riffle. 1994. Nocturnal melatonin levels in men exposed to magnetic fields: A replication study. In: Abstracts of the Annual Review of Research on Biological Effects of Electric and Magnetic Fields from the Generation, Delivery and Use of Electricity, Albuquerque, New Mexico, November 6–10, A-51, pp. 51–52. Frederick, Maryland: W/L Associates, Ltd.

Grandolfo, M., M.H. Repacholi. 1993. Risk assessment and IRPA/INIRC guidelines on protection against electromagnetic fields and waves. In: *Electricity and Magnetism in Biology and Medicine,* M. Blank, ed., pp. 77–80. San Francisco: San Francisco Press.

Greene, J.J., W.J. Skowronski, J.M. Mullins, R.M. Nardone. 1991. Delineation of electric and magnetic field effects of extremely low frequency electromagnetic radiation on transcription. *Biochem. Biophysic. Res. Commun.* 174:742–749.

Grissom, C.B. 1995. Magnetic field effects in biology: A survey of possible mechanisms with emphasis on radical-pair recombination. *Chem. Rev.* 95:3–24.

Guénel, P., P. Paskmark, J.B. Andersen, E. Lynge. 1993. Incidence of cancer in persons with occupational exposure to electromagnetic fields in Denmark. *Brit. J. Ind. Med.* 50:758–764.

Haggren, W., S.M. Yellon, J.L. Phillips, W.R. Adey. 1992. Effect of magnetic field exposure in adult Djungarian hamsters on melatonin rhythms and molecular markers. In: Abstracts of the First World Congress for Electricity and Magnetism in Biology and Medicine, Lake Buena Vista, Florida, June 14-19, p. P-119.

Hardeland, R., R.J. Reiter, B. Poeggeler, D.-X. Tan. 1993. The significance of the metabolism of the neurohormone melatonin: Antioxidative protection and formation of bioactive substances. *Neurosci. Biobehav. Rev.* 17:347–357.

Harkins, T.T., C.B. Grissom. 1994. Magnetic field effects on B_{12} ethanolamine ammonia lyase: Evidence for a radical mechanism. *Science* 263:958–960.

Harland, J.D., R.P. Liburdy. 1994. Inhibition of melatonin's and tamoxifen's action in MCF-7 cells by magnetic fields *Mol. Biol. Cell* 5:19a, Abstract 107.

Herschman, H.R., D.W. Brankow. 1987. Colony size, cell density and nature of the tumor promoter are critical variables in expression of a transformation phenotype (focus formation) in co-cultures of UV-TDTx and C3H10T½ cells. *Carcinogenesis* 8:993–998.

Huff, J. 1993. Issues and controversies surrounding qualitative strategies for identifying and forecasting cancer causing agents in the human environment. *Pharmacol. & Toxicol. Suppl.* 1:12–27.

Huggins, C., N.C. Yang. 1962. Induction and extinction of mammary cancer. *Science* 137:257–262.

Johann, S., T. Lederer, S. Mikorey, W. Kraus, G. Blumel. 1993. Influence of electromagnetic fields on morphology and mitochondrial activity of breast cancer cell line MCF-7. *Bioelectrochem. Bioenerg.* 30:127–132.

Karabakhtsian, R., N. Broude, N. Shalts, S. Kochlastyi, R. Goodman, A.S. Henderson. 1994. Calcium is necessary in the cell response to EM fields. *FEBS Lett.* 349:1–6.

Kato, M., K. Honma, T. Shigemitsu, Y. Shiga. 1993. Effects of exposure to a circularly polarized 50-Hz magnetic field on plasma and pineal melatonin levels in rats. *Bioelectromagnetics* 14:97–106.

Kato, M., K. Honma, T. Shigemitsu, Y. Shiga. 1994. Horizontal or vertical 50-Hz, 1-μT magnetic fields have no effect on pineal gland or plasma melatonin concentration of albino rats. *Neurosci. Lett.* 168:205–208.

Kavaliers, M., K.P. Ossenkopp, D.M. Tysdale. 1991. Evidence for the involvement of protein kinase C in the modulation of morphine-induced analgesia and the inhibitory effects of exposure to 60 Hz magnetic fields in the snail, *Cepaea nemoralis. Brain Res.* 554:65–71.

Khalil, A.M., W. Qassem. 1991. Cytogenetic effects of pulsing electromagnetic field of human lymphocytes in vitro: Chromosomal aberrations, sister chromatid exchanges and cell kinetics. *Mutat. Res.* 247:141–146.

Kraybill, H.F., M.A. Mehlmann. 1977. *Environmental Cancer.* New York: Wiley & Sons.

Kumlin, T., J. Juutilainen, J. Jönne, J., H. Komulainen, V.-M. Kosma, S. Lang, M. Pasanen, T. Rytomaa, K. Servomaa. 1995. A study of the possible cancer promoting effects of 50 Hz magnetic fields on UV-initiated skin tumors in ODC-transgenic mice. In: Abstracts of the 17th Annual Bioelectromagnetics Society Meeting, Boston, Massachusetts, p. 211.

Kwee, S., P. Raskmark. 1995. Changes in cell proliferation due to environmental non-ionizing radiation. 1. ELF electromagnetic fields. *Bioelectrochem. Bioenerg.* 36:109–114.

Lacy-Hulbert, A., R.C. Wilkins, T.R. Hesketh, J.C. Metcalfe. 1995a. Cancer risk and electromagnetic fields. *Nature* 375:23

Lacy-Hulbert, A., R.C. Wilkins, T.R. Hesketh, J.C. Metcalf, J.C. 1995b. No effect of 60 Hz electromagnetic fields on *myc* or b-actin expression in human leukemic cells. *Radiat. Res.* 144:9–17.

Lerchl, A., K.O. Nonaka, R.J. Reiter. 1991. Pineal gland "magnetosensitivity" to static magnetic fields is a consequence of induced electric currents (eddy currents). *J. Pineal. Res.* 10:109–116.

Liburdy, R.P. 1992a. Biological interactions of cellular systems with time-varying magnetic fields. *Ann. N.Y. Acad. Sci.* 649:74–95.

Liburdy, R.P. 1992b. Calcium signaling in lymphocytes and ELF fields: Evidence for an electric field metric and a site of interaction involving the calcium ion channel. *FEBS Lett.* 301:53–59.

Liburdy, R.P. 1992c. ELF fields and the immune system: Signal transduction, calcium metabolism, and mitogenesis in lymphocytes with relevance to carcinogenesis. In: *Interaction Mechanisms of Low-Level Electromagnetic Fields in Living Systems*, B. Norden and C. Ramel, eds., pp. 217–239. New York: Oxford University Press.

Liburdy, R.P. 1994. Cellular interactions with electromagnetic fields: Experimental evidence for field effects on signal transduction and cell proliferation. In: *On the Nature of Electromagnetic Field Interactions with Biological Systems*, A.H. Frey, ed., pp. 99–126. Austin, Texas: R. G. Landes Co.

Liburdy, R.P. 1995. Cellular studies and interaction mechanisms of extremely low frequency fields. *Radio Sci.* 30:179–203.

Liburdy, R.P., J. Walleczek. 1989. The influence of magnetic fields on calcium metabolism in the lymphocyte. In: Abstracts of the Annual Review of Research on Biological Effects from Electric and Magnetic Fields, Portland, Oregon, September 13–17, A-2. Frederick, Maryland: W/L Associates, Ltd.

Liburdy, R.P., M.G. Yost. 1993. Time-varying and static magnetic fields act in combination to alter calcium signal transduction in the lymphocyte. In: *Electricity and Magnetism in Biology and Medicine*, M. Blank, ed., pp. 331–334. San Francisco: San Francisco Press.

Liburdy, R.P., J.D. Harland, D.E. Callahan. 1993a. Effects of 60 Hz electric and magnetic fields on Con-A binding and calcium signal transduction in rat thymocytes. *FASEB J.* 7 (# 4649): A805.

Liburdy, R.P., T.R. Sloma, R. Sokolic, P. Yaswen. 1993b. ELF magnetic fields, breast cancer, and melatonin: 60 Hz fields block melatonin's oncostatic action on ER^+ breast cancer cell proliferation. *J. Pineal Res.* 14:89–97.

Liburdy, R.P., D.E. Callahan, J. Harland, E. Dunham, T.R. Sloma, P. Yaswen. 1993c. Experimental evidence for 60 Hz magnetic fields operating through the signal transduction cascade: Effects on calcium influx and c-*myc* mRNA induction. *FEBS Lett.* 334:301–308.

Liburdy, R.P., D.E. Callahan, T.R. Sloma, P. Yaswen. 1993d. Intracellular calcium, calcium transport, and c-*myc* mRNA induction in lymphocytes exposed to 60 Hz magnetic fields: The cell membrane and the signal transduction pathway. In: *Electricity and Magnetism in Biology and Medicine*, M. Blank, ed., pp. 311–314. San Francisco: San Francisco Press.

Liburdy, R.P., D.E. Callahan, J.D. Harland. 1993e. Protein shedding and ELF magnetic fields: Antibody binding at the CD3 and CD20 receptor sites of human lymphocytes. In: *Electricity and Magnetism in Biology and Medicine*, M. Blank, ed., pp. 651–653. San Francisco: San Francisco Press.

Lindström, E., P. Lindström, A. Berglund, K. Hansson Mild. 1993. Intracellular calcium oscillations induced in a T-cell line by a weak 50 Hz magnetic field. *J. Cell. Physiol.* 156:395–398.

Lindström, E., A. Berglund, K. Hansson Mild, P. Lindström, E. Lundgren. 1995a. CD45 phosphatase in Jurkat cells is necessary for response to applied ELF magnetic fields. *FEBS Lett.* 370:118–122.

Lindström, E., P. Lindström, A. Berglund, E. Lundgren, K.Hansson Mild. 1995b. Intracellular calcium oscillation in a T-cell line after exposure to extremely low frequency magnetic fields with variable frequencies and flux densities. *Bioelectromagnetics* 16:41–47.

Litovitz, T.A., D. Krause, J.M. Mullins. 1991. Effect of coherence time of the applied magnetic field on ornithine decarboxylase activity. *Biochem. Biophys. Res. Commun.* 178:862–865.

Litovitz, T.A., C.J. Montrose, W. Wang. 1992. Dose–response implications of the transient nature of electromagnetic-field-induced bio-effects. *Bioelectromagnetics Suppl.* 1:237–246.

Loomis, D.P., D.A. Savitz, and C. V. Ananth. 1991. Electromagnetic field exposure and male breast cancer. *Lancet* 33:737.

Loomis, D.P., D.A. Savitz, C.V. Ananth. 1994. Breast cancer mortality among female electrical workers in the United States. *J. Natl. Cancer Inst.* 86:921–925.

Löscher, W., M. Mevissen. 1995. Linear relationship between flux density and tumor copromoting effect of prolonged magnetic field exposure in a breast cancer model. *Cancer Lett.* 96:175–180.

Löscher, W., M. Mevissen, W. Lehmacher, A. Stamm. 1993. Tumor promotion in a breast cancer model by exposure to a weak alternating magnetic field. *Cancer Lett.* 71:75–81.

Löscher, W., U. Wahnschaffe, M. Mevissen, A. Lerchl, A. Stamm. 1994. Effects of weak alternating magnetic fields on nocturnal melatonin production and mammary carcinogenesis in rats. *Oncology* 51:288–295.

Luben, R.A. 1991. Effects of low-energy electromagnetic fields (pulsed and DC) on membrane signal transduction processes in biological systems. *Health Phys.* 61:15–28.

Luben, R.A. 1993. Effects of low-energy electromagnetic fields (EMF) on signal transduction by G protein linked receptors. In: *Electricity and Magnetism in Biology and Medicine*, M. Blank, ed., pp. 57–62. San Francisco: San Francisco Press.

Luben, R.A. 1994. Membrane signal transduction as a site of electromagnetic field actions in bone and other tissues. In: *On the Nature of Electromagnetic Field Interactions with Biological Systems*, A.H. Frey, ed., pp. 83–98. Austin, Texas: R.G. Landes Co.

Lyle, D.B., J. Doshi, T.A. Fuchs, J.P. Casamento, Y. Sei, P.K. Arora, M.L. Swicord. 1993. Intracellular calcium signaling in Jurkat E6.1 cells exposed to an induced 1 mV/cm, 60 Hz sinusoidal electric field. In: *Electricity and Magnetism in Biology and Medicine*, M. Blank, ed., pp. 307–310. San Francisco: San Francisco Press.

Maltin, L. 1993. A practical guide to shielding of DC and low frequency magnetic fields. In: Abstracts of the 15th Annual Bioelectromagnetics Society Meeting, June 13–17, Los Angeles, California, Invited Presentation. Frederick, Maryland: The Bioelectromagnetics Society.

Marcu, K.B., S.A. Bossome, A.J. Patel. 1992. MYC function and regulation. *Annual Rev. Biochem.* 61:809–860.

Marino, C., F. Antonini, B. Avella, L. Galloni, L., P. Scacchi. 1995. 50 Hz magnetic field effects on tumoral growth in *in vivo* systems. In: Abstracts of the 17th Annual Bioelectromagnetics Society Meeting, Boston, Massachusetts, pp. 171–172.

Matanoski, G.M., P.N. Breyese, E.A. Elliot. 1991. Electromagnetic field exposure and male breast cancer. *Lancet* 33:737

Mattsson, M.O., U. Rehnhom, K.H. Mild. 1993. Gene expression in tumor cells after exposure to a 50 Hz sinusoidal magnetic field. In: *Electricity and Magnetism in Biology and Medicine*, M. Blank, ed., pp. 500–502. San Francisco: San Francisco Press.

McCann, J., F. Dietrich, C. Rafferty, A.O. Martin. 1993. A critical review of the genotoxic potential of electric and magnetic fields. *Mutat. Res.* 297:61–95.

McCormick, D.L., B.M. Ryan, J.C. Findlay, G.A. Boorman. 1994. Exposure to 60 Hz magnetic fields and lymphoma development in PIM transgenic mice. In: Abstracts of the Annual Review of Research on Biological Effects of Electric and Magnetic Fields from the Generation, Delivery and Use of Electricity, Albuquerque, New Mexico, November 6–10, pp. 44–45. Frederick, Maryland: W/L Associates, Ltd.

McLauchlan, K.A., U.E. Steiner. 1991. The spin-correlated radical pair as a reaction intermediate. *Mol. Phys.* 73:241–263.

McLean, J.R.N., M.A.Stuchly, R.E.J. Mitchel, D. Wilkinson, H. Yang, M. Goddard, D.W. Lecuyer, M. Schunk, E. Callary, D. Morrison. 1991. Cancer promotion in a mouse-skin model by a 60-Hz magnetic field: II. Tumor development and immune response. *Bioelectromagnetics* 12:273–287.

McLean, J.R.N., A. Thansandote, D.W. Lecuyer, C. Davidson, M.J. Goddard, R. Burnett. 1993. The effect of magnetic fields on tumor co-promotion in SENCAR mouse skin. In: Abstracts of the 15th Annual Bioelectromagnetics Society Meeting, Los Angeles, California, June 13–17, p. 153. Frederick, Maryland: The Bioelectromagnetics Society.

McLean, J.R.N., A. Thansandote, D.W. Lecuyer, J. Kim, J. 1995. The effect of 60 Hz magnetic fields on co-promotion of chemically induced skin tumours on SENCAR mice: A discussion of three studies. In: Abstracts of the 17th Annual Bioelectromagnetics Society Meeting, Boston, Massachusetts, p. 212.

Mevissen, M., A. Stamm, S. Buntenkötter, R. Zwingelberg, U. Wahnschaffe, W. Löscher. 1993. Effects of magnetic fields on mammary tumor development induced by 7,12-dimethylbenz(a)anthracene in rats. *Bioelectromagnetics* 14:131–143.

Mevissen, M., M. Kietzmann, W. Löscher. 1995. *In vivo* exposure of rats to a weak alternating magnetic field increases ornithine decarboxylase activity in the mammary gland by a similar extent as the carcinogen DMBA. *Cancer Lett.* 90:207–214.

Mikhail, E.L., W.Z. Fam. 1991. Development of lymphoma in third-generation mice exposed to 60-Hz magnetic field. In: Abstracts of the 13th Annual Bioelectromagnetics Society Meeting, Salt Lake City, Utah, p. 24.

Mikhail, E.L., W.Z. Fam. 1993. Incidence of lymphoma in CFW mice exposed to low-frequency electromagnetic fields. In: *Electricity and Magnetism in Biology and Medicine*, M. Blank, ed., pp. 389–392. San Francisco: San Francisco Press.

Mikorey-Lechner, S., S. Johann, G. Blumel, W. Kraus. 1993. Effect of low frequency electromagnetic fields on a breast cancer cell line incubated with various cytostatic agents. In: *Electricity and Magnetism in Biology and Medicine*, M. Blank, ed., pp. 382–388. San Francisco: San Francisco Press.

Moller, H. 1993. Occurrence of carcinogens in the external environment: Epidemiological investigations. *Pharmacol. Toxicol.* 72 (Suppl. 1):39–45.

Monti, M.G., L. Pernecco, M.S. Moruzzi, R. Battini, P. Zaniol, B. Barbiroli. 1991. Effect of ELF pulsed electromagnetic fields on protein kinase C activation process in HL-60 leukemia cells. *J. Bioelectr.* 10:119–130.

Monti, M.G., L. Pernecco, M.S. Moruzzi, R. Battini, P. Zaniol, B. Barbiroli. 1993. Extremely low frequency electromagnetic fields stimulate activation of protein kinase C in HL-60 leukemia cells by increasing membrane transport of calcium. In: *Electricity and Magnetism in Biology and Medicine*, M. Blank, ed., pp. 522–524. San Francisco: San Francisco Press.

Morgan, M.G. 1993. Possible health risks from power-frequency fields: Issues in risk perception, communication, assessment, and management. In: *Electricity and Magnetism in Biology and Medicine*, M. Blank, ed., pp. 12–16. San Francisco: San Francisco Press.

Morgan, N.G. 1989. *Cell Signaling*. New York: The Guilford Press.

Murphy, J.C., D.A. Kaden, J. Warren, A. Sivak. 1993. Power frequency electric and magnetic fields—A review of genetic toxicology. *Mutat. Res.* 296:221–240.

Nair, I. 1993. Scientific uncertainty, risk assessment, and standard-setting. In: *Electricity and Magnetism in Biology and Medicine*, M. Blank, ed., pp. 81–84. San Francisco: San Francisco Press.

Olcese, J.M. 1990. The neurobiology of magnetic field detection in rodents. *Progr. Neurobiol.* 35:325–330.

Phillips, J.L., W. Haggren, W.J. Thomas, T. Ishida-Jones, W.R. Adey. 1992. Magnetic field-induced changes in specific gene transcription. *Biochim. Biophys. Acta* 1132:140–144.

Polk, C. 1992. Dosimetry of extremely-low-frequency magnetic fields. *Bioelectromagnetics Suppl.* 1:209–235.

Putney, J.W. 1993. Excitement about calcium signaling in inexcitable cells. *Science* 262:676–678.

Putney, J.W., S.J. Bird. 1993. The signal for capacitative calcium entry. *Cell* 75:199–201.

Putney, J.W., S.J. Bird. 1994. The inositol phosphate-calcium signaling system in nonexcitable cells. *Endocr. Rev.* 14:610–631.

Rannug, A., B. Holmberg, K.H. Mild. 1993a. A rat liver foci promotion study with 50-Hz magnetic fields. *Environment. Res.* 62:223–229.

Rannug, A., T. Ekström, K.H. Mild, B. Holmberg, I. Gimenez-Conti, T.J. Slaga. 1993b. A study on skin tumour formation in mice with 50 Hz magnetic field exposure. *Carcinogenesis* 14:573–578.

Rannug, A., B. Holmberg, T. Ekström, K.H. Mild. 1993c. Rat liver foci study on coexposure with 50 Hz magnetic fields and known carcinogens. *Bioelectromagnetics* 14:17–27.

Rannug, A., B. Holmberg, T. Ekström, K.H. Mild, I. Gimenezconti, T.J. Slaga. 1994. Intermittent 50 Hz magnetic field and skin tumour promotion in SENCAR mice. *Carcinogenesis* 15:153–157.

Reiter, R.J. 1992. Changes in circadian melatonin synthesis in the pineal gland of animals exposed to extremely low frequency electromagnetic radiation: A summary of observations and speculation on their implications. In: *Electromagnetic Fields and Circadian Rythmicity*. M.C. Moore-Ede, S.S. Campbell, and R.J. Reiter, eds., pp. 13–17. Boston: Birkhauser.

Reiter, R.J. 1993. Static and extremely low frequency electromagnetic field exposure: Reported effects on the circadian production of melatonin. *J. Cell. Biochem.* 51:394–403.

Reiter, R.J. 1995. Oxidative processes and antioxidative defence mechanisms in the aging brain. *FASEB J.* 9:526–533.

Reiter, R.J., A. Lerchl. 1993. Regulation of mammalian pineal melatonin production by the electromagnetic spectrum. In: *Melatonin. Biosynthesis, Physiological Effects, and Clinical Applications*, H.-S. Yu and R.J. Reiter, eds., pp. 107–127. Boca Raton, Florida: CRC Press.

Reiter, R.J., B.A. Richardson. 1990. Magnetic fields effects on pineal indoleamine metabolism and possible biological consequences. *FASEB J.* 6:2283–2287.

Reiter, R.J., B. Poeggeler, D.-X. Tan, L.-D. Chen, L.C. Manchester, J.M Guerrero. 1993. Antioxidant capacity of melatonin: A novel action not requiring a receptor. *Neuroendocrinol. Lett.* 15:103–116.

Reiter, R.J., D.-X. Tan, B. Poeggeler, A. Menendez-Pelaez, L.D. Chen, S. Saarela. 1994. Melatonin as a free radical scavenger: Implications for aging and age-related diseases. *Ann N.Y.Acad Sci.* 719:1–12.

Reiter, R.J., D. Melchiorri, E. Sewerynek, B. Poeggeler, L. Barlow-Walden, J. Chuang, G.G. Ortiz, D. Acuna-Castroviejo. 1995. A review of the evidence supporting melatonin's role as an antioxidant. *J. Pineal Res.* 18:1–11.

Rose, R.C., A.M. Bode. 1993. Biology of free radical scavengers: An evaluation of ascorbate. *FASEB J.* 7:1135–1142.

Rosen, G.M., S. Pou, C.L. Ramos, M.S. Cohen, B. Britigan. 1993. Free radicals and phagocytic cells. *FASEB J.* 9:200–209.

Rosenthal, M., G. Obe. 1989. Effects of 50 Hz electromagnetic fields on proliferation and on chromosomal alterations in human peripheral lymphocytes untreated or pretreated with chemical mutagens. *Mutat. Res.* 210:329–335.

Roy, S., Y. Noda, V. Eckert, M. Traber, A. Mori, R. Liburdy, L. Packer. 1995. The phorbol 12-myristate 13-acetate (PMA)-induced oxidative burst in rat peritoneal neutrophils is increased by a 0.1 mT (60 Hz) magnetic field. *FEBS Lett.* 376:164–166.

Russo, J., J. Saby, W.M. Isenberg, I.H. Russo. 1977. Pathogenesis of mammary carcinoma induced in rats by 7,12-dimethylbenz[a]anthracene. *J. Natl. Cancer Inst.* 59:435–445.

Saffer, J.D., S.J. Thurston. 1995a. Cancer risk and electromagnetic fields. *Nature* 375:22.

Saffer, J.D., S.J. Thurston. 1995b. Short term exposures to 60 Hz magnetic fields do not alter *myc* expression in HL60 or Daudi cells. *Radiat. Res.* 144:18–25.

Sagan, L.A. 1992. Epidemiological and laboratory studies of power frequency electric and magnetic fields. *J. Am. Med. Assoc.* 268:625–629.

Savitz, D.A., A. Ahlbom. 1994. Epidemiologic evidence on cancer in relation to residential and occupational exposures. In: *Biological Effects of Electric and Magnetic Fields*, D.O. Carpenter and S. Ayrapetyan, eds., pp. 233–261. San Diego: Academic Press.

Scaiano, J.C., N. Mohtat, F.L. Cozens, J. McClean, A. Thansandote. 1994a. Application of the radical pair mechanism to free radicals in organized systems: Can the effects of 60 Hz be predicted from studies under static fields? *Bioelectromagnetics* 15:549–554.

Scaiano, J.C., F.L. Cozens, J. McClean. 1994b. Model for the rationalization of magnetic fields effects in vivo. Application of the radical-pair mechanism to biological systems. *Photochem. Photobiol.* 59:585–598.

Scarfi, M.R., F. Bersani, A. Cossarizza, D. Monti, G. Castelani, R. Cadossi, G. Franceschetti, C. Franceschi. 1991. Spontaneous and mitomycin-C induced micronuclei in human lympocytes exposed to extremely low frequency pulsed magnetic fields. *Biochem. Biophys. Res. Commun.* 176:194–200.

Scarfi, M.R., F. Bersani, A. Cossarizza, D. Monti, O. Zeni, M.B. Lioi, G. Franceschetti, M. Carpi, C. Franceschi. 1993. 50 Hz AC sinusoidal electric fields do not exert genotoxic effects (micronucleus formation) in human lymphocytes. *Radiat. Res.* 135:64–68.

Scarfi, M.R., M.B. Lioi, O. Zeni, G. Franceschetti, C. Franceschi, F. Bersani. 1994. Lack of chromosomal aberration and micronucleus induction in human lymphocytes exposed to pulsed magnetic fields. *Mutat. Res.* 306:129–133.

Selmaoui, B., Y. Touitou. 1995. Sinusoidal 50-Hz magnetic fields depress rat pineal NAT activity and serum melatonin. Role of duration and intensity of exposure. *Life Sci.* 57:1351–1358.

Shaw, I.C., H.B. Jones. 1994. Mechanisms of non-genotoxic carcinogenesis. *Trends Pharmacol. Sci.* 15:89–93.

Shen, Y.H., B.J. Shao, H. Chiang, Y.D. Fu. 1995. The effects of ELF (50 Hz) magnetic field exposure on thymic lymphoma/leukemia in ICR mice. In: Abstracts of the 17th Annual Bioelectromagnetics Society Meeting, Boston, Massachusetts, pp. 129–130.

Shore, R.E. 1988. Electromagnetic radiations and cancer. Cause and prevention. *Cancer* 62 (Suppl.):1747–1754.

Stevens, R.G. 1987. Electric power use and breast cancer: A hypothesis. *Am. J. Epidemiol.* 125:556–561.

Stevens, R.G., S. Davis, D.B. Thomas, L.E. Anderson, B.W. Wilson. 1992. Electric power, pineal function, and the risk of breast cancer. *FASEB J.* 6:853–860.

Stuchly, M.A., D.W. Lecuyer, R.D. Mann. 1983. Extremely low frequency electromagnetic emissions from video display terminals and other devices. *Health Phys.* 45:713–722.

Stuchly, M.A., D.W. Lecuyer, J. Mclean. 1991. Cancer promotion in a mouse-skin model by a 60-Hz magnetic field: I. Experimental design and exposure system. *Bioelectromagnetics* 12:261–271.

Stuchly, M.A., J.R.N. McLean, R. Burnett, M. Goddard, D.W. Lecuyer, R.E.J. Mitchel. 1992. Modification of tumor promotion in the mouse skin by exposure to an alternating magnetic field. *Cancer Lett.* 65:1–7.

Tenforde, T.S. 1991. Biological interactions of extremely-low-frequency electric and magnetic fields. *Bioelectrochem. Bioenerg.* 25:1–17.

Tenforde, T.S. 1992. Biological interactions and potential health effects of extremely-low-frequency magnetic fields from power lines and other common sources. *Ann. Rev. Public Health* 13:173–196.

Tenforde, T.S. 1993. Cellular and molecular pathways of extremely low frequency electromagnetic field interactions with living systems. In: *Electricity and Magnetism in Biology and Medicine*, M. Blank, ed., pp. 1–8. San Francisco: San Francisco Press.

Tenforde, T.S., W.T. Kaune. 1987. Interaction of extremely low frequency electric and magnetic fields with humans. *Health Phys.* 53:585–606.

Thomson, R.A.E., S.M. Michaelson, Q.A. Nguyen. 1988. Influence of 60-Hertz magnetic fields on leukemia. *Bioelectromagnetics* 9:149–158.

Trosko, J.E. 1990. Toxicological implications of altered gap junctions. In: *In Vitro Toxicology*, D. Brusick and M.O. Bradley, eds., pp. 1–115. New York: Mary Ann Lkiebert, Inc.

Trump, B.F., I.K. Berezesky. 1995. Calcium-mediated cell injury and cell death. *FASEB J.* 9:219–228.

Tuffet, S., R. de Seze, J.-M. Moreau, B. Veyret. 1993. Effects of a strong pulsed magnetic field on the proliferation of tumor cells in vitro. *Bioelectrochem. Bioenerg.* 30:151–160.

Tynes, T., A. Andersen. 1990. Electromagnetic fields and male breast cancer. *Lancet* 336:1596.

Ubeda A., M.A. Trillo, D.E. House, C.F. Blackman. 1995. A 50-Hz magnetic field blocks melatonin-induced enhancement of junctional transfer in normal C3H/10T½ cells. *Carcinogenesis* 16(12):2945–2949.

Vainio, H., J. Wilbourn. 1993. Cancer etiology: Agents causally associated with human cancer. *Pharmacol. Toxicol.* Suppl.1:4–11.

Vijayalaxmi, R.J. Reiter, E. Sewerynek, B. Poeggeler, B.Z. Leal, M. Meltz. 1995. Marked reduction of radiation-induced micronuclei in human blood lymphocytes pretreated with melatonin. *Radiat. Res.* 143:102–106.

Walleczek, J. 1992. Electromagnetic field effets on cells of the immune system: The role of calcium signaling. *FASEB J.* 6:3177–3185.

Walleczek, J., R.P. Liburdy. 1990. Nonthermal 60 Hz sinusoidal magnetic-field exposure enhances $^{45}Ca^{2+}$ uptake in rat thymocytes: Dependence on mitogen activation. *FEBS Lett.* 271:157–160.

Walleczek, J., P.L. Miller, W.R. Adey. 1993. Simultaneous dual-sample fluorimetric detection of real-time effects of ELF electromagnetic fields on cytosolic free calcium and divalent cation flux in human leukemic T-cells (Jurkat). In: *Electricity and Magnetism in Biology and Medicine*, M. Blank, ed., pp. 303–306. San Francisco: San Francisco Press.

Welsch, C.W. 1985. Host factors affecting the growth of carcinogen-induced rat mammary carcinomas: A review and tribute to Charles Brenton Huggins. *Cancer Res.* 45:3415–3443.

Wertheimer, N., E. Leeper. 1982. Adult cancer related to electrical wires near the home. *Int. J. Epidemiol.* 11:345–355.

Wilson, B.W., C.W. Wright, J.E. Morris, R.L. Buschbom, D.P. Brown, D.L. Miller, R. Sommers-Flannigan, L.E. Anderson. 1990. Evidence for an effect of ELF electromagnetic fields on human pineal gland function. *J. Pineal Res.* 9:259–269.

Yasui, M., T. Kikuchi, M. Ogawa, Y. Otaka, M. Tsuchitani, H. Iwata. 1993a. Life span exposure test of rats to 50-Hz sinusoidal alternating magnetic fields. II. Chronic carcinogenicity evaluation. In: Abstracts of the 15th Annual Bioelectromagnetics Society Meeting, Los Angeles, California, June 13–17, p. 153–154. Frederick, Maryland: The Bioelectromagnetics Society.

Yasui, M., T. Kikuchi, Y. Otaka, M. Kato, M. 1993b. Life span exposure test of rats to 50 Hz sinusoidal alternating magnetic fields. In: *Electricity and Magnetism in Biology and Medicine*, M. Blank, ed., pp. 839–841. San Francisco: San Francisco Press.

Yost, M.G., R.P. Liburdy. 1992. Time-varying and static magnetic fields act in combination to alter calcium signal transduction in the lymphocyte. *FEBS Lett.* 296:117–122.

22 Magnetic Fields, Melatonin, Tamoxifen, and Human Breast Cancer Cell Growth

ROBERT P. LIBURDY
JOAN D. HARLAND
Life Science Division, Lawrence Berkeley National Laboratory, UC Berkeley, Berkeley, California

CONTENTS

INTRODUCTION
BACKGROUND
MATERIAL AND METHODS
  Cells, Hormones, and Drugs
  Magnetic Field Exposure System
  Cell Culture Techniques
  Statistical Analyses
RESULTS
  Inhibition of Melatonin Action by a 12-mG, 60-Hz Magnetic Field
  Inhibition of Tamoxifen Action by a 12-mG, 60-Hz Magnetic Field
  The Magnetic Field is Associated with the Field Blocking Effect
DISCUSSION
ACKNOWLEDGMENTS
REFERENCES

INTRODUCTION

This chapter reviews experimental evidence obtained in our laboratory indicating that environmental-level magnetic fields [12 mG (=1.2 μT), 60 Hz] can interfere with the growth-regulating actions of the hormone melatonin and the cancer drug tamoxifen in cell culture.

In studies in our laboratory over the past several years, we have observed that 12-mG, 60-Hz magnetic fields can act to block the growth inhibition of physiological levels (10^{-9} M) of melatonin on MCF-7 human breast cancer cells in vitro. Composite data over this period suggest that the static DC magnetic field is apparently not critical for the blocking effect of such fields on melatonin action. Interestingly, the same 12-mG, 60-Hz magnetic fields appear to inhibit the cytostatic action of pharmacological doses (10^{-7} M) of tamoxifen. Regarding the magnetic field metric for this interaction, the 12-mG magnetic field (B), not the associated induced electric field (E) due to Faraday's Law of Current Induction, is associated with the field effect. Thus, the magnetic field appears to be the operative exposure metric.

Performing cell culture studies requires carefully controlling the magnetic field inside of cell culture incubators. A stray magnetic field can significantly confound the reproducibility of data, both within and across laboratories. Therefore, we developed a special exposure system to generate uniform, 60-Hz magnetic fields using four-square Merritt coils enclosed in specialized mu-metal chambers to eliminate stray, time-varying AC and static DC magnetic fields.

Recently, an independent replication of the 12-mG inhibition of melatonin action has been reported; this study is discussed herein. It is of mechanistic interest that, according to our data, a 12-mG magnetic field inhibits tamoxifen action, because this raises the possibility that the estrogen receptor may be a possible biochemical site for this field interaction. Further studies of the type described here, employing a well-characterized exposure system and cellular model system, will shed light on magnetic field interactions with biological systems.

BACKGROUND

Experimental evidence from cellular, animal, and human laboratory studies exists which suggests that environmental-level electric and magnetic fields (EMF) might represent a potential risk factor for human breast cancer via a field effect that depresses or time-shifts melatonin secretion into the blood (Pool 1990; Wilson et al. 1981, 1983, 1986; Welker et al. 1983; Yellon 1993; Graham et al. 1993, 1994; Kato et al. 1994a, b; Löscher et al. 1994). Also, some recent epidemiologic studies have raised the possibility that EMF exposure may be a potential risk factor for breast cancer (Tynes and Anderson 1990; Matanoski et al. 1991; Demers et al. 1991; Loomis et al. 1994).

That low-frequency, time-varying EMF may depress or time-shift melatonin secretion has been reported by several investigators. This effect was first reported by B. Wilson in rats (Wilson et al. 1981, 1983, 1986), and has since been observed in cultured pinealocytes (Welker et al. 1983), hamsters (Yellon 1993), rats (Kato et al. 1994a; Löscher et al. 1994), and in some human volunteers exposed to 200-mG, 60-Hz magnetic fields at night (Graham et al. 1993, 1994). Suppression of melatonin has been ascribed to an effect of these fields on the pineal gland, which produces melatonin. Melatonin has a variety of biological functions, including circadian rhythm control, endocrine function inhibition, immune function enhancement, and oncostatic properties (Maestroni 1993; Reiter in press; Guerrero and Reiter 1992). Relevant to the latter is the observation that melatonin is reported to inhibit 7,12-dimethlybenz(a)anthracene (DMBA)-induced rat mammary gland carcinogenesis (Subramanian and Kothari 1991). Consistent with an in vivo model of interaction involving melatonin, recent animal studies have reported that magnetic fields can enhance DMBA breast cancer growth in rats (Mevissen et al. 1993; Löscher et al. 1993). In addition, D. Blask and coworkers have reported that melatonin inhibits the in vitro growth of MCF-7 cells, an estrogen receptor-positive human mammary tumor line, further supporting the oncostatic properties of melatonin (Hill and Blask 1988; Cos and Blask 1990; Cos et al. 1991). Other groups have subsequently reported on the oncostatic action of melatonin in MCF-7 cells (Molis et al. 1994 and references therein, 1995; Cos and Sanchez-Barceló 1994, 1995; Crespo et al. 1994). One possible mechanism envisioned for EMF effects, then, is a field-related depression of melatonin, leading to increased breast cancer risk (Stevens et al. 1992).

In our laboratory, we have addressed the possibility of a more direct, but complementary mechanism for an effect of EMF on breast cancer; namely, the interaction of the field with the target cell to alter melatonin's biological action. In support of this hypothesis, we recently reported that environmental-level, 12-mG, 60-Hz magnetic fields block melatonin's natural growth-inhibitory action on MCF-7 cells in culture, while having no effect on untreated cell growth (Liburdy et al. 1993a, b). These two modes of field action—depression of pineal gland melatonin secretion and blocking of melatonin's action on target cells—raise the possibility of a synergistic effect in vivo.

It is significant that our melatonin finding recently has been independently replicated (Blackman et al. 1996). Replication studies are difficult to execute and require commitment, careful attention to detail, and should follow three basic rules:

1. In cellular experiments, the same cells should be obtained from the originating laboratory and the same serum employed.

2. The same protocols should be followed, and these protocols should be well-defined and made available from the originating laboratory.

3. Similar or identical exposure systems as used in the originating laboratory should be employed.

Although there were slight variations from our methods in the protocols employed in the replication study reported by C. Blackman of the U.S. Environmental Protection Agency (EPA), such as using a Helmholtz coil instead of a four-square Merritt coil, there was apparently enough detail in the protocols to identify the important variables in the MCF-7 experiments. This study, we believe, is the first such true replication of a key magnetic field-induced bioeffect.

To conduct the studies reviewed here, we designed and implemented a special exposure system that (1) generates a uniform magnetic field for exposure of cells in culture, and (2) employs a mu-metal shielding chamber to eliminate the confounding presence of spurious, time-varying AC and static DC magnetic fields generated by commercial incubators (Liburdy et al. 1993b; Liburdy 1994a, 1995). This exposure system (operating at 2 mG, 60 Hz) is used in our laboratory to grow and maintain MCF-7 cells prior to their use in higher-field exposures. This process assures us that the past EMF history of the cells is well-characterized before use in experiments.

In considering a possible mechanism for magnetic field effects, we asked whether such fields decrease the growth-inhibitory action of the drug tamoxifen. Tamoxifen is the most widely used anti-estrogen therapy for the control of breast cancer, and, importantly, is known to bind to and probably act via the estrogen receptor (Coezy et al. 1982; Martin et al. 1988). Our observation that a 12-mG, 60-Hz magnetic field can inhibit tamoxifen action in culture raises the possibility of estrogen receptor involvement in this field interaction. Such an observation opens an avenue for future study that may shed light on possible biochemical sites with which magnetic fields may interact.

MATERIALS AND METHODS

Cells, Hormones, and Drugs

The MCF-7 cell is an epithelial-like cell derived from the pleural effusion of a mammary adenocarcinoma (ATCC HTB-22) (Soule et al. 1973). Melatonin-sensitive MCF-7 cells at passage #18 were a generous gift of Dr. David Blask of the Mary Imogene Bassett Hospital Research Institute, Cooperstown, New York. Cells were maintained in Dulbecco's Modified Eagle's Medium (DMEM; 1.0 g/L glucose, #D8788, Sigma Chemical Co., St. Louis, Missouri) supplemented with 10% fetal bovine serum (#101, Lot #10786, Tissue Culture Biologicals, Tulare, California), penicillin (200 units/mL), and streptomycin (100 μg/mL) (penicillin/streptomycin: University of California–San Francisco Cell Culture Facility). Use of high-glucose DMEM or some serum lots was observed to diminish melatonin sensitivity. Cells were grown as a monolayer at 37°C in a humid atmosphere, with 5% CO_2. Melatonin (N-acetyl-5-methoxytryptamine; #M5250) and tamoxifen (#T9262) were purchased from Sigma Chemical Co. Melatonin and tamoxifen solutions were prepared before use by dissolving crystals in minimum ethanol, followed by dilution in media.

Magnetic Field Exposure System

The cell culture exposure system we developed and use in our laboratory has been described previously (Liburdy et al. 1993b; Liburdy 1994a, 1995). To address the engineering issue of contaminating magnetic fields present inside commercial cell culture incubators, we designed an exposure system that generates a uniform magnetic field environment free of stray, time-varying magnetic or electric fields associated with operating the incubator. Special features are: (1) a perforated Plexiglas platform table, within (2) a double-wound, four-coil Merritt exposure system (plastic frame wound with double-wrap, bifilar cable, in the Merritt's turn ratio of 26/11/11/26), placed inside (3) a ventilated mu-metal chamber to eliminate extraneous time-varying and static magnetic fields, within (4) a water-jacketed Queue incubator (Queue Systems Inc., Parkersburg, West Virginia, Model 2710), maintained at 37°C ± 0.1°C. We chose the four-square Merritt coil, because it provides the largest uniform exposure volume (Merritt et al. 1983; Kirschvink 1992b) (Fig. 1). We placed these exposure coils inside a mu-metal chamber (Fig. 2). This chamber (Magnetic Shield Corp., Perfection Mica Co., Bensenville, Illinois) has ventilation holes on the top and bottom, and is constructed of nickel and trace metals. This design allows effective shielding of cells inside from spurious magnetic fields generated during operation of the incubator so that the interior static magnetic field levels are approximately > 10 mG, and AC magnetic field levels are essentially not measureable at extremely low frequency (ELF) using our dosimetry probes (see next paragraph). Signal generators were used to drive the coils (Dynascan Corp., Chicago, Illinois; B & K Precision Model 3020); coils were shielded with aluminum or copper foil to eliminate the electric field associated with each current-carrying coil. Figure 3 shows the complete exposure system in place inside a commercial incubator.

    Field dosimetry was performed using a commercially available fluxgate magnetometer (Hewlett Packard Model 428B fluxgate meter, Cupertino, California), calibrated by the Magnetic Field Measurements Group at Lawrence Berkeley Laboratory, or by us in our laboratory using a calibration coil we designed. Field readings were taken before, during, and after most experiments, and yielded values within approximately ± 5%. We also have performed measurements using a Multiwave II System (Electric Research and Management Inc., State College, Pennsylvania); cross-calibration of our Hewlett Packard fluxgate probes with a Multiwave II Bartington probe gave values within approximately ± 15%. Merritt coils generated very uniform field

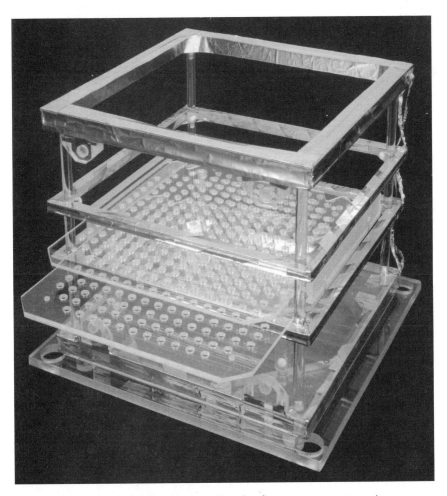

FIG. 1. Cell culture exposure coil. A Plexiglas frame was constructed to accommodate four square coils that are wound in a specific turn ratio, and that are separated according to a special relationship described by Merritt et al. (1983). The frame is essentially a cube with an edge length of approximately 35 cm. The volume between the two central coils is associated with a very uniform (< 2% variation) magnetic field when the coil is energized (Liburdy 1995; Kirschvink 1992b). In the design we employed, the coil frame can be physically rotated about the platform for holding the cell culture plates by 90°, so as to re-orient the magnetic field vector from a perpendicular to a parallel direction with respect to the cell culture plate. Refer to Figure 8 and text.

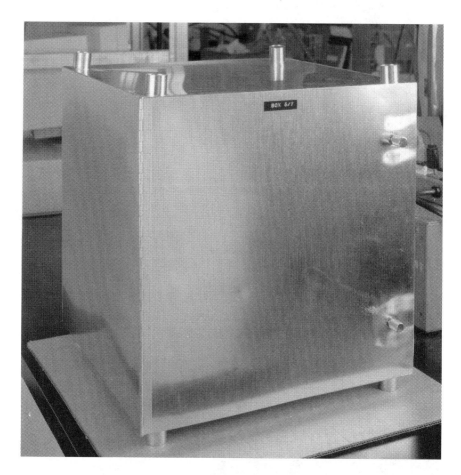

FIG. 2. Mu-metal chamber. This chamber is a cube that was constructed from Co-Netic™ AA alloy (~ 80% nickel) that is approximately 1.016 mm thick with an edge length of approximately 40 cm (Magnetic Shield Corp., Bensenville, Illinois). The chamber was butt-seam welded and hydrogen annealed after fabrication, and has a hinged door that can be secured to the chamber. Four ventilation holes on the top and bottom are approximately 2.54 cm in diameter, and have an extension tube of 2.45 cm in length; these holes are located in the corners of the cube form.

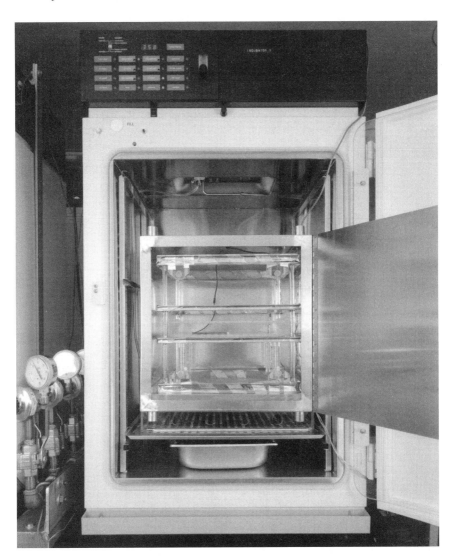

FIG. 3. Cell culture exposure system. Shown is the combination of the four-square Merritt coil and the mu-metal chamber, which are both placed inside a commercial cell culture incubator. Also shown is a thermistor temperature probe, which is threaded through one of the ventilation holes into the mu-metal chamber and placed inside the chamber at the position where cell culture plates are typically located.

values (Merritt et al. 1983; Kirschvink 1992b) over the central volume where our cells were placed; static DC fields were reduced to approximately 0.1 mG by the mu-metal shields. We performed 2-mG and 12-mG field exposures simultaneously using three identical exposure systems. This approach permitted experiments to be conducted on same-passage cells that were exposed to (1) 2-mG magnetic fields oriented perpendicular to Petri dishes, (2) 12-mG magnetic fields oriented perpendicular to Petri dishes, and (3) 12-mG magnetic fields oriented parallel to Petri dishes. Coils were energized during the entire period of cell growth. Temperature was monitored continuously and recorded daily, using thermistor probes (YSI Inc., Yellow Springs, Ohio) placed inside the mu-metal chambers and located next to the cell culture plate area.

Cell Culture Techniques

We passaged MCF-7 cells on Falcon 60-mm plates (Becton Dickinson, New Jersey). For drug/hormone sensitivity assays, cells were harvested in 0.2% ethylenediaminetetreacetic acid (EDTA) phosphate buffer (2 g/L Na_2-EDTA, 8 g/L NaCl, 0.2 g/L KH_2PO_4, 1.15 g/L Na_2HPO_4), separated into a single-cell preparation by passing three times through a 25-gauge needle, and seeded at 0.1×10^5 cells/35-mm dish in 1.5 mL of media. By 4 hours, the cells had attached and media was changed, with or without drug/hormone additions. Cell growth was followed up to days 5–8. Cells were maintained continuously in original culture media and exposure conditions until counting. On counting days, cells were detached with 0.2 mL trypsin solution at 37°C (0.50 g/L trypsin, 0.5 g/L EDTA, 1.0 g/L glucose, and 0.58 g/L $NaHCO_3$), diluted with 0.8 ml PBS, and counted by hemacytometer. Three plates for each treatment category were counted per counting day.

Melatonin sensitivity of MCF-7 cells is affected by several factors, including source of fetal bovine serum, schedule of media change, MCF-7 cell passage number, cell density at time of harvesting, cell seeding density, and thoroughness of single-cell preparation at the time of seeding. Although several groups have reported that melatonin exhibits oncostatic properties in MCF-7 cells (Molis et al. 1994 and references therein; Cos and Sanchez-Barceló 1994, 1995; Crespo et al. 1994), we note that one group of investigators has reported that an MCF-7 subclone studied in their laboratory failed to respond to melatonin (L'Hermite-Baleriaux and de Launoit 1992). We have prepared extensive written protocols for our procedures that are available upon request.

Statistical Analyses

Data shown here were tested for statistical significance using the SigmaPlot Student t-test (Jandel Corporation, Corte Madera, California). The multifactor analysis of variance program in Statgraphics (Manugistics Inc., Rockville, Maryland) also was used to analyze data in Figure 5 across melatonin doses. Error bars in the figures represent the standard error of the mean.

RESULTS

Inhibition of Melatonin Action by a 12-mG, 60-Hz Magnetic Field

We have observed that exposure to a 12-mG, 60-Hz field and a 135- to 145-mG, DC magnetic field blocks the growth-inhibitory action of melatonin on MCF-7 breast cancer cells (Liburdy et al. 1993b). In Figure 4, experimental data are presented showing the effect of 60-Hz, 2-mG or 12-mG magnetic fields on melatonin's growth inhibition of MCF-7 cells using mu-metal shielded cultures. Effect of the field is shown for the day (5, 6, or 7) of maximum melatonin effect. Across seven experiments, treatment with the physiological dose of 10^{-9} M melatonin in 2-mG magnetic fields resulted in an approximate 26% inhibition of MCF-7 cell growth ($p < 0.00001$; 100% is defined as growth in the absence of hormone). Exposure to 12-mG magnetic fields, however, blocked melatonin's action. This result confirms our previously reported observations (Liburdy et al. 1993a, b), and also suggests that static magnetic fields ($\leq$ 145 mG) may not play a role in this effect. We note that two preliminary reports in abstract form indicate results consistent with these 60-Hz effects (Blask et al. 1993a, b). More importantly, these findings have been independently replicated at the EPA (Blackman et al. 1996).

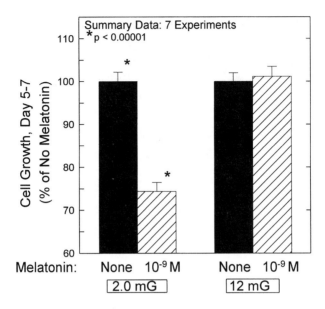

FIG. 4. Comparison of melatonin inhibition of MCF-7 cell growth in the presence of 2-mG or 12-mG fields; summary data from seven experiments. Cells were seeded at 0.1×10^5/plate and grown in media containing no melatonin or 10^{-9} M melatonin in an incubator with a background 60-Hz magnetic field of 2 mG, or a 60-Hz magnetic field of 12 mG. In all experiments, cultures were mu-metal shielded (Liburdy 1994b, 1995). In a 2-mG background field, melatonin exhibited an average 26% inhibition of MCF-7 cell growth on days 5–7 (see text); in a 12-mG field, melatonin had no significant effect on cell growth.

In his studies, Dr. Blackman received MCF-7 cells from our laboratory, as well as extensive written protocols describing our laboratory procedures. Dr. Blackman conducted three experiments in which he measured cell growth (cell counts) on day 7 for cells in three categories, as detailed in Table 1. This data represents an independent replication of our earlier findings (Liburdy et al. 1993b). In follow-on control studies, Dr. Blackman evaluated cell growth of MCF-7 cells in the absence of melatonin in a 12-mG versus 2-mG, 60-Hz magnetic field (using mu-metal shielded chambers). This experiment addressed the question of whether the 12-mG field may influence MCF-7 cell growth, per se. When Dr. Blackman assessed the growth of five independent plates of

TABLE 1
Cell Growth in Replicate Studies by Blackman et al. (1996)

	Control	Melatonin	Melatonin & B field
B field	(< 2 mG)	(< 2 mG)	(12 mG)
Mean[a]	1.38[b]	1.15[b]	1.39
SE	0.15	0.14	0.14
n	9	9	9

[a] The mean is expressed $\times 10^6$ cells.
[b] The means were significantly different (p < 0.001).

cells cultured in the absence of melatonin at < 2 mG or 12 mG, he observed no statistically significant difference between the magnetic field-treated cell cohorts (p = 0.713). Thus, the magnetic field by itself, in the absence of melatonin, produced no effect on growth of MCF-7 cells. This finding is consistent with our control data.

To test whether melatonin-mediated growth inhibition was blocked by 12-mG magnetic fields over a broad range of concentrations, we conducted studies at 10^{-11}–10^{-5} M melatonin. Figure 5 reveals that a 12-mG magnetic field can significantly inhibit melatonin's action across the concentration range of 10^{-11}–10^{-7} M (p < 0.02). This 12-mG effect on melatonin is reproducible in our laboratory; to date in 100% (seven out of seven) of our experiments showing significant melatonin inhibition at 2 mG, we have observed blocking by the 12-mG field.

Inhibition of Tamoxifen Action by a 12-mG, 60-Hz Magnetic Field

Extending our melatonin studies to tamoxifen, we tested the effects of 60-Hz, 2- and 12-mG fields on the growth-inhibitory action of tamoxifen over a range of doses, from 10^{-6}–10^{-8} M. This range includes

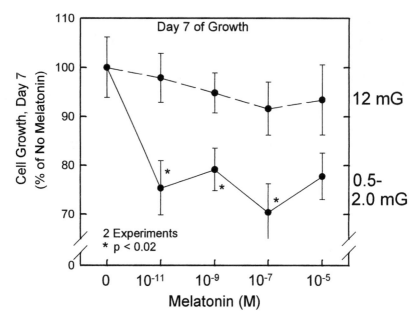

FIG. 5. Effect of a 12-mG versus a 0.5- to 2-mG (environmental background) magnetic field on inhibition of MCF-7 cell growth by melatonin, across a range of doses. Cell growth was determined by counting on day 7; all numbers are expressed as percentage of control (untreated) growth. Results are the means ± SE of two experiments. The Student t-test shows a significant effect of the 12-mG field versus the 2-mG field at each individual melatonin dose for 10^{-11}–10^{-7} M melatonin ($p < 0.02$) (comparison of 0.5–2.0 mG versus 12 mG at individual melatonin doses); multifactor analysis of variance shows a significant 12-mG blocking effect ($p < 0.0001$) across the entire concentration range of hormone.

tamoxifen's pharmacological dose of 150 ng/mL, corresponding to 4 × 10^{-7} M (Swain and Lippman 1990).

Figure 6 shows cell growth data (day 7) for experiments involving a 2-mG versus a 12-mG magnetic field; cell growth is shown normalized to 100% for MCF-7 cells in the absence of tamoxifen. In a 2-mG field, tamoxifen inhibited MCF-7 cell growth in a dose-dependent manner; there was approximately 68% inhibition at 10^{-6} M tamoxifen, decreasing to 38% and 1% at 10^{-7} and 10^{-8} M, respectively. These data agree

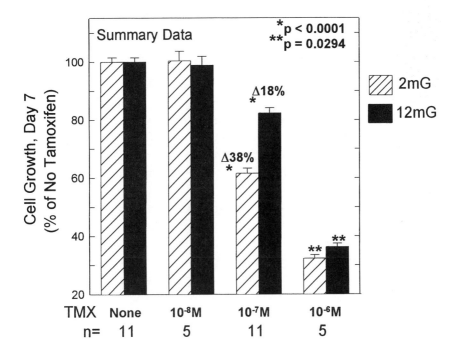

FIG. 6. Effect of a 12-mG versus a 2-mG magnetic field on inhibition of MCF-7 cell growth on day 7 by 10^{-8}–10^{-6} M tamoxifen (TMX). In all experiments, cells were grown within mu-metal shields. Results are the means of 5 or 11 experiments.

with previous reports of tamoxifen's in vitro growth-inhibitory activity on MCF-7 cells (Lippman et al. 1976).

The growth inhibitory action of 10^{-7} tamoxifen was seen to be reduced or partially blocked by the presence of a 12-mG magnetic field. In a 12-mG field, only an 18% reduction of cell growth by day 7 was observed compared to a 38% reduction in the presence of a 2-mG field. However, the 12-mG field has only a slight effect on the action of 10^{-6} M tamoxifen (from 68% inhibition to 64%; p = 0.0294). This dose-dependent effect may be due to a threshold response, or to toxicity of the higher dose of tamoxifen. As with melatonin, the field interaction requires the presence of tamoxifen; but it differs from that for mela-tonin (Fig. 5), which appears to be essentially constant across doses of 10^{-5}–10^{-11} M.

It could be argued that this result represents a temporary field effect that is observed perhaps only on day 7. However, this 12-mG blocking effect was seen on both days of tamoxifen sensitivity during MCF-7 exponential growth (compare Figs. 7A and 7B). Furthermore, these results are reproducible in our laboratory: In 10 of 11 experiments in which we have seen tamoxifen significantly inhibit MCF-7 cell growth, we have observed a significant ($p < 0.05$) blocking effect by the 12-mG magnetic field.

These data support an effect of a 12-mG, environmental-level mag-netic field on tamoxifen's growth-inhibitory action in vitro at pharma-cological doses. Recently, follow-on studies have been performed in our laboratory in which the experimenter was blinded to tamoxifen drug treatment; a similar 12-mG magnetic field effect was observed as shown in Figure 6 for tamoxifen at 10^{-7} M.

The Magnetic Field is Associated with the Field Blocking Effect

An important question to address, and one of significant mechanistic importance, is referred to in our laboratory as the "E versus B" ques-tion. This question relates to whether either the magnetic field (B) or the induced electric field (E) component is responsible for the blocking effect of both melatonin and tamoxifen. According to Faraday's Law of Current Induction, a time-varying magnetic field will induce in an object an electric field proportional to the radius of the cross-sectional area perpendicular to the incident magnetic field (Bassen et al. 1992; Liburdy 1992a, 1994b). Therefore, in order to differentiate E-field and B-field effects on cell growth, we simultaneously exposed MCF-7 cells in three matched incubators to either a 2-mG magnetic field, a 12-mG magnetic field, or a second 12-mG magnetic field rotated 90° (B-field vector parallel to culture dish). As shown in Figure 8, rotating the 12-mG field 90° reduces the effective induced E field nearly 5.6-fold from an induced E field [root mean square (RMS)—average] compo-nent of 1.98 μV/m to 0.353 μV/m by reducing the cross-section seen by the B field when rotated, while maintaining a constant 12-mG B field

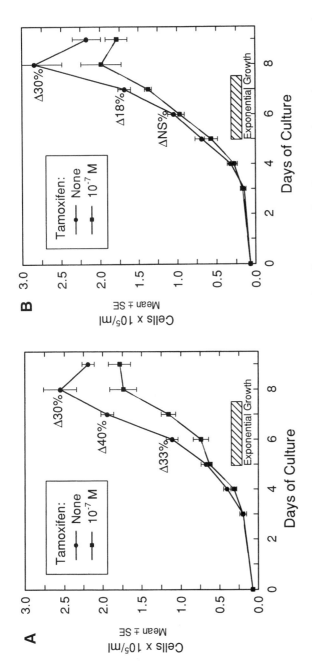

FIG. 7. Growth curve of MCF-7 cells in the presence or absence of 10^{-7} M tamoxifen. Exponential growth occurs on days 5, 6, and 7. Panel A: Growth in a 2-mG magnetic field. Tamoxifen shows 33% and 40% inhibition on days 6 and 7, respectively. Panel B: Growth in a 12-mG magnetic field. Tamoxifen exhibits 0% and 18% inhibition on days 6 and 7, respectively.

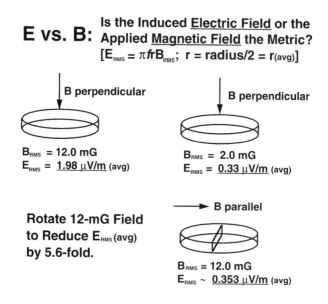

E vs. B: Is the Induced <u>Electric Field</u> or the Applied <u>Magnetic Field</u> the Metric?
$$[E_{RMS} = \pi f r B_{RMS};\ r = radius/2 = r_{(avg)}]$$

B perpendicular

B perpendicular

B_{RMS} = 12.0 mG
E_{RMS} = 1.98 μV/m (avg)

B_{RMS} = 2.0 mG
E_{RMS} = 0.33 μV/m (avg)

Rotate 12-mG Field to Reduce E_{RMS} (avg) by 5.6-fold.

B parallel

B_{RMS} = 12.0 mG
E_{RMS} ~ 0.353 μV/m (avg)

FIG. 8. Estimated values of average induced E (electric) fields in 2-mG (perpendicular), 12-mG (perpendicular), and 12-mG (parallel) magnetic field exposure systems, based on Faraday's Law of Current Induction. The magnetic B field exposure (B_{RMS}) at two different orientations remains the same for the MCF-7 monolayer culture; however, the average induced E field [E_{RMS}(avg)], which depends on the cross-sectional area of the culture media containing electrolytes seen by the B field, is reduced approximately 5.6-fold when the 12-mG field is rotated 90° from the B perpendicular to the B parallel orientation.

(M. Misakian, personal communication[1]). The induced E field is expressed as the RMS value of the sinusoidally varying induced E field computed according to Faraday's Law of Current Induction using the average radius of the Petri dish, radius/2. The induced E field in the parallel orientation is essentially uniform over the surface of the dish upon which the cells are located [E_{RMS} = ~ 0.353 μV/m(avg.)].[1] This is

---

[1] The calculated electric fields in the Petri dishes do not take into account the presence of cell proximity effects as described by Drs. M. Stuchly and W. Xi in, "Modeling induced currents in biological cells exposed to low frequency magnetic fields," *Phys. Med. Biol.* 39:1319–1330, 1994.

different from the case in which the magnetic field is in the perpendicular orientation, where E varies according to the radius of the dish via Faraday's Law; the average electric field corresponds to radius/2, as indicated in Figure 8. To reduce E, we could instead have reduced dish radius, but this method would introduce potential biological complications due to alterations in surface/volume ratios and cell distribution. Such alterations have been shown in modeling studies to have a significant effect on the induced current density in cell monolayers exposed to a perpendicular 60-Hz magnetic field (M. Misakian, personal communication; see footnote on p. 686). Addressing the E versus B question is important from a mechanistic point of view: Magnetic fields can penetrate cells, but electric fields induced by environmental-level magnetic fields cannot penetrate beyond the cell membrane. Therefore, induced electric fields most likely interact directly with the cell at the membrane level (Liburdy 1992a, b).

The results are presented in Figures 9 and 10 for melatonin and tamoxifen, respectively. As we have reported previously (Liburdy et al. 1993b), magnetic fields did not affect MCF-7 cell growth significantly in the absence of melatonin. However, across three experiments, growth was significantly inhibited by 10^{-9} M melatonin, for an average of 32% inhibition on day 7 in a 2-mG magnetic field ($p < 0.0001$). In the 12-mG field oriented perpendicular to the plane of cells, melatonin's activity was blocked nearly completely ($p = 0.6493$); in the 12-mG magnetic field rotated 90° relative to the plane of the plate, melatonin's action was still blocked significantly ($p = 0.1101$). These data suggest that the 12-mG magnetic field component is the operative one for melatonin blocking effects.

In Figure 10, the analogous experiment for tamoxifen shows similar results. With 10^{-7} M tamoxifen in a 2-mG magnetic field, MCF-7 cell growth was significantly inhibited on day 7 by an average of 40% across four experiments ($p < 0.0001$). In a 12-mG magnetic field, the MCF-7 cell growth was still significantly blocked ($p = 0.0032$), but was reduced to an average of 15% inhibition. Similar results were seen in the 12-mG magnetic field rotated 90°, with an average of 17% inhibition (no significant difference from 12-mG perpendicular field; $p = 0.7506$). Thus, the 12-mG magnetic field component is associated with blocking tamoxifen as well as melatonin inhibition of MCF-7 cell growth.

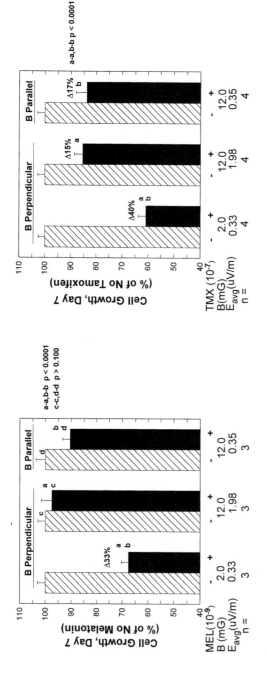

FIG. 9.   Effect of the 60-Hz magnetic field orientation on melatonin's cytostatic action in MCF-7 cells. Cells were counted after 7 days in culture with or without melatonin (MEL) treatment in a 2-mG perpendicular field, a 12-mG perpendicular field, or a 12-mG parallel field. All values are expressed as a percent of the untreated culture cell counts in the same field. The cells in the 2-mG field show an average of 33% inhibition by 10^{-9} M melatonin; in the 12-mG perpendicular and 12-mG parallel fields, inhibition is reduced to 2% and 9%, respectively.

FIG. 10.   Effect of 60-Hz magnetic field orientation on tamoxifen (TMX) cytostatic action in MCF-7 cells on day 7. The cells in the 2-mG field show an average of 40% inhibition; the 12-mG perpendicular and parallel cultures show 15% and 17% inhibition, respectively.

Discussion

In studies in our laboratory, reviewed here, we have observed that environmental-level, 12-mG, 60-Hz magnetic fields partially block tamoxifen's cytostatic action, and completely block melatonin's cytostatic action on human breast cancer cells in vitro. We believe these findings may represent the first experimental report of environmental-level EMF interfering with the cytostatic action of a hormone or drug in vitro.

The tamoxifen data raise the possibility that the estrogen receptor may be a site for magnetic field interaction with the cell, since tamoxifen is an anti-estrogen that specifically binds to the estrogen receptor (Coezy et al. 1982; Martin et al. 1988). This hypothesis is speculation, and we caution that tamoxifen is reported to alter the metabolism of cells that are estrogen receptor-negative, which implies that this drug is multifactorial in action. In addition, we find differences in dose–response relationships between the magnetic field effect for tamoxifen versus melatonin, suggesting possible differences in an interaction mechanism between the two compounds. Finally, unlike many EMF effects reported in the literature, we find that the magnetic field itself, not the induced electric field, is associated with this effect (Liburdy 1995).

For both tamoxifen and melatonin, there are a number of possible levels at which a magnetic field interaction might take place: at the membrane, at the estrogen receptor, at various other signal-transduction molecules, at the nuclear membrane, or during transcription or translation necessary for regulation of cell growth and division. At each level, the magnetic field, which penetrates the cell, could act specifically or nonspecifically. For example, at the MCF-7 cell membrane, magnetic fields could alter either drug/hormone entry, or calcium (Ca^{+2}) entry, influencing downstream signal-transduction events to overcome cytostatic effects. In support of this latter hypothesis, some magnetic field exposures have been reported to elevate intracellular Ca^{+2} levels in cells (Liburdy 1995, 1994b, 1992a–c; Liburdy et al. 1993c, d; Walleczek and Liburdy 1990), and intracellular Ca^{+2} concentration plays a role in estrogen receptor expression in MCF-7 (Ree et al. 1991). The regulation of MCF-7 cell growth is complex; "crosstalk" occurs between the two signal-transduction mechanisms of the estrogen receptor and of calcium-dependent signaling regulated by growth factors at the cell surface (Philips et al. 1993).

Far more is known about the mechanism of tamoxifen activity in MCF-7 cells than that of melatonin. Melatonin may bind to a specific receptor, and several groups are investigating this possibility (Acuña-Castroviejo et al. 1994; Menendez-Pelaez and Reiter 1993; Ebisawa et al. 1994), but this putative binding site has not yet been isolated in MCF-7 cells. Melatonin has been reported to suppress the transcription of the estrogen receptor gene in MCF-7 cells (Molis et al. 1994); thus, there may be an indirect link between melatonin, the estrogen receptor, and melatonin's oncostatic properties. Tamoxifen, on the other hand, is an anti-estrogen that specifically binds to the estrogen receptor (Swain and Lippman 1990). It is thought that tamoxifen inhibits MCF-7 cell growth by inducing an alternate conformational change in the estrogen receptor (different from that caused by estradiol), which allows the receptor complex to bind to its DNA-binding regions but not transcribe its estrogen receptor response genes (Martin et al. 1988). Therefore, while the magnetic field could interfere with tamoxifen entry through the cell membrane, our data could also be explained by a field-associated modulation of tamoxifen binding to the estrogen receptor. However, the 12-mG field does not affect MCF-7 cell growth in the absence of tamoxifen, suggesting that the magnetic field may alter tamoxifen but not estradiol binding to the estrogen receptor, or may differentially affect binding of the estrogen receptor complex to its DNA-binding domain. Alternatively, the field could alter estrogen receptor gene expression in the cell, allowing the cell to overcome tamoxifen inhibition of cell growth at intermediate tamoxifen doses but not at higher ones. This possibility would explain the minimal field effect seen at 10^{-6} M tamoxifen. It would be interesting to test magnetic field effects on ICI 164,384 (a pure anti-estrogen), because tamoxifen has partial agonist activities (Chalbos et al. 1993; Gottardi et al. 1989); the field may favor tamoxifen's agonist activity.

In contrast, the mechanism of melatonin's cytostatic effect is as-yet unknown, but melatonin may also interact with the estrogen receptor. Melatonin blocks estradiol's mitogenic effect in MCF-7, and estradiol partially rescues MCF-7 from melatonin inhibition (Cos et al. 1991; Danforth et al. 1983). The differential magnetic field effect on melatonin versus tamoxifen (dose-independent versus dose-dependent) could be due to differences in the mechanism of interaction with the two compounds, in the mechanism of the two compounds themselves, or in toxicity. If tamoxifen is highly toxic at 10^{-6} M, in contrast to melatonin, magnetic field interactions could not rescue the killed cells.

Our observation that the magnetic field, not the electric field, is associated with blocking of both melatonin and tamoxifen has some importance regarding mechanisms. Induced E fields in the cell culture media interact initially at the level of the cell membrane, as they cannot penetrate beyond the cell membrane at power-line frequencies (Liburdy 1992a, b). The B field, however, while able to act at the cell membrane, penetrates the cell, providing more extensive possibilities for a site of interaction.

The question of E or B fields as the operative component is important from a second standpoint—that of environmental dosimetry in recommending safe exposure levels for humans. Most previous studies of biological effects of EMF have found the E field (Liburdy 1995), and not the B field to be the operative metric, and investigators have argued that an induced E field biological effect is unlikely at milligauss magnetic field strengths, since the resultant induced E field is less than the "thermal noise limit" within the cells (minimum response threshold of 10^{-4} V/m) (Weaver and Astumian 1990). However, we note that our in vitro model system is not a true representation of in vivo conditions.

One biophysical model that could explain how a magnetic field interacts with biological systems is the presence of a magnetic sensor within the cell (such as magnetite). Such a sensor could theoretically translate magnetic fields in the milligauss range into biomechanical effects (Kirschvink et al. 1992, 1993; Kirschvink 1992a; Polk 1994). Depending where such a sensor is physically located, effects on ion channels, receptors, or protein–protein interactions might be influenced. Currently, there is no direct experimental evidence for the presence of magnetite in MCF-7 cells.

A second biophysical model for magnetic field interaction with target molecules relates to magnetochemistry and radical pair recombination. Strong static magnetic fields (1000–1500 G) recently have been shown to alter a kinetic parameter, Vmax/Km, of a biochemical reaction, most likely through modification of intersystem crossing rates between singlet and triplet spin states in the spin-correlated radical pair (Harkins and Grissom 1994). Recently, in a collaborative effort between Dr. L. Packer's laboratory and ours, a report has suggested that specialized cells (such as neutrophils) which generate large quantities of free radicals upon activation ("respiratory burst") produce significantly more free radical species when activated in the presence of a 1-G, 60-Hz magnetic field (Roy et al. 1995). Although these studies are of interest, the fields involved are orders of magnitude higher than those employed in our studies. Regarding free radicals and melatonin, we note the interesting recent observations based on in vivo and in vitro experimental evidence that melatonin can act as a strong radical scavenger (Reiter et al. 1993).

Recently, a hypothesis was discussed that weak, low-frequency EMF may couple to biological systems via a mechanism involving stochastic resonance (Weisenfeld and Moss 1994). Although speculative, as the authors state, if stochastic resonance is relevant, the effects of a weak magnetic field might be amplified to have biological ramifications.

The studies reported here open the door for future studies to test possible mechanisms of field interaction, including studies to measure drug and hormone uptake and localization within the cell, ligand–receptor binding, binding to estrogen receptor response elements, estrogen receptor expression, cell-cycle kinetics, and signal-transduction parameters (such as G-proteins, intracellular Ca^{+2}, c-*myc*, and c-*erb*). A fruitful line of research would be to extend the findings reported here to other estrogen receptor-positive mammary lines in order to determine the generality of the effect. Estrogen receptor-negative cells could be evaluated as well as controls. Certain biophysical questions also need further attention, such as assessing a dose threshold for magnetic field strengths, frequency dependence, exposure time dependence, and reversibility. Such studies could lead to a better understanding of the mechanism of environmental magnetic field modulation of hormone/drug interactions at the cellular level.

ACKNOWLEDGMENTS

The helpful comments of many colleagues during the preparation of this chapter are most gratefully acknowledged. We also thank

Elizabeth Dunham, Cathleen Heffernan, Maureen Seeley, and Valorie Eckert for technical assistance in these studies. Aspects of this chapter have been reported in abstract form (Harland and Liburdy 1994) and can be found in manuscript(s) submitted for publication in peer-review journals. Research was supported in part by the the Office of Utility Technologies of the Office of Energy Efficiency and Renewal Energies, U.S. Department of Energy, under contract DE-AC03-76SF00098; the National Institutes of Health, National Institute of Environmental Health Sciences, through Project CA07279; and by the Department of Army, U.S. Medical Research and Development Command, through Project 2198.

REFERENCES

Acuña-Castroviejo, D., R.J. Reiter, A. Menendez-Pelaez, M.I. Pablos, A. Burgos. 1994. Characterization of high-affinity melatonin binding sites in purified cell nuclei of rat liver. *J. Pineal Res.* 16:100–112.

Bassen, H., T. Litovitz, M. Penafiel, R. Meister. 1992. ELF in vitro exposure systems for inducing uniform electric and magnetic fields in cell culture media. *Bioelectromagnetics* 13:183–198.

Blackman, C.F., S.G. Benane, D.E. House, J.P. Blanchard. 1996. Independent replication of the 12 mG magnetic field effect on melatonin and MCF-7 cells in vitro. In: Abstracts of the 18th Annual Bioelectromagnetics Society Meeting, June 9–14, 1996, Victoria, Canada, #A-1-2, pp. 1–2.

Blask, D.E., S.T. Wilson, K. Valenta. 1993. Alterations in the growth response of human breast cancer cells to the inhibitory action of a physiological concentration of melatonin in incubators with different ambient 60 Hz magnetic fields. In: Abstracts of the Annual Review of Research on Biological Effects of Electric and Magnetic Fields from the Generation, Delivery, and Use of Electricity, Savannah, Georgia, October 31–November 4, 1993. Abstract A-28.

Blask, D.E., S.T. Wilson, J.D. Saffer, M.A. Wilson, L.E. Anderson, B.W. Wilson. 1993. Culture conditions influence the effects of weak magnetic fields on the growth-response of MCF-7 human breast cancer cells to melatonin *in vitro*. In: Abstracts of the Annual Review of Research on Biological Effects of Electric and Magnetic Fields from the Generation, Delivery, and Use of Electricity, Savannah, Georgia, October 31–November 4, Abstract P-45, p. 65.

Chalbos, D., A. Phillips, F. Galtier, H. Rochefort. 1993. Synthetic anti-estrogens modulate induction of pS2 and cathepsin-D messenger ribonucleic acid by growth factors and adenosine 3´5´-monophosphate in MCF-7 cells. *Endocrinology* 133:571–576.

Coezy, E., J.-L. Borgna, H. Rochefort. 1982. Tamoxifen and metabolites in MCF-7 cells: Correlation between binding to estrogen receptor and inhibition of cell growth. *Cancer Res.* 42:317–323.

Cos, S., D.E. Blask. 1990. Effects of the pineal hormone melatonin in the anchorage-independent growth of human breast cancer cells (MCF-7) in a clonogenic culture system. *Cancer Lett.* 50:115–119.

Cos, S., E.J. Sanchez-Barceló. 1994. Differences between pulsatile or continuous exposure to melatonin in MCF-7 human breast cancer cell proliferation. *Cancer Lett.* 85:105–109.

Cos, S., E.J. Sanchez-Barceló. 1995. Melatonin inhibition of MCF-7 human breast-cancer cells growth: Influence of cell proliferation rate. *Cancer Lett.* 93:207–212.

Cos, S., D.E. Blask, A. Lemus-Wilson, A.B. Hill. 1991. Effects of melatonin on the cell cycle kinetics and estrogen-rescue of MCF-7 human breast cancer in culture. *J. Pineal Res.* 10:36–42.

Crespo, D., C. Fernandez-Viadero, R. Verduga, V. Overjero, S. Cos. 1994. Interaction between melatonin and estradiol on morphological and morphometric features of MCF-7 human breast cancer cells. *J. Pineal Res.* 16(4):215–222.

Danforth, D.N., L. Tamarkin, M. Lippman. 1983. Melatonin increases estrogen receptor binding activity of human breast cancer cells. *Nature* 305:323–325.

Demers, P., D.B. Thomas, K.A. Rosenblatt, L.M. Jimenez, A. McTiernan, H. Stalsberg, A. Stemhagen, W.D. Thompson, M.G. McCrea-Curnen, W. Satariano, D.F. Austin, P. Isacson, R.S. Greenberg, C. Key, L. Kolonel, D.W. Weat. 1991. Occupational exposure to electromagnetic fields and breast cancer in men. *Amer. J. Epidemiol.* 134:340–347.

Ebisawa, T., S. Karne, M.R. Lerner, S.M. Reppert. 1994. Expression cloning of a high-affinity melatonin receptor from Xenopus dermal melanophores. *Proc. Natl. Acad. Sci. USA* 91:6133–6137.

Gottardis, M.M., R.J. Wagner, E.C. Borden, V.C. Jordan. 1989. Differential ability of antiestrogens to stimulate breast cancer cell (MCF-7) growth in vitro and in vivo. *Cancer Res.* 49:4765–4769.

Graham, C., M.R. Cook, H.D. Cohen, D.W. Riffle, S.J. Hoffman, F.J., McClernon, D. Smith, M.M. Gerkovich. 1993. EMF suppression of nocturnal melatonin in human volunteers. In: Abstracts of the Annual Review of Research on Biological Effects of Electric and Magnetic Fields from the Generation, Delivery, and Use of Electricity, Savannah, Georgia, October 31–November 4, A-31. Frederick, Maryland: W/L Associates, Ltd.

Graham, C., M.R. Cook, H.D. Cohen, D.W. Riffle. 1994. Nocturnal melatonin levels in men exposed to magnetic fields: A replication study. In: Abstracts of the Annual Review of Research on Biological Effects of Electric and Magnetic Fields from the Generation, Delivery and Use of Electricity, Albuquerque, New Mexico, November 6–10, A-51, pp. 51–52. Frederick, Maryland: W/L Associates, Ltd.

Guerrero, J.M., R. Reiter. 1992. A brief survey of pineal gland–immune system interrelationships. *Endocrine Res.* 18: 91–113.

Harkins, T.T., C.B. Grissom. 1994. Magnetic field effects on B_{12} ethanolamine ammonia lyase: Evidence for a radical mechanism. *Science* 263:958–960.

Harland, J.D., R.P. Liburdy. 1994. Inhibition of melatonin's and tamoxifen's action in MCF-7 cells by magnetic fields *Mol. Biol. Cell* 5:19a, Abstract 107.

Hill, S.M., D.E. Blask. 1988. Effects of pineal hormone melatonin on the proliferation and morphological characteristics of human breast cancer cells (MCF-7) in culture. *Cancer Res.* 48:6121–6126.

Kato, M., K. Honma, T. Shigemitsu, Y. Shiga. 1994a. Circularly polarized 50-Hz magnetic field exposure reduces pineal blood melatonin concentrations of Long-Evans rats. *Neurosci. Lett.* 166:59–62.

Kato, M., K. Honma, T. Shigemitsu, Y. Shiga. 1994b. Horizontal or vertical 50-Hz, 1-μT magnetic fields have no effect on pineal gland or plasma melatonin concentration of albino rats. *Neurosci. Lett.* 168:205–208.

Kirschvink, J.L. 1992a. Constraints on biological effects of weak extremely low frequency electromagnetic fields: comment. *Phys. Rev. A* 46(4):2178–2184.

Kirschvink, J.L. 1992b. Uniform magnetic fields and double-wrapped coil systems: Improved techniques for the design of bioelectromagnetic experiments. *Bioelectromagnetics* 13:401–411.

Kirschvink, J.L., A. Kobayashi-Kirschvink, J.C. Diaz-Ricci, S. Kirschvink. 1992. Magnetite in human tissues: A mechanism for the biological effects of weak ELF magnetic fields. *Bioelectromagnetics* Suppl. 1:101–114.

Kirschvink, J.L., J. Diaz Ricci, M.H. Nesson, S.J. Kirschvink. 1993. *Magnetite Based Magnetoreceptors: Ultrastructural, Behavioral, and Biophysical Studies.* Technical Report TR-102008, Palo Alto, California: Electric Power Research Institute (EPRI).

L'Hermite-Baleriaux, M., Y. de Launoit. 1992. Is melatonin really an in vitro inhibition of human breast cancer cell proliferation? *In Vitro Cell. & Devel. Biol.* 28A:583–584.

Liburdy, R.P. 1992a. Biological interactions of cellular systems with time-varying magnetic fields. *Ann. N.Y. Acad. Sci.* 649:74–95.

Liburdy, R.P. 1992b. Calcium signalling in lymphocytes and ELF fields: Evidence for an electric field metric and a site of interaction involving the calcium ion channel. *FEBS Lett.* 301:53–59.

Liburdy, R.P. 1992c. ELF fields and the immune system: Signal transduction, calcium metabolism, and mitogenesis in lymphocytes with relevance to carcinogenesis. In: *Interaction Mechanisms of Low-Level Electromagnetic Fields in Living Systems*, B. Norden and C. Ramel, eds., pp. 217–239. New York: Oxford University Press.

Liburdy, R.P. 1994a. Cell culture incubators, ELF fields, and important considerations for cell culture exposure and propagation: An exposure system for in vitro bioelectromagnetics research. In: Abstracts of the 16th Annual Bioelectromagnetics Meeting, Copenhagen, Denmark, June 12–17, Abstract P-198.

Liburdy, R.P. 1994b. Cellular interactions with electromagnetic fields: Experimental evidence for field effects on signal transduction and cell proliferation. In: *On the Nature of Electromagnetic Field Interactions*, A.H.Frey, ed, pp. 99–125. Austin, Texas: R.G. Landes Co.

Liburdy, R.P. 1995. Cellular studies and interaction mechanisms of extremely low frequency fields. *Radio Sci.* 30:179–203.

Liburdy, R.P., R. Sokolic, R., P. Yaswen. 1993a. ELF magnetic fields and melatonin-induced growth inhibition of ER$^+$ breast cancer cells. In: *Electricity and Magnetism in Biology and Medicine*, M. Blank, ed., pp. 398–399. San Francisco: San Francisco Press.

Liburdy, R.P., T.S. Sloma, R. Sokolic, P. Yaswen. 1993b. ELF magnetic fields, breast cancer, and melatonin: 60 Hz fields block melatonin's oncostatic action on ER$^+$ breast cancer cell proliferation. *J. Pineal Res.* 14:89–97.

Liburdy, R.P., D.E. Callahan, J. Harland, E. Dunham, T.R. Sloma, R. Yaswen. 1993c. Experimental evidence for 60 Hz magnetic fields operating through the signal transduction cascade: Effects on calcium influx and c-MYC mRNA induction. *FEBS Lett.* 334:301–308.

Liburdy, R.P., D.E. Callahan, T.R. Sloma, P. Yaswen. 1993d. Intracellular calcium, calcium transport, and c-MYC mRNA induction in lymphocytes exposed to 60 Hz magnetic fields: The cell membrane and the signal transduction pathway. In: *Electricity and Magnetism in Biology and Medicine*, M. Blank, ed., pp. 311–314. San Francisco: San Francisco Press.

Lippman, M.E., G. Bolan, K. Huff. 1976. The effects of estrogen and antiestrogen on hormone-responsive human breast cancer in long-term tissue culture. *Cancer Res.* 36:4595–4601.

Loomis, D.P., D.A. Savitz, C.V. Ananth. 1994. Breast cancer mortality among female electrical workers in the United States. *J. Natl. Cancer. Inst.* 86:921–925.

Löscher, W., M. Mevissen, W. Lehmacher, A. Stamm. 1993. Tumor promotion in a breast cancer model by exposure to a weak alternating magnetic field. *Cancer Lett.* 71:75–81.

Löscher, W., U. Wahnschaffe, M. Mevissen, A. Lerchl, A. Stamm. 1994. Effects of weak alternating magnetic fields on nocturnal melatonin production and mammary carcinogenesis. *Oncology* 51:288–295.

Maestroni, G.J.M. 1993. The immunoneuroendocrine role of melatonin. *J. Pineal Res.* 14:1–10.

Martin, P.M., Y. Berthois, E.V. Jensen. 1988. Binding of antiestrogens exposes an occult antigenic determinant in the human estrogen receptor. *Proc. Natl. Acad. Sci. USA* 85:2533–2537.

Matanoski, G.M., P.N. Breysse, E.A. Elliot. 1991. Electromagnetic field exposure and male breast cancer. *Lancet* 337:737.

Menendez-Pelaez, A., R.J. Reiter. 1993. Distribution of melatonin in mammalian tissues: The relative importance of nuclear versus cytosolic localization. *J. Pineal Res.* 15:59–69.

Merritt, R., G. Purcell, G. Stroink. 1993. Uniform magnetic field produced by three, four, and five square coils. *Rev. Sci. Instrum.* 54:879–882.

Mevissen, M., A. Stamm, S. Burtenkotter, R. Zwingelberg, U. Wahnschaffe, W. Löscher. 1993. Effects of magnetic fields on mammary tumor development induced by 7,12-dimethylbenz(a)anthracene in rats. *Bioelectromagnetics* 14:131–143.

Molis, T.M., L.L. Spriggs, S.M. Hill. 1994. Modulation of estrogen receptor mRNA expression by melatonin in MCF-7 human breast cancer cells. *Mol. Endocrinol.* 8:1681–1690.

Molis, T.M., L.L. Spriggs, Y. Jupiter, S.M. Hill. 1995. Melatonin modulation of estrogen-regulated proteins, growth factors, and proto-oncogenes in human breast cancer. *J. Pineal Res.* 18(2):93–103.

Philips, A., D. Chalbos, H. Rochefort. 1993. Estradiol increases and anti-estrogens antagonize the growth factor-induced Activator Protein-1 activity in MCF-7 breast cancer cells without affecting c-*fos* and c-*jun* synthesis. *J. Biol. Chem.* 268:14103–14108.

Polk, C. 1994. Effects of extremely low frequency magnetic fields on biological magnetite. *Bioelectromagnetics* 15:261–270.

Pool, R. 1990. Is there an EMF–cancer connection? *Science* 249:1096–1098.

Ree, A.H., B.F. Landmark, S.I. Walaas, L. Lahooti, L. Eikvar, W. Eskild, V. Hansson. 1991. Down-regulation of messenger ribonucleic acid and protein levels for estrogen receptors by phorbol ester and calcium in MCF-7 cells. *Endocrinology* 129(1):339–344.

Reiter, R. *The Pineal Gland and Melatonin: Regulation and Role in Oxidative Defense, Cancer and Aging.* Boca Raton, Florida: R.G. Landes Co., CRC Press Inc. (in press).

Reiter, R.J., B. Poeggeler, D.-X. Tan, L.-D. Chen, L.C. Manchester, J.M Guerrero. 1993. Antioxidant capacity of melatonin: A novel action not requiring a receptor. *Neuroendocrinol. Lett.* 15:103–116.

Roy, S., Y. Noda, V. Eckert, M. Traber, A. Mori, R. Liburdy, L. Packer. 1995. The phorbol 12-myristate 13-acetate(PMA)-induced oxidative burst in rat peritoneal neutrophils is increased by a 0.1 mT (60 Hz) magnetic field. *FEBS Lett.* 376:164–166.

Soule, H.D., J. Vasquez, A. Long, S. Albert, M. Brennan. 1973. A human cell line from a pleural effusion derived from a breast carcinoma. *J. Natl. Cancer Inst.* 51:1409–1416.

Stevens, R.G., S. Davis, D.B. Thomas, L.E. Anderson, B.W. Wilson. 1992. Electric power, pineal function, and the risk of breast cancer. *FASEB J.* 6:853–860.

Subramanian, A., L. Kothari. 1991. Suppressive effect by melatonin on different phases of 9,10-dimethyl-1-1,2-benzanthracene (DMBA)-induced rat mammary gland carcinogenesis. *Anti-Cancer Drugs* 2:297–303.

Swain, S.M., M.E. Lippman. 1990. Endocrine therapies of cancer, Chapter 4. In: *Cancer Chemotherapy: Principles and Practice*, p. 84. Philadelphia: J. B. Lippincott Co.

Tynes, T., A. Andersen. 1990. Electromagnetic fields and male breast cancer. *Lancet* 336:1596.

Walleczek, J., R.P. Liburdy. 1990. Nonthermal 60 Hz sinusoidal magnetic-field exposure enhances $^{45}Ca^{2+}$ uptake in rat thymocytes: Dependence on mitogen activation. *FEBS Lett.* 271:157–160.

Weaver, J.C., R.D. Astumian. 1990. The response of living cells to very weak electric fields: The thermal noise limit. *Science* 247:459–462.

Welker, H.A., P. Semm, R.P. Willig, J.C. Commentz, W. Wiltschko, L. Volrath. 1983. Effects of an artificial magnetic field on serotonin N-acetyl transferase activity and melatonin content of the rat pineal gland. *Exp. Brain Res.* 50:426–432.

Wiesenfeld, K., F. Moss. 1994. Stochastic resonance and the benefits of noise: From ice ages to crayfish and squids. *Nature* 373:33–36.

Wilson, B.W., L.E. Anderson, D.I. Hilton, R.D. Phillips. 1981. Chronic exposure to 60-Hz electric fields: Effects on pineal function in the rat. *Bioelectromagnetics* 2:371–380.

Wilson, B.W., L.E. Anderson, D.J. Hilton, R.D. Phillips. 1983. Chronic exposure to 60-Hz electric fields: Effects on pineal function in the rat (erratum). *Bioelectromagnetics* 4:293.

Wilson, B.W., E.K. Chess, L.E. Anderson. 1986. 60 Hz electric field effects on pineal melatonin rhythms: time course of onset and recovery. *Bioelectromagnetics* 7:239–242.

Yellon, S.M. 1993. Replication studies of the effect of an acute 60 Hz magnetic field exposure on the nighttime melatonin rhythm in the adult Djungarian hamster. In: Abstracts of the Annual Review of Research on Biological Effects of Electric and Magnetic Fields from the Generation, Delivery, and Use of Electricity, Savannah, Georgia, October 31–November 4, A-29. Frederick, Maryland: W/L Associates, Ltd.

23 Epidemiologic Studies of EMF and Breast Cancer Risk: A Biologically Based Overview

THOMAS C. ERREN

Institut und Poliklinik für Arbeits- und Sozialmedizin der
Universität zu Köln, Germany

CONTENTS

INTRODUCTION
CLASSIFICATION OF EXPOSURE AND DISEASE
POSTULATED LINKS BETWEEN ELF EMF AND HORMONE-
  DEPENDENT CANCER
MATERIALS AND METHODS
EPIDEMIOLOGIC DATA ON ELF EMF AND BREAST CANCER
DISCUSSION OF THE EPIDEMIOLOGIC EVIDENCE FOR AN
  ELF EMF–BREAST CANCER LINK
IMPLICATIONS FOR RESEARCH
CONCLUDING REMARKS
ACKNOWLEDGMENTS
REFERENCES

INTRODUCTION

Electric and magnetic fields (EMF) associated with the electric power
we ordinarily use in houses, offices, and factories are ubiquitous. A

possible link of extremely low frequency (ELF) EMF to cancer became a substantial scientific concern in 1979, when an epidemiologic study suggested an association of 60-Hz magnetic fields with an increase in childhood cancer incidence (Wertheimer and Leeper 1979). Wertheimer and Leeper's investigation sparked off intense interest; subsequently, EMF have been associated with bioeffects in some experiments and with various cancers in epidemiologic studies. Interestingly, a specific carcinogenic mechanism that implies ELF EMF has been proposed only for cancer of the breast (Stevens 1987). Epidemiologic evidence that breast cancer in men and women may be related to employment in various electrical occupations, or to residential exposures to ELF EMF, has been discussed controversially. This chapter (1) reviews biological theories that postulate a link between ELF EMF and breast cancer; (2) considers whether existing epidemiologic data indicate an elevated breast cancer risk in men and women; and (3) suggests a possible approach to future research on the topic.

Electric and magnetic fields are produced when alternating current (AC) flows back and forth, thus changing its strength and direction rhythmically (World Health Organization 1987). While electric fields are generated by fixed electric charges, magnetic fields build up when a current flows. In North America, the AC frequency is 60 Hz (Hertz = cycles/sec); in Europe and many other countries of the world the frequency is 50 Hz. The electromagnetic spectrum spans an enormous range of frequencies of at least 23 orders of magnitude, including ELF EMF (up to 100 Hz), radio waves, microwaves, infrared, visible light, ultraviolet rays, X-rays and gamma rays (up to $10 \ e^{23}$ Hz) (World Health Organization 1984). Depending on its frequency or energy, electromagnetic radiation interacts with matter in different ways. High-energy X-rays may ionize when absorbed by a molecular system and cause disease such as cancer. Low-energy ELF EMF can influence cellular processes and certain endocrine, immune, and reproductive processes (Morgan and Nair 1992). An important distinction between the electric and magnetic components of ELF EMF is the fact that magnetic fields pass through many materials while the electric energy is shielded by most conducting matter. Given this "protection" from electric field components, research has focused on the potential biological relevance of magnetic fields (Wertheimer and Leeper 1979).

CLASSIFICATION OF EXPOSURE AND DISEASE

Epidemiologic studies of EMF health effects are prone to errors arising from misclassification of exposure. These errors may be similar in subgroups being compared (nondifferential), or they may vary (differential). The primary difficulty stems from the fact that there is little clue as to what the specific agent(s) in the ELF EMF mixture is(are). While investigators have chosen various estimators in search of a biophysically relevant ELF EMF component, it is questionable whether any exposure indicator has assessed the putative agent accurately. The resulting misclassification of study participants with respect to what constitutes exposure is likely to be random. As a consequence, estimates of relative risk of disease associated with the exposure may be biased toward the null value, and any true association between ELF EMF and the endpoint in question may be underestimated and may go undetected. Also, it must be noted that if ELF EMF pose a carcinogenic risk, then the risk ratios for the true effect of exposure generally tend to be underestimated because the reference groups are not unexposed to the ubiqitious EMF. On the other hand, if a relevant ELF EMF component is identified, differential recall of past exposure can lead to a bias away from the null value. In this case, positive associations may not reflect a real cause–effect relationship. Given the difficulty of accurate exposure assessment and the possible recall problems, both the direction and magnitude of errors due to misclassification of exposure are unpredictable.

Misclassification of disease is not a concern when the effect in question is breast cancer. Unlike other malignancies such as nervous system tumors, leukemia, or lymphoma, breast cancer is likely to be correctly classified in either gender, irrespective of the diagnostic source.

In sum, the uncertainty of what may constitute a relevant ELF EMF exposure is critical with regard to classification of exposure, and limits an understanding of confounding and effect modification. For pragmatic reasons, this review discusses the different exposure estimators that have been used in various studies, but does not attempt to analyze the effect of varying exposure assessment, possible confounding, or effect modification.

POSTULATED LINKS BETWEEN ELF EMF AND HORMONE-DEPENDENT CANCER

The interaction of ELF EMF with biological systems has been studied extensively during the last 15 years, and leading researchers in bioelectromagnetics agree that ELF EMF have cellular, immune, and neuroendocrine effects despite relatively low energies (Morgan and Nair 1992). A credible hypothesis has been formulated to explain a possible relation between ELF EMF and breast cancer. Cohen et al. (1978) suggested that low melatonin levels may elevate breast cancer risks. The pineal gland's secretion of melatonin follows a circadian rhythm with high levels at night. The authors suggested that "environmental lighting" and "undefined environmental stimuli," among other possible factors, may result in a low melatonin concentration. A few years later, studies in rats demonstrated that ELF EMF may suppress the pineal gland's production of melatonin, and that reduced melatonin may increase dimethyl-benz(a)anthracene (DMBA)-induced mammary carcinogenesis (Stevens 1987). Based on the experimental evidence, Stevens postulated a "functional pinealectomy" by chronic exposure to ELF EMF as an etiologic factor for breast cancer in rats (Fig. 1). The disturbed interaction of reduced "oncostatic" melatonin and high levels of both estrogen and prolactin then increases oncogenesis via accelerated stem cell turnover. Yet another mechanism hypothesizes that reduced melatonin levels mediate the release of existing DMBA-induced cancer cells from a quiescent state (Stevens 1993). Furthermore, melatonin has been identified as a very potent hydroxyl radical scavenger that considerably inhibits DNA attack through free radicals. Conversely then, melatonin levels that are hypothetically suppressed by ELF EMF result in less protection against oxidative damage (Reiter et al. 1993).

The central step of any melatonin-mediated carcinogenesis in humans was experimentally indicated in 1993 (Graham et al. 1993). When a subgroup of male volunteers with low baseline melatonin levels was exposed to ELF EMF, nocturnal melatonin blood levels

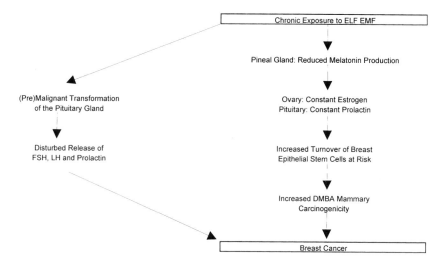

FIG. 1. Hypothetical hormone-mediated mammary carcinogenesis. Model adapted from Stevens (1987) and modified by findings of Floderus et al. (1994): Proposed "functional pinealectomy" by chronic exposure to ELF EMF as an etiologic factor for breast cancer in rats. Hypothetically, long-term exposure to ELF EMF causes a (pre)malignant transformation of the pituitary gland, which may result in cancer of hormonal target organs like the breast and/or cancer of the gland itself.

were significantly suppressed. However, Graham et al. later reported in an abstract that they were unable to confirm these findings in a larger study (Graham et al. 1994).

Recent epidemiologic findings of excessive breast cancer cases and tumors of the pituitary gland in Swedish railway workers are consistent with the general notion that ELF EMF may affect interrelated hormone-dependent organs (Floderus et al. 1994). The pituitary gland lies at the nexus of the central nervous system and the hormonal system, and its follicle stimulating hormone (FSH), luteinizing hormone (LH), and prolactin are involved in hormone-dependent carcinogenesis of both the breast and the prostate. Disturbed prolactin release by the pituitary constitutes one step in the malignant cascade of mammary carcinogenesis that ELF EMF may trigger (Fig. 1). If a malignant transition of the pituitary gland is confirmed in subsequent studies, this would support the concept of a hormone-mediated pathway between ELF EMF and cancer. Hypothetically, high-level exposure to magnetic fields causes a (pre)malignant transition of the pituitary gland. This may result in cancer of hormonal target organs like the breast, and/or cancer of the gland itself. Interestingly, a morphological link along the axis of hormone-dependent organs has been postulated earlier. When Cohen et al. suggested a role of the pineal gland in the etiology of breast cancer, they considered the correlation between pineal calcification and the incidence of breast cancer as the strongest evidence (Cohen et al. 1978).

MATERIALS AND METHODS

Since the hypothesis of Stevens and Cohen et al. is credible, this review focuses on the epidemiologic evidence for an association between ELF EMF and breast cancer. Cancers of the central nervous system, leukemia, and lymphoma are beyond the scope of this biologically based overview, because no specific pathomechanism has been hypothesized to explain an association between ELF EMF and these cancers. The scientific literature has been searched, using MEDLINE, to identify studies, published up to April 1996, that present data on ELF EMF and breast cancer. Tables 1 and 2 and Figures 2 and 3 refer to 20 studies in chronological order of publication. Six of them (Olin et al. 1985; Vagerö et al. 1985; McDowall 1986; Milham 1988; Guberan and Usel 1989; Schreiber et al. 1993) recorded no cases of breast cancer during the periods of observation.

To examine whether there is an ELF EMF effect on breast cancer, the risk estimates from independent studies for the maximally exposed category were combined. Summary estimates of relative risks (RRs) were derived for selected groups of studies using the method described by Greenland (1987). Weighted means (b') of the natural logarithms of published RR estimates were calculated, using the inverse of the corresponding variance estimates as weights ($w = 1/V$). Any one value of V was taken as the square of the difference between the logarithms of the published upper (L_u)

TABLE 1

Cohort Studies That Provide Data on ELF EMF and Breast Cancer

First author	Sample size	Exposure estimate	Variables controlled for	Risk estimate	95% confidence limits
Vageroe 1983	54,624 m 18,478 f	job title	age, locale (social class)	null hypothesis of no difference was accepted	
Olin 1985	1,254 m	job title		$RR = 0^a$	
Vageroe 1985	2,918 m, f	work history	age, sex	m: $SMR = 0^a$ f: $SMR = 0.6^b$	0.3, 1.3
McDowall 1986	7,631 m, f	distance	age, sex, locale, social class	m: $SMR = 0^a$ f: $SMR = 1.06^b$	0.66, 1.60
Milham 1988	67,829 m	amateur radio operators		$SMR = 0^a$	

continued

TABLE 1 (continued)

Cohort Studies That Provide Data on ELF EMF and Breast Cancer

First author	Sample size	Exposure estimate	Variables controlled for	Risk estimate	95% confidence limits
Guberan 1989	1,948 m	job title	age, socioeconomic status (SES)	SMR = 0[a]	
Matanoski 1991	50,582 m	job title + field measurement		SIR = 6.5[b]	0.79, 23.5
Tynes 1992	37,945 m	job title + type of exposure		SIR = 2.07[b, c]	1.07, 3.61
Schreiber 1993	1,775 m 1,774 f	distance + field measurement	sex	m: SMR = 0[a] f: SMR = 1.15[b]	0.63, 1.93
Guenel 1993	Intermittent exposure: 154,000 m 79,000 f	job title + potential exposure	sex	m: SMR = 1.22 f: SMR = 0.96	0.77, 1.83 0.91, 1.01
	continuous exposure: 18,000 m 4,000 f	screening field measurement		m: SMR = 1.36[b] f: SMR = 0.88[b]	0.16, 4.91 0.68, 1.15

continued

TABLE 1 (continued)

Cohort Studies That Provide Data on ELF EMF and Breast Cancer

First author	Sample size	Exposure estimate	Variables controlled for	Risk estimate	95% confidence limits
Floderus 1994	36,207,540 person-years among male railway workers	job title + magnetic field measurement		SIR = 4.9[b]	1.6, 11.8
Theriault[d] 1994	4,151 cancer cases among 223,292 men [1970–1989]	job title field measurement estimation of historical exposure	occupational carcinogens SES (smoking)	SIR = 0.85[b]	0.34, 1.75
Savitz 1995	2,656,436 person-years among 138.905 men	work history + magnetic field measurement	occupational carcinogens age, race, social class, working status	SMR = 0.80[b]	0.29, 1.74

[a] The risk estimate was inferred from the studies with null results.
[b] Presentation in figures 2 and 3.
[c] Since the (presumably smaller) RR for the maximally exposed was not reported, the overall SIR for breast cancer in the cohort was used.
[d] Theriault et al. calculated an SIR in the cohort.
m = male   f = female

TABLE 2

Case–Control Studies That Provide Data on ELF EMF and Breast Cancer

First author	Sample size	Exposure estimate	Variables controlled for	Risk estimate	95% confidence limits
Wertheimer 1987	1,179 m, f	wire code + exposure at workplace	age, sex, locale, SES	f: OR = 1.64[a]	1.16, 2.33
Vena 1991	382 f	electric blanket use	age, SES, education	overall: OR = 0.97 most frequent use: OR = 1.31[a]	0.70, 1.35 0.88, 1.95
Demers 1991	227 m	job title	Religion, education, diagnostic X-rays, Quete-let index	any exposed job: OR = 1.8 electricians, telephone line - men, electric power workers: OR = 6.0[a]	1.0, 3.7 1.7, 21
Loomis 1992	250 m	job title	age	OR = 2.2[a]	0.6, 7.8

continued

TABLE 2 (continued)
Case–Control Studies That Provide Data on ELF EMF and Breast Cancer

First author	Sample size	Exposure estimate	Variables controlled for	Risk estimate	95% confidence limits
Rosenbaum 1994	71 m	job title	age, race, county, year of diagnosis	OR = 0.7[a]	0.3, 1.9
Vena 1994	290 f	electric blanket use	age, SES, education	overall: OR = 1.18	0.83, 1.68
				most frequent use: OR = 1.43[a]	0.94, 2.17
Loomis[b] 1994	27,814 breast cancer cases, 68 women exposed	job title	age, race, social class	OR = 1.38[a]	1.04, 1.82

[a] Presentation in Figures 2 and 3.
[b] Proportional mortality analysis
m = male f = female
SES = socioeconomic status

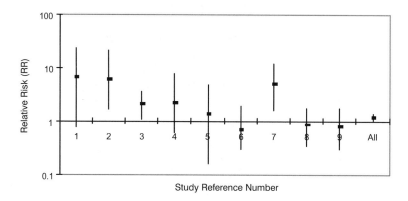

FIG. 2. ELF EMF and breast cancer in men. The relative risk (RR) and 95% confidence limits contributed by the referenced studies are displayed in order of publication on a logarithmic scale. 1 = Matanoski et al. 1991; 2 = Demers et al. 1991; 3 = Tynes et al. 1992; 4 = Loomis 1992; 5 = Guénel et al. 1993; 6 = Rosenbaum et al. 1994; 7 = Floderus et al. 1994; 8 = Thériault et al. 1994; 9 = Savitz and Loomis 1995. "All" indicates the combined RR and 95% confidence interval (CI). RRs with confidence limits that do not overlap the line are statistically significant.

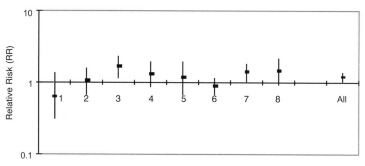

FIG. 3. ELF EMF and breast cancer in women.The RR and 95% confidence limits contributed by the referenced studies are displayed in order of publication on a logarithmic scale. 1 = Vagerö et al. 1985; 2 = McDowall 1986; 3 = Wertheimer and Leeper 1987; 4 = Vena et al. 1991; 5 = Schreiber et al. 1993; 6 = Guénel et al. 1993; 7 = Loomis et al. 1994; 8 = Vena et al. 1994. "All" indicates the combined RR and 95% CI. RRs with confidence limits that do not overlap the line are statistically significant.

and lower (L_l) 95% confidence limits for the measure of RR concerned, divided by 3.92; i.e., V = $\{[\ln(L_u)–\ln(L_l)]/3.92\}^2$. The weighted mean was then exponentiated to provide a summary estimate of RR [RR = exp(b')].

The degree of homogeneity in the k individual results contributing to any one summary RR was evaluated by calculating the statistic suggested by Greenland (1987): $[\chi^2 = \Sigma^k w(b–b')^2]$. Under the null hypothesis that all k studies are providing estimates of the same RR parameter, this statistic is distributed as $\chi2$ with (k–1) degrees of freedom.

Pooled summaries were calculated by grouping study results according to gender. Furthermore, summary RRs were estimated for case–control studies and cohort studies that provided nonzero Standardized Mortality Ratios (SMRs) or Standardized Incident Ratios (SIRs). Results from the analyses of the various groupings of studies are summarized in Table 3. Of the 20 studies that provide data on the risk of breast cancer in men and/or women, 19 were used to calculate pooled summary RR estimates: six case–control studies (Wertheimer and Leeper 1979; Vena et al. 1991; Demers et al. 1991; Loomis 1992; Rosenbaum et al. 1994; Vena et al. 1994), five cohort studies involving SMRs (Vagerö et al. 1985; McDowall 1986; Schreiber et al. 1993; Guénel et al. 1993; Savitz and Loomis 1995), four cohort studies using SIRs (Matanoski et al. 1991; Tynes and Anderson 1992; Floderus et al. 1994; Thériault et al. 1994), and one proportionate mortality study (Loomis et al. 1994). The study by Vagerö et al. (1983) was not included because it was not possible to derive the RR and 95% confidence interval (CI) from the data presented.

A summary RR for men is based on nine studies (Matanoski et al. 1991; Demers et al. 1991; Tynes et al. 1992; Loomis 1992; Guénel et al. 1993; Floderus et al. 1994; Rosenbaum et al. 1994; Thériault et al. 1994; Savitz and Loomis 1995). Six other cohort studies in men, in which no breast cancer cases were observed, were considered separately (Olin et al. 1985; Vagerö et al. 1985; McDowall 1986; Milham 1988; Guberan and Usel 1989; Schreiber et al. 1993). The likely effect of their omission from the summary RR calculations

TABLE 3
Statistics for Analysis of ELF EMF and Breast Cancer by Gender and by Study Design

	Men[a]	Women[b]
Sum of weights	36.67	221.55
Weighted sum	19.17	37.93
Summary b'	0.52	0.17
RR = exp b'	1.69	1.19
Standard error of b'	0.17	0.07
95% confidence interval for RR	1.22–2.33	1.04–1.35
Homogeneity chi-squared	20.22	13.99
Homogeneity degrees of freedom	8	7
Homogeneity p-value[c]	$0.005 < p < 0.01$	$0.05 < p < 0.1$

[a] Matanoski 1991; Demers 1991; Tynes 1992; Loomis 1992; Guénel 1993; Rosenbaum 1994; Floderus 1994; Thériault 1994; Savitz 1995.
[b] Vagerö 1985; McDowall 1986; Wertheimer 1987 Vena 1991; Schreiber 1993; Guénel 1993; Loomis 1994; Vena 1994.
[c] heterogenous at $p < 0.10$
RR = relative risk.

	Cohort men[a]/women[b]	Case–control men[c]/women[d]
Sum of weights	27.40 / 94.66	9.28 / 77.82
Weighted sum	14.58 / - 7.92	4.59 / 30.03
Summary b'	0.53 / - 0.08	0.49 / 0.39
RR = exp b'	1.70 / 0.92	1.64 / 1.47
Standard error of b'	0.19 / 0.1	0.33 / 0.11
95% confidence interval for RR	1.17–2.48 / 0.75–1.13	0.86–3.12 / 1.18–1.83
Homogeneity chi-squared	12.65 / 2.42	7.56 / 0.72
Homogeneity degrees of freedom	5 / 3	2 / 2
Homogeneity p-value[e]	$0.025 < p < 0.05$/ $0.25 < p < 0.5$	$0.01 < p < 0.025$ / $0.5 < p < 0.75$

[a] Matanoski 1991; Tynes 1992; Guénel 1993; Floderus 1994; Thériault 1994; Savitz 1995.
[b] Vagerö 1985; McDowall 1986; Schreiber 1993; Guénel 1993.
[c] Demers 1991; Loomis 1992; Rosenbaum 1994.
[d] Wertheimer 1987; Vena 1991; Vena 1994.
[e] heterogenous at $p < 0.10$.
RR = relative risk.

(because the method used requires nonzero estimates of risk in all contributing data sets) was assessed as follows:

Arbitrarily small, but nonzero, values were attributed to the RRs and the corresponding lower 95% confidence limits. Upper 95% confidence limits were calculated on the assumption that breast cancer risks are distributed as Poisson variables, and that the expected number of deaths under the null hypothesis can be approximated by multiplying the man-years of observation concerned by the overall (age adjusted to the 1970 U.S. standard population) U.S. male breast cancer incidence rate of 0.9/100,000 over the years 1986–1990 (Miller et al. 1993). With these assumptions, the variability in the summary estimates of RR for men, now based on 15 studies, was assessed approximately. Eight studies were used to calculate a pooled RR for women (Vagerö et al. 1985; McDowall 1986; Wertheimer and Leeper 1987; Vena et al. 1991; Schreiber et al. 1993; Guénel et al. 1993; Loomis et al. 1994; Vena et al. 1994).

EPIDEMIOLOGIC DATA ON ELF EMF AND BREAST CANCER

A cohort study published by Vagerö et al. (1983) examined the incidence of cancer in the electronics industry. The subjects were 54,624 male and 18,478 female workers identified by the Swedish Cancer Environment Registry between 1961 and 1973. The 1,855 cases of cancer among men and 1,009 cases among women were compared to the cancer incidence of the general working population. Exposure was crudely assessed as belonging to the electronics, telecommunications, or electrical manufacturing industry. This branch of industry, as a whole, showed a slightly higher overall incidence of cancer (RR = 1.15; 95% CI: 1.10 –1.20). From the results presented it appears that, for breast cancer, the null hypothesis of no difference was accepted by the authors.

In the study by Olin et al. (1985), a small sample of 1,254 male electrical engineers was observed over nearly five decades and there was no reported case of male breast cancer.

In a retrospective cohort study of 2,918 persons in the telecommunications industry (2,051 men, 867 women), Vagerö et al. (1985) analyzed the cancer morbidity from 1958–1979 using the Swedish

Cancer Registry. This relatively small study of limited power reported no breast cancer case in males, while in women the SMR was 0.6 (95% CI: 0.3–1.3). The authors concluded that their assessment of exposure was critical. The cohort, as a whole, was classified by very broad exposure categories, and a detailed exposure description of the cases was difficult. Since it was impossible to apply an appropriate job exposure matrix, nondifferential misclassification may have diluted the SMR.

McDowall (1986) analyzed the mortality of 7,631 persons identified from the 1971 Population Census of East Anglia as residing in the vicinity of electricity transmission facilities. Exposure levels were assessed by proximity to electric lines and substations with regard to distances suggested earlier (Wertheimer and Leeper 1979). The 7,631 study participants were followed to the end of 1983, and 814 deaths were reported. Mortality of the study population was compared with regional and national mortality rates. Among the 409 men who died during the study period, no breast cancer case was detected, and 22 cases in women were in line with the expected regional levels (SMR 1.06; 95% CI: 0.66–1.60).

In an effort to approximate the effects of residential and occupational exposure to EMF, Wertheimer and Leeper (1987) extended the analysis of their 1982 study of adult cancer and High Current Configurations (HCC). In addition to the electrical wiring configuration near the home, study participants were allocated to a Denver/exposed subgroup if it was thought likely that they were employed or had been employed. The analysis of matched pairs showed an exposure odds ratio (OR) of 1.64 for breast cancer in women who had a higher exposure to ELF EMF (p ≤ 0.01). Dr Wertheimer (personal communication 1996) has pointed out that, although not quoted in the paper, the 95% CI for this estimate is easily calculable from the information provided as (1.16, 2.33).

In an attempt to investigate a group likely to have been exposed excessively to ELF EMF, Milham (1988) analyzed Washington State and California amateur radio licensees. 67,829 "exposed" males accounted for 232,499 person-years "at risk." Between 1979 and 1984, 2,485 deaths occurred, of which 741 were attributed to malignant neoplasms, with no breast cancer case mentioned.

In Switzerland, Guberan and Usel (1989) conducted a cohort study of 1,916 painters and 1,948 electricians who were identified through the 1970 census as residents in the Canton of Geneva. They were followed up to 1984. For the electricians, there was neither an overall nor site-specific significant excess risk for cancer. The overall mortality did not differ from the expected, with 137 observed and 139 expected deaths (SMR = 0.99; 90% CI: 0.85–1.14). No case of breast cancer was mentioned. The authors reported an insufficiently low power due to small numbers of expected deaths. Exposure assessment was inappropriately dichotomized into "electricians" and "car electricians." The high loss to follow-up of 27% is critical in terms of the "healthy worker survivor effect" (Arrighi and Hertz-Picciotto 1994). No information about the 27% of the cohort which was lost to follow-up was provided. Therefore, it is possible that affected workers had left the company, and that this resulted in a systematic underestimation of the true risk.

Matanoski et al. (1991) matched workers who were actively employed in a state-wide telephone company between 1976 and 1980 to the cancer registry of the respective state. Person-time experience and cancer were only considered if the individual was employed during the study period. The current jobs of 50,582 workers were used to allocate exposure categories. Personal magnetic field monitoring in a sample indicated higher mean exposures for cable splicers and central office technicians. Two cases of male breast cancer under age 65 were identified in central office technicians exposed to a complex field environment. The SIR was 6.5 (95% CI: 0.79–23.5, Poisson assumption).

Vena et al. (1991) did a case–control study of postmenopausal women from 1987–1989 in western New York and determined the use of electric blankets in the previous 10 years in 382 cases and 439 randomly selected community controls. The authors adjusted for age and education, and found no excess risk associated with daily use as compared with nonuse (OR = 0.97; 95% CI: 0.70–1.35). Continuous use of an electric blanket throughout the night was associated with an OR of 1.31 (95% CI: 0.88–1.95). When adjusted for age, education, other regressor variables such as the Quetelet index [weight (kg)/height (m^2)], and risk factors related to socioeconomic status and the use of electric blankets (age at menarche, age at first pregnancy, number of pregnancies, benign breast disease), there was an OR of 1.46 (95% CI: 0.96–2.20). The power analysis showed that only RRs above 2.1 would be detectable (presumably at the 5% significance level). In view of the slightly elevated risk estimate for the most frequent electric blanket users, the authors recommended further investigation. The authors noted that the findings cannot be generalized to risk for premenopausal breast cancer.

In a population-based case–control study, Demers et al. (1991) investigated breast cancer in men who were occupationally exposed to ELF EMF. They identified, via 10 population-based cancer registries of the Surveillance, Epidemiology, and End Results program of the National Cancer Institute, 227 incident cases with diagnosis between 1983 and 1987. Exposure or probable exposure to EMF was determined for cases and controls. Occupations were categorized into five subgroups to adjust for the type of ELF EMF and probability of exposure. Comparison with 300 randomly selected controls showed an OR of 1.8 (95% CI: 1.0–3.7) for any exposed job. High risks were reported among electric power and utility occupations (OR 6.0; 95% CI: 1.7–21), and in communications and broadcasting jobs (OR 2.9; 95% CI: 0.8–10).

In Norway, Tynes et al. (1992) identified 37,945 male electrical workers from a 1960 census cohort for which occupational data were available. The workers were classified by exposure categories that included information about job categories and the anticipated ELF EMF exposure type. Cancer incidence among the 37,945 electrical workers during the follow-up period from 1961–1985 was provided by the Cancer Registry of Norway and was compared with the national incidence rates for economically active men in 1960. The SIR for breast cancer based on 12 observed cases was 2.07 (95% CI: 1.07–3.61). The risk for breast cancer was highest among electrical transport workers who were exposed to intermediate magnetic fields and weak EMF (four observed cases accounted for an SIR of 3.96; 95% CI: 1.08–10.14).

In a case–control study, Loomis (1992) analyzed breast cancer mortality in male electrical and telephone workers. Occupational data were generated and classified with respect to ELF EMF exposure from death registration certificates from 24 states in the United States between 1985 and 1989. Each of 250 breast cancer deaths was matched by year of death to 10 controls who died from any other cause. Three cases younger than 65 years old at death had held electrical occupations (OR 2.2; 95% CI: 0.6–7.8). The single telephone worker who died of breast cancer was 9 times the expected number (95% CI: 0.9–88.7). The authors noted that the rare occurrence of male breast cancer implies unstable statistical estimates and, hence, limits conclusions from this study.

A retrospective cohort study undertaken in the Netherlands by Schreiber et al. (1993) examined residential exposure to ELF EMF from two 150-kV power lines and one transformer substation. The 3,549 persons (1775 men, 1774 women) included in the study had lived in close proximity to the power sources for at least 5 consecutive years. There was no significant association of exposure to ELF EMF with breast cancer (no male breast cancer case; 14 female cases yielded an SMR of 1.15, 95% CI: 0.63–1.93). The small number of person-years at risk in this study restricts its power to detect moderate but real excess risks that may have been present. For instance, the power to identify relative risks equal to 1.5 or 2.0 (presumably at the 5% significance level) was only 20% and 40%, respectively.

Guénel et al. (1993) analyzed the incidence of cancer over a study period from 1970–1987 in a cohort af 2.8 million economically active persons in Denmark aged 20–64 years in 1970. Exposure assessment was based on classification by industry and occupation in 1970, potential exposure to ELF EMF, and several field measurements. 154,000 men (79,000 women) were categorized as intermittently exposed and 18,000 men (4,000 women) as continously exposed to ELF EMF. For men with a probable intermittent magnetic exposure there was a disease excess for breast cancer of 1.22 (95% CI: 0.77–1.83); with continuous exposure to magnetic fields, the relative cancer incidence was 1.36 (95% CI: 0.16–4.91). The numbers for women were 0.96 (95% CI: 0.91–1.01) and 0.88 (95% CI: 0.68–1.15), respectively. The authors concluded that an ELF

EMF-associated excess risk for breast cancer might be present in men.

Rosenbaum et al. (1994) used a case–control design to study male breast cancer in workers who were exposed to heat and EMF. The comparison of 71 histologically confirmed cases of primary breast cancer reported to the New York State Tumor Registry from 1979–1988 and 256 controls yielded an OR of 0.7 (95% CI: 0.3–1.9) for males believed to have had EMF exposure. Comparing the 71 cases with controls drawn from a voluntary cancer screening clinic was critical in terms of selection bias. Exposure to ELF EMF was assessed by job titles only and it was impossible to determine the duration of any given job. In addition, occupational data were available for 63 of the 71 (89%) cases as compared to 99% of the controls. For 6 of the 63 cases, ELF EMF exposure was indicated by job title, and for 8 cases of male breast cancer no job information was available. Selection bias, the critical exposure assessment, and the "healthy worker effect" may have contributed to an OR smaller than 1.0.

In a re-analysis of 1961–1979 incidence data, Floderus and Toernquist (1994) studied selected cancers in Swedish railway workers. All men 20–64 years of age and employed in the industry in 1960 were included in the study and accounted for a total of 36,207,540 person-years at risk. Due to structural changes of the railway industry, a large proportion of men probably experienced high levels of ELF EMF only during 1960–1970. Follow-up was therefore divided into two 10-year periods (1961–69: 17,150,940 person-years; 1970–79: 19,056,600 person-years). For the first decade, elevated RRs for breast cancer (RR = 4.9; 95% CI: 1.6–11.8) and tumors of the pituitary gland (RR = 3.2; 95% CI: 1.6–6.2) were reported in workers with extremely high exposures to ELF EMF. The inclusion of the pituitary gland was based on an a priori hypothesis. An investigation of a cluster of so-called "brain tumors" associated with EMF in a case–control study showed that some of the tumors were in fact malignancies of the pituitary gland (Floderus et al. 1993). Consequently, the investigators included tumors of the pituitary gland in their re-analysis. It should be noted that the railway magnetic field frequency in Sweden of 16.66

Hz, by definition, falls in the range of ELF EMF but is different from the frequencies examined in other studies.

Loomis et al. (1994) considered proportionate mortality from breast cancer among women in electrical occupations. The authors analyzed a large data set from 24 states based on U.S. mortality information for the years 1985–1989. The final analysis referred to 68 cases of breast cancer and 199 controls in persons who had electrical occupations. These data were compared with 27,814 women with breast cancer and 110,750 controls who had occupations other than "electrical." According to the authors, women in electrical occupations were proportionally more likely to die from breast cancer than women with other occupations (OR 1.38; 95% CI: 1.04–1.82). The estimated excess risk is small and may be attributable to low mortality rates from other causes among those with electrical occupations. Note also that the putative cause of death was based on death certificates, and that this may have introduced biases.

Thériault et al. (1994) used a case–control design to analyze the cancer risks among three cohorts of workers in electric utilities in Canada and France. Among 223,292 men there were 4,151 incident cancer cases between 1970 and 1989. Breast cancer showed no increase in risk with increasing exposure to magnetic fields; there were 7 cases of breast cancer observed compared to an expected 8.25 such cancers in the cohort. The authors calculated an SIR of 0.85 for breast cancer in the cohort. From the data presented it is possible to derive an approximate 95% CI with 0.34 for the lower limit and 1.75 for the upper limit (Rothman and Boice 1979). Controls were recruited from the same utilities. At one utility with as many as 170,000 workers, follow-up of workers after termination of employment, and hence after cancer diagnosis, was not possible. The number of men lost to follow-up and diagnosis would be of particular interest because there may have been selective migration of "pre-diseased" workers from the utility. Thus, a "healthy worker survivor effect" may have led to an underestimate of the true risks, even though the controls were taken from the same cohort. Such attenuation of adverse effects is more problematic when analyzing small rather than large excess risks. It would have been useful to attempt to control for a possible healthy worker survivor effect by adjusting for varying length of follow-up (Arrighi and Hertz-Picciotto 1994). Nevertheless, the authors were able to identify an elevated risk for acute nonlymphoid leukemia and acute myeloid leukemia in workers who had more than the median cumulative exposure to magnetic fields (OR 3.15; 95% CI: 1.20–8.27 and OR 2.36; 95% CI: 1.00–5.58, respectively), and a not significant risk for brain cancer (OR 1.95; 95% CI: 0.76–5.00). These findings suggest that the healthy worker survivor effect is unlikely to have seriously distorted estimates from this study.

In the course of a case–control study, Vena et al. (1994) investigated the use of electric blankets in 290 premenopausal breast cancer cases and 289 age-matched, randomly selected community controls from 1986–1991 in western New York State. The authors adjusted for age, education, and other risk factors as described previously (Vena et al. 1991). The ORs ranged from 1.18 for any use of electric blankets during 10 years prior to the study period (95% CI: 0.83–1.68) to 1.43 for those women who indicated use throughout the night (95% CI: 0.94–2.17). Study limitations discussed by Vena et al. include recall bias and misclassification of electric blanket use, statistical power, and low response rates among cases and controls. Exposure classification was assessed solely by "....limited information on blanket use...." (Vena et al. 1994, p. 977). Although it has been suggested that electric blankets considerably increase the ELF EMF exposure only when used throughout the night (Del Pizzo 1990), only 8% of study individuals were highly exposed by that criterion, and no other possible sources of ELF EMF exposure were taken into account. The study had 80% power to detect an OR of 2.0 at the 5% significance level, but only 28% power to detect an OR of 1.5 at that level for the highest use category. It is remarkable that only 290 out of 456 identified cases participated in the study, due to physician and/or patient refusal. The choice of controls for this study also is questionable. Because cases were newly diagnosed in hospitals, it might have been more appropriate to take controls from patients in the same institutions in which the cases were detected (Miettinen 1985). The authors concluded that additional studies, with more comprehensive exposure assessment and more individuals in high exposure categories, are needed to clarify various uncertainties regarding a possible ELF EMF effect on breast cancer risks.

In the course of a historical cohort study, Savitz and Loomis (1995) investigated mortality between 1950 and 1986 in 138,905 male employees at five electric power companies in the United States involving 2,656,436 person-years at risk. A moderate association was found between occupational magnetic field exposure and brain cancer, but not with leukemia. SMRs were also reported for other causes of death, including malignant neoplasms of the breast (SMR 0.90; 95% CI: 0.29–1.74). However, an analysis of breast cancer with regard to cumulative career magnetic field exposure or exposure in any other time window was beyond the authors' scope. A small increase in total mortality and total cancers with increasing cumulative magnetic field exposure was discussed in terms of a diminution of the healthy worker effect. Since the endpoint of interest here is cancer, it is noteworthy that this occupational cohort's mortality from cardiovascular disease and nonmalignant respiratory disease was more depressed than the overall cancer mortality when compared with the population at large (implying that the relative SMR for cancer was higher than 1.0). With regard to exposure assessment, the investigators linked individual work histories to 2,842 work-shift field measurements and approximated exposure to potentially carcinogenic chemicals in the electric power companies.

DISCUSSION OF THE EPIDEMIOLOGIC EVIDENCE FOR AN ELF EMF–BREAST CANCER LINK

The current knowledge about a role of ELF EMF in breast cancer is equivocal. Six of nine recent studies in men suggest that the relative risk of breast cancer is increased by exposure to ELF EMF (Fig. 2.). Three of the latter excess risks were significant at the 5% level. However, when evaluating the studies that present data about ELF EMF and breast cancer in men, it is important to note that, while lung cancer and breast cancer are the two most common female cancers in industrialized countries, male breast cancer is an extremely rare disease: The age-adjusted, 5-year incidence rate of breast cancer for

1986–1990 in the United States was 0.9/100,000 in men as compared with 108.4/100,000 in women (Miller et al. 1993). Analyzing a very rare disease may present various pitfalls: A random distribution of a rare disease in space and time includes aggregations of events that have no causal relation with a putative hazard. Furthermore, estimates that are obtained from small numbers may be subject to wide fluctuations and yield unstable results. It can be critical to place confidence in findings that are based on few cases.

On the other hand, identifying an apparently excessive number of extremely rare male breast cancer cases may correctly instigate epidemiologic research and conclusions. Therefore, even a few studies that suggest an association between this cancer in men and a biologically plausible causal factor justify further investigation. In these situations it may be helpful to pool results from various studies that on their own would provide only imprecise estimates of possible effects, and to thus derive a summary estimate of the relative risk and its statistical significance (Table 3.). The combined evidence from the nine independent studies in men (Matanoski et al. 1991; Demers et al. 1991; Tynes et al. 1992; Loomis 1992; Guénel et al. 1993; Floderus et al. 1994; Rosenbaum et al. 1994; Thériault et al. 1994; Savitz and Loomis 1995), each in itself with small numbers of cases, suggests that exposure to ELF EMF increases breast cancer risks significantly, by about 70% of the background risk (RR = 1.69; 95% CI: 1.22–2.33).

However, the individual results contributing to this weighted average vary substantially (Fig. 2.), and this heterogeneity in the data is confirmed by a formal test of significance ($p < 0.01$). It is clear, moreover, from Figure 2, that this heterogeneity is not due to just one particular study. Summary RRs calculated from various combinations of eight of the nine studies fluctuate above and below unity, depending on which particular data set is removed. These observations are not surprising given the differences in study design, lengths of follow-up, and variation in background breast cancer rates. Probably most important is the fact that the measures and intensities of exposure in the different studies varied substantially, and therefore contributed to the heterogeneity of results (Hertz-Picciotto and Neutra 1994). It is not clear which of the various exposure indices reflect(s) actual exposure to the hypothesized hazard most realistically.

Nevertheless, Figure 2 shows that all nine studies contributing to the summary RR for men provided estimates of 95% CIs that include the summary RR figure (1.69). Yet the heterogeneity in the results cautions that, while they might be interpreted collectively as indicating the existence of an effect, the pooled statistics do not appropriately reflect the variability and the range of individual estimates of RR. The estimate of summary RR and the associated CIs are thus not interpretable securely as estimates of universal parameters relevant to men in general.

In a recent editorial, Dr. Trichopoulos (1994) pointed out that findings of no association between ELF EMF and breast cancer among men are not considered adequately in the controversy. Trichopoulos' comments, as cited by Taubes (1994), suggest a "one-sided reference bias" (Sackett 1979) that warrants further investigation. In support of his critique, the author concluded that many studies which considered occupational exposure to ELF EMF and cancers of all types in men did not record a single case of breast cancer (Olin et al. 1985; Vagerö et al. 1985; McDowall 1986; Milham 1988; Guberan and Usel 1989; Schreiber et al. 1993). In Table 4, the crude incidence of male breast cancer of 0.9/100,000 during 5 years in the United States is applied to the person-years of observation in these studies, and the approximated expected number of cases, assuming RRs of 1, 1.4, and 4, respectively, are calculated. A basic premise in these calculations is that the background incidence of breast cancer in the various studies is similar to that in the United States. Table 4 illustrates that none of these studies was likely to observe even a single case of male breast cancer due to its very rare occurrence and the limited study size and follow-up, even if a 40% increase in risk due to ELF EMF effect were present. Even a four-fold increase in risk would have been expected to result in just one or two cases in the most powerful of these studies (Milham 1988). In addition, it must be noted that in Table 4, all person-years of observation are considered at risk. When we assume a latency interval between exposure to ELF EMF and disease manifestation,

TABLE 4
Evaluation of Studies in Which No Breast Cancer Cases Were Found in Men

First author	Year of publication	Person-years of observation	Approximated expected number[a]	Approximated number if RR = 1.4	Approximated number if RR = 4
Olin	1985	61,446	0.11	0.15	0.44
Vageroe	1985	64,108	0.12	0.16	0.46
McDowall	1986	91,572	0.16	0.23	0.66
Milham	1988	232,499	0.42	0.59	1.67
Guberan	1989	29,220	0.05	0.07	0.21
Schreiber	1993	36,540	0.07	0.09	0.26

[a] Approximated number of male breast cancer cases = person-years of observation × crude incidence
RR = relative risk.

When the effect in question is breast cancer, the epidemiologic data are equivocal. While an association between ELF EMF and breast cancer is supported in men, the evidence is less convincing in women. With conflicting empirical evidence, a causal interpretation depends more on a credible pathophysiologic mechanism. A melatonin-mediated carcinogenesis of the breast has yet to be substantiated, but such a hypothesis links ELF EMF to hormone-dependent cancer. Hence, targeted research on biological mechanisms centered upon a melatonin effect on breast cancer is recommended to either support or discard a causal link between ELF EMF and breast cancer.

The objective is to further clarify an intriguing scientific problem: If a biological mechanism were to be elucidated, this would have considerable relevance for public health policy and research. On the other hand, refutation of a melatonin-mediated ELF EMF effect on carcinogenesis seems equally important if that hypothesis is false in view of the practice to support imperfect data by an unproven hypothesis, and vice versa (Trichopoulos 1994).

ACKNOWLEDGMENTS

Thomas Erren expresses appreciation for valuable comments from Dr. Michael Jacobsen, Dr. Raymond Neutra, Dr. Allan Smith, and Dr. Peter Morfeld. The author acknowledges the hospitality of the members of the Division of Public Health Biology/Epidemiology, University of California at Berkeley, for providing excellent working conditions during his postgraduate study. This work was supported by a grant from the German Academic Exchange Service (DAAD).

REFERENCES

Arrighi, H.M., I. Hertz-Picciotto. 1994. The evolving concept of the healthy worker survivor effect. *Epidemiology* 5:189–196.

Cohen, M., M. Lippman, B. Chabner. 1978. Role of pineal gland in aetiology and treatment of breast cancer. *Lancet* 2(8094):814–816.

Del Pizzo, V. 1990. A model to assess personal exposure to ELF magnetic fields due to common household sources. *Bioelectromagnetics* 11:139–147.

Demers, P., D.B. Thomas, K.A. Rosenblatt, L.M. Jimenez, A. McTiernan, H. Stalsberg, A. Stemhagen, W.D. Thompson, M.G. McCrea-Curnen, W. Satariano, D.F. Austin, P. Isacson, R.S. Greenberg, C. Key, L. Kolonel, D.W. Weat. 1991. Occupational exposure to electromagnetic fields and breast cancer in men. *Amer. J. Epidemiol.* 134:340–347.

Doll, R., A.B. Hill. 1950. Smoking and carcinoma of the lung: Preliminary report. *Br. Med. J.* 2:739.

Floderus, B., T. Persson, C. Stenlund, et al. 1993. Occupational exposure to electromagnetic fields in relation to leukemia and brain tumors. *Cancer Causes & Control* 4:465–476.

Floderus, B., S. Toernquist, C. Stenlund. 1994. Incidence of selected cancers in Swedish railway workers, 1961–79. *Cancer Causes & Control* 5:189–194.

Graham, C., M.R. Cook, H.D. Cohen, D.W. Riffle, S.J. Hoffman, F.J., McClernon, D. Smith, M.M. Gerkovich. 1993. EMF suppression of nocturnal melatonin in human volunteers. In: Abstracts of the Annual Review of Research on Biological Effects of Electric and Magnetic Fields from the Generation, Delivery, and Use of Electricity, Savannah, Georgia, October 31–November 4, A-31. Frederick, Maryland: W/L Associates, Ltd.

Graham, C., M.R. Cook, H.D. Cohen, D.W. Riffle. 1994. Nocturnal melatonin levels in men exposed to magnetic fields: A replication study. In: Abstracts of the Annual Review of Research on Biological Effects of Electric and Magnetic Fields from the Generation, Delivery and Use of Electricity, Albuquerque, New Mexico, November 6–10, A-51, pp. 51–52. Frederick, Maryland: W/L Associates, Ltd.

Greenland, S. 1987. Quantitative methods in the review of epidemiologic literature. *Epidemiol. Rev.* 9:1–30.

Guberan, E., M. Usel. 1989. Disability, mortality, and incidence of cancer among Geneva painters and electricians: A historical prospective study. Br. J. Ind. Med. 46:16–23.

Guénel, P., P. Raskmark, J.B. Andersen, E. Lynge. 1993. Incidence of cancer in persons with occupational exposure to electromagnetic fields in Denmark. *Brit. J. Ind. Med.* 50(8):758–764.

Hertz-Picciotto, I., R.R. Neutra. 1994. Resolving discrepancies among studies: The influence of dose on effect size. *Epidemiology* 5:156–163.

Lee, D.H.K., I.J. Selikoff. 1979. Historical background to the asbestos problem. *Environ. Res.* 18:300–314.

Loomis, D.P. 1992. Cancer of breast among men in electrical occupations. *Lancet* 339:1482–1483.

Loomis, D.P., D.A. Savitz, C.V. Ananth. 1994. Breast cancer mortality among female electrical workers in the United States. *J. Natl. Cancer Inst.* 86:921–925.

Matanoski, G.M., P.N. Breyese, E.A. Elliot. 1991. Electromagnetic field exposure and male breast cancer. *Lancet* 33:737

McDowall, M.E. 1986. Mortality of persons resident in the vicinity of electricity transmission facilities. *Br. J. Cancer* 53:271–279.

Miettinen, O. 1985. The "case–control" study: Valid selection of subjects. *J. Chron. Dis.* 38:543–548.

Milham, S. Jr. 1988. Increased mortality in amateur radio operators due to lymphatic and hematopoietic malignancies. *Am. J. Epidemiol.* 127:50–54.

Miller, B.A., L.A.G. Ries, B.F. Hankey, et al. (eds). 1993. SEER Cancer Statistics Review: 1973–1990. National Cancer Institute. NIH Pub. No. 93-2789.

Morgan, M.G., I. Nair. 1992. Alternative functional relationships between ELF EMF field exposure and possible health effects: Report on an expert workshop. *Bioelectromagnetics* 13:335–350.

Neutra, R. 1993. Testimony of Raymond Richard Neutra before the Sub Committee on Energy and Power United States House of Representatives. Abstract.

Olin, R., D. Vagerö, A. Ahlbom. 1985. Mortality experience of electrical engineers. *Br. J. Ind. Med.* 42:211–212.

Poole, C., D. Trichopoulos. 1991. Extremely low-frequency electric and magnetic fields and cancer. *Cancer Causes & Control* 2:267–276.

Reingold, A.L. 1982. Toxic shock syndrome surveillance in the United States, 1980 and 1981. *Ann. Intern. Med.* 96:875.

Reiter, R.J., B. Poeggeler, D.-X. Tan, et al. 1993. Melatonin suppression by magnetic fields and the relation to cancer: A theoretical hypothesis to explain the interactions. Abstracts of the Annual

Review of Research on Biological Effects of Electric and Magnetic Fields from the Generation, Delivery, and Use of Electricity, Savannah, Georgia, October 31–November 4, pp. 99–100. Frederick, Maryland: W/L Associates, Ltd.

Rosenbaum, P.F., J.E. Vena, M.A. Zielezny, A.M. Michalek. 1994. Occupational exposures associated with male breast cancer. *Am. J. Epidemiol.* 139(1):30–36.

Rothman, K.J., J.D. Boice. 1979. Epidemiologic Analysis with a Programmable Calculator. NIH Publication No. 79-1649, Washington D.C.: U.S. Department of Health.

Sackett, D.L. 1979. Bias in analytic research. *J. Chron. Dis.* 32:51–63.

Sasco, A.J., A.B. Lowenfels, P. Pasker-de Jong. 1993. Review article: Epidemiology of male breast cancer. A meta-analysis of published case–control studies and discussion of selected aetiological factors. *Int. J. Cancer* 53:538–549.

Savitz, D.A., D.P. Loomis. 1995. Magnetic field exposure in relation to leukemia and brain cancer mortality among electric utility workers. *Am. J. Epidemiol.* 141:123–134.

Schreiber, G.H., G.M.H. Swaen, et al. 1993. Cancer mortality and residence near electricity transmission equipment: A retrospective cohort study. *Int. J. Epidemiol.* 22:9–15.

Stevens, R.G. 1987. Electric power use and breast cancer: A hypothesis. *Am. J. Epidemiol.* 125:556–561.

Stevens, R.G. 1993. Biologically based epidemiological studies of electric power and cancer. *Environ. Health Perspect. Suppl.* 4:93–100.

Taubes, G. 1994. Breast cancer link claimed, criticized. *Science* 264:1658.

Thériault, G., M. Goldberg, B. Armstrong, et al. 1994. Cancer risks associated with occupational exposure to magnetic fields among electric utility workers in Ontario and Quebec, Canada, and France: 1970–1989. *Am. J. Epidemiol.* 139:550–572.

Trichopoulos, D. 1994. Are electric or magnetic fields affecting mortality from breast cancer in women ? Editorial. *J. Natl. Cancer Inst.* 86(12):885–886.

Tynes, T., A. Anderson, et al. 1992. Incidence of cancer in Norwegian workers potentially exposed to electromagnetic fields. *Am. J. Epidemiol.* 136:81–88.

these studies may have been even less likely to encounter a single breast cancer case.

Nevertheless, the question arises how inclusion of the six studies with null results (Table 4) in the pooled analysis might have altered the estimates recorded in Table 3. Results from some approximations along these lines confirm the expected attenuation in the RR estimate. The effect of including these particular six studies, involving in total 515,390 additional man-years of observation, might reduce the estimate from 1.7 to about 1.4 (if each of the null results is treated as having yielded RR estimates and lower 95% confidence limits equal to 10^{-5}, rather than zero). But the approximate 95% CI for this revised pooled estimate (1.09, 2.07) still excludes unity. It appears, therefore, that if statistical significance at the 5% level is regarded as a sensible criterion for distinguishing between real effects and purely random fluctuations, then the collective evidence from the 15 studies in men considered here supports the contention that exposure to ELF EMF increases risks of breast cancer in men.

It has been suggested that demonstration of an effect of ELF EMF on breast cancer risks in men would indicate that a similar effect is likely to occur in women (Trichopoulos 1994). The pooled RR from eight studies in women (Table 3) does indeed indicate a 19% excess ELF EMF-associated risk for women, and this is statistically significant at the 5% level (RR = 1.19; 95% CI: 1.04, 1.35). In this case, however, and in contrast to the results from men, the heterogeneity in the data ($\chi^2_7 = 13.987$, p ≈ 0.051) is due essentially to just one study (Wertheimer and Leeper 1987); exclusion of that data set would reduce the summary RR to 1.12, and this estimate is not distinguishable from unity at the 5% level (95% CI: 0.98, 1.30). Moreover, there are no strong contraindications to pooling the seven studies that contribute to the latter results ($\chi^2_6 = 3.306$, p ≈ 0.77). In this respect, therefore, and in the magnitude of the estimated excess ELF EMF-associated risk (19% in women, as compared with 39% in men), the gender-specific results differ substantially.

There are at least three possible reasons why the studies considered suggest an increased breast cancer risk in men but less conin women. Thus, causality cannot be inferred from overall conflicting data at this point.

IMPLICATIONS FOR RESEARCH

Biological coherence is a major criterion for inferring causality from statistical associations. In fact, there are more epidemiologic studies that link cancer to ELF EMF than to environmental tobacco smoke (ETS). It was the experimental evidence that smoke constituents can cause cancer, and a good understanding of the carcinogenic mechanism and of dose–response relationships, that led the Environmental Protection Agency (EPA) to list ETS as a probable human carcinogen (Neutra 1993). To date, many epidemiologic studies on ELF EMF have been conducted without focus on a specific biological understanding of possible disease mechanisms. When there are strong relationships between an exposure and disease, [for instance, cigarette smoke and lung cancer (Doll and Hill 1950), occupational asbestos and pleural mesothelioma (Lee and Selikoff 1979), or superabsorbent tampons and toxic shock syndrome among young women (Reingold 1982)], a lack of biological rationale may be overcome. In the case of ELF EMF, however, the assessment of broad proxies of what was suspected to be hazardous has neither confirmed nor refuted adverse health effects. This suggests that future research should address specifically those biological mechanisms that are consistent with epidemiologic findings suggesting an association between ELF EMF and cancer (Poole and Trichopoulos 1991).

A prime candidate for investigation is a melatonin-mediated effect of ELF EMF on breast cancer. Provided that very large cohorts are available, this malignancy can be investigated in either gender. Targeted research on melatonin may provide evidence to support the hypothesized pathophysiology. Conversely, the study of very large cohorts would be able to refute the hypothesized carcinogenic role of melatonin if there is little or no association between ELF EMF and cancer.

Although there are difficulties in enumerating and following up sufficiently large cohorts, the effect of ELF EMF on hormone-dependent cancer could nevertheless be investigated in a "prospective case–referent study." The standard case–control study cannot directly address the question of whether there is a melatonin-mediated carcinogenesis of the breast. Unless blood samples taken over a prolonged period are available, it is not feasible to correlate exposures to ELF EMF with melatonin levels retrospectively. Given the universal exposure to ELF EMF in the ambient environment, a prospective case–referent study may specifically test a melatonin-mediated carcinogenesis. Subjects would be characterized on the basis of whether they have breast cancer or not, and exposure to ELF EMF and melatonin levels would be assessed prospectively in both cases and referents. If EMF have a melatonin-mediated effect on breast cancer, it is not likely that the effect ceases or is obscured once the cancer is manifest. Consequently, the hormone levels may differ within cases, depending on the etiology, and between cases and referents, depending on the exposure. In occupational settings, people may be exposed to quantitatively higher and qualitatively different EMF. However, if there is a melatonin-mediated effect on breast tissue, the investigation of cases and referents exposed to nonoccupational "low-level" ELF EMF may provide insight into exposure thresholds and other facets of dose–response relationships.

Limitations of the suggested study arise from the possibility that onset and/or treatment of breast cancer may invariably change the hormonal imbalances that we seek to identify and quantify. Nonetheless, lacking promising alternatives and basic research data with regard to hormone-dependent carcinogenesis, the suggested prospective case–referent study could provide a novel approach to further research.

CONCLUDING REMARKS

Due to the universal exposure to hypothetically carcinogenic ELF EMF, there is broad public concern and scientific interest. The first generation of epidemiologic studies has generated scientific controversy since 1979. In summary, there are rather small and inconsistent associations between ELF EMF and cancer in general, and little is known about confounding or effect modification.

When the effect in question is breast cancer, the epidemiologic data are equivocal. While an association between ELF EMF and breast cancer is supported in men, the evidence is less convincing in women. With conflicting empirical evidence, a causal interpretation depends more on a credible pathophysiologic mechanism. A melatonin-mediated carcinogenesis of the breast has yet to be substantiated, but such a hypothesis links ELF EMF to hormone-dependent cancer. Hence, targeted research on biological mechanisms centered upon a melatonin effect on breast cancer is recommended to either support or discard a causal link between ELF EMF and breast cancer.

The objective is to further clarify an intriguing scientific problem: If a biological mechanism were to be elucidated, this would have considerable relevance for public health policy and research. On the other hand, refutation of a melatonin-mediated ELF EMF effect on carcinogenesis seems equally important if that hypothesis is false in view of the practice to support imperfect data by an unproven hypothesis, and vice versa (Trichopoulos 1994).

ACKNOWLEDGMENTS

Thomas Erren expresses appreciation for valuable comments from Dr. Michael Jacobsen, Dr. Raymond Neutra, Dr. Allan Smith, and Dr. Peter Morfeld. The author acknowledges the hospitality of the members of the Division of Public Health Biology/Epidemiology, University of California at Berkeley, for providing excellent working conditions during his postgraduate study. This work was supported by a grant from the German Academic Exchange Service (DAAD).

REFERENCES

Arrighi, H.M., I. Hertz-Picciotto. 1994. The evolving concept of the healthy worker survivor effect. *Epidemiology* 5:189–196.

Cohen, M., M. Lippman, B. Chabner. 1978. Role of pineal gland in aetiology and treatment of breast cancer. *Lancet* 2(8094):814–816.

Del Pizzo, V. 1990. A model to assess personal exposure to ELF magnetic fields due to common household sources. *Bioelectromagnetics* 11:139–147.

Demers, P., D.B. Thomas, K.A. Rosenblatt, L.M. Jimenez, A. McTiernan, H. Stalsberg, A. Stemhagen, W.D. Thompson, M.G. McCrea-Curnen, W. Satariano, D.F. Austin, P. Isacson, R.S. Greenberg, C. Key, L. Kolonel, D.W. Weat. 1991. Occupational exposure to electromagnetic fields and breast cancer in men. *Amer. J. Epidemiol.* 134:340–347.

Doll, R., A.B. Hill. 1950. Smoking and carcinoma of the lung: Preliminary report. *Br. Med. J.* 2:739.

Floderus, B., T. Persson, C. Stenlund, et al. 1993. Occupational exposure to electromagnetic fields in relation to leukemia and brain tumors. *Cancer Causes & Control* 4:465–476.

Floderus, B., S. Toernquist, C. Stenlund. 1994. Incidence of selected cancers in Swedish railway workers, 1961–79. *Cancer Causes & Control* 5:189–194.

Graham, C., M.R. Cook, H.D. Cohen, D.W. Riffle, S.J. Hoffman, F.J., McClernon, D. Smith, M.M. Gerkovich. 1993. EMF suppression of nocturnal melatonin in human volunteers. In: Abstracts of the Annual Review of Research on Biological Effects of Electric and Magnetic Fields from the Generation, Delivery, and Use of Electricity, Savannah, Georgia, October 31–November 4, A-31. Frederick, Maryland: W/L Associates, Ltd.

Graham, C., M.R. Cook, H.D. Cohen, D.W. Riffle. 1994. Nocturnal melatonin levels in men exposed to magnetic fields: A replication study. In: Abstracts of the Annual Review of Research on Biological Effects of Electric and Magnetic Fields from the Generation, Delivery and Use of Electricity, Albuquerque, New Mexico, November 6–10, A-51, pp. 51–52. Frederick, Maryland: W/L Associates, Ltd.

Greenland, S. 1987. Quantitative methods in the review of epidemiologic literature. *Epidemiol. Rev.* 9:1–30.

Guberan, E., M. Usel. 1989. Disability, mortality, and incidence of cancer among Geneva painters and electricians: A historical prospective study. Br. J. Ind. Med. 46:16–23.

Guénel, P., P. Raskmark, J.B. Andersen, E. Lynge. 1993. Incidence of cancer in persons with occupational exposure to electromagnetic fields in Denmark. *Brit. J. Ind. Med.* 50(8):758–764.

Hertz-Picciotto, I., R.R. Neutra. 1994. Resolving discrepancies among studies: The influence of dose on effect size. *Epidemiology* 5:156–163.

Lee, D.H.K., I.J. Selikoff. 1979. Historical background to the asbestos problem. *Environ. Res.* 18:300–314.

Loomis, D.P. 1992. Cancer of breast among men in electrical occupations. *Lancet* 339:1482–1483.

Loomis, D.P., D.A. Savitz, C.V. Ananth. 1994. Breast cancer mortality among female electrical workers in the United States. *J. Natl. Cancer Inst.* 86:921–925.

Matanoski, G.M., P.N. Breyese, E.A. Elliot. 1991. Electromagnetic field exposure and male breast cancer. *Lancet* 33:737

McDowall, M.E. 1986. Mortality of persons resident in the vicinity of electricity transmission facilities. *Br. J. Cancer* 53:271–279.

Miettinen, O. 1985. The "case–control" study: Valid selection of subjects. *J. Chron. Dis.* 38:543–548.

Milham, S. Jr. 1988. Increased mortality in amateur radio operators due to lymphatic and hematopoietic malignancies. *Am. J. Epidemiol.* 127:50–54.

Miller, B.A., L.A.G. Ries, B.F. Hankey, et al. (eds). 1993. SEER Cancer Statistics Review: 1973–1990. National Cancer Institute. NIH Pub. No. 93-2789.

Morgan, M.G., I. Nair. 1992. Alternative functional relationships between ELF EMF field exposure and possible health effects: Report on an expert workshop. *Bioelectromagnetics* 13:335–350.

Neutra, R. 1993. Testimony of Raymond Richard Neutra before the Sub Committee on Energy and Power United States House of Representatives. Abstract.

Olin, R., D. Vagerö, A. Ahlbom. 1985. Mortality experience of electrical engineers. *Br. J. Ind. Med.* 42:211–212.

Poole, C., D. Trichopoulos. 1991. Extremely low-frequency electric and magnetic fields and cancer. *Cancer Causes & Control* 2:267–276.

Reingold, A.L. 1982. Toxic shock syndrome surveillance in the United States, 1980 and 1981. *Ann. Intern. Med.* 96:875.

Reiter, R.J., B. Poeggeler, D.-X. Tan, et al. 1993. Melatonin suppression by magnetic fields and the relation to cancer: A theoretical hypothesis to explain the interactions. Abstracts of the Annual

Review of Research on Biological Effects of Electric and Magnetic Fields from the Generation, Delivery, and Use of Electricity, Savannah, Georgia, October 31–November 4, pp. 99–100. Frederick, Maryland: W/L Associates, Ltd.

Rosenbaum, P.F., J.E. Vena, M.A. Zielezny, A.M. Michalek. 1994. Occupational exposures associated with male breast cancer. *Am. J. Epidemiol.* 139(1):30–36.

Rothman, K.J., J.D. Boice. 1979. Epidemiologic Analysis with a Programmable Calculator. NIH Publication No. 79-1649, Washington D.C.: U.S. Department of Health.

Sackett, D.L. 1979. Bias in analytic research. *J. Chron. Dis.* 32:51–63.

Sasco, A.J., A.B. Lowenfels, P. Pasker-de Jong. 1993. Review article: Epidemiology of male breast cancer. A meta-analysis of published case–control studies and discussion of selected aetiological factors. *Int. J. Cancer* 53:538–549.

Savitz, D.A., D.P. Loomis. 1995. Magnetic field exposure in relation to leukemia and brain cancer mortality among electric utility workers. *Am. J. Epidemiol.* 141:123–134.

Schreiber, G.H., G.M.H. Swaen, et al. 1993. Cancer mortality and residence near electricity transmission equipment: A retrospective cohort study. *Int. J. Epidemiol.* 22:9–15.

Stevens, R.G. 1987. Electric power use and breast cancer: A hypothesis. *Am. J. Epidemiol.* 125:556–561.

Stevens, R.G. 1993. Biologically based epidemiological studies of electric power and cancer. *Environ. Health Perspect. Suppl.* 4:93–100.

Taubes, G. 1994. Breast cancer link claimed, criticized. *Science* 264:1658.

Thériault, G., M. Goldberg, B. Armstrong, et al. 1994. Cancer risks associated with occupational exposure to magnetic fields among electric utility workers in Ontario and Quebec, Canada, and France: 1970–1989. *Am. J. Epidemiol.* 139:550–572.

Trichopoulos, D. 1994. Are electric or magnetic fields affecting mortality from breast cancer in women ? Editorial. *J. Natl. Cancer Inst.* 86(12):885–886.

Tynes, T., A. Anderson, et al. 1992. Incidence of cancer in Norwegian workers potentially exposed to electromagnetic fields. *Am. J. Epidemiol.* 136:81–88.

Vagerö, D., R. Olin, et al. 1983. Incidence of cancer in the electronics industry: Using the new Swedish Cancer Environment Registry as a screening instrument. *Br. J. Ind. Med.* 40:188–192.

Vagerö, D., A. Ahlbom, R. Olin. 1985. Cancer morbidity among workers in the telecommunications industry. *Br. J. Ind. Med.* 42:191–195.

Vena, J.E., S. Graham, R. Hellmann, et al. 1991. Use of electric blankets and risk of postmenopausal breast cancer. *Am. J. Epidemiol.* 134:180–185.

Vena, J.E., J.L. Freudenheim, J.R. Marshall, et al. 1994. Risk of premenopausal breast cancer and use of electric blankets. *Am. J. Epidemiol.* 140:974–979.

Wertheimer, N., E. Leeper. 1979. Electrical wiring configuration and childhood cancer. *Am. J. Epidemiol.* 109:273–284.

Wertheimer, N., E. Leeper. 1987. Magnetic field exposure related to cancer suptypes. Ann. N.Y. Acad. Sci. 502:43–54.

World Health Organization. 1984. Extremely low frequency (ELF EMF) fields. Environmental Health Criteria 35, WHO, Geneva.

World Health Organization. 1987. Magnetic fields. Environmental Health Criteria 69, WHO, Geneva.

PART V
Synthesis and Conclusions

24 Synthesis and Conclusions

RICHARD G. STEVENS
BARY W. WILSON
LARRY E. ANDERSON
Pacific Northwest National Laboratory,
Richland, Washington

CONTENTS

THE MYSTERY OF BREAST CANCER
BREAST CANCER AND USE OF ELECTRIC POWER
PLAUSIBILITY
THE BUILT ENVIRONMENT
FUTURE DIRECTIONS
PROSTATE CANCER
CONCLUSION
REFERENCES

THE MYSTERY OF BREAST CANCER

Even as breast cancer rates increase in industrialized countries, under-standing of the environmental and lifestyle factors affecting breast cancer risk remains elusive. For reasons that are not understood, risk is higher in industrialized nations than in developing countries. At first appearance, a connection between electric power and breast cancer seems tenuous. However, consideration of the potential for disruption

739

of melatonin rhythms by exposure to light at night (LAN) and/or anthropogenic electric and magnetic fields (EMF) provides an impetus for investigating the possibility.

In this book, investigators from a wide array of disciplines have contributed information and insights that allow a clearer evaluation of the biological rationale, the circumstantial case, and the limited direct evidence bearing on the "Melatonin Hypothesis"; i.e., that certain aspects of the use of electric power may be implicated in the high rates of breast cancer in industrialized societies (Stevens et al. 1992; Stevens and Davis 1996). At the foundation of this hypothesis is the body of evidence suggesting that LAN, and perhaps anthropogenic EMF, can affect neuroendocrine function and, specifically, the production of melatonin by the pineal gland. This Melatonin Hypothesis has grown out of work initiated at Pacific Northwest National Laboratory, and has been developed and extended by the work of many of the authors in this volume.

BREAST CANCER AND USE OF ELECTRIC POWER

There is active investigation, in both laboratory and epidemiological studies (as described in previous chapters), of the relationship between exposure to EMF and breast cancer. However, there is very limited direct evidence of a relationship between light and breast cancer, and very little ongoing work.

Early experiments wherein rats were initiated with high doses (20–30 mg) of dimethylbenzathracene (DMBA) and exposed to extended or constant-light photoperiods yielded mixed results (Jull 1966; Hamilton 1969; Aubert et al. 1980). Later, Shah et al. (1984) reported that constant light increased DMBA-induced mammary tumorigenesis in rats. They used a more modest dose of 10 mg DMBA per 100 g body weight of the rats; a typical female rat weighs ~150 g at the dosing age of 55 days. At 55 days of age, rats exposed to constant light from birth showed a greater concentration of terminal end buds and alveolar buds in mammary tissue than did rats raised on a 10-hour light:14-hour dark regimen. Constant-light animals also showed greater DNA synthesis activity in the mammary tissue, and higher levels of circulating prolactin. A suggested mechanism for these results is that reduced melatonin resulted in increased circulating estrogen and prolactin, and, consequently, increased turnover of the breast epithelial stem cells, thus increasing the risk of malignant transformation (Shah et al. 1984; Mhatre et al. 1984).

An interesting epidemiological study bearing on LAN and breast cancer was published in 1991. If LAN increases risk of breast cancer in sighted women, Hahn (1991) reasoned that profoundly blind women, who do not perceive LAN, would be at reduced risk. He analyzed more than 100,000 hospital discharge records published by the National Hospital Discharge Survey. He identified those women with a primary diagnosis of breast cancer, and a comparison group with diagnoses of stroke or cardiovascular disease. He then determined the prevalence of a secondary diagnosis of profound, bilateral blindness in the women with breast cancer and in the comparison group. Among the comparison group, 0.26% were also blind, which is approximately that expected on the basis of national surveys of nonhospitalized women. Among the women with breast cancer, however, only 0.15% were also blind, consistent with Hahn's prediction. Hahn adjusted for diabetes and marital status as best he was able, but the adjustment depended on the reliability of the data in the hospital records.

PLAUSIBILITY

The Melatonin Hypothesis is based principally on three lines of evidence: (1) light effects on melatonin production, (2) EMF effects on melatonin production, and (3) the role of melatonin in breast cancer etiology. The best understood aspect of this triad of evidence is effects of light on melatonin. It is clear from many published studies that:

1. Light of sufficient intensity suppresses the normal nocturnal melatonin peak in all people (excluding the blind) so far tested.

2. There are large differences among people in their light sensitivity at night.

3. There appears to be a melatonin dose response to light.

Whether ambient nighttime light levels or brief exposure to bright light at night affect melatonin in any significant proportion of the population at large remains unclear, and is the subject of current research.

Also of importance, but as yet undetermined, is the extent to which chronic exposure to artificial lighting during the day can disrupt long-term melatonin rhythms.

The effect of melatonin on development of mammary cancer in experimental animals has been shown to be strong; however, the role of melatonin in human breast cancer remains unclear. Melatonin inhibits the development of both DMBA- and N-nitroso-N-methylurea (NMU)-induced mammary cancer in rats, whereas pinealectomy enhances tumor development. This observation does not define the mechanism by which melatonin affects breast cancer at the cellular or tissue level. Other evidence has shown melatonin to be oncostatic to certain subclones of MCF-7 breast cancer cells, and to affect estrogen and prolactin levels in some animal species, as well as the development of the breast epithelial tissue at risk. Whatever the mechanism of action may be, melatonin can have a strong influence on mammary cancer in rats. For humans, however, the evidence is sparse and exceedingly difficult to gather. There is a report that women with ER$^+$ breast cancer have lower nighttime melatonin levels than control women or women with ER$^-$ breast cancer (Tamarkin et al. 1983), but the disease itself may well affect melatonin production.

Stored serum banks are often used to test etiologic hypotheses for hormones or micronutrients, but are virtually useless for studies of melatonin because the blood is typically drawn during the day, when melatonin is at its lowest concentration. Use of stored pre-diagnosis morning urine samples may make epidemiological studies of melatonin and breast cancer possible. There is some evidence that the level of 6-hydroxy-melatonin sulfate (6-OHMS), the primary metabolite of melatonin, in the morning void urine reflects the total nocturnal production of melatonin very well (Arendt et al. 1985).

The most limited aspect of the Melatonin Hypothesis is the evidence for EMF effects on melatonin production. In animals, at least six independent laboratories have published results of studies wherein a low-intensity electric or magnetic field suppressed nighttime melatonin. Few of the experiments are directly comparable in that some labs have used 50- or 60-Hz magnetic fields, some have used rapid changes in Earth-strength static magnetic fields, and some have used 60-Hz electric fields. There have been conflicting reports, and some carefully executed experiments have shown no effects. To date, reported experiments have shown either suppression or no effect; there are no reports to our knowledge, either published or presented in abstract form, of a stimulation of melatonin by a low-intensity EMF exposure. Therefore, the weight of evidence is that under some circumstances in certain experimental settings, EMF can suppress melatonin. Three laboratories have performed experiments in humans, with inconsistent results; none of these data have yet been published. If effects are found in the laboratory, this does not necessarily mean there are effects in the typical home and work environment of people. Several studies are currently addressing that possibility by use of portable meters, and assessment of melatonin by assay of its primary urinary metabolite, 6-OHMS.

Additional studies that will provide direct evidence supporting or refuting the Melatonin Hypothesis also are being conducted. These include epidemiological studies designed to test the hypothesis in humans, and laboratory experiments to replicate the Löscher/ Mevissen results (Löscher et al. 1993; Mevissen et al. 1996). A very recent study of occupational EMF exposure and risk of breast cancer in women that was published just as this book was going to press has also added some support for the hypothesis (Coogan et al. 1996). If the direct evidence accumulates to the point of strongly supporting a LAN and/or EMF-induced elevation of risk of breast cancer in women, then understanding the mechanism would offer possible mitigation strategies. A role for melatonin would provide an appealing mechanism. However, additional biomolecular studies would be needed to determine whether a melatonin mechanism, or some other as-yet unsuspected mechanism, was responsible.

THE BUILT ENVIRONMENT

The generation and distribution of electric power has made possible our modern life and building environments. Among the most profound environmental consequences of electrification is exposure to LAN, and to light during the day of a different character than sunlight. We have come in our evolutionary past from an environment with dark nights and bright, full-spectrum days to an environment with lighted nights in homes during sleep and dim, spectrum-restricted "days" inside buildings where most people work. Indeed, the "built environment" is the predominant environment in the industrialized world. Since the vast majority of people in industrialized societies work in buildings, and virtually all people sleep in buildings, the long-term health effect of the indoor lighted environment deserves attention, particularly in terms of chronic disruption of melatonin rhythms (Bullough et al. in press). As stated by Brainard et al. (1988), "...lighting for everyday use is currently arranged for the optimum visual effectiveness. An additional consideration may now be necessary: what intensity and spectrum of illumination are optimal for proper regulation of the circadian and neuroendocrine apparatus?"

FUTURE DIRECTIONS

Future directions include: (1) epidemiological studies of the lighted environment and risk of breast cancer; (2) short-term experiments in humans to examine the effects of different lighting schemes on performance and melatonin, particularly in simulated night-shift settings (Wehr et al. 1995); and (3) animal experiments examining the effects of different lighting conditions (varying frequency profile, intensity, and timing) on hormone levels and organ weights (Saltarelli and Coppola 1979).

PROSTATE CANCER

Prostate cancer in men is also increasing in industrialized societies, and is thought to have a hormonal etiologic component. There is very little work on the possible role of melatonin in the pathogenesis of prostate cancer, but some does exist (Philo and Berkowitz 1988). Therefore, an investigation of EMF, LAN, and prostate cancer in men deserves consideration based on a similar line of reasoning to that advanced for breast cancer in women (Stevens 1993).

CONCLUSION

Apart from electric power, and its products LAN and anthropogenic EMF, other factors in modern life that might disrupt melatonin rhythms should be studied. There have been a number of reports of an association of alcohol consumption and risk of breast cancer (Hiatt and Bawol 1984; Longnecker et al. 1988; Blot 1992), consistent with a role for melatonin (Stevens and Hiatt 1987). In addition, shift work and certain aspects of diet may have an effect; shift work for the obvious reason of disrupting melatonin rhythms (Touitou et al. 1990; Dollins et al. 1993), and diet from the perspective of variations in tryptophan content (Fernstrom 1985) and the fat–protein–carbohydrate ratios (Fernstrom and Wurtman 1974; Fernstrom et al. 1979).

At this writing, the Melatonin Hypothesis remains speculative. Although the indirect evidence provides a rationale, the direct evidence is inadequate to draw a conclusion on the subject. Direct evidence is being gathered at a rapid pace, and might well lead to resolution within 5 years because, sadly, breast cancer is so common in the industrialized world that many large studies can be conducted simultaneously.

REFERENCES

Arendt, J., C. Bojkowski, C. Franey, J. Wright, V. Marks. 1985. Immunoassay of 6-hydroxymelatonin sulphate in human plasma and urine. *J. Clin Endocrinol. & Metabol.* 60:1166–73.

Aubert, C., P. Janiaud, J. Lecalvez. 1980. Effect of pinealectomy and melatonin on mammary tumour growth in Sprague-Dawley rats under conditions of lighting. *J. Neural Transm.* 47:121–130.

Blot, W.J. 1992. Alcohol and cancer. *Cancer Res. Suppl.* 52:2119s–2123s.

Brainard, G.C., A.J. Lewy, M. Menaker, R.H. Fredrickson, L.S. Miller, R.G. Weleber, V. Cassone, D. Hudson. 1988. Dose–response relationship between light irradiance and the suppression of plasma melatonin in human volunteers. *Brain Res.* 454:212–218.

Bullough, J., M.S. Rea, R.G. Stevens. Light and magnetic fields in a neonatal intensive care unit. *Bioelectromagnetics* (in press).

Coogan, P.F., R.W. Clapp, P.A. Newcomb, T.B. Wenzl, G. Bodgan, R. Mittendorf, J.A. Baron, M.P. Longnecker. 1996. Occupational exposure to 60-Hz magnetic fields and risk of breast cancer in women. *Epidemiology* 7:459–464.

Dollins, A.B., H.J. Lynch, R.J. Wurtman, et al. 1993. Effects of illumination on human nocturnal serum melatonin levels and performance. *Physiol Behav.* 53:153–160.

Fernstrom, J.D. 1985. Dietary effects on brain serotonin synthesis: Relationship to appetite regulation. *Am. J. Clin. Nutr.* 42:1072–1082.

Fernstrom, J.D., R.J. Wurtman. 1974. Nutrition and the brain. *Scientific American* 230:84–91.

Fernstrom, J.D., R.J. Wurtman, B. Hammerstrom-Wiklund, et al. 1979. Diurnal variations in plasma concentrations of tryptophan, tyrosine, and other neutral amino acids: Effect of dietary protein intake. *Am. J. Clin. Nutr.* 32:1912–1922.

Hahn, R.A. 1991. Profound bilateral blindness and the incidence of breast cancer. *Epidemiology* 2:208–210.

Hamilton, T. 1969. Influence of environmental light and melatonin upon mammary tumour induction. *Br. J. Surg.* 56:764–766.

Hiatt, R.A., R.D. Bawol. 1984. Alcoholic beverage consumption and breast cancer. *Am. J. Epidemiol.* 120:676–683.

Jull, J.W. 1966. The effect of infection, hormonal environment, and genetic constitution on mammary tumor induction in rats by 7,12-dimethylbenz(a) anthracene. *Cancer Res.* 26:2368–2373.

Longnecker, M.P., J.A. Berlin, M.J. Orza, T.C. Chalmers. 1988. A meta-analysis of alcohol consumption in relation to risk of breast cancer. *J. Am. Med. Assoc.* 260:652–656.

Löscher, W., M. Mevissen, W. Lehmacher, A. Stamm. 1993. Tumor promotion in a breast cancer model by exposure to a weak alternating magnetic field. *Cancer Lett.* 71:75–81.

Mevissen, M., A. Lerchl, M. Szamel, W. Löscher. 1996. Exposure of DMBA-treated rats in a 50-Hz, 50-μT magnetic field: Effects on mammary tumor growth, melatonin levels, and T lymphocyte activation. *Carcinogenesis* 17:903–910.

Mhatre, M.C., P.N. Shah, H.S. Juneja. 1984. Effects of varying photoperiods on mammary morphology, DNA synthesis, and hormone profile in female rats. *J. Natl. Cancer Inst.* 72:1411–1416.

Philo, R., A.S. Berkowitz. 1988. Inhibition of Dunning tumor growth by melatonin. *J. Urol.* 139:1099–1102.

Saltarelli, C.G., C.P. Coppola. 1979. Influence of visible light on organ weights in mice. *Lab Animal Sci.* 29:319–322.

Shah, P.N., M.C. Mhatre, L.S. Kothari. 1984. Effect of melatonin on mammary carcinogenesis in intact and pinealectomized rats in varying photoperiods. *Cancer Res.* 44:3403–3407.

Stevens, R.G. 1993. Biologically based epidemiological studies of electric power and cancer. *Environ. Health Perspect.* 101(Suppl. 4):93–100.

Stevens, R.G., S. Davis. 1996. The melatonin hypothesis: Electric power and breast cancer. *Environ. Health Persp.* 104 (Suppl. 1):135–140.

Stevens, R.G., R.A. Hiatt. 1987. Alcohol, melatonin, and breast cancer. *New Engl. J. Med.* 317:1287.

Stevens, R.G., S. Davis, D.B. Thomas, L.E. Anderson, B.W. Wilson. 1992. Electric power, pineal function, and the risk of breast cancer. *FASEB J.* 6:853–860.

Tamarkin, L., D. Danforth, A. Lichter, E. De Moss, M. Cohen, B.Chabner, M. Lippman. 1983. Decreased nocturnal plasma melatonin peak in patients with estrogen receptor positive breast cancer. *Science* 216:1003–1005.

Touitou, Y., Y. Motohashi, A. Reinberg, et al. 1990. Effect of shift work on the nighttime secretory patterns of melatonin, prolactin, cortisol, and testosterone. *Eur. J. Appl. Physiol.* 60:288–292.

Wehr, T.A., H.A. Giesen, D.E. Moul, E.H. Turner, P.J. Schwartz. 1995. Suppression of men's responses to seasonal changes in day length by modern artificial lighting. *Am. J. Physiol.* 269:R173–R178.

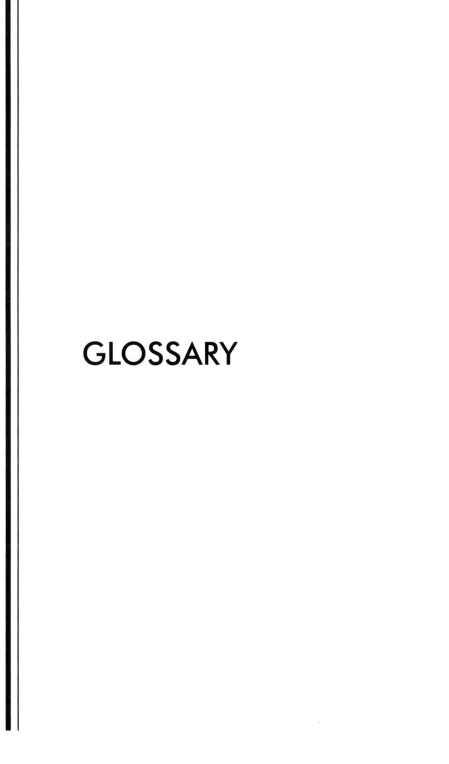

GLOSSARY

Glossary

2-IMLT	2-[^{125}I]iodomelatonin
6-OHMS	6-hydroxy melatonin sulfate
A	ampere
AC	alternating current
ANOVA	analysis of variance
AP-1	activator protein-1
B_H	the intensity of the horizontal component of a magnetic field
B_V	the intensity of the vertical component of a magnetic field
cAMP	cyclic AMP (adenosine 3´:5´-cyclic phosphate)
cf.	confer
CI	confidence interval
Con-A	concanavalin A
cpm	counts per minute
CPRS	Comprehensive Psychopathological Rating Scale
CRE	cAMP response element
CREB	cAMP regulatory element binding protein
CREM	cAMP response element modulator
DC	direct current
DENA	diethylnitrosoamine
df	degrees of freedom
DHEA	dehydroepiandrosterone-sulfate
DMBA	7,12-dimethylbenz(a)anthracene
DMEM	Dulbecco's Modified Eagle's Medium
DST	dexamethasone suppression test
E_2	estradiol
EAL	ethanolamine ammonia lyase
ECG	electoencephalogram
EDTA	ethylenediaminetetraacetic acid
ELF	extremely low frequency
EMF	electric and magnetic fields
ENU	N-ethyl-N-nitrosourea

EPA	U.S. Environmental Protection Agency
ER	estrogen receptor
ER$^+$	estrogen receptor positive
ER$^-$	estrogen receptor negative
eV	electron volts
F	output of analysis of variance statistical test
FBS	fetal bovine serum
FRA-2	FOS-related antigen-2
FSH	follicle stimulating hormone
G	Gauss
GAPDH	glyceraldehyde-6-phosphate dehydrogenase
GnRH	gonadotropin releasing hormone
GPDH	glyceraldehyde 3-phosphate dehydrogenase
GSH	reduced glutathione
GST	glutathione S-transferase
HCC	High Current Configurations
HIOMT	hydroxyindole-O-methyltransferase
HPA	hypothalamic–pituitary–adrenal
HPBL	human peripheral blood lymphocytes
HPG	hypothalamic–pituitary–gonadal
ICER	inducible cAMP early regulator
IGF-1	insulin-like growth factor
IL-1	interleukin 1
IL-2	interleukin 2
INIRC	International Non-Ionizing Radiation Committee
IPR	ion parametric resonance
IRPA	International Radiation Protection Association
J-J	Japanese women in Japan
LA-J	Japanese women in Los Angeles
LA-W	Caucasian women in Los Angeles
LAN	light at night
LH	luteinizing hormone
LPS	lipopolysaccharide
MAO	monoamine oxidase
NAT	N-acetyltransferase
NGF	nerve growth factor
NMMA	N-monomethyl-L-arginine
NMU	N-nitroso-N-methylurea
NNO	normalized neurite outgrowth
NO	nitric oxide
NOS	nitric oxide synthase

• OH	hydroxyl radical
ODC	ornithine decarboxylase
OR	odds ratio
p	probability value (0.01 = 1 in 100)
PB	Phenobarbitol
PCR	polymerase chain reaction
PHA	phytohemagglutinin
PKC	protein kinase C
PMA	12-myristate 13-acetate
r	correlation coefficient
R	roentgen
RDC	Research Diagnostic Criteria
RF	radio frequency
RIA	radioimmunoassay
RMS	root mean square
RoC	rate of change
RR	relative risk
RT-PCR	reverse transcription–polymerase chain reaction
S	siemen
S-NAT	seratonin N-acetyltransferase
SCE	sister-chromatid exchange
SD	single domain
SD	standard deviation
SE	standard error
SEM	standard error of mean
SHBG	sex-hormone-binding globulin
SIDS	sudden infant death syndrome
SIR	Standardized Incident Ratio
SMR	Standardized Mortality Ratio
SPM	superparamagnetic
ST	signal transduction
t	t test
T	Tesla
TGF	transforming growth factor
TPA	12-O-tetradecanoylphorbol-13-acetate
UERM	urinary excretion rates of melatonin
UV	ultraviolet
V	volt
VDT	video-display terminal
W	watt

INDEX

Index

12-*O*-tetradecanoylphorbol-13-acetate (TPA), 560, 600, 627, 635, 641
6-hydroxy melatonin sulfate (6-OHMS), 340, 644, 742, 743
7,12 dimethylbenz(a)anthracene (DMBA), 192, 194, 359, 386, 563, 575, 600, 635, 640, 672, 704, 740

A
activator-protein 1 (AP-1), 303
adduct formation, carcinogen-induced, 198
age, differences in melatonin levels, 35
alcohol consumption, 18, 745
alternating current (AC), 54
appliances, 58, 60, 68, 100, 102

B
baboon, 432
behavioral studies, 112, 134, 144, 162
    magnetoreception, 112
beta-adrenergic stimulation, 383, 385
binding sites of melatonin in breast cancer, 206
bioeffects causal-mechanism theories
    coherence, 74, 84, 464
    ion parametric resonance, 74, 90, 106, 174
    ionization, 57
    magnetite, 74, 118, 691
    transient signal-to-noise, 88
breast cancer, 1, 9
    birth cohorts, 10
    estrogen receptor, 11, 190, 564, 614, 670
    incidence, 20, 325, 715
    male, 715
    mortality, 10
    screening, 11
breast cancer cells, MCF-7, 83, 199
    growth inhibition by melatonin, 204
breast epithelial stem cells, 556

C
c-*fos*, 210, 303, 607
calcium, intracellular, 304, 598
carcinogenesis, 14, 192, 305,
    epigenetic pathway, 589
    initiation, 37, 191, 302, 575, 587
    promotion, 37, 193, 560, 588
cell culture incubators, 670, 674
cell membrane potential, 70
cell proliferation (mitogenesis), 591
circadian rhythm, 26, 113, 236, 303, 481, 504, 671, 704
    entrainment, 114, 133, 153, 159, 286, 303
    retinal photoreceptors, 113, 141, 159, 286, 341, 343
circular polarization, 364
cocarcinogenesis models with known carcinogens, 624, 627
    lymphoma/leukemia, 597
    skin cancer, 634
color vision, 286
compass orientation, 114, 124, 129, 132, 343
copromoter, 586
corticosterone, 395
cortisol, 235, 240, 399, 403, 408, 480, 482
    levels during depression, 235
culture conditions, 191, 202, 209
cyclic AMP (cAMP), 27, 138, 234, 251, 299, 595

D
data acquisition, 82, 93
depression, 35, 137, 235, 251, 273, 276, 285
    light therapy, 245, 276
    melatonin levels, 237, 240, 251, 254, 257, 276, 281
dietary fat, 1, 15, 22, 24
diethylnitrosoamine (DENA), 640
direct current (DC), 51, 58, 65, 88, 95, 678

dopamine, 138, 534, 542
dose, 52
dose metrics, 82
dosimetry, 51, 55
    induced fields, 65, 484
    scaling factors, 67, 575
    skin depth, 72
    static fields, 55

E
Earth-strength magnetic fields, 112, 136
electric fields, 55, 66, 159, 339, 393, 418, 436, 454, 531, 575, 592, 600, 604, 609, 647, 674, 686, 702
    induced current, 64, 69, 365, 687
electromagnetic spectrum, 51
elliptical polarization, 418
EMF, 1, 51
endogenous clock, 306, 504
endogenous melatonin, 194, 196, 207, 320, 480, 544
entrainment, 114, 133, 153, 159, 286, 299
    role of light, 269, 285, 298
enzymes, critical in pineal melatonin synthesis, 298
epidemiologic studies, 701
estradiol, 13, 17, 192, 205, 220, 319, 323, 325, 327, 329, 480, 542, 563, 690
estrogen, 11, 40, 208, 216, 320, 327, 480, 482, 496, 556, 558, 564, 612, 614, 670, 689, 704, 741
estrogen-growth response system, 205
estrogen receptor status, 11
    and tamoxifen, 614, 618, 673, 684, 687, 691
estrogen receptor-positive breast cancer, 612
estrous cycle of sheep, 394, 397, 400, 402, 417
exogenous melatonin, 196-197, 207, 480, 481
exposure systems, 94, 344, 347, 506, 535, 591, 613, 616, 672, 678, 686
    Merritt coil, 310, 507, 674
eye, 56, 119, 147, 153-154, 159, 236, 274, 277, 281, 283, 369

F
Faraday's Law of Current Induction, 87, 670, 684, 686, 687
field characteristics, 87, 532
follicle stimulating hormone (FSH), 319, 320, 329, 534, 541, 705
free radicals, 27, 37, 38, 75, 213, 591, 618, 692, 704

G
gap junction communication, 181, 591
gene expression, 27, 252–253, 298, 301, 576, 589, 591, 595, 603, 606, 608, 624, 648, 690
    pineal, 297
    and protein synthesis, 591, 603
geomagnetic field, 57, 63, 90, 103, 112, 116, 118, 124, 339, 488, 534, 621, 632
    spatial irregularities, 126, 128
    temporal variation, 113–114, 127, 133, 135, 146, 154
glutathione (GSH), 197–198, 213, 216
gonadotropin releasing hormone (GnRH), 541–542
granular vesicles, 363
growth factors, 191, 199, 205, 216, 302, 608, 643, 690, 698

H
hypothalamic-pituitary-gonadal (HPG) axis, 528, 533, 540

I
immune system, 329, 392, 395, 481, 542, 567, 576, 590, 635
    immunomodulation, 320, 580
induced electric field and bioeffects, 73
interferon gamma, 481

J
jet lag, 36, 236, 254, 519

L
latitude, 126, 234, 238, 397
light, measurement techniques, 287
light sensitivity, 120, 493, 741
light therapy, 245, 247, 276, 282
light-at-night, 484

low-melatonin syndrome, 240
luteinizing hormone (LH), 320, 329, 534, 541, 544, 705

M

magnetic field exposure, 38, 60
magnetic field orientation, 360, 431, 463, 688
magnetic fields, power-frequency 59, 88
magnetite, 74, 118, 120, 133, 144, 156, 691
  axial sensitivity, 123, 145, 155
  polar sensitivity, 123, 146, 155
  single-domain (SD) particles, 120, 145, 155
  superparamagnetic (SPM) particles, 118, 121, 145, 155
magnetophosphenes, 73, 341
magnetoreception, 11, 342, 558
mammary ductal system, 198
  differentiating effect of melatonin, 205
MCF-7 ER+ breast cancer cells, 205
melatonin duration, 404, 407
melatonin rhythm, 29, 33, 36, 194, 196, 242, 252, 286, 305, 339, 482, 510, 514, 528, 531
  factors affecting, 744
melatonin suppression, 199, 270, 274, 280, 282, 285, 351, 354, 357, 361, 364, 369, 431, 451, 453, 462, 490
menstrual cycle, 320, 480, 482, 530, 541
mitogenesis (*see* cell proliferation)
monoamine oxidase, 245

N

N-acetyltransferase (NAT), 28, 300, 312, 340, 505, 531, 644
N-ethyl-N-nitrosourea (ENU), 642
N-nitroso-N-methylurea (NMU), 192, 194, 196, 206, 563, 575, 637, 742
nerve growth factor, 174
neurite outgrowth, 173
nitric oxide, 213, 220
norepinephrine, 28, 30, 32, 141, 299, 534, 536, 540

O

occupational exposure, 96, 100, 305, 586, 716, 725, 745
ocular physiology for melatonin regulation, 276, 279, 283, 285
ornithine decarboxylase (ODC), 88, 560, 567, 572, 590, 608, 630, 644

P

parameters of melatonin status, 320
parietal eye photoreceptors, 153
phase-advance theory of manic-depressive illness, 236
Phenobarbitol (PB), 640
photoperiod, 133, 195, 306, 308, 354, 405, 437, 470, 504, 512, 514, 516, 534, 541
  neuroendocrine response to, 533, 540
photoreceptors, 113, 116, 119, 123, 141, 147, 149, 153, 159, 278, 285, 341, 378
pineal gland, 1, 25
pinealectomy, 192, 195, 219, 481, 534, 542, 564, 643, 704, 742
pituitary gland, 39, 705, 720
progesterone, 190, 204, 212, 220, 325, 399, 403, 408, 418, 480, 541
prolactin, 40, 192, 194, 199, 205, 220, 325, 395, 480, 482, 534, 537, 539, 556, 558, 563, 704, 740
propranolol, 32, 481
protein kinase C (PKC) activation, 300, 597
  and calcium mobilization, 623
puberty, 33–34, 394–395, 397, 403, 408, 417, 517, 530

R

radical pair reactions, 112
  effect of magnetic fields, 598, 604, 611, 614, 634, 639
receptor–ligand binding, 594, 608, 623
reproduction, 39, 282, 486, 504, 506, 528, 533, 542, 544
retina, 29, 141, 143, 159, 234, 272, 279, 284, 299, 311, 341, 367, 465, 505, 507, 531, 544
risk factors, breast cancer, 9

S
screening, 11
season, 234, 239, 354, 394, 405, 504, 518, 543, 566
seasonal affective disorder, 236, 252, 298
serotonin, 28, 31, 235, 299, 363, 542
sex, effects on melatonin, 35
sheep, 301, 306, 392, 454, 465, 481, 504, 510
signal transduction, 210, 220, 271, 278, 591, 594
sleep deprivation, 236
sleep disorders, 36, 519
stray fields, 70, 345, 594
stress, 245, 395, 410, 419, 437, 530, 540
superior cervical ganglion, 28, 277, 299, 367
suprachiasmatic nuclei, 26, 28, 32, 39, 234, 244, 251, 253, 277, 282, 299, 303, 304, 309, 311, 338, 341, 504-505, 507

T
T lymphocytes, 396, 420, 567, 577, 596, 598, 602, 616
tamoxifen, 11, 190, 201, 204, 613, 618, 670, 673, 682, 687
testosterone, 40, 481, 534, 747

tissue properties
    conductivity, 63
    inhomogeneity, 67–68
    membranes, 68, 88, 207, 620
    permittivity, 63
transcription, 30, 208, 210, 299, 304, 306, 590, 604, 689
transient signal-to-noise, 88
transmission lines, 59, 360, 393, 397, 400, 418
trigeminal nerve, 134, 144, 157, 161
tryptophan, 27, 381
    role in melatonin synthesis, 378
tumor promoter, 560, 610, 635, 651
tumor, spontaneous development, 624, 634

U–Z
ultraviolet, -51
urinary excretion rates of melatonin, 321
Vitamin A, 17
wavelength for melatonin regulation, 273, 278
Zeitgebers, circadian entrainment, 162